Clinical Pharmacology in Athletic Training

Michelle A. Cleary, PhD, ATC
Chapman University

Thomas E. Abdenour, DHSc, ATC, CES
Certified Athletic Trainer

Michael Pavlovich, PharmD, FAPhA
Westcliff Compounding Pharmacy

HUMAN KINETICS

Library of Congress Cataloging-in-Publication Data

Names: Cleary, Michelle A., 1970- author. | Abdenour, Thomas E., author. | Pavlovich, Michael, 1964- author.
Title: Clinical pharmacology in athletic training / Michelle A. Cleary, Thomas E. Abdenour, Michael Pavlovich.
Description: Champaign, IL : Human Kinetics, [2022] | Includes bibliographical references and index.
Identifiers: LCCN 2021022727 (print) | LCCN 2021022728 (ebook) | ISBN 9781492594185 (paperback) | ISBN 9781492594192 (epub) | ISBN 9781492594208 (pdf)
Subjects: MESH: Sports Medicine--methods | Drug Therapy--methods | Pharmaceutical Preparations
Classification: LCC RC1210 (print) | LCC RC1210 (ebook) | NLM QT 261 | DDC 617.1/027--dc23
LC record available at https://lccn.loc.gov/2021022727
LC ebook record available at https://lccn.loc.gov/2021022728

ISBN: 978-1-4925-9418-5 (print)

This publication is written and published to provide authoritative information relevant to the subject matter presented as of the date of publication. The authors have made every effort to ensure the accuracy of the information herein, particularly in regard to drug selection and dose. As new scientific research is conducted, recommended treatments and therapies may change. Appropriate information sources (including current package inserts and other product information) should be consulted, especially for new or unfamiliar drugs or procedures. It is the responsibility of every practitioner to evaluate the appropriateness of options in the context of actual clinical situations and with due consideration to new developments. This publication is a reference designed as a supplement to, not a substitute for, the expertise, skill, knowledge, and judgment of health care providers in patient care. It is published and sold with the understanding that the authors and publisher are not engaged in rendering legal, medical, or other professional services by reason of their authorship or publication of this work. If medical or other expert assistance is required, the services of a competent professional should be sought.

The web addresses cited in this text were current as of June 2021, unless otherwise noted.

Senior Acquisitions Editor: Joshua J. Stone; **Acquisitions Editor:** Jolynn Gower; **Developmental and Managing Editor:** Amanda S. Ewing; **Copyeditor:** Joy Hoppenot; **Proofreader:** Leigh Keylock; **Indexer:** Nan N. Badgett; **Permissions Manager:** Dalene Reeder; **Graphic Designer:** Dawn Sills; **Cover Designer:** Keri Evans; **Cover Design Specialist:** Susan Rothermel Allen; **Photograph (cover):** monsitj/iStockphoto/Getty Images; **Photographs (interior):** © Human Kinetics, unless otherwise noted; **Photo Asset Manager:** Laura Fitch; **Photo Production Specialist:** Amy M. Rose; **Photo Production Manager:** Jason Allen; **Senior Art Manager:** Kelly Hendren; **Illustrations:** © Human Kinetics, unless otherwise noted; **Printer:** Walsworth

Printed in the United States of America 10 9 8 7 6 5 4 3 2 1

The paper in this book was manufactured using responsible forestry methods.

Human Kinetics
1607 N. Market Street
Champaign, IL 61820
USA

United States and International
Website: **US.HumanKinetics.com**
Email: info@hkusa.com
Phone: 1-800-747-4457

Canada
Website: **Canada.HumanKinetics.com**
Email: info@hkcanada.com

E7960

Tell us what you think!
Human Kinetics would love to hear what we can do to improve the customer experience. Use this QR code to take our brief survey.

This work is dedicated to the athletic trainers who have come before and those who will come after. May we continue to be proud of our evolving profession and strive for recognition and appreciation for our hard work.

—Michelle Cleary

I dedicate this to Christine and our children and my parents and siblings for their unwavering belief in me.

—Tom Abdenour

Contents

Preface

Clinical Pharmacology in Athletic Training guides the athletic training (AT) student's and practicing clinician's clinical application of therapeutic medications to the assessment and management of injured or ill patients. The authors integrate a comprehensive foundational knowledge of pharmacology with the skills that will allow readers to safely administer both prescription and over-the-counter drugs in the treatment of the physically active patient. This text is the first to be written specifically for the graduate professional-level health care student and to incorporate content that addresses the *Commission on Accreditation of Athletic Training Education (CAATE) 2020 Standards for Accreditation of Professional Athletic Training Programs*. It includes the educational competencies that address appropriate pharmacological agents for the management of the patient's condition, including indications, clinical concerns, dosing, interactions, and adverse reactions. The text's focus on clinical applications addresses the AT's role in administering medications or other therapeutic agents by the appropriate route of administration on the order of a physician or other provider with legal prescribing authority. Its overarching theme of interprofessional practice will allow the AT to collaborate with other health professionals in a manner that optimizes the quality of care provided to individual patients. The practicing AT must be prepared to meet the needs of the physically active patient in a constantly evolving health care setting.

Health care professionals, including ATs, who provide medications for physically active patients have a responsibility to meet both legal and ethical requirements. AT students and practicing clinicians need a functional understanding of pharmacology to work effectively in their respective settings. The purpose of this text is to introduce therapeutic medications to graduate students in the health professions and serve as a reference of pharmacology for practicing clinicians. It reviews medications commonly prescribed for the sports medicine patient and describes the components of drug classification by mechanism of action. This text emphasizes the AT's responsibility to advocate for the patient and communicate effectively and appropriately with clients or patients, family members, coaches, administrators, and other health care professionals about the needs of the patient. The authors' aim is to emphasize the day-to-day use of these medications rather than provide a complete breakdown of pharmacology.

This text provides the latest information on over-the-counter and prescription medications commonly used in athletics. Throughout the text, generic drug names are presented in *italics*. Generic drug names are written in lower case, while the trade name of each drug begins with a capital letter as appropriate. The terms "drug" and "medication" are used interchangeably throughout the text.

After reading this text, the AT student should be able to do the following:

- Describe the legal and ethical responsibilities of the AT in administering both prescription and over-the-counter medications.
- Describe the various forms of drugs and the storage considerations for each.
- Differentiate between enteral and parenteral routes of drug administration.
- Describe mechanisms of drug action.
- Differentiate the phases of drug activity—specifically the pharmaceutical, pharmacokinetic, and pharmacodynamics—including drug action, drug-response relationship, factors altering drug responses, and predictable and unpredictable adverse drug responses.
- Describe unintended adverse effects of drug administration and how various factors, such as age, body mass, and concurrent medications, can alter drug responses.
- List the common medications used to treat pain, including nonopioid and opioid analgesics and anesthetics.
- Differentiate between mechanisms of action for steroidal and nonsteroidal drugs used to treat pain.
- List drugs used to treat infection, including antibiotics, antivirals, and other antimicrobials used to treat dermatological infections.
- Describe the characteristics of drugs used to affect the respiratory, cardiovascular, meta-

bolic, gastrointestinal, muscular, nervous, and reproductive systems.
- Describe the characteristics of performance-enhancing drugs, supplements, and cannabinoids.

Organization

Part I reviews pharmacodynamics and pharmacokinetic principles and discusses the patients' rights of drug administration. The text explains the legal aspects of the AT's role in administering drugs as well as the AT's responsibilities and scope of practice related to medication management. It provides a basic overview of the Food and Drug Administration (FDA) approval process and the FDA classifications for newly approved drugs. It introduces the AT student to the chemical, generic, brand, and official names of commonly used drugs and provides appropriate online reference materials for identifying current drug information as well as resources for prevention of poisoning, abuse, and overdoses.

Part II of this text describes medications commonly used to treat pain, inflammation, and infections. In each chapter, drug profile summaries provide ready access to the indications, contraindications, side effects, and adverse reactions for each type of medication. The chapters in part III are organized in a linear fashion, beginning with a brief overview of the conditions related to the body system. A basic knowledge of human anatomy, physiology, health, and wellness is expected, and foundational information on these topics are not included. Each chapter provides an in-depth description of the signs and symptoms to be treated with each class of medication, as well as the route of administration, factors altering drug responses, predictable drug responses, and unpredictable adverse drug responses.

Special Features

The following special features aid in the learning process:

- Chapter objectives set the stage for the main topics covered in the chapter.
- Key terms are set in bold throughout the text to indicate terms of special importance. A glossary of definitions is included at the back of the book.
- Red Flag sidebars highlight warnings and precautions of certain medications or medicolegal issues.
- Evidence in Pharmacology sidebars highlight recent research regarding medications.
- Clinical Application sidebars present real stories from the field of athletic training.
- Case studies highlight specific applications of therapeutic medication. Questions for analysis prompt readers to think critically about the case studies.
- Chapters in parts II and III conclude with a table of drugs described in the chapter that summarizes the medication's type, generic and brand names, pronunciation, common indications, and other special considerations for the AT.

Instructor Ancillaries in HK*Propel*

Several instructor ancillaries are available online in HK*Propel*:

- **Presentation package**—The presentation package includes more than 380 PowerPoint slides of text, artwork, and tables from the book that instructors can use for class discussion and demonstration. The slides in the presentation package can be used directly in PowerPoint or printed for transparencies or handouts for distribution to students. Instructors can easily add, modify, and rearrange the order of the slides as well as search for images based on key words.
- **Test package**—The test package contains a bank of 550 questions in multiple-choice and true-or-false format. The files may be downloaded for integration with a learning management system or printed as paper-based tests.

The instructor pack also includes suggested answers to the end-of-chapter case study questions.

Instructor ancillaries are free to adopting instructors, including an ebook version of the text that allows instructors to add highlights, annotations, and bookmarks. Please contact your sales manager for details about how to access instructor resources in HK*Propel*.

Acknowledgments

The evolution of the athletic training profession has brought us to this point, where a book on clinical pharmacology is standard in graduate athletic training programs. I look forward to seeing how the future of the profession continues to unfold. As the primary author of this book, I could not have had a better writing partner than Tom Abdenour, the consummate clinician and lifelong learner who kept our project moving forward. I am humbly in gratitude for Mike Pavlovich for his passion and expertise, so necessary in a project of this magnitude. The constant support of my best friend and partner in life, my husband Geoff Maloney, has been the foundation for my work. I am eternally grateful to him and to other family members and friends who have supported me over the years. My mom, Roberta McCaw, has always encouraged me to think outside the box and ask the question "Why?" My dad, Jack Cleary, has been a driving force, pushing me to succeed and achieve my goals. He always made me feel that I deserved to lead a fabulous life full of hard work, fun, and adventure. Although much of the work on this book took place during the COVID-19 pandemic, this text was one positive thing that came out of that nerve-racking experience. Finally, I am grateful to my colleagues at Chapman University in the physician assistant studies program, Chair Mike Burney, and Dean Janeen Hill, who have allowed me the time, support, and encouragement I needed to make this project come to life. My gratitude goes to everyone who has encouraged, supported, and mentored me throughout my life and career. Thank you.

—Michelle Cleary

First and foremost, I would like to acknowledge my partners in crime, Michelle Cleary and Mike Pavlovich: Michelle for her vision of what this could look like based on her prior works and Mike for his long-term advocacy for athletic trainers. Both of these professionals have made me a better athletic trainer. None of this would have been possible without the steady hand of my many mentors, starting with my brother, Mike Abdenour, AT-Retired, as well as the many people who have influenced my career in one fashion or another. I would like to thank the external reviewers for taking time out of their extremely busy schedules to review our work. Your feedback of what our colleagues need to know and how to present it was very much appreciated. Last but not least, the support from our Human Kinetics team was beyond valuable. In particular, we are grateful for Amanda Ewing, Jolynn Gower, Ray Vallese, and the late Joshua Stone, as well as the many people behind the scenes at HK. We appreciated everyone's skills and guidance and, most importantly, your patience as we put this together. Thank you all!

–Tom Abdenour

In full appreciation for all the athletic trainers who have so readily and openly invited me into their practices and provided the opportunity for my own professional growth over many years. I especially want to thank Tom Abdenour and Michelle Cleary for including me in their monumental undertaking.

–Mike Pavlovich

PART I

Foundational Pharmacology Concepts

Part I of this text provides the athletic training (AT) student and other health care professionals (HCPs) with foundational concepts relating to the clinical use of medicines or drugs in the physically active population. This text focuses on providing a working knowledge of pharmacology, which is the body of knowledge concerned with the action of chemicals on biologic systems. Medical pharmacology relates to the use of chemicals in the prevention, diagnosis, and treatment of disease. Chapter 1 reviews the legal aspects of drug administration and regulation, as well as the discovery and development of new drugs. Chapter 2 relates to the role of the AT as part of the sports medicine team, while chapter 3 focuses on drug names and basis for classification. Pharmacokinetics (chapter 4) describes the effects of the body on drugs (e.g., absorption, distribution, metabolism, and excretion, or ADME). Pharmacodynamics (chapter 5) refers to the actions of the drug on the body, such as mechanism of action and therapeutic and toxic effects. Toxicology is the area of pharmacology concerned with the undesirable effects of chemicals on biologic systems and is discussed throughout the text. Chapter 6 outlines how prescribers determine dosage and different routes of drug administration. This foundational knowledge is applied in subsequent chapters.

1

Legal Aspects of Therapeutic Medication Management

OBJECTIVES

After reading this chapter, you will be able to do the following:

- Describe how athletic trainers deliver health care services under the direction of a licensed physician
- Explain the legal requirements for athletic training practice as it relates to therapeutic medications
- Differentiate between administering, dispensing, and storing medications in the athletic training clinic
- Identify drugs according to the current schedule of the Controlled Substances Act
- Describe the prescribing authority of various health care providers (prescribers)
- Discuss legislation that affects athletic trainers traveling with medications domestically and internationally

Several health care providers (HCPs) have prescribing authority, and the athletic trainer (AT) may collaborate with each while providing medical services in a variety of settings. HCPs with the authority to prescribe medications, or prescribers, must follow federal and state laws when prescribing medications in a legal and ethical manner. The AT is usually the health care provider on the front lines or the primary care provider for athletes and other physically active people. In this capacity, the AT must advocate for the patient and serve as a liaison between the patient and the prescriber. All members of the sports medicine team have a duty to inform an athlete of the risks of participating considering the athlete's condition, and HCPs should prescribe medication to enable continued participation only if doing so is consistent with the athlete's health interests.[12]

This chapter introduces the legal aspects of managing therapeutic medications and the roles of the HCPs who function together to provide legal and ethical health care to athletes and physically active people. The clinical aspects of administering medications to patients and appropriate procedures for administering medications in the athletic training setting are discussed in chapter 2.

Health Care Providers With Prescribing Authority

A **prescription drug** or **medication** is a pharmaceutical drug that legally requires a medical prescription to be dispensed. In contrast, **over-the-counter (OTC) drugs** can be obtained without a prescription. Substance control is important because of the potential for misuse, from drug abuse to practicing medicine without a license and without sufficient education. Different jurisdictions have different definitions of what constitutes a prescription drug. Some states require **prescribers** (table 1.1) to register with a regulatory agency, such as a state board of pharmacy, in order to dispense controlled or non-controlled prescription medications (or both). Due

TABLE 1.1 Summary of Health Care Providers With Prescribing Authority

Prescriber	Definition	Prescriptive authority*
Doctor of Medicine (MD) Doctor of Osteopathic Medicine (DO)	Physicians who practice medicine or surgery	Have the broadest prescriptive authority, including controlled or scheduled substances.
Physician Assistant (PA)	Practice medicine in collaboration with or under the indirect supervision of a physician	Have limitations on prescription authority in some states and for controlled substances.
Nurse Practitioner (NP) Doctor of Nursing Practice (DNP)	Examine patients, diagnose illnesses, prescribe medication, and provide treatments	Have prescription power with limitations for controlled substances (in some states); some states permit independent practice or require a written agreement with a physician in order to provide care.
Doctor of Clinical Pharmacy (PharmD)	Pharmacists who assess and manage patients' medication therapy	Some states allow prescriptive authority under protocol with a medical provider that includes prescriptive privileges and laboratory monitoring.
Doctor of Podiatric Medicine (DPM) Podiatrists	Diagnose and treat conditions affecting the foot, ankle, and structures of the leg	Can prescribe or administer restricted medications; limited to scope of practice.
Doctor of Optometry (OD)	Optometrists who examine the eyes and visual systems and perform medical diagnosis and management of eye disease	Can prescribe medications to treat certain eye diseases and issue glasses and contact lens prescriptions for corrective eyewear.
Doctor of Dental Surgery (DDS) Doctor of Medicine in Dentistry (DMD)	Dentists who treat various conditions that arise in the mouth, teeth, head, and neck	Can prescribe medications such as antibiotics, fluorides, analgesics, local anesthetics, sedatives or hypnotics, and other medications related to dentistry.
Clinical Psychologist (PhD or PsyD)	Medical psychologists who have undergone specialized training	May prescribe drugs to treat emotional and mental disorders, according to protocols, with an MD or DO.
Doctor of Chiropractic (DC)	Focus on manipulation of the musculoskeletal system, especially the spine	May have the ability to write a prescription, depending on scope of practice laws in a specific jurisdiction.

*Prescriptive authority regulates not only the HCP but also the type of medications that can be prescribed within their scope of practice. Only specifically authorized HCPs can prescribe controlled or scheduled drugs (MD, DO, and some PAs, DNPs, and pharmacists).

Note. National or local (i.e., state or provincial) legislation governs who can write a prescription, and all prescribers must be appropriately licensed, certified, or registered.

to the variability in state laws, it is imperative that all members of the sports medicine team be aware of the regulations in the states in which they practice.[4]

In addition to ATs, other HCPs must follow state and federal laws regarding administering and dispensing of medications, particularly in the youth sport setting. The secondary school setting is unique in that most patients are minors; in many states, this changes how the AT can practice. In most states, an AT is not permitted to furnish OTC medications to minors under any circumstance. In school systems, most states allow the school's physician, school nurse, parent or guardian, and the affected student to administer medication.

The Sports Medicine Team

The care of an injured or ill patient may be the responsibility of one HCP or an **interprofessional health care team** of many providers. Depending on the location of patient care and the patient receiving it, the sports medicine team may include ATs, physicians (MD or DO), pharmacists (PharmD), physical therapists (DPT), nurses (various levels: RN or NP), physician assistants (PAs), chiropractors (DC), and athletic training students. Various members of the sports medicine team may manage different medications within their scope of practice, making it necessary to follow proper **protocols** for storing, packaging, transporting, tracking, administering, and dispensing both OTC and prescription medications. Even for nonprescription (i.e., OTC) drugs, it is essential that the sports medicine team understand and remain in compliance with all current federal and state laws and institutional regulations concerning medication management in the sports medicine setting.

Role of the Directing Physician

Within the sports medicine team, the team physician or directing physician takes a leadership role. Team physicians are usually primary care or family practice physicians or orthopedic surgeons who are hired by professional teams, colleges, and universities to provide medical care for their athletes.[12] Medications may be prescribed by the team or institution's physician or a patient's personal physician. The directing physician is ultimately responsible for ensuring that records and medications, including sample medications, are distributed from or stored at the sports medicine facility or related location. The utility of dispensing sample medications is controversial, and their use has been prohibited in many hospital systems. Both the Accreditation Association for Ambulatory Health Care and the Joint Commission, organizations that accredit many collegiate student health centers and hospitals, have developed specific standards that must be followed for the use of sample medications. The physician must also supervise the disposal of expired medications and should review all protocols for the distribution of OTC medications. Although the athlete is ultimately responsible for avoiding prohibited medications and obtaining therapeutic-use exemption waivers (discussed in chapter 21), the physician should be familiar with medications that are banned or restricted by any relevant sports governing body.[4]

Role of the Athletic Trainer

Unless explicitly authorized by individual state practice acts, ATs cannot legally dispense prescription medications, even under **standing orders** or with permission from a physician, because this places both parties at risk for legal liability.[2] Although dispensing cannot be authorized, ATs may be permitted to administer OTC medications and certain emergency prescription drugs, such as *epinephrine* autoinjectors and *naloxone*, depending on their state practice acts. Athletic trainers should know how and when to use emergency medications (refer to *Acute and Emergency Care in Athletic Training*[15]) and must follow state and federal laws and regulations concerning the legal administration of medications.[2,4]

RED FLAG

Administering and Dispensing Medication

Drug **administration** refers to giving a single dose of medication for immediate use (or within 24 hours), whereas drug **dispensing** involves preparing, labeling, or providing multiple doses of a medication for future use. Once the physician administers the initial dose, the remainder of the prescription is likely to be referred to a local pharmacy with the expectation that it will be filled. These steps can cause time delays and added expense or increase the risk that the medication is not delivered to the patient.

Current state and federal laws prohibit physicians from delegating the duty of prescription drug dispensing to providers not licensed to do so, including ATs.[13] However, in some states, physicians can delegate the authority to dispense medications to other HCPs who are drug prescribers, including nurse practitioners and physician assistants. Certain states also permit ATs limited designation to administer medications under certain conditions, such as during an emergency.[10]

A **formulary** is a list of medications used by a health care entity. ATs must have the formulary when traveling with individual athletes and teams. Although there is widespread belief that ATs are not permitted to dispense OTC medication, it is challenging to find regulations prohibiting this practice. Ultimately, the decision to dispense OTC medication is dictated by existing state laws and practice acts and written policies and procedures established in consultation with the directing or collaborating physician. It is important to document all dispensed OTC medications in the proper format. Further, the AT must not administer any medication to minors or children (<18 years old). Adult athletes (>18 years) should sign an Assignment of Benefits and Athlete-to-AT Agency form (figure 1.1), which is important for providing legal authority for pharmacological (and other) treatments. Statements such as these create a chain of command for the transport of medications on the athlete's behalf. To determine appropriate use in a particular institution or clinic, this form must always be discussed with the administration, including the athletic director, team physician, legal counsel, and risk management office.

Athletic trainers work in a variety of clinical settings, each of which has unique circumstances concerning both OTC and prescription medications. For example, international, Olympic, and professional teams and most intercollegiate athletic conferences have requirements regarding the availability and use of both OTC and prescription medications. Athletic trainers working in emerging settings (e.g., dance companies, acrobatic troupes, orchestras, and live theaters) may also be confronted with unique considerations, such as having appropriate locations for the storage and dispensing of medications. When traveling within the United States or internationally with their patients, ATs must fully understand the local government laws and regulations (see additional details in Traveling With Prescription Medications).[3,4] When administering medications, the AT must do the following:[2,4,5]

- Understand the federal and state laws regarding medication administration, dispensation, and storage.
- Know and understand the regulations regarding medication and the athletic training practice acts in both the home state and the states she may visit with patients.
- Act as a resource for questions or concerns about any medication the patient is given.
- Develop policies and procedures for maintaining safe storage and inventory of medications. This includes appropriate documentation of any distributed medications.
- Understand the role of an athletic training student, who is a student enrolled in classes while matriculating through a professional education program accredited by the Commission on Accreditation of Athletic Training Education. Best practices, therefore, prevent a noncertified or unlicensed student from administering or furnishing any medications. This guideline should be outlined in the clinic or facility's policies and procedures.
- Understand the role of volunteer student aides (those not currently enrolled in an accredited athletic training program). Student aides should not be involved in managing any medication.
- Follow all requirements of standing orders with the directing physician.

I authorize the athletic trainer listed below, under supervision and protocol of the team physician, to act as my caretaker and agent to receive, procure, store, transport, and issue any medications prescribed for me. While any medications are in my custody, I am responsible for their proper storage and will take necessary precautions to keep them out of the reach of children.

FIGURE 1.1 A portion of an Assignment of Benefits and Athlete-to-AT Agency form.

RED FLAG

Athletic Training Students and OTC Medication

Under no circumstances should athletic training students be involved in the conveyance of OTC medication to a patient. The temptation is to rationalize the availability of these medications, which are used regularly and do not require a physician prescription. Despite enthusiasm to assist a staff athletic trainer, the student must not be authorized to manage OTC medications for any purpose, such as restocking inventory or conveying medication to a patient. Conversely, a staff athletic trainer should not delegate this responsibility to a student due to liability and professional ethics concerns.

Federal and State Laws

The sports medicine team must be aware of federal and state regulations regarding the administration and dispensation of drugs or medications, as well as the regulations specific to each profession (e.g., AT, physician, pharmacist, school nurse). A **drug** is considered any substance (other than food and water) that is consumed, inhaled, injected, smoked, absorbed via a patch on the skin (transdermal), or dissolved under the tongue (sublingual) to create a physiological (and often psychological) change within the body. All members of the sports medicine team should be mindful of laws and regulations set forth by various state boards of medicine, state boards of athletic training, or related governing boards.[4] Various U.S. federal agencies regulate how medication is dispensed and administered:[4,11]

- **Food and Drug Administration (FDA)**—Regulates the safety, efficacy, and security of drugs, including appropriate labeling.
- **Drug Enforcement Administration (DEA)**—Enforces federal laws related to controlled substances.
- **Occupational Safety and Health Administration (OSHA)**—Oversees concerns related to contamination of and exposure to hazardous drugs.

U.S. Food and Drug Administration

The FDA is the administrative body that oversees the drug research and development process in the United States and grants approval for marketing new drug products. It has no jurisdiction over supplements. To receive FDA approval for marketing, the originating institution or company must submit evidence of a drug's safety and effectiveness. If a drug has not been shown through adequately controlled testing to be safe and effective for a specific use, it cannot be marketed in interstate commerce for this use.[11] Unfortunately, "safe" can mean different things to the patient, the HCP, and society. Complete absence of risk is impossible to demonstrate, but this fact may not be understood by members of the public, who frequently assume that any medication sold with the approval of the FDA should be free of serious side effects. This confusion is a major factor in litigation and dissatisfaction with aspects of drugs and medical care.[11]

Drug Legislation

Drug regulation in the United States reflects several health events that precipitated major shifts in public opinion. For example, the Federal Food, Drug, and Cosmetic Act (1938) was largely a reaction to deaths associated with the use of a preparation of *sulfanilamide* that was marketed before it and its vehicle had been adequately tested. Serious adverse effects were also attributed to *thalidomide*, an agent introduced in Europe in 1957 and marketed as a nontoxic hypnotic. It was promoted as being especially useful as a sleep aid during pregnancy. In 1961, reports were published suggesting that *thalidomide* was responsible for a dramatic increase in the incidence of a rare birth defect (**phocomelia**) involving shortening or complete absence of the arms and legs. Epidemiologic studies provided strong evidence for the association of this defect with *thalidomide* use by women during the first trimester of pregnancy, and the **teratogenic drug** was withdrawn from sale worldwide. An estimated 10,000 children were born with birth defects because of maternal exposure to this 1 agent. The tragedy led to the requirement for more extensive testing of new drugs for teratogenic effects and stimulated passage of the Kefauver-Harris Amendment of 1962 (see sidebar). Despite its disastrous fetal **toxicity** and effects in pregnancy, *thalidomide* is a relatively safe drug for people other than the fetus. Even the most serious risk of toxicities may be avoided or managed if understood. Despite its toxicity to the unborn fetus, *thalidomide* is now approved by the FDA for limited use as a potent immunoregulatory agent and to treat certain forms of leprosy.[11]

Relevant Legislation Regulating Drugs in the United States

- **Pure Food and Drug Act (1906)**—Prohibited mislabeling and adulteration of foods and drugs (but did not establish requirement for efficacy or safety).
- **Harrison Narcotics Tax Act (1914)**—Established regulations for the use of opium, opioids, and *cocaine* (marijuana added in 1937).
- **Food, Drug, and Cosmetic Act (1938)**—Required that new drugs be tested for safety as well as purity.
- **Kefauver-Harris Amendment (1962)**—Required proof of efficacy as well as safety for new drugs.
- **Controlled Substances Act (1971)**—Placed all substances that were in some manner regulated under existing federal law into 1 of 5 schedules. This placement is based on the substance's medical use, potential for abuse, and safety or dependence liability.
- **Dietary Supplement and Health Education Act (1994)**—Amended the Food, Drug, and Cosmetics Act of 1938 to establish standards for dietary supplements but prohibited the FDA from applying drug efficacy and safety standards to supplements.

Drug legislation in the United States underwent major revisions as of May 1, 1971, when the Controlled Substances Act (CSA) was enacted. This law requires that every person who manufactures, dispenses, prescribes, or administers any controlled substance be registered annually with the Attorney General; this registration function is the responsibility of the DEA.[1] The Controlled Substances Act places all substances that were in some manner regulated under existing federal law into 1 of 5 schedules (see Drug Schedules later in this chapter) based on 3 factors:[6]

1. **Potential for abuse**—How likely is this drug to be abused?
2. **Accepted medical use**—Is this drug used as a treatment in the United States?
3. **Safety and potential for addiction**—Is this drug safe? How likely is this drug to cause addiction? What kinds of addiction?

When prescribing medication to athletes or patients, prescribers must comply with all relevant laws regarding possessing and dispensing drugs, including **controlled substances**.[12] Any HCP responsible for possessing, storing, and distributing controlled substances must be registered with the DEA to perform these functions. He must maintain accurate inventories, records, and security of the controlled substances.[6] For these reasons, increasingly, athletic training clinics and facilities and many on-campus health care facilities do not allow controlled substances to be stored or distributed from the facility.

Evidence in Pharmacology

Heroin and *Cocaine*

Heroin and *cocaine* are illicit drugs that are highly addictive. Abuse of either can be lethal; however, the federal government views them differently. The Controlled Substance Act classifies *heroin* as a Schedule I drug and *cocaine* as a Schedule II drug.[14] The significant difference between the two is that *heroin* has no value or role as a prescription medication, whereas *cocaine* can be used as a local anesthetic for the oral, nasal, and laryngeal cavities.[8]

Drug Schedules

Drugs, substances, and certain chemicals used to make drugs are classified into 5 schedules depending on the drug's acceptable medical use and its potential for abuse or dependency (table 1.2). The abuse rate is a determinate factor in the scheduling of the drug; for example, Schedule I drugs have a high potential for abuse and the potential to create severe psychological or physical dependence and do not have an FDA-approved medical use (indication). Schedule II through V drugs do have an FDA-approved indication. The lower the number, the higher the potential for abuse and dependence. Schedule V drugs represent the least potential for abuse of the controlled substances. **Noncontrolled substances** are prescription medications with less risk of abuse or addiction that have the purpose of

TABLE 1.2 Drug Schedules, Definitions, and Examples Based on the Controlled Substances Act

Schedule	Definition of drugs (substances or chemicals)	Examples
Schedule I	Drugs with no currently accepted medical use and a high potential for abuse	*Heroin*, lysergic acid diethylamide (LSD), marijuana (cannabis), 3,4-methylenedioxymethamphetamine (ecstasy), *methaqualone* (Quaalude), and peyote
Schedule II	Drugs with a high potential for abuse, with use potentially leading to severe psychological or physical dependence	*Cocaine, methamphetamine, methadone, hydromorphone* (Dilaudid), *meperidine* (Demerol), *oxycodone* (OxyContin), *fentanyl, hydrocodone* (e.g., Vicodin), *dextroamphetamine* (Dexedrine), *amphetamine* and *dextroamphetamine* (Adderall), and *methylphenidate* (Ritalin) *Codeine* (pure) and any drug for non-parenteral administration containing the equivalent of more than 90 mg of *codeine* per dosage unit
Schedule III	Drugs with a moderate to low potential for physical and psychological dependence	*Ketamine*, anabolic steroids, and *testosterone* Products containing <90 mg of *codeine* per dosage unit (e.g., Tylenol with *codeine*)
Schedule IV	Drugs with a low potential for abuse and low risk of dependence	*Tramadol* (Ultram), *alprazolam* (Xanax), *diazepam* (Valium), *lorazepam* (Ativan), *zolpidem* (Ambien), *eszopiclone* (Lunesta), and *zaleplon* (Sonata)
Schedule V	Drugs with lower potential for abuse than Schedule IV; consist of preparations containing limited quantities of certain narcotics	Lomotil, Motofen, Lyrica, *gabapentin* Cough preparations with <200 mg of *codeine* or per 100 mL (e.g., Robitussin-AC) Schedule V drugs are generally used for antidiarrheal, antitussive, and analgesic purposes.

Drugs listed are intended for general reference; this is not a comprehensive listing of all controlled substances.
A substance need not be listed as a controlled substance to be treated as a Schedule I substance for criminal prosecution.[6]
Synthetic THC and THC analogs are FDA approved (see chapter 20 for a full discussion) and available as *dronabinol* (Marinol, Syndros) and *nabilone* (Cesamet).

treating various medical conditions. A listing of drugs and their schedule can be found on the DEA website or CSA Scheduling by Alphabetical Order.[7]

Traveling With Prescription Medications

Physicians, ATs, and other HCPs who travel outside of their state of licensure must be careful to ensure that they are properly handling and dispensing medications according to legislation for the state they are visiting. Moreover, physicians should not delegate to ATs the responsibility to dispense controlled substances.[12] The sports medicine team (whether they travel or not) should be aware of the following:[3,10]

- To dispense or administer a drug, the prescriber (e.g., physician assistant or nurse practitioner) must be licensed or otherwise authorized by the state in which the dispensing or administering occurs.

- A DEA license is the property and responsibility of the prescriber, not the institution. The prescriber is responsible for the acquisition, storage, dispensing, and disposal of all controlled substances within the athletic training facility.
- A prescriber can transport controlled substances only between physical locations at which she is registered by the DEA and only within the state that has granted authorization numbers for distributing and administering controlled substances.
- Orders written for a team rather than an individual patient are not permissible.
- An AT may be granted very limited responsibility for administering prescription drugs. This varies by state; local law must be considered.
- Coaches absolutely cannot distribute prescription medications under any circumstance.
- The HCP does not need to be licensed to deliver OTC medication, but the OTC drugs must be delivered with federally required packaging and labeling (described in chapter 2). Penalties for noncompliance with these regulations include a fine of $10,000 to $25,000 USD per violation (where each pill may count as a violation), possible loss of DEA privileges, and possible medical board sanctions.
- Students should never administer, distribute, or dispense OTC or prescription medications.

In summary, the AT should never carry controlled substances across state lines and must beware of transporting these drugs, even within the home state.[10]

In the past, states did not provide legal protection for ATs or sports medicine professionals who were traveling to another state with an athletic team solely to provide care for that team. Fortunately, to address the multiple concerns associated with this lack of protection, in 2017, Congress passed the Sports Medicine Licensure Clarity Act, which allows ATs and sports medicine providers to engage in the treatment of injured athletes across state lines without the fear of incurring great professional loss. This legislation provides the following:[10]

- ATs and sports medicine professionals who travel to other states with an athletic team to provide care for that team will receive legal protection.
- For the purposes of liability, health care services provided by a covered AT or sports medicine professional to an athlete, an athletic team, or a staff member of an athlete or athletic team in a secondary state will be deemed to have occurred in the professional's primary state of licensure.

Clinical Application

International Travel

When traveling internationally with medications, the AT should consider these recommendations:

- Prior to starting the trip, the AT should consult with the host organizing committee, host team, or the sport's nongovernmental organization (NGO) regarding local laws that need to be followed.
- When possible, the team physician should carry the medication and travel with it in his name.
- The AT should travel with as little inventory as possible.
- The AT should be aware of any particular regulations relative to transporting or administering the medication, regardless if it is controlled, noncontrolled, or over the counter.
- Medications available by prescription in 1 nation may not be available in another.
- The AT should be certain that any medication prescribed by a local physician is not going to cause a positive drug test.

Drug Development, Studies, and Standards

Coronavirus disease 2019 (COVID-19), the infectious disease caused by severe acute respiratory syndrome coronavirus 2 (SARS-CoV-2), was first identified in December 2019 and resulted in a global pandemic. The COVID-19 pandemic thrust vaccine research into the public conversation and frequent news media reports. Establishing a new drug, such as a COVID-19 vaccine, is an arduous and rigorous process. The approval process includes multiple steps, some of which routinely require many years to complete.

Drug Development

Drug development is the process of bringing a new pharmaceutical drug to the market once a lead compound has been identified through the process of drug discovery (figure 1.2). The approval process includes preclinical research on microorganisms and animals. Next, the company must file for regulatory status with the FDA for an investigational new drug (IND) to initiate **clinical trials** on humans. Often, 4 to 6 years of clinical testing are necessary to accumulate and analyze all required data. In each phase of the clinical trials, volunteers or patients must be informed of the investigational status of the drug as well as the possible risks and allowed to decline or consent to participating and receiving the drug.[11]

Drug Studies

Drug studies in humans can begin only after an IND is reviewed by the FDA and a local institutional review board (IRB). The IRB is a panel of scientists and nonscientists in hospitals and research institutions that oversees clinical research to ensure that the study is acceptable, participants have given consent and are fully informed of their risks, and researchers take appropriate steps to protect patients from harm.[9] If successful, the final step is obtaining regulatory approval with a new drug application (NDA) to market the drug. A drug that is approved is considered by the FDA to be safe and effective when used as directed.[9,11]

Drug Standards

Several organizations worldwide publish reference texts describing drug standards (lists of the known value, strength, quality, and ingredients of various drugs) for quality and strength. Before official standards were published, drugs, particularly those from plant sources, could vary in strength from being ineffective to providing almost a fatal dose, depending on the quality of the plant, the soil, and the growing conditions. The most prominent drug standards in the United States are as follows:[1]

- **United States Pharmacopeia–National Formulary**—The United States Pharmacopeia and the National Formulary have been combined into 1 official volume, the United States Pharmacopeia–National Formulary (USP–NF). The USP–NF includes a list of approved drugs and defines them with respect to source, chemistry, physical properties, tests for identity, method of assay, storage, and dosage. The formulary also provides directions for compounding and general use.
- **Physicians' Desk Reference or Prescriber's Digital Reference**—Revised annually and readily supplied to all hospitals and physicians, the Physicians' Desk Reference (PDR) is a widely used reference source and is now found on the Internet as the Prescriber's

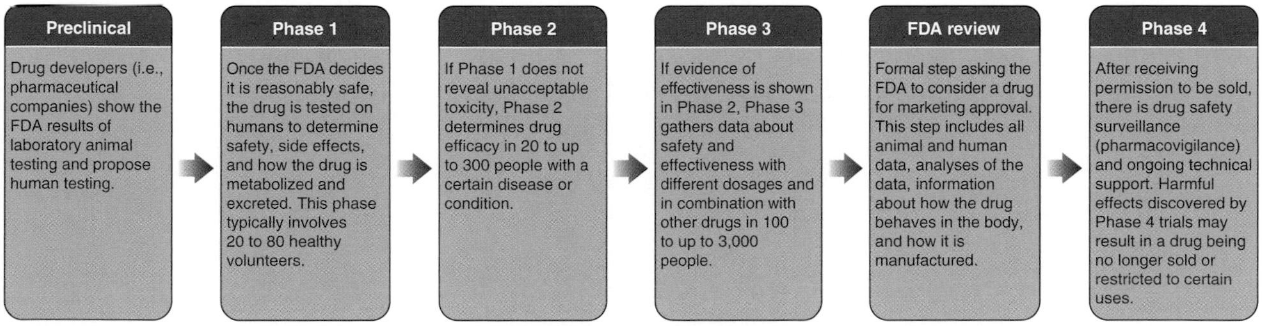

Preclinical
Drug developers (i.e., pharmaceutical companies) show the FDA results of laboratory animal testing and propose human testing.
Phase 1
Once the FDA decides it is reasonably safe, the drug is tested on humans to determine safety, side effects, and how the drug is metabolized and excreted. This phase typically involves 20 to 80 healthy volunteers.
Phase 2
If Phase 1 does not reveal unacceptable toxicity, Phase 2 determines drug efficacy in 20 to up to 300 people with a certain disease or condition.
Phase 3
If evidence of effectiveness is shown in Phase 2, Phase 3 gathers data about safety and effectiveness with different dosages and in combination with other drugs in 100 to up to 3,000 people.
FDA review
Formal step asking the FDA to consider a drug for marketing approval. This step includes all animal and human data, analyses of the data, information about how the drug behaves in the body, and how it is manufactured.
Phase 4
After receiving permission to be sold, there is drug safety surveillance (pharmacovigilance) and ongoing technical support. Harmful effects discovered by Phase 4 trials may result in a drug being no longer sold or restricted to certain uses.

FIGURE 1.2 Steps in FDA clinical trials for new drugs.

Digital Reference. The PDR is not intended as an official standard. Each manufacturer supplies information for inclusion, usually by trade name, and gives the accepted uses, side effects, and doses for commercially available pharmaceutical agents.[1]

Summary

A practicing AT should be familiar with many concepts of pharmacology and very knowledgeable about the content areas included in this text. The most critical of these concepts is how to oversee the use of prescription and OTC medications in accordance with national and state athletic training standards as well as with federal, state, and local regulations. HCPs, the directing or team physician, and ATs must comply with these regulations when managing medication. ATs should have functional knowledge of both controlled and noncontrolled substances and recognize the limits of transporting these medications while traveling with a team. The practicing AT must be able to navigate the various websites pertaining to a medication's indications, contraindications, and prescription parameters. The following chapters describe the role of the AT in administering medications as well as foundational concepts in pharmacology that are essential for the AT to understand and apply to clinical practice.

Case Studies

Case Study 1

The local university replaced its retiring long-term team physician with a recent graduate of a family practice sports medicine fellowship. One of the initial changes the new team physician made was to mandate that the athletic training clinic have a DEA license apart from the university's student health service. This license would be mandatory if the clinic stored controlled substances. The physician felt it was a good practice to have it even though there were currently no narcotics in the inventory. The athletic director felt this was a good idea and approved the $731 fee that covered the clinic for 3 years.

Questions for Analysis

1. Why did the student health service DEA license need to be replaced?
2. The retiring physician stored prescription medication in the satellite athletic training clinic at the off-campus arena. Is that covered by the new DEA license? Explain your answer.

Case Study 2

Rich took a new job as an athletic trainer in an airplane manufacturing plant after working several years at the local university. The factory's athletic training clinic had a small stock of prescription medications that the industrial setting physician could administer as needed. Rich evaluated an assembly line worker with a lower back strain and felt that a muscle relaxant was indicated. He gave the worker 8 tablets and told him to follow up with the physician in a few days.

Questions for Analysis

1. Is it appropriate for the clinic to stock prescription medication such as muscle relaxants? Explain your answer.
2. Is what Rich did within his professional scope and standards? Explain your answer.

2

Administering Medications in the Athletic Training Setting

OBJECTIVES

After reading this chapter, you will be able to do the following:

- Recognize the guidelines regarding medication administration that athletic trainers and other sports medicine clinicians must adhere to
- Implement policies and procedures for medication administration in the athletic training clinic
- Identify the key components of a physician's prescription pad and common Latin abbreviations
- Identify potential errors in prescribing medication
- List the information included in a medication order or prescription
- List strategies for avoiding or preventing a medication error

Physically active people use both prescription and over-the-counter (OTC) medications as part of their medical care. Medications for musculoskeletal inflammation, pain, and asthma and oral antibiotics are some of the drugs most prevalently used by elite athletes.[1,11,32] Since the 1970s, athletic trainers (ATs) have been advised that they need to be knowledgeable of medications involved with injury care; have legal, ethical, and moral responsibilities to the patient; and should avoid administering harmful drugs.[24] As the profession of athletic training evolved, management of medication by ATs became more prevalent. Changes in federal and state mandates have allowed physicians more convenience in ordering, storing, dispensing, and administering medications in the athletic training setting.[27] However, ATs who administer medications must comply with legal and ethical requirements and realize that failure to do so could have serious consequences, both for themselves and the prescribing physician with whom they are collaborating.[17,31,35] This chapter provides students with a functional understanding of basic indications and contraindications of medications that are stored, ordered, furnished, or otherwise managed for their patients.

Athletic Training Clinic

The most common sports medicine facilities include, but are not limited to, the traditional athletic training clinic, on-site practice or game facilities, and treatment spaces within a performance venue; ancillary facilities associated with travel (e.g., bus, plane, hotel) must be adapted to deliver athletic training services.[4,8] The traditional athletic training clinic typically serves as the primary health care location for those participating in secondary school and collegiate athletic programs and professional sports teams. Local, state, and federal entities issue often overlapping regulations and standards to ensure the quality of facilities that deliver health care services.[8] As discussed in chapter 1, federal law requires any facility that receives, stores, administers, or dispenses controlled substances to maintain a valid registration from the U.S. Drug Enforcement Administration (DEA).[10] Athletic training facilities that dispense noncontrolled substances (such as oral antibiotics) must provide these medications in a properly labeled and packaged container. For these activities, DEA registration is not necessary.[5,20]

As required by the Board of Certification (BOC), policies and procedures are a critical element of therapeutic medication administration. When written properly, clear expectations (policies) and instructions (procedures) allow for a policy to be implemented and provide standardization in day-to-day operational activities. Sound policies and procedures relating to medication administration dictate that these are living documents that bring structure to the sports medicine program.

Clear policies and procedures communicate the expectations of the organization and provide guidance for a straightforward policy framework. This practice allows for fewer misunderstandings about what to do in specific situations and establishes transparency and consistency in the way the organization operates and makes decisions relating to patient care. With the rapid pace of new and updated laws, it is important to adhere to and communicate ever-changing regulations and best practice. A policies and procedures document, when kept current, helps ATs ensure compliance with all medication-related laws and simplifies the process of communicating change throughout the organization. Policies and procedures should be reviewed and approved annually, and a copy should then be forwarded to administrators and the organization's risk management office.[9]

Evidence in Pharmacology

Treating Patients Who Are Minors

Many ATs employed in the secondary and middle school settings care for patients younger than 18 years old. The Council on School Health recommends that school districts establish polices for administration of medications at school.[7] A simple approach for ATs is the presumption that minors are not to be provided any medication without consent from the parent or guardian.[23] It is also important for the intercollegiate AT to ensure that incoming freshmen younger than 18 years old have written consent and authorization for treatment from a parent or guardian. This practice covers administration of medications by the athletic training staff, team physicians, and others involved in patient care.[7]

Guidelines for Administering Medications

Guidelines for administering medications in the athletic training setting have been published since 1992 emphasizing the schedule classification of drugs, the role of documentation, and the mandate to follow federal and state laws.[35] Nevertheless, serial studies conducted shortly after these guidelines were first published identified concerns of AT compliance with state and federal regulations regarding prescription and OTC medication management.[21,22] In the initial study, essentially half of the ATs surveyed admitted to marginal adherence to federal regulations, citing that they had allowed athletic training students to distribute medications and had not tracked dissemination of OTC medication.[22] The follow-up study identified a lack of proper medication storage equipment and OTC distribution that was facilitated without tracking, but assistant ATs seemed to be more compliant with federal regulations than head ATs.[21] Current educational standards have specific competencies relating to therapeutic medications that all entry-level ATs should know.

Evidence in Pharmacology

CAATE Standards for Therapeutic Medications

Educational standards from the Commission on Accreditation of Athletic Training Education (CAATE) stipulate that an entry-level AT should be able to do the following:[6]

- Educate patients regarding appropriate pharmacological agents for the management of their condition, including indications, contraindications, dosing, interactions, and adverse reactions
- Administer medications or other therapeutic agents by the appropriate route of administration on the order of a physician or other provider with legal prescribing authority

The CAATE standards are subject to periodic review and update. It is recommended that clinicians, faculty members, and researchers consult the most up-to-date standards regarding the expectations of an entry-level AT.

Administrative Principles for Prescription Medications

If considering incorporating prescription medications into the athletic training clinic, members of the medical staff must follow sound administrative principles.[27] These principles apply to prescription medications, particularly controlled substances. The athletic training staff should do the following:[5,6,8,9,27]

- **Develop a medication policy and procedures manual for the athletic training clinic.** This is the road map or framework for managing medications and establishing protocols for dispensing medication, managing inventory, keeping records, and so on. Policies should be reviewed annually and adjusted accordingly.[19,30]
- **Understand state and federal regulations policies as they apply to athletic training.** Federal guidelines supersede state and local statutes relative to managing medications. To store, receive, administer, and dispense controlled substances, the medical director or lead team physician should be the physician of record who registers the athletic training facility with the DEA. Thus, the address of the athletic training clinic will be on record with the DEA. The address of a physician's off-campus office is insufficient to meet this requirement. DEA permits are site specific and may not be transferred. Many facilities choose not to have controlled substances in the athletic training clinic.
- **Establish a chain of command.** A hierarchy of responsible team physicians and ATs should be established based on which people will be managing medications. Duties for responsibilities, such as ordering drugs and inventory tracking, should be delineated. Athletic training students are never allowed in this chain of command.
- **Keep proper records.** Maintaining legible, accurate, and complete records is a necessity. Records should cover the name of the patient receiving the medication, when it was dispensed, and a log of the lot number of the batch. Records must be stored in accordance with state and federal laws for 3 years. It is incumbent on the AT to have a functional record management system that meets his needs.
- **Destroy expired medications.** Expired or damaged prescription and OTC medications must be rotated out of stock. Expired medications should never be dispensed. A **reverse distributor** should be used to dispose of expired inventory. Any returned medication should be added to a destruction container immediately on return.
- **Correctly label all medications.** A medication must be exclusive to the patient for whom it was intended. Medications should not be shared among teammates or given to anonymous patients.
- **Securely lock medications and controlled substances.** All medications should be stored in locked cabinets, with access limited to ATs and team physicians. Controlled substances should have a higher level of security scrutiny. For example, they should be stored in an area that only physicians can access. Medica-

tion cabinets must be placed in a physician's office within the athletic training facility and not in the general traffic areas.

- **Provide sample medications.** These are prepackaged medications with a limited number of doses that are convenient to administer. Samples may help reduce costs, but they must be properly documented with a paper trail when being brought into the athletic training facility. This level of documentation acknowledges when the samples were incorporated into the clinic as well as the patient receiving the medication. Samples are owned by a licensed physician and must not leave the facility.

Managing Prescription Medication in the Athletic Training Facility

Specific guidance for ATs managing medications in their work setting emanated from the original *Consensus Statement on Managing Prescription and Non-Prescription Medications in the Athletic Training Facility*, which was issued by the National Athletic Trainers' Association (NATA) in 2009.[23] Among other critical points, the statement reinforces that ATs must adhere to all state and federal statutes relative to administering medication. The following guidelines cover personnel, infrastructure, and tracking of medications in the athletic training facility:[23]

- **Personnel**—For facilities in a traditional athletic training setting
  - **Athletic trainer**—Only a staff AT should have access to prescription or OTC medications.
  - **Physician**—The team physician or directing physician is ultimately responsible for all phases of managing prescription medications.
  - **Pharmacist**—Pharmacists who work with the athletic medicine department should be approved by the team physician.
  - **Administrator or Director of Sports Medicine**—This person administratively supervises the sports medicine staff or directing physician, who should understand the means by which the athletic medicine's medication is managed.
- **Packaging**—If more than 1 dose is being administered to a patient, the dose should be dispensed in a secure single package provided by the pharmacy (described further in the Drug Packaging section).
- **Labeling**—Medications should be kept in the original package from the pharmacist and a label with specific patient information and directions should be added at the time it is dispensed.
- **Distribution**—Physicians are the only personnel allowed to distribute prescription medications. Only sports medicine personnel may distribute OTC medications. Athletic training students must never administer, dispense, or otherwise give out or furnish *any* medications.
- **Documentation**—Individual records of prescription medications must be maintained in a medication documentation form. Ultimately, this information must be transferred to the patient's individual medical record, regardless if it is a digital or paper file. OTC distribution must also be documented.
- **Inventory control**—Periodic reconciliation (e.g., monthly, bimonthly, semiannually) of prescription medications brought into inventory and distributed to patients must be maintained.
- **Disposal**—Medications that have expired or have been returned by patients need to be disposed of in a destruction container in accordance with state regulations and coordinated with the designated pharmacy or reverse distributor.
- **Emergency medications**—The team or directing physician is responsible for determining which emergency medications are available in the athletic training facility for any individual needs.

Drug Orders

In emergencies, the prescriber might give the AT a verbal order for medication; if the prescriber is not present at the athletic training clinic, she may give the AT an order over the telephone. If an athletic training clinic is involved with prescription medications, policies are needed for the various types of medication orders. Such policies should be communicated with staff as well as athletes or patients (figure 2.1). The policy determines the person authorized to take drug orders—usually the

RED FLAG

Documentation

Athletic trainers involved in managing medications must be diligent with documenting how medicines are distributed. Over-the-counter medications are not immune from proper documentation even though they are readily available to patients. Ignoring documentation of OTCs is not safe and can go beyond the scope of state or national laws.[5] The BOC also recommends maintaining and retaining records of OTC medication distribution. Tracking the medication's lot number is important in case of the unlikely event of a product recall or an adverse event associated with the medication.[9]

Head AT or Director of Sports Medicine. The AT taking the verbal order is responsible for writing it on the order form in the medical record, including the names of both the clinician and the prescriber. Best practice is that a note be written to indicate that the order was read back to the prescriber for validation. The prescriber must then cosign this order, usually within 24 hours, for the order to be valid.[12] Medication orders may be classified into 1 of 4 types:[12]

1. **Standing order**—Indicates that the drug is to be administered until discontinued or for a certain number of doses; facility policy must dictate that most standing orders expire after a certain number of days. A renewal order must be written by the physician before the drug may be continued.
2. **Stat order**—One-time order to be given immediately.
3. **Single order**—One-time order to be given at specified time.
4. **PRN order**—Given as needed based on patient need.

Some facilities also have a "now order" classification, where the health care provider (HCP) has 1.5 hours to give the medication. This is different from a stat order, which must be given within minutes. The athletic training clinic's policy must clearly define each of these types of orders and how they are carried out. The AT must be familiar with common abbreviations used in pharmacology[12] to avoid medication errors (further described in the Preventing Medication Errors section).

Drug Packaging

Packaging prescription medications in the athletic training setting can pose several concerns. Historically, tablets or capsules were transferred from a stock bottle to a small pill envelope.[25] This process is considered repackaging and does not meet standards set by the U.S. Food and Drug Administration

UNIVERSITY OF XYZ ATHLETIC MEDICINE

USE OF MEDICATION NOTICE

The University of XYZ athletic medicine staff is committed to providing the best overall care for your injuries or illnesses. At times, this includes prescribing and/or administering medication. As a part of this process, we want you to be sufficiently informed about any medications prescribed or recommended for your medical conditions or injuries.

Use of prescription or over-the-counter medication is voluntary. Some medications pose a risk of long-term side effects if overused. These risks are statistically minimal, particularly if the medication is used in accordance with recommended dose guidelines. However, there are certain medications that present a risk of addiction or complications if abused.

If you have a question or concern regarding any medication prescribed or recommended by a member of our athletic medicine staff, please contact a team physician or your athletic trainer.

John Doe, MD
Director of Athletic Medicine
University of XYZ

FIGURE 2.1 Sample use of medication notice.

(FDA).[28] The U.S. Department of Health and Human Services considers repackaging as "the act of taking a finished drug product from the container in which it was distributed by the original manufacturer and placing it into a different container without further manipulation of the drug."[34] Additionally, the FDA expresses concerns that the stability, safety, and efficacy of a drug could be affected by repackaging. To minimize repackaging concerns, medications must be administered to the patient in the original container from the pharmacy.[28]

Legally, a traditional-style medication bottle or blister pack with a specific number of doses may be packaged by the manufacturer, dispensed by the pharmacy, and then administered to the patient in its original and unaltered state. A standardized prescription label is affixed to the package in the pharmacy, or a physician can add specific instructions for use. An instruction form should be attached specifically for the prescription. A copy of this form should be added to the patient's file or its data entered directly into the patient's electronic medical or health record.[28]

Filling a Prescription

The appropriate process of furnishing a prescription medication to a patient in an athletic training setting is no different than for any patient consulting with a prescriber. By law, only a prescriber can administer or dispense controlled substances. Remember that although these terms may seem synonymous, they are distinct and not interchangeable.

The prescription label (figure 2.2) is the documented record of instructions from the physician to the patient. This form meets the criteria of dispensing medication from a pharmacist, as noted previously. The core components of the prescription must be on file with the pharmacist and in the patient's medical record. Requirements of a prescription are as follows:[29]

- Prescriber's name, address, phone, and licensure information
- Patient's name
- Patient's identifying data (e.g., home address, date of birth)
- Date the prescription was written
- Specific medication name, strength, and number of doses
- Specific instructions for use:
    - Frequency
    - Route of administration
    - Number of refills
    - Warnings associated with the medication

Fortunately, modern advances in electronic prescribing (e-prescribing) streamline the prescription process and dramatically reduce prescription errors. In this process, the prescriber initially enters the prescription where it is verified and processed in an electronic format, resulting in a labeled medication product, supportive documentation, and an updated, sharable patient electronic medication profile.[14]

Historically, Latin abbreviations have been used to communicate critical instructions regarding dosing frequency and method of delivery to the

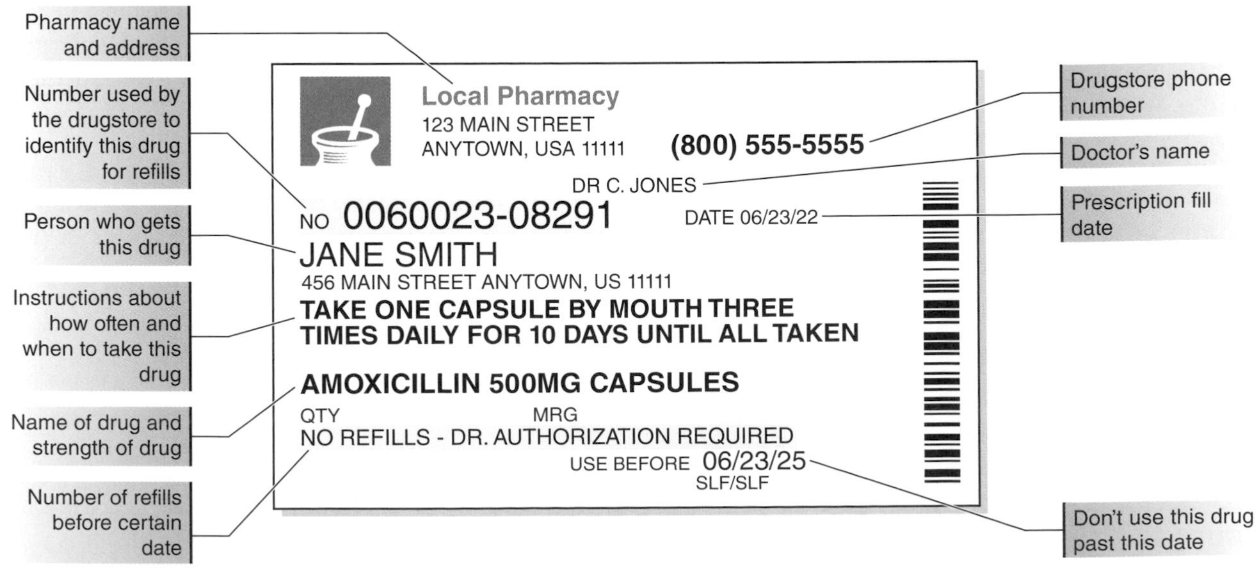

FIGURE 2.2 Sample prescription form label.

pharmacist. Prescribers have moved away from these abbreviations for the most part, but still rely on shorthand notations for various other components of the prescription. The more common prescription instructions pertain to the medication's measurement quantity, frequency of taking a medicine, and the drug release technology.[2] The AT should be familiar with common medical abbreviations relating to sports medicine (table 2.1). Clinicians should be careful to avoid the common mistake of confusing QID and Q1d, where the first is "4 times per day" and the second is "every day."[2]

TABLE 2.1 Common Medical Abbreviations Used in Sports Medicine Prescriptions

Abbreviation	Definition	Category
AAA	Apply to affected area	Instructions
AC	Before meals	Time
Amp	Ampoule	Dosage form
ATC	Around the clock	Frequency
BID	Twice daily	Frequency
CC	Chief complaint	Other
CR	Controlled release	Drug-release technology
ER	Extended release	Drug-release technology
g	Gram	Measurement
gtt	Drops	Measurement
Hr or h	Hour	Time
IM	Intramuscular	Route of administration
IR	Immediate release	Drug-release technology
IV	Intravenous	Route of administration
LA	Long acting	Drug-release technology
mEq/L	Milliequivalent/liter	Measurement
mL	Milliliter	Measurement
PC	After meals	Time
PO	By mouth	Route of administration
PR	Rectally	Route of administration
PRN	As needed	Frequency
SL	Sublingually	Route of administration
Q2h	Every 2 hours	Frequency
Q3h	Every 3 hours	Frequency
Q4h	Every 4 hours	Frequency
Q6h	Every 6 hours	Frequency
Q12h	Every 12 hours	Frequency
Q1d or QD	Every day	Frequency
QID	Four times per day	Frequency
SR	Sustained release	Drug-release technology
Susp	Suspension	Dosage form
Tbsp	Tablespoon	Measurement
TID	Three times daily	Frequency
XL or XR or XT	Extended release	Drug-release technology

Sloppy handwriting and reliance on Latin abbreviations contribute to medication errors.[3] However, contemporary medical practices, such as the computer physician order entry (CPOE) and minimal use of verbal prescriptions, can be useful in reducing the risk for medication errors. These practices enhance correct spelling of patient names and provide prescription instructions in a legible, understandable mode. On some occasions, a physician may not have access to electronic transmission modes. For example, an athletic training clinic may not have the appropriate digital connection to transmit the prescription. In cases such as this, a prescription will likely be written on a traditional prescription pad. Thus, it is vital to ensure that all information transmitted is accurate and easy to follow.[3]

The preponderance of communication between the physician or provider and pharmacist in the United States is in English. However, when working with patients for whom English is a second language, the physician or pharmacist may need to convey prescription information in the patient's native language.[18]

Preventing Medication Errors

A medication error is any preventable event that may cause or lead to inappropriate medication use or patient harm while the medication is in the control of the HCP, patient, or consumer. Such events may be related to professional practice, health care products, procedures, and systems, including prescribing; order communication; product labeling, packaging, and nomenclature; compounding; dispensing; distribution; administration; education; monitoring; and use.[26] Some of the factors associated with medication errors include the following:[16]

- Medications with similar names or similar packaging
- Medications that are not commonly used or prescribed
- Commonly used medications to which many patients are allergic (e.g., antibiotics, opiates, and nonsteroidal anti-inflammatory drugs)
- Simultaneous use of multiple drugs to treat a single ailment or condition or simultaneous use of multiple drugs by 1 patient (**polypharmacy**)
- Medications that require testing to ensure that proper (i.e., nontoxic) therapeutic levels are maintained (e.g., *lithium*, *warfarin*, *theophylline*, and *digoxin*)

Errors in drug administration can be prevented through various means. As previously mentioned, using electronic formats for written prescriptions eliminates a handwritten prescription that can be misinterpreted or lost. Sports medicine practitioners

Clinical Application

Advising Patients on Taking Medications

The AT should reinforce the following information to the patient when administering OTC or prescription medications:

- Reiterate that the patient must exercise care when taking any medication (both prescription and OTC) and follow the prescriber or manufacturer instructions
- Clarify the basic nature of how the medication works and why it is being prescribed
- Remind the patient that the prescriber or pharmacist is available to answer specific questions or clarify elements of the prescription
- Reinforce medication contraindications or special instructions (i.e., take with food)
- Confirm that the patient understands the information provided
- Document any patient feedback or concerns
- Ask if the patient has questions regarding his understanding of the medication or the physician's rationale for prescribing it

should apply these rights of medication administration (figure 2.3) to promote medication safety:[13,15,17,33]

1. **Right patient**—Ask the patient their name. Is there a medication prescribed to someone with a similar or same name? Could there be confusion when another HCP is involved?
2. **Right drug**—Carefully examine the packaging, particularly if this is a new or different medication for the patient. Is the drug name on the label consistent with the physician's orders? Is the product description on the pharmacy label consistent with the product in the package? Check the contents against the original packaging; do not repackage medications.
3. **Right dose**—Confirm the information listed on pharmacy package by comparing it with the prescriber's orders. Has the medication been properly administered? Have there been omissions, treatment completed, wrong strength, or double dose?
4. **Right route**—Confirm the intended route of administration by comparing the pharmacy label with the prescriber's orders. Is the drug to be given orally? Or instead by injection or intravenously?
5. **Right time**—Ensure that the drug is administered at the correct time. Has the patient skipped a dose? Was the drug administered late? Should the drug be taken with food instead of on an empty stomach?
6. **Right documentation**—Has the patient been documented to have received the drug? Always record the administration of the drug in the medication log and in the patient's medical record.

RED FLAG

Patients With Similar Names

Pharmacists must have accurate patient information when filling a prescription to ensure that the right patient receives the intended medication. Some sons have the same first and last name as their fathers. Patients may share the same last name with their in-laws. Confusion around names could cause pharmacists to provide patients with the wrong medication. Preventing this type of medication error requires specific identification information. Identifying a patient by both name and birth date is the easiest way to ensure that a prescription is matched to the correct patient.

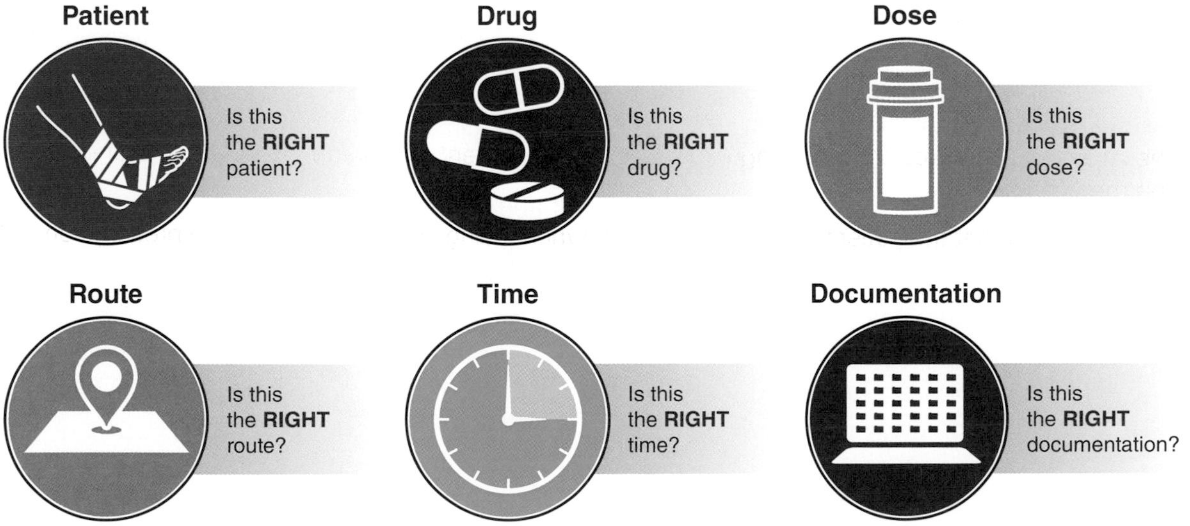

FIGURE 2.3 The rights of medication administration.

Summary

Medicines can play a vital role in restoring or maintaining any patient's well-being. If an athletic training facility opts to administer OTC or prescription medications, the AT administration and staff must adhere to strict state and federal guidelines. A policies and procedures manual should be developed to guide ATs in the administration of medications in the sports medicine clinic. Prescribers and clinicians must give clear and specific instructions on the appropriate use and administration of each medication. Best practices in patient care and preventing medical errors involve following simple procedures, such as the rights of medication administration, collaborating with prescribers, advising patients on their use of medication, and monitoring the patient for adverse effects. Finally, although documentation of medication transactions can be challenging for busy ATs, it is necessary.

Case Studies

Case Study 1

Smitty is a professional hockey player who reported nasal congestion and a painful left ear. The symptoms occurred during cold and flu season, and he was one of several players with similar symptoms. He was referred to the team physician, who prescribed a decongestant. Smitty acknowledged that he was confused by the label's directions of "take 1 tab PO QID." Based on his own interpretation, he consumed a full day's dose all at once rather than taking 1 tablet 4 times daily. Within an hour of taking all of the tablets, Smitty complained that he was slightly dizzy. Evaluation determined that his blood pressure was mildly elevated compared to his preparticipation physical exam reading.

Questions for Analysis

1. What is the difference between QID and QD?
2. What is the lesson for the patient? For the AT?

Case Study 2

Ahmad is a lineman at the local power company whose job description includes climbing power poles with a 15-lb (7-kg) utility belt. Ahmad reported lower back strain after losing his footing and slipping down a wet power pole. He was diagnosed with mechanical lower back pain absent of obvious disc pathology. At the conclusion of the exam, the physician gave Ahmad an envelope containing several days' worth of 800 mg *ibuprofen* tablets and provided verbal instructions on their use. The physician acknowledged that the medication was prescription strength but equated it to a comparable quantity of over-the-counter *ibuprofen* and thus did not deem it important to document the dosage or provide Ahmad with any written directions.

Questions for Analysis

1. Was it appropriate for the physician to provide the medication in that manner? Explain your answer.
2. The physician decided to not record the amount of 800 mg *ibuprofen* he provided because *ibuprofen* comes in OTC strength. Is this a valid argument? Explain your answer.

3

Drug Names, Classification, and Safety

OBJECTIVES

After reading this chapter, you will be able to do the following:

- Develop strategies for recognizing, documenting, and communicating important information about common medications in sports medicine
- Describe the differences between generic and trade names of drugs
- Define the major terms in the dose–response relationship
- Identify the major classifications of adverse drug reactions
- Describe collaboration with a drug information expert, the pharmacist
- Develop strategies for health care professionals to provide effective and culturally sensitive responses and recommendations to a patient
- Outline the steps in the medication use process
- Describe how the expanding integration of information technology has changed the methods of searching, analyzing, and providing drug information to patients and health care professionals

The content of this textbook is organized in a logical way that minimizes the amount of information to memorize and maximizes the athletic trainer's (AT) ability to continue to learn.[24] Although many medications have complex-sounding names, the graduate AT student does not need to know every name of every medication she might encounter during the course of patient care. However, the AT must be able to recognize, document, and communicate important information about various medications that patients may be taking.[11,24]

This chapter discusses how drugs are named according to generic names, trade names, and classes of drugs. Drugs are described according to a common mechanism of action and chemical structure. Additionally, this chapter addresses the clinical application of pharmacologic interventions in terms of medication errors, adverse drug effects, and allergic drug reactions. Finally, it describes the medication use process, the clinical pharmacist's role in drug safety, and appropriate resources of drug information to be used by the practicing athletic trainers (ATs) when caring for patients using therapeutic medications.

Drug Names

All drugs have a generic and trade name.

- The **generic name** can sometimes be an abbreviated version of the drug's chemical name; for example, the drug with the chemical name acetylsalicylic acid (ASA) is commonly known as *aspirin*. The generic (nonproprietary) name is registered with the U.S. Food and Drug Administration (FDA) and listed in a directory of medications in the **United States Pharmacopeia–National Formulary** (USP–NF).
- A drug's **trade name** (or brand name) is proprietary and legally protected by patents and exclusivity; for example, there are many brand names for *aspirin*, including Bufferin. The patent owner (usually a pharmaceutical company) has exclusive rights for marketing the product for a limited time after approval of the new drug.[6,15]

Generic drug names are written in lower case, and trade names always begin with a capital letter. In this text, when applicable, the generic name is listed first in *italics* and the capitalized trade name appears next in parentheses.[11] Table 3.1 provides examples of generic and trade names of several common drugs, including their indications for use.

Several important terms are related to generic and trade name drugs:

- **Bioequivalence**—Requirement by the FDA that generic medications meet the same standards for safety and efficacy as their brand-name counterparts.
- **Patent**—Property rights granted during the development of a drug.
- **Exclusivity**—Delays and prohibitions on the approval of generic competitor drugs; promotes a balance between new drug innovation and greater public access to drugs that result from generic drug competition. Currently, the term of the exclusivity of a new patent is 20 years, after which the generic drug can be produced.

Currently, more than half of the prescriptions written in the United States are for generic drugs.[10] In the United States, most pharmacists have the authority to substitute generic drugs for brand-name medications when the drug is dispensed to the patient. However, the prescriber can request that the pharmacist not substitute a generic for a branded medication by indicating this on the prescription ("do not substitute" or "dispense as written").[10,11]

Drug Classes

Medications are commonly classified as a **drug class**, which is a set of medications and other compounds with similar characteristics:[15,29]

- **Same mechanism of action**—Bind to the same biological target to produce the same effect or action
- **Similar chemical structures**—Grouped together and named by the chemical compound that they have in common
- **Same therapeutic indication**—Based on the indication for treating the same symptom, condition, or disease

Many drugs can be classified in more than 1 class. Therefore, part II of this text focuses on the therapeutic effects of medications that are common in the sports medicine setting:

- **Drugs to treat pain:** nonopioid analgesics and anesthetics (chapter 7), opioid analgesics (chapter 8)
- **Drugs to treat inflammation:** anti-inflammatories—steroidal and nonsteroidal (chapter 9)
- **Drugs to treat infection:** antibiotics (chapter 10)

TABLE 3.1 Examples of Generic and Trade Names

Generic name	Trade name	Indication
albuterol	Ventolin, Proventil, ProAir	Asthma
nitroglycerin	Nitrostat	Angina
metaxalone	Skelaxin	Muscle spasm or pain
azithromycin	Zithromax	Infection

Additionally, drugs can be categorized by the body system they are used to treat, which are presented in part III of this text.

Drug Safety

Drug safety involves assessment of risk versus benefit to the patient. Any drug prescribed must be approved by the FDA, which conducts extensive testing to determine its safety and effectiveness.

Drug Efficacy Versus Effectiveness

A drug (or any medical treatment) should be used only when the patient will benefit from the treatment. Benefit to the patient is determined by the ability of the drug to produce the desired result (efficacy) and the likelihood of adverse effects (safety). Cost is also commonly balanced with benefit of using the drug.[18]

Efficacy is the capacity of the drug to produce an effect (e.g., reduce hypertension). It can be accurately assessed only in ideal conditions (i.e., when patients are selected by proper criteria and strictly adhere to the dosing schedule). Thus, efficacy is measured under expert supervision in a group of patients who are most likely to have a response to a drug, such as in a controlled clinical trial.[18]

Effectiveness differs from efficacy in that it considers how well a drug works in real-world use; often, a drug that is efficacious in clinical trials is not very effective in actual use. For example, a drug may have high efficacy in reducing hypertension but may have low effectiveness because it causes so many **adverse effects** that patients stop taking it. Effectiveness also may be lower than efficacy if clinicians inadvertently prescribe the drug inappropriately (e.g., giving a fibrinolytic drug to a patient thought to have an ischemic stroke, but who actually had an unrecognized cerebral hemorrhage, which was revealed on a CT scan). Thus, effectiveness tends to be lower than efficacy.[9,18] Potency and efficacy are further discussed in chapter 5.

Safe and Efficacious Medication Use

Athletic trainers have a multitude of responsibilities within their scope of practice, including collaborating with pharmacists regarding safe and effective medication therapy. All clinicians aim to maximize patient safety while minimizing medication mishaps, such as medication errors and adverse drug events (see Adverse Drug Effects and Therapeutic Monitoring). Given the sheer amount of information involved and available when taking care of patients today, safe and effective medication use can be reasonably obtained only when clinicians effectively manage the information and related information systems involved in support of the medication use process.[12]

RED FLAG

Patient Compliance

Patient satisfaction with the AT has a significant effect on their compliance behavior. Patients are more likely to follow instructions and recommendations when their expectations for the patient–provider relationship and for their treatment are met. These expectations include not only clinical but also interpersonal competence; thus, cultivating good interpersonal and communication skills is essential.[6,18]

Therapeutic Index

When a provider prescribes medications to patients, it is ideal to have large differences between the dose that is efficacious and the dose that causes adverse effects (see Adverse Drug Effects and Therapeutic Monitoring). A large difference is considered a wide **therapeutic index** (TI), therapeutic ratio, or **therapeutic window**. Medications with very high TI (e.g., *penicillin*) are extremely safe in the absence of a known allergic response in a given patient. On the other hand, in medications with a narrow TI, factors that are usually clinically inconsequential (e.g., food–drug interactions, drug–drug interactions, small errors in dosing) can have harmful clinical effects. For example, the anticoagulant *warfarin* has a narrow TI and interacts with many drugs and foods. Insufficient anticoagulation increases the risk of complications resulting from treatment of the disorder with anticoagulation drugs (e.g., increased risk of stroke), whereas excessive anticoagulation increases risk of bleeding.[9,18] Select antibiotics are also subject to a food–drug interaction. Calcium and casein in milk decrease the bioavailability of both *ciprofloxacin* (500 mg) tablets and *tetracycline*; when *azithromycin* is taken with food, its absorption is decreased, resulting in a reduction in bioavailability of up to 43%.[5] The therapeutic effect must always be balanced by the lethality (toxic effect) of the drug, yielding a **margin of safety**.

Preventable Causes of Drug-Related Problems

- **Drug interactions**—Use of a drug results in a drug–drug, drug–food, drug–supplement, or drug–disease interaction, leading to adverse effects or decreased efficacy.
- **Inadequate monitoring**—A medical problem is being treated with the correct drug, but the patient is not adequately monitored for complications, effectiveness, or both.
- **Inappropriate drug selection**—A medical problem that requires drug therapy is being treated with a less-than-optimal drug.
- **Inappropriate treatment**—A patient is taking a drug for no medically valid reason.
- **Lack of patient adherence**—The correct drug for a medical problem is prescribed, but the patient is not taking it as directed.
- **Overdosage**—A medical problem is being treated with too much of the correct drug.
- **Poor communication**—Drugs are inappropriately dosed, duplicated, continued, or stopped when care is poorly transitioned between providers or facilities.
- **Underprescribing**—A medical problem is being treated with too little of the correct drug.
- **Untreated medical problem**—A medical problem requires drug therapy, but either no drug is being used to treat that problem or nonpharmacological interventions are needed. For example, prediabetes may be an untreated medical problem (and may be caused by other medications) that may not require a medication. Diet and exercise are commonly prescribed.

Adapted from Buxton (2017); Lynch (2019).

Number Needed to Treat

The **number needed to treat (NNT)** is an epidemiological term accounting of the likely benefits of a therapeutic medication (or any other intervention). The NNT is the number of patients who need to be treated in order for 1 patient to benefit. For example, consider a drug that decreases the mortality of a certain disease from 10% to 5%, an absolute risk reduction of 5% (1 in 20). That means that of 100 patients, 90 would live even without treatment, and thus would not benefit from the drug. Also, 5 of the 100 patients will die even though they take the drug and thus also would not benefit from it. Only 5 of the 100 patients (1 in 20) would benefit from taking the drug; thus, 20 patients need to be treated for 1 to benefit, and the NNT is 20. The NNT can be simply calculated as the inverse of the absolute risk reduction; if the absolute risk reduction is 5% (0.05), the NNT = 1 / 0.05 = 20. The NNT can also be calculated for adverse effects; in this case, it is sometimes called the **number needed to harm (NNH)**.[18]

Absolute Versus Relative Risk

Importantly, NNT is based on changes in **absolute risk**; it cannot be calculated from changes in relative risk. **Relative risk** is the proportional difference between 2 risk levels. For example, a drug that decreases mortality from 10% to 5% decreases absolute mortality by 5% but decreases relative mortality by 50% (i.e., a 5% death rate indicates 50% fewer deaths than a 10% death rate). Most often, benefits are reported in the literature as relative risk reductions because these make a drug look more effective than the absolute risk reductions. (Taking the previous example, a 50% reduction in mortality sounds much better than a 5% reduction.) In contrast, adverse effects are usually reported as absolute risk increases because they make a drug appear safer. For example, if a drug increases the incidence of bleeding from 0.1% to 1%, the increase is more likely to be reported as 0.9% than 1,000%.[18]

Adverse Drug Effects and Therapeutic Monitoring

Pharmacology intersects with toxicology when the physiological response to a drug becomes an adverse drug event.[13,20,28] An **adverse drug effect** or **event (ADE)** is an injury that results from medication use. Some ADEs are caused by preventable errors. ADEs that are not preventable are often the result of an **adverse drug reaction (ADR)**, which is an undesirable response associated with use of a drug that either compromises therapeutic efficacy, enhances toxicity, or both.[2,13,20,28] ADRs can be manifested as diarrhea or constipation, rash, headache, or other nonspecific symptoms. One of the challenges presented by ADRs is that prescribers may attribute the adverse effects to the patient's underlying condition and fail to recognize contributing factors such as the patient's age or number of other medications taken.[13] Potential ADEs (near misses or close calls) are medication errors that do not cause any harm to the patient because they are intercepted before they reach the patient or because the patient is able to physiologically absorb the error without any harm.[13]

Most adverse drug reactions are dose dependent; others are allergic or idiosyncratic.[18,19] ADRs may obviously result from drug use or be too subtle to identify as drug related. Subtle ADRs can cause functional deterioration, changes in mental status, failure to thrive, loss of appetite, confusion, and depression. The types of ADRs are as follows:[18,19]

- **Dose-dependent**—When drugs have a narrow TI (e.g., hemorrhage with oral anticoagulants), ADRs are a particular concern. ADRs may result from decreased drug clearance in patients with impaired renal or hepatic function or from drug–drug interactions.
- **Allergic**—These ADRs are not dose related and require prior exposure to the medication. **Drug allergies** develop when a drug acts as an antigen or allergen. After a patient is sensitized, subsequent exposure to the drug produces 1 of several different types of allergic reaction. Clinical history and appropriate skin tests can sometimes help predict allergic ADRs. These reactions are detailed in the sections that follow.
- **Idiosyncratic**—These are unexpected ADRs that are not dose related or allergic. They occur in a small percentage of patients who take a drug. **Idiosyncrasy** is an imprecise term that has been defined as a genetically determined abnormal response to a drug, but not all idiosyncratic reactions have a pharmacogenetic cause. The term may become obsolete as specific mechanisms of ADRs become known.

Classification of Adverse Drug Reactions

ADRs can range from mild to severe (table 3.2). Serious ADRs are those that can cause disability or birth defects, are life threatening, and result in hospitalization or death.[13,28] Severe or lethal ADRs may be specifically mentioned in black box warnings in the prescribing information provided by the manufacturer.[19]

TABLE 3.2 Classification of Adverse Drug Reactions (ADRs)

Severity	Description	Examples
Mild	No antidote or treatment is required; hospitalization is not prolonged.	Antihistamines (some): drowsiness Opioids: constipation
Moderate	Change in treatment (e.g., modified dosage, addition of a drug), but not necessarily discontinuation of the drug. Hospitalization may be prolonged or specific treatment may be required.	Hormonal contraceptives: venous thrombosis NSAIDs: hypertension and edema
Severe	Potentially life threatening. Requires discontinuation of the drug and specific treatment of the ADR.	ACE inhibitors: angioedema Tricyclic antidepressants: abnormal heart rhythm Sulfonamides: Stevens-Johnson syndrome
Lethal	Directly or indirectly contributes to a patient's death.	*Acetaminophen* overdosage: liver failure Anticoagulants: hemorrhage

NSAID = nonsteroidal anti-inflammatory drug; ACE = angiotensin-converting enzyme

Based on Hughes (2008); Smith (2019); Tam (2015).

Clinical Application

FDA Black Box Warning

The FDA has multiple platforms for communicating medication safety information to providers and the public: mandated label changes, safety communications, and the **black box warning (BBW)**, one of its strongest warnings.[13,23] The BBW is verbiage on a medication's packaging that is surrounded by a black box (figure 3.1); it must be included in all print and broadcast advertisements. The FDA may issue the warning at the time when the manufacturer applies for approval in the regulatory process or in the early marketing phase if safety concerns are identified. The BBW is generally issued by the FDA based on clinical data or adverse events such as death or cardiovascular events that have been recorded secondary to using the medication. In addition to acknowledging risks of the medication, this warning lists updated information regarding practice guidelines or specific at-risk patient populations.[13,23]

WARNING
Cardiovascular Risk
May increase risk of serious and potentially fatal cardiovascular thrombotic events, MI (heart attack), and stroke; risk may increase with duration of use; possible increased risk with cardiovascular disease or cardiovascular disease risk factors; contraindicated for CABG peri-operative pain.

GI Risk
Increased risk of serious GI adverse events include bleeding, ulcer, and stomach or intestine perforation, which can be fatal; may occur at any time during use and without warning symptoms; elderly patients at greater risk for serious GI events.

FIGURE 3.1 Sample black box warnings from the FDA.

RED FLAG

Black Box Warnings

Teriparatide is an osteoanabolic medication for the treatment of women with osteoporosis that has effectively reduced fracture risk in this vulnerable population. However, based on animal research, the patient is at a remote risk of developing an osteosarcoma secondary to using this medication. *Teriparatide* comes with an FDA black box warning indicating that the risk of osteosarcoma[3] is roughly 3 per 1,000,000. An off-label application of the medication has been incorporated into the treatment of bone stress injuries in elite athletes. Any provider who prescribes *teriparatide* to an athlete must explain the BBW risk to the patient and his advocates, such as his agent, family, or personal medical staff.[3]

Managing Adverse Drug Reactions

The severity of ADRs and whether the ADE is related to the patient's drug therapy should be monitored.[27] The health care practitioner (HCP) should be familiar with the drug and the relevant literature concerning ADEs. Important and timely information for HCPs on prescription and over-the-counter drugs is available online (see Drug Information Resources). Sometimes it can be difficult to determine whether the patient's ADE is related to the drug, due to progression of the disease or other pathology, or due to some unknown source. The HCP may be involved in determining if the observed ADE is due to the drug or another factor by doing the following:[18,27]

- Checking that the correct drug product and dose were ordered and given to the patient
- Verifying that the onset of the ADE occurred after the drug was taken and not before
- Determining the time interval between the beginning of drug treatment and the onset of the event

Clinical Application

High-Alert Medications

Under no circumstances should the AT or another HCP modify or change a patient's medication. If the AT or HCP suspects an adverse drug reaction, the patient must be immediately referred to the prescriber or, in severe cases, transported by EMS to the emergency department. Medication errors can be considered a sentinel event when they are associated with high-alert medications. According to the Institute for Safe Medication Practices, **high-alert medications** are those likely to cause significant harm when used in error. The top 5 high-alert medications are as follows:[14]

1. *Insulin*
2. Opiates and narcotics
3. Injectable potassium chloride (or phosphate) concentrate
4. Intravenous anticoagulants (*heparin*)
5. Sodium chloride solutions above 0.9%

- Referring the patient to the prescriber and monitoring the patient's status, looking for improvement
- Collaborating with the prescriber and monitoring the patient for recurrence of the ADE

Allergic Drug Reactions

Immunologically mediated adverse drug reactions, also known as allergic or **drug hypersensitivity reactions (DHR)**, result from an overresponse of the immune system to the standard dose of a drug. The hyperresponse of the immune system to the antigenic drug leads to tissue damage manifesting as an organ-specific or generalized systemic reaction. Although some reactions are relatively well defined, the majority are due to mechanisms that are either unknown or poorly understood. Adverse drug effects not proven to be immune mediated that resemble allergic reactions in their clinical presentation are referred to as allergic-like or **pseudoallergic reactions**. Drug hypersensitivity reactions are responsible for 6% to 10% of adverse reactions to medications. The true frequency of allergic drug reactions is difficult to determine because many reactions are not reported and others may be difficult to distinguish from nonallergic adverse events.[26] Factors that influence the likelihood of allergic drug reactions include the following:[17]

- Chemical composition of the drug
- Whether the drug contains proteins of nonhuman origin
- Route of drug administration
- Sensitivity of the patient as determined by genetics or environmental factors (For some drugs, genetic predisposition has been identified as a risk factor for allergic-mediated **dermatologic reactions**.)

Managing Drug Allergy or Drug Hypersensitivity Reactions

Symptoms of these reactions can involve asthma and rhinitis, urticaria or angioedema, anaphylaxis, aseptic meningitis, or pneumonitis (figure 3.2). Dermatologic or skin reactions represent the most frequently recognized and reported form of allergic drug reaction.[17] Up to 20% of people with asthma are sensitive to *aspirin* and other nonsteroidal anti-inflammatory drugs (NSAIDs).[17,26] In susceptible patients, *aspirin* and other NSAIDs can produce 2 general types of reactions: urticaria or angioedema and rhinosinusitis or asthma[17,26] The most common reactions to *penicillin* include urticaria, pruritus, and angioedema.[26] Prescribers may consider the following actions when managing allergic reactions to drugs:[17,26]

- Discontinuation of the medication or agent when possible
- Treatment of the adverse clinical signs and symptoms
- Substitution, if necessary, of another agent

Evidence in Pharmacology

Angioedema

Angioedema can occur secondary to taking certain medications, particularly ACE inhibitors or NSAIDs. It presents as an allergic reaction, such as from food or other allergens, or a nonallergic reaction as the result of an increase in bradykinin levels in the body that does not respond to the usual and customary treatment for histamine-mediated allergens. Angioedema and urticaria are the most common **side effects** of NSAIDs and aspirin.

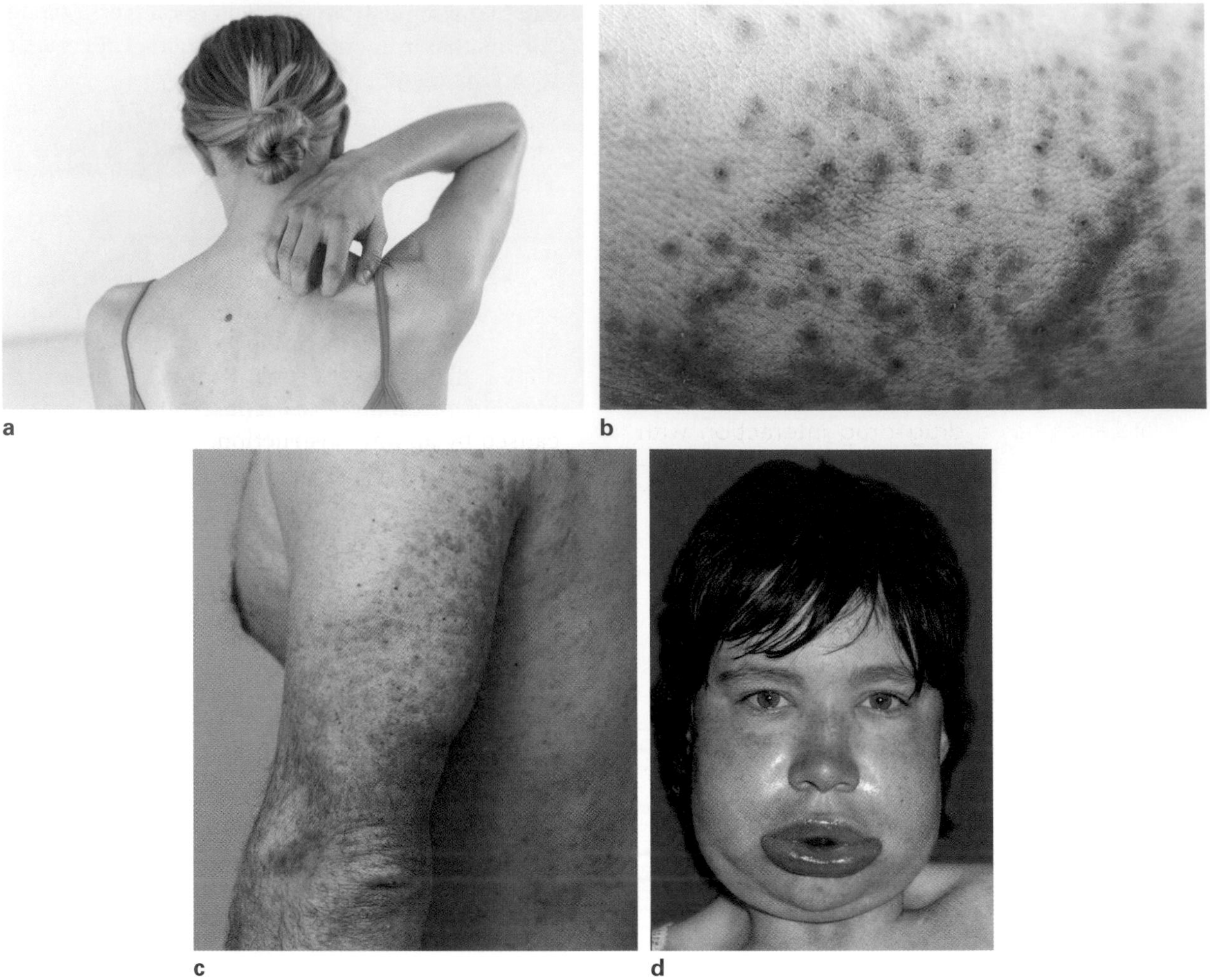

FIGURE 3.2 Common signs of drug allergy or hypersensitivity reactions: *(a)* itching, *(b)* skin rash, *(c)* urticaria, *(d)* angioedema.

a BSIP/Universal Images Group via Getty Images; *b* Cavallini James/BSIP/Universal Images Group via Getty Images; *c* BSIP/UIG Via Getty Images; *d* Clinical Photography, Central Manchester University Hospitals NHS Foundation Trust, UK/Science Source

Managing Anaphylactic Drug Reactions

Anaphylaxis is an acute, life-threatening allergic reaction involving multiple organ systems that generally begins within 30 minutes (and almost always within 2 hours) of exposure to the inciting allergen.[17,26] A consensus panel on allergy has defined anaphylaxis as highly likely when one of the following scenarios is present:[17]

- Acute onset of a reaction (minutes to several hours) that involves the skin (mucosal tissue) and respiratory tract or a decrease in blood pressure
- Rapid onset of a reaction after exposure to a likely allergen that involves 2 organ systems (respiratory tract, skin) and causes a decrease in blood pressure or persistent gastrointestinal symptoms
- Decrease in blood pressure alone after exposure to a known allergen
- Other presentations that may indicate anaphylaxis, such as acute chest pain or arrhythmia without dermatologic manifestations (Here, the potential exists for false-positive results.)

Medications are the second most common overall cause of anaphylaxis (after food allergy) and the primary cause of anaphylaxis in adults. The most common classes of drugs that produce anaphylaxis are the following:

- Antibiotics, especially β-lactam antibiotics (including *penicillin* and cephalosporins)
- Anti-inflammatories, such as *aspirin* and NSAIDs[16,17]

RED FLAG

Drug–Drug Interactions

Jardiance has a drug–drug interaction with *methylprednisolone* that is important to consider when treating diabetic patients with an acute lumbar spine injury. When combined with *methylprednisolone*, Jardiance's effectiveness diminishes, which could affect the patient's blood glucose management.[8] This is important to remember for an athletic trainer treating a patient's lower back conditions with *methylprednisolone*; he should investigate whether the patient is diabetic and happens to be taking Jardiance.

Anaphylaxis requires prompt treatment to restore respiratory and cardiovascular function. *Epinephrine* is the drug of choice for counteracting bronchoconstriction and peripheral vasodilation. IV fluids should be administered aggressively to restore intravascular volume.[17,26] The risk of fatal anaphylaxis is greatest within the first few hours. Late phase or biphasic reactions can occur 1 to 72 hours after the initial presentation, with most occurring within 6 hours. Because of the possibility of a biphasic reaction, patients should be observed for at least 8 hours after an anaphylactic reaction.[7] Fatal anaphylaxis most often results from asphyxia caused by airway obstruction, either at the larynx or within the lungs.[17,26]

Medication Use Process

To ensure that the correct medication goes to the proper patient as well as for purposes of identification and record keeping, the prescription order may be electronically transmitted to the pharmacy (figure 3.3).[6,12,21] For medications whose dosage involves a calculation with a patient's pertinent factors, such as weight, age, or body surface area,

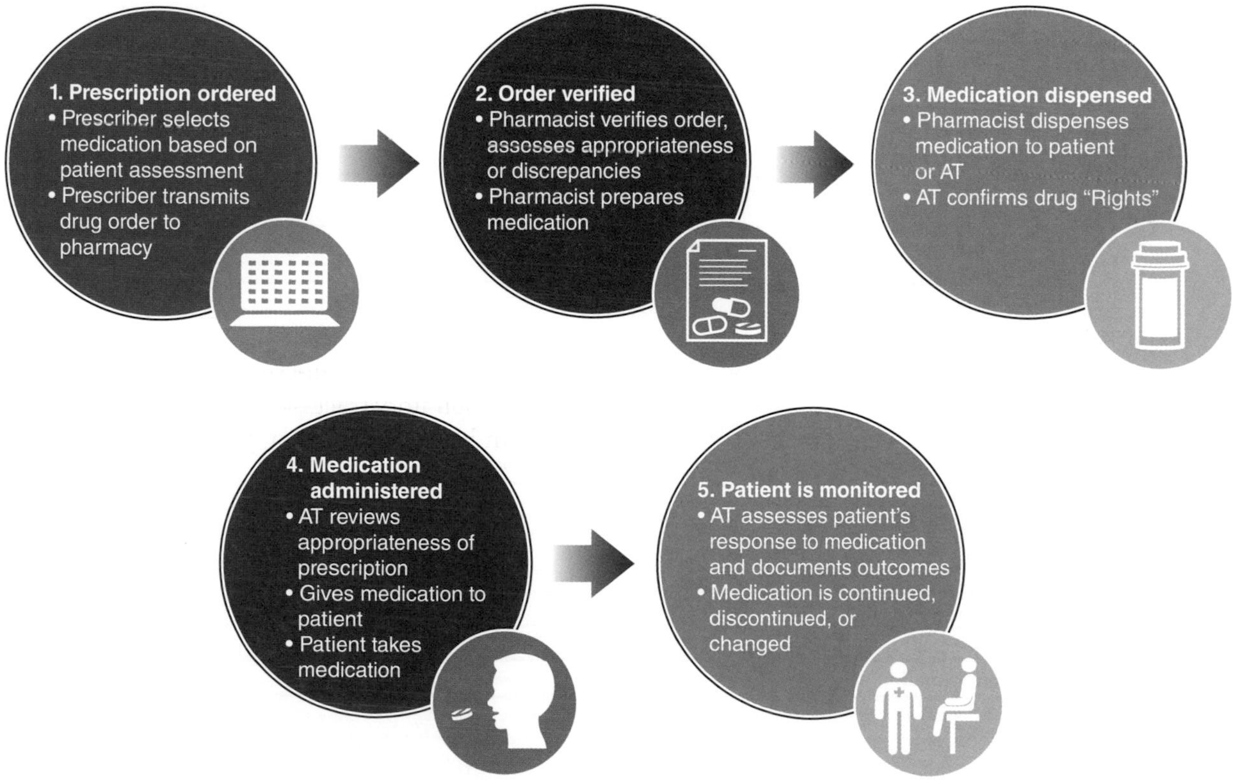

FIGURE 3.3 Steps in the medication use process.

pharmacists verify the drug order, including the calculated dose and the dosage formula used, such as "240 mg every 8 hours."[6] As described in chapter 2, before administering a dose of medication to the patient, the AT should confirm the rights of medication administration. Once the patient takes the medication, the AT should monitor her for adverse drug reactions and document the administration of the medication in her medical record and the facility drug log.

Pharmacist's Role in the Medication Use Process

Consulting with a pharmacist provides the AT with an additional measure of safety because the pharmacist can confirm that the correct medication is being dispensed for the prescribed regimen. The pharmacist provides the most accurate and correct drug information (figure 3.4) to the patient, including a reminder of the intended purpose of the medication, such as "for relief of pain" or "to relieve itching." Additionally, the pharmacist reinforces the correct route of administration by the choice of the first word of the directions. For example, directions begin with the words "take" or "give" for oral dosages; "apply" for externally applied products; "insert" for suppositories; "place" or "instill" for eye, ear, or nose drops; and "inhale" for aerosols.[6,12]

Improving Patient Adherence

Adherence is the extent to which the patient follows a regimen prescribed by a health care professional. The patient is the final and most important determinant of how successful a therapeutic regimen will be and should be engaged as an active participant who has a vested interest in its success. Whatever term is used—*compliance*, *adherence*, *therapeutic alliance*, or *concordance*—prescribers must promote a collaborative interaction between the AT and patient in which each brings an expertise that helps to determine the course of therapy. The patient's quality-of-life beliefs may differ from the HCP's therapeutic goals. Using **cultural competence**, the AT must honor the patient's wishes and advocate for his best interest.

Drug Information Resources

Since new drugs are continuously being introduced, it is necessary for the AT to develop an approach to lifelong learning as well as a framework for finding quality drug information and providing accurate and correct information to patients. **Pharmacy health literacy** is the degree to which ATs are able to obtain, process, and understand basic health and medication information and the pharmacy services needed to make appropriate health care decisions. The quantity of medical information and literature

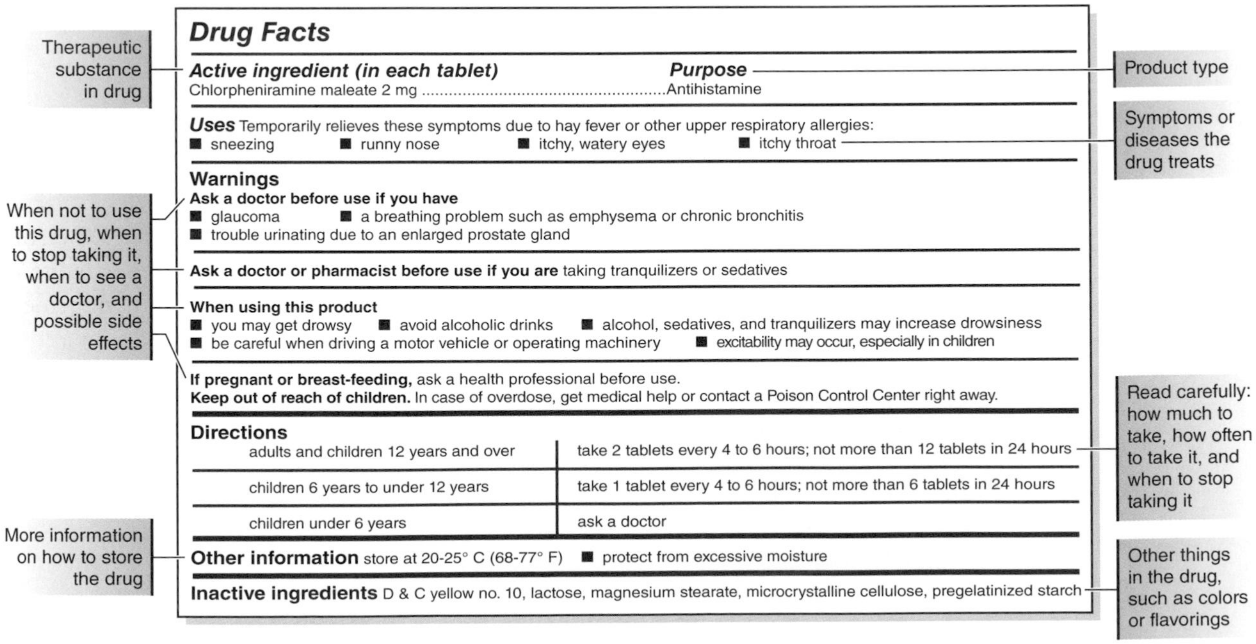

FIGURE 3.4 Sample drug facts label.

Clinical Application

Suggestions for Improving Patient Adherence

Here are some suggestions for talking to patients and improving adherence Note that none of these suggestions guarantees 100% adherence.[6,27]

- Provide culturally sensitive, respectful communication; ask how patient takes medicine.
- Develop a collaborative relationship between the prescriber and patient; encourage pharmacist involvement.
- Provide and encourage use of patient-specific materials such as patient hand-outs (available from dependable resources, see Drug Information Resources section).
- Reinforce information from prescriber. Use precise, clear instructions, giving the most important information first.
- Simplify instructions whenever possible.
- Assess the patient's literacy, language, and comprehension and modify educational counseling as needed. Be culturally aware and sensitive. To improve compliance, don't rely on the patient's knowledge of disease alone.
- Enlist support and assistance from family members and caregivers.
- Use behavioral techniques such as goal setting, self-monitoring, cognitive restructuring, skills training, contracts, and positive reinforcement.

available is growing at an astounding rate. The U.S. National Library of Medicine (NLM) processes about 1 billion online searches per year from users seeking medical and health-related information via PubMed.[22] As the medical literature expands, access to drug information resources for ATs and the public continues to grow. Yet many patients lack the necessary skills to use this information effectively. ATs must ensure that drug information is correctly interpreted and appropriately applied.[21]

Evidence in Pharmacology

Health Literacy

Only 12% of adults have proficient health literacy (e.g., can interpret the prescription label correctly). People with limited health literacy, such as non-native English speakers, are more likely to make medication errors, since they are more likely to misinterpret the prescription label information. Evidence demonstrates an association between low health literacy and poor health outcomes.[1]

Regardless of their specialty, ATs and other HCPs with the responsibility for overseeing the safe use of medications must strive to develop a functional understanding of applied pharmacotherapy. Whether working in a secondary school, university, military base, industrial factory, or outpatient clinic, ATs and other HCPs must apply their skills and knowledge for the optimal care of patients. Pharmacists are the true experts on all aspects of therapeutic medications. These specialists should not be relegated to the role of information dispenser or gatekeeper. Instead, pharmacists should be consulted and allowed to extend their knowledge of drugs and therapeutics to the clinical management of individual patients or the care of large populations.[21] It is impossible to acquire all available and useful resources in all areas of clinical practice. It is also difficult to choose only 1 resource for a practice setting, because each resource may possess different levels of accuracy, comprehensiveness, currency, and ease of use. Differences in practice setting, available funding, patient populations seen, and types of information most commonly needed all affect which resources should be made available and used.[22]

Clinical Application

Accessing High-Quality Drug Information

In clinical practice, providing inaccurate and outdated information may lead to suboptimal patient outcomes and harm; thus, HCPs should be cautious when using information from various online or mobile-enabled media. Current standards and regulations on mobile applications for drug information are not adequate. Until there are tighter regulations over all medical- and health-related mobile apps, clinicians must be vigilant in choosing and using high-quality apps for patient care.[22]

As new therapies become available to treat many conditions, ATs, other HCPs, and especially pharmacists are daily asked to provide responses to numerous drug information requests from a variety of people. It is tempting to just select the easiest, most familiar resources without ensuring or checking the original source of the information; however, doing so may increase the possibility of missing new resources or finding incomplete, incorrect, or outdated information.[22]

High-quality electronic resources allow users to quickly access information and perform multiple searches simultaneously. They contain the most current information available on the given topic. Additionally, many electronic networked resources allow use of the same resource at more than 1 location. This allows multiple HCPs to access information from a variety of physical locations rather than restricting the information to medical libraries or a pharmacy.[22] Many textbooks are now being combined into an electronic package available on the Internet and as e-books. The combination of multiple resources in 1 package may make selection of resources for a practice site much easier, but it is also more costly. As these combination packages increase in popularity with students and universities, the expectations that practitioners have for access to resources in work settings will also likely continue to increase.[22] Many of the major databases available electronically also offer products for mobile devices.[12,22]

Formulating a Response to Questions From Patients

The constantly evolving resources affect access to drug and medical information for both HCPs and patients. Due to this access and the current trend among patients in using online information, HCPs are faced with answering health- and medication-related questions as they occur, and it is important to stay current and vigilant on the latest information regarding medical practice and treatment. Patients must realize that not all published information is accurate or reliable. Some resources are more accurate, more current, and easier to use than others.[22]

Formulating effective responses and recommendations requires the use of a structured, organized approach whereby critical factors are systematically considered and thoughtfully evaluated. The steps in responding to patients are

1. organizing relevant patient information,
2. gathering information about the disease states and affected body systems,
3. collecting medication information,
4. obtaining pertinent background information, and
5. identifying other relevant factors that can potentially influence outcomes.

Once these data are collected and carefully assembled, they must be critically analyzed and evaluated in the proper context. Responses and recommendations are synthesized by integrating information from diverse sources through the use of logic and deductive reasoning.[21]

Summary

The AT must have a working knowledge of drug names, classes, and common adverse drug reactions. Concepts relating to drug safety include balancing therapeutic benefits and adverse effects of a medication and determining the effectiveness of the medication in treating the condition or disease state. The medication-use process includes obtaining relevant patient information, gathering information about indications and contraindications, collecting medication information, obtaining high-quality patient drug information, and identifying other relevant factors that can potentially influence outcomes. Once these data are collected and carefully assembled, they must be critically analyzed and evaluated in the proper context. Responses and recommendations should be synthesized by integrating information from diverse sources through the use of logic and deductive reasoning.[21] The constantly evolving online resources available on drug information affect not only HCP access to information but also patient access to medical information.

Clinical Application

Using High-Quality Drug Information Resources

The following resources are available online. Readers are encouraged to do a basic Internet search to access applicable websites. Note that the following list is not comprehensive; it reflects high-quality resources recommended on the Internet. It is impossible to compile a comprehensive list of all resources that are useful in all areas of practice.

PHYSICIANS' DESK REFERENCE OR PRESCRIBERS' DIGITAL REFERENCE (PDR)

This is the oldest reference for drug information. It compiles the official prescribing information (i.e., package insert) for current medications. It is available online or as a mobile application (mobilePDR) and is available without subscription after a free registration via the website. The reference includes contact information for manufacturers and a list of poison control centers. A patient-friendly version allows viewing and printing information on more than 2,300 medications.

DRUGS.COM

This online resource includes drug monographs, a tablet and capsule identifier, interactions checker, and news related to medication approvals or recalls. The professional version provides more detailed information sourcing from reliable sources, such as Micromedex, Stedman's Medical Dictionary, and the FDA. Drugs are searchable, either using a keyword or looking through an alphabetical list. The information is also available through a mobile application. One limitation of this resource is the inclusion of commercial advertisements on each page of the website.

EPOCRATES

This family of electronic resources includes both mobile and online products. These resources include drug information (e.g., monographs, interaction checker, safety data, tablet identification) and diseases (epidemiology, prognosis, treatment). It is also available as a mobile application.

MEDSCAPE (PUBLISHED BY WEBMD)

This electronic database references more than 125 medical journals and textbooks. It is a free subscription service that allows HCPs to register their information preferences to receive the latest information within a particular specialty area. It includes clinical information as well as financial, managed care, and medical practice information. It also provides simplified monographs for drug information and dose calculation. This resource is available as a mobile application.

U.S. FOOD AND DRUG ADMINISTRATION

The FDA website provides comprehensive, up-to-date information on medications, food and dietary supplements, medical devices, and other medical products. It provides updates on drug recalls, medication safety information, adverse drug events, drug approvals, changes to drug labeling, medication guides, and documents exchanged between the manufacturer and the FDA during the drug approval process.

Case Studies

Case Study 1

Benicio is a 28-year-old professional athlete with a history of knee inflammation. He was recently prescribed an NSAID that he had used successfully in the past. At that time, his treatment included therapeutic modalities and strength work in addition to the medication. As the AT finished his treatment in Benicio's hotel room after their pregame meal, he noticed that the medication was on the nightstand next to Benicio's bed. Benicio had an unusual limp during the game and did not play particularly well. After the game, he acknowledged to the AT that he neglected to take the NSAID prior to the game.

Questions for Analysis

1. Should the AT have done something to ensure that Benicio complied with taking the medication prior to the game?
2. Should the AT discuss a medication adherence plan for Benicio with the team physician?

Case Study 2

Sofia is a 60-year-old woman who was diagnosed with osteoporosis. She recently sustained a vertebral fracture and was prescribed *teriparatide* (Forteo). When her physician demonstrated the self-administration injection technique, he told Sofia that the medication had an FDA warning about bone cancer. This alarmed her. The physician put her mind at ease, noting that the risk was minimal, and explained the nature of the research behind the black box warning. This helped Sofia, and she agreed to take the medication.

Questions for Analysis

1. What is the FDA black box warning?
2. What did the physician do to ease Sofia's mind?

4

Pharmacokinetics

OBJECTIVES

After reading this chapter, you will be able to do the following:

- Compare the differences between pharmacokinetics and pharmacodynamics
- Delineate the common routes of medication administration in sports medicine
- Describe the concept of bioavailability and the quantity of a drug that reaches the systemic circulation
- Trace the path of an oral medication from administration to excretion, including the first-pass mechanism
- Reinforce the need for thorough medication review for all injury or illness conditions that are being treated pharmacologically

Clinical **pharmacokinetics** is the discipline that describes the absorption, distribution, metabolism, and elimination (ADME) of drugs in patients requiring drug therapy.[2,18] These concepts, including biotransformation, are the effects of bodily processes on a drug. Understanding and employing pharmacokinetic principles can increase the probability of therapeutic success and reduce the occurrence of adverse drug effects in the body.[6] A successful drug must be able to cross the physiologic barriers (e.g., skin, cell membrane, blood-brain barrier, or lining of intestines) that limit the access of foreign substances to the body. Drug absorption may occur by several mechanisms that allow drugs to pass through these barriers. After absorption, the drug is distributed within the body, by such systems as blood and lymphatic vessels, to reach its target tissue in an appropriate concentration. The drug's ability to act on its target tissues is also limited by several processes within the patient. These processes include metabolism, in which the body transforms drugs through enzymatic degradation (primarily in the liver), and excretion, in which the drug is eliminated from the body primarily by the kidneys and in the feces.

Clinical Application

Pharmacokinetics Concepts

The sage advice from physician to patient to "take 2 aspirin and call me in the morning" has served as the punch line of many jokes. However, why was the advice to take 2 aspirin, rather than 3 aspirin or only 1? Some key components of the answer to this question involve the pharmacological concepts of pharmacokinetics and pharmacodynamics, principles that are rooted in physiology, biochemistry, and molecular biology.[7] Both the athletic training clinician and graduate student should have a foundational understanding of these concepts, however extensive and detailed they may be.

Pharmacokinetics describes the *effects of the body on a drug* (ADME), whereas pharmacodynamics relates to the *effects of a drug on the body*, such as mechanism of action and therapeutic effects. This chapter presents a broad overview of the pharmacokinetic processes of absorption, distribution, metabolism, and excretion (figure 4.1), with a conceptual emphasis on basic principles that, when applied to a clinical situation, should enable the AT student or clinician to understand the pharmacokinetic basis of drug therapy.[1,14,16,22] Chapter 5 describes the clinical importance of pharmacodynamics, which is applied in subsequent chapters.

Biopharmaceutics

Biopharmaceutics is the study of the physical and chemical properties of drugs and their proper dosage as related to the onset, duration, and intensity of drug action. Another definition of biopharmaceutics is the study of the effects of physicochemical properties of a drug and its drug product (dosage form) **in vitro** and the bioavailability of that drug **in vivo** to produce a desired therapeutic effect. The interrelationship between the physical and chemical properties of the drug, the dosage form (drug product) in which the drug is given, and the route of administration on the rate and extent of systemic drug absorption are all aspects of biopharmaceutics.[16,18] Using knowledge of pharmacokinetic parameters, the prescriber's goal is to design optimal drug regimens, including the route of administration, dose, frequency, and duration of treatment.[22] After the drug is liberated from its dosage form (see the section Drug Liberation), biopharmaceutics (figure 4.2) relates the physicochemical properties of the drug to its **disposition**, or fate, in the body and to its pharmacological effect.[13]

Drug Liberation

The first step of the pharmacokinetic process is for the drug to be dissolved in the body fluid to be absorbed through biological membranes. For the drug to dissolve, it must be **liberated**, or released, from its dosage form; a drug in the solid state must dissolve to its molecular form in body fluids. Once a drug molecule has been liberated from its dosage form, it begins its journey to the drug receptor target. For most drug products, the **active ingredient** is dispersed within its **formulation**, either in its molecular form or as solid particles.[9,13] The ability of a drug to be liberated and dissolved in body fluids depends on the dosage form, the solubility of the active ingredients, and the intended site of action. For instance, the antibiotic *vancomycin* is essentially not absorbed in the intestine when administered by mouth, so it would not be helpful in treating an infection of the bloodstream; however, for a patient with a localized enteric bacterial condition in the intestines, taking this antibiotic by mouth would be effective for eradicating the offending bacteria. On the other hand, oral *vancomycin* is not appropriate for treating systemic or localized infections that occur outside of the gastrointestinal tract—for example, *methicillin*-resistant *Staphylococcus aureus* (MRSA) in peripheral tissues.

Dosage Forms

Dosage forms of drugs include the familiar tablets, capsules, and suspensions, as well as many others (see the sidebar for examples).[9] Drugs that are

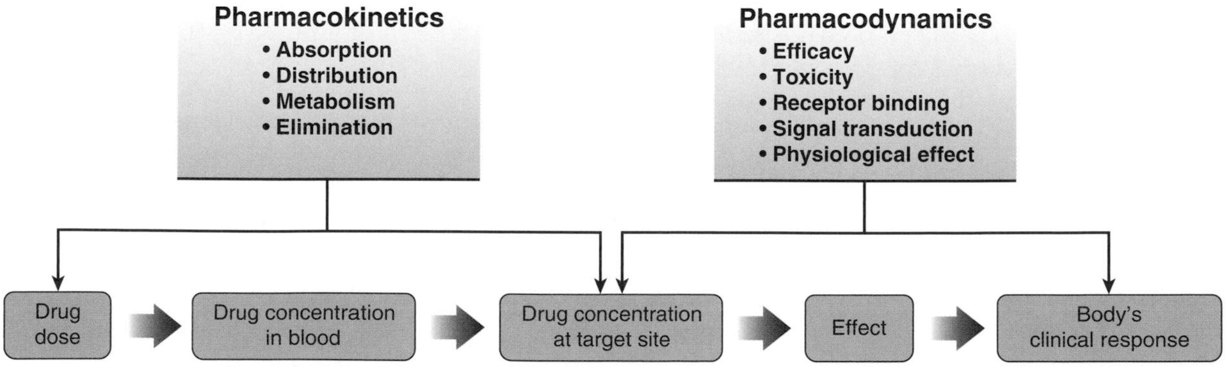

FIGURE 4.1 Schematic diagram of the relationship between pharmacokinetics and pharmacodynamics of a drug.

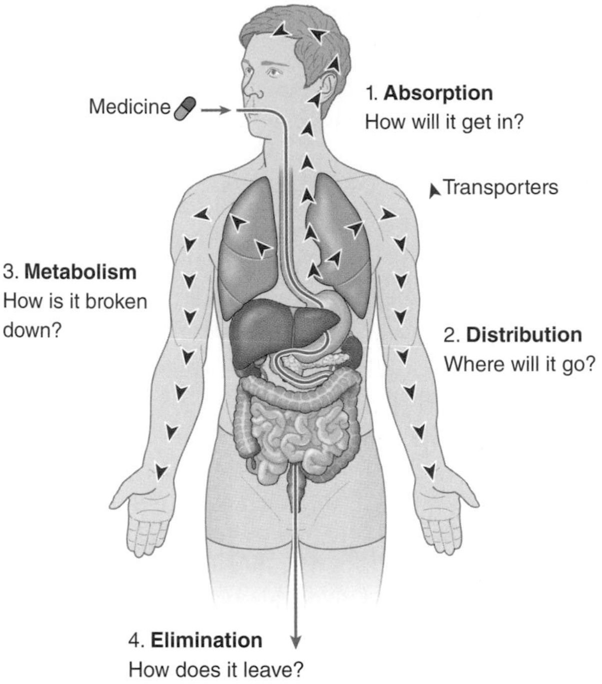

FIGURE 4.2 Schematic representation of biopharmaceutics: drug absorption, distribution, metabolism, and elimination.

Examples of Drug Dosage Forms and the Common State of the Drug Within Them

- **Tablet**—Crystals in a compressed powder
- **Capsules, powder filled**—Crystals in a noncompressed powder
- **Capsules, liquid filled**—Molecules or crystals in vegetable oil
- **Suppository**—Crystals in waxy, water-**miscible**, or water-immiscible base
- **Solution**—Molecules dissolved in fluid
- **Suspension**—Crystals in a lattice matrix held in an aqueous or nonaqueous liquid
- **Ointment**—Crystals or molecules in a semisolid oily base
- **Cream**—Crystals or molecules in a water-miscible semisolid cream base
- **Gel**—Crystals or molecules in a water-miscible semisolid gel base
- **Aerosol**—Crystals or molecules suspended in a gas, liquid, or semisolid

administered as aqueous solutions are ready to be absorbed into the body fluids. Several examples include a drug administered in an oily or fat base (e.g., ointment applied to the skin, oil injected into a muscle, or suppository that melts in the rectum) that must separate in the aqueous biological fluid (e.g., plasma) and dissolve. A drug in an aqueous suspension must dissolve into suspended crystals in the body fluid. A drug in a compressed tablet must dissolve in a process of tablet **disintegration**, which fully exposes the drug crystals to the gastrointestinal fluids for **dissolution**.[9,13]

Drug Solubility

All medication must be dissolved in body fluid before it can enter body tissues. **Solubility** is the concentration of solute in a solution at equilibrium; it is a fundamental drug property that can be expressed with descriptive terms such as "freely soluble" and "practically insoluble." Among the many factors that can affect a drug's solubility are temperature, drug and solvent **polarity**, hydrogen bonding, particle size, and state of ionization (a charge on the particle).[17] To achieve the best possible drug action, medications are formulated to dissolve at an optimal rate. Solubility of the drug is also affected by the form of the medication; for example, solutions are more rapidly absorbed than capsules or tablets because the active ingredient is already dissolved in liquid. In certain medications with an active ingredient that does not dissolve in an aqueous base, an anhydrous (containing no water) base may be used. Water taken with a tablet helps not only with swallowing but also in dissolving the medication.[4]

All human cells are limited by a phospholipid bilayer membrane structure, which has a **hydrophobic** (lipid) core and 2 hydrophilic surfaces (inside and outside the cell). Cell membranes are bilayer structures formed from phospholipids that allow **lipid-soluble (lipophilic)** drug molecules to enter the cell. **Water-soluble (hydrophilic)** drug molecules require special transport proteins to enter the cell. A drug that is very lipophilic (lipid soluble) easily diffuses from the blood vessel into the extravascular tissue space, facilitating entry to the cell. For example, some organs (such as the brain) have a cell membrane with high lipid content; thus, lipid-soluble agents rapidly dissolve in high concentrations.[9] Drugs that are hydrophilic (water soluble) require a membrane channel, pore, or transport protein to enter the target cell (further described in chapter 5).

Drug targets are generally macromolecules located in tissues and fluids throughout the body. Additionally, blood-borne pathogens and other bacteria may be at the site of the drug target. For most drug products, the targets are in tissues and cells that are accessed from the bloodstream;[19] however, some targets can be accessed without drug absorption into the bloodstream.

Drug Absorption

In pharmacokinetics, **absorption** is the movement of drug molecules from the site of administration to the bloodstream. The rate and extent of drug absorption of each of these processes will differ. The step with the slowest rate is the **rate-limiting step**, which ultimately dictates how quickly a drug enters the bloodstream. In general, the rate of dissolution or rate of absorption is the rate-limiting step.[13] The rate of the drug absorbed into the body depends on these processes:[1,4,6,8,11,22]

- **Dosage forms**—Determine how the drug is liberated in the body fluids (described previously in this chapter)
- **Solubility of the drug**—Formulation and physicochemical properties determine how the drug dissolves in body fluid (described previously in this chapter)
- **Route of administration**—Determines how the drug is administered and what barriers it must cross to be absorbed
- **Plasma drug concentration**—How much of the drug is available for therapeutic effects; depends on first-pass metabolism and bioavailability
- **Mechanisms of absorption**—Transport of the drug molecules across cell membranes

Mechanisms of Drug Absorption

Absorption involves the way a drug enters the body, passes into the circulation, and then enters cells (figure 4.3). Absorption of drugs is based on many factors, such as the size of the drug molecules and availability of a transmembrane carrier protein for a specific drug. In passive transport processes, drugs move into cells down their concentration **gradient** (i.e., from a region of high concentration to a region of low concentration). Some drugs are actively transferred into and out of cells with the aid of drug transporters, or membrane-bound proteins. The mechanisms of drug absorption include the following:[1,6,13,15,16]

- **Passive diffusion**—The drug passes through cell membrane lipid bilayers. This is the most common way that drugs cross biological membranes. It favors drugs that are lipophilic.
- **Facilitated diffusion**—The drug is passively moved with its concentration gradient.
- **Paracellular transport**—The drug diffuses between cells, which is the typical way that drugs pass through tissues.
- **Active transport**—The drug is actively moved against its concentration gradient, requiring energy in the form of adenosine triphosphate (ATP).

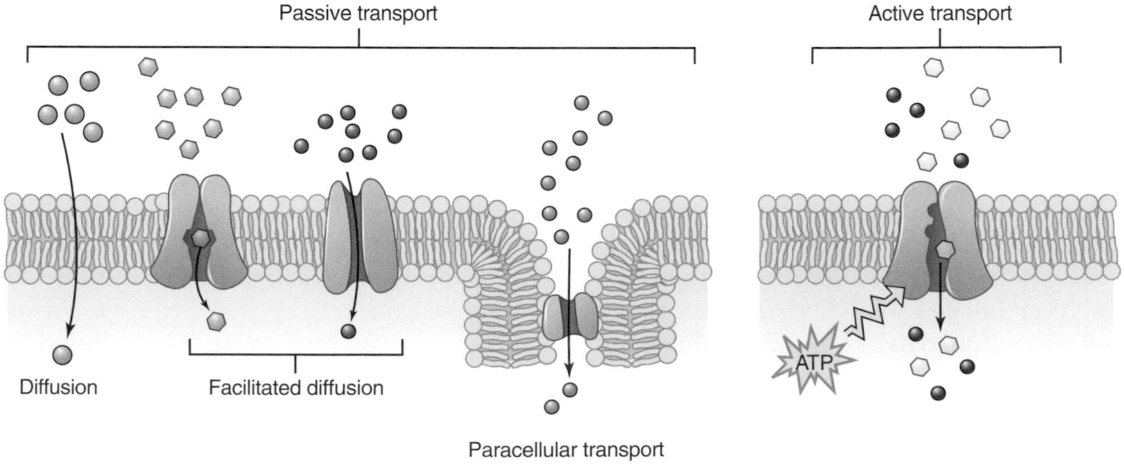

FIGURE 4.3 The variety of ways drugs are transported across cellular barriers in their passage throughout the body.

Evidence in Pharmacology

IV Fluid Administration for Dehydration

Fluid consumption while exercising in hot weather is essential for preventing dehydration and subsequent heat illness. If water or a sports drink is insufficient to restore normal hydration status after sport, a physician may opt for administration of intravenous (IV) saline. For any medication administered intravenously, 100% of that drug is absorbed into the systemic circulation. In athletic-related dehydration, administration of fluid is critical. Although the guideline is that an IV is not necessary if the patient can drink fluids, it offers a modality for rapid rehydration.

The Blood-Brain Barrier

The central nervous system (CNS) presents special challenges to pharmacologic therapy. Unlike most other anatomic regions, the CNS is particularly well insulated from foreign substances. The **blood-brain barrier (BBB)** uses specialized tight junctions to prevent the passive diffusion of most drugs from the systemic to the cerebral circulation. Therefore, drugs designed to act in the CNS must either be sufficiently small and hydrophobic to traverse biological membranes easily or use existing transport proteins in the blood-brain barrier to penetrate CNS structures. Hydrophilic drugs that are unable to target facilitated or active transport proteins in the blood-brain barrier cannot penetrate the CNS.

Route of Administration

After a drug is dissolved in body fluid, the molecules must pass through membrane barriers to be transferred to the target location. For most drug routes (figure 4.4), the transporting fluid is the blood. Drugs that are injected through intramuscular and subcutaneous routes enter the bloodstream directly through capillaries and the lymphatic system. Drugs administered to the mucosal sites of the lungs, nasal cavity, mouth, vagina, and rectum must cross varying types of epithelia.[13] This section focuses on drug absorption after oral and intravenous routes of administration.

For drugs administered through the enteral administration (e.g., oral route), absorption primarily occurs through the single layer of cells that line the stomach and the upper small intestine (duodenum and jejunum). Absorption through the upper small intestines is usually far greater than through the stomach, primarily because the small intestine has a larger surface area (i.e., more epithelial villi and enterocyte microvilli) and the pH is generally better suited for absorption.[1,4,6,8,11,13,22] Advantages and disadvantages of enteral drug administration are further discussed in chapter 6.

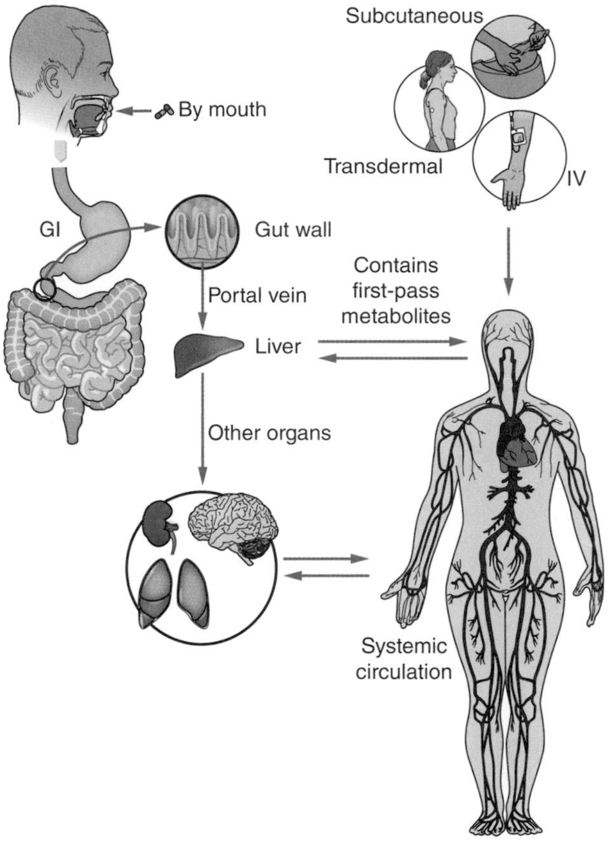

FIGURE 4.4 Absorption is the process of the movement of drug molecules from the site of administration to the systemic circulation.

First-Pass Metabolism

Drugs that are administered by the enteral route are metabolized before reaching the systemic circulation. As the drug is absorbed through the gastrointestinal tract, it enters the hepatic portal circulation (figure 4.5) and is metabolized in the liver before entering the systemic circulation. This process is referred to as **first-pass metabolism** or the **first-pass effect**. Drugs with high first-pass metabolism are administered in doses sufficient to ensure that enough active drug reaches the desired site of action.[1,6,16] The stomach has a relatively large epithelial surface, but its thick mucus layer and short

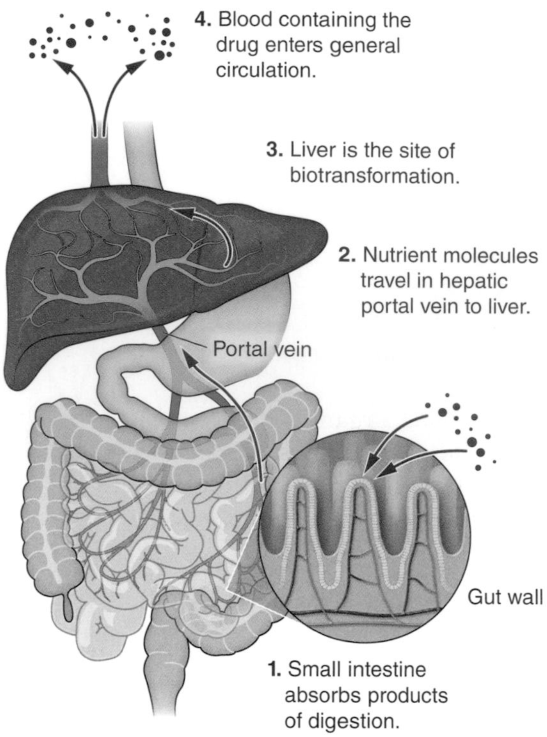

FIGURE 4.5 Drugs administered through the oral route must first pass through the hepatic portal system, where they are metabolized in the liver before entering the systemic circulation.

transit time limit absorption. Because most absorption occurs in the small intestine, gastric emptying is often the rate-limiting step. Food, especially fatty food, slows gastric emptying. This explains why taking some drugs on an empty stomach speeds absorption. After traversing the gastrointestinal epithelium, drugs are carried by the portal system to the liver before entering the systemic circulation. The portal circulation protects the body from the systemic effects of ingested toxins by delivering these substances to the liver for detoxification, potentially complicating drug delivery. In this process, liver enzymes may inactivate a fraction of the ingested drug.

The amount of drug metabolized in the liver can significantly limit the amount of active drug that enters the systemic circulation.[13] Any drug that exhibits significant first-pass metabolism must be administered in a sufficient quantity to ensure that an effective concentration of active drug exits the liver into the systemic circulation and then reaches the target organ. To be absorbed, a drug administered orally must survive encounters with low pH and numerous GI secretions, including potentially degrading enzymes. Peptide drugs (e.g., *insulin*) are particularly susceptible to degradation and thus are not administered orally.

Bioavailability

Bioavailability is the proportion (percent or fraction) of the drug administered and the quantity of drug that reaches the systemic circulation.[1,2,22] Bioavailability depends on

- the route by which the drug is administered,
- the chemical form of the drug, and
- patient-specific factors, such as gastrointestinal motility and hepatic function.[1]

An intravenous drug that is administered directly into the systemic circulation is 100% bioavailable.[8,13] The drug is then distributed to other body compartments and eliminated or excreted. In contrast, other routes of administration (e.g., oral, subcutaneous, and intramuscular) demonstrate slower entry of the drug into the systemic circulation and may have a lower bioavailability (figure 4.6). The **area under the curve (AUC)** is proportional to the total amount of drug absorbed by the body (assuming linear pharmacodynamics with *elimination rate constant*. Drugs that are administered orally are incompletely absorbed or undergo first-pass metabolism in the liver and require a longer period of time to reach a peak concentration of drug in the plasma.[1,16,22]

Plasma Concentration

Drug absorption is necessary to establish adequate levels of the drug in the plasma. Plasma drug concentration is determined by 2 rate processes:

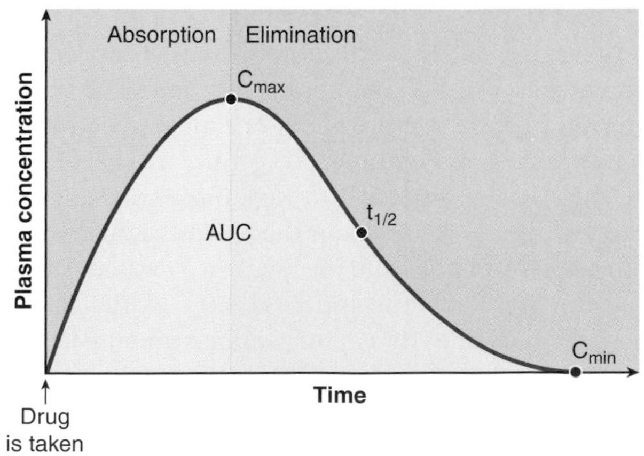

FIGURE 4.6 Bioavailability and area under the curve (AUC) after administration of a single dose of a hypothetical drug administered by oral, subcutaneous, intramuscular, or intravenous routes. C_{max} = maximum plasma concentration; $t_{1/2}$ = half plasma concentration; C_{min} = lowest plasma concentration.

1. The rate at which a drug appears in plasma
2. The rate at which a drug is eliminated from plasma

Additionally, the drug must also reach its target receptors in concentrations sufficient to have the desired therapeutic effect on a physiologic process. Drug distribution is achieved primarily through the circulatory system, with a minor component distributed by the lymphatic system. The concentration of a drug in the plasma is typically used to define and monitor therapeutic drug levels, since the effect of the drug in the target tissue often correlates well with the plasma drug concentration.[1,9,14,16]

The rate of appearance of the drug in plasma (input) depends on the route of administration and the rates of ADME processes for the drug. The plasma concentration curve (also called a plasma concentration vs. time curve or a blood concentration curve) is a graph demonstrating the plasma drug concentration (Y-axis) as a function of time (X-axis) after dosing. The shape of a plasma concentration curve depends on the route of administration. A drug that is administered intravenously (as an IV **bolus**) involves direct administration of the entire drug dose into the bloodstream, so there is no absorption step. Plasma concentration reaches a maximum instantaneously. Intravenous administration can also be an infusion, where the drug solution is slowly dripped into a vein; in this case, the input rate is the infusion rate. Plasma concentration rises gradually as the drug is infused, so long as the rate of administration is greater than the rate of elimination.[14,16] Figure 4.7 shows typical plasma concentration curves after a single IV bolus or oral dose of a drug, respectively. Note that for IV bolus administration, the **maximum plasma concentration** (C_{max}) occurs immediately after dosing. For oral administration, the maximum plasma concentration is reached at a certain time after administration (t_{max}).

Drug Distribution

Following absorption or systemic administration into the bloodstream, a drug is distributed through the bloodstream into interstitial and intracellular fluids. Initially, the liver, kidney, brain, and other well-perfused organs receive most of the drug; delivery to muscle, most viscera, skin, and fat is slower. Thus, distribution of the drug (figure 4.8) is determined by its movement between the blood, or vascular, **compartment** (central compartment) and the interstitial (extracellular) fluid that surrounds the cells of the target tissue (peripheral compartment).[1,6,16] A drug's entry into the systemic circulation and distribution to its target cell or tissue are influenced by several factors:[9,13,14]

- Physicochemical properties of the drug, such as size, charge, and lipophilicity
- Cardiac output and blood flow between the compartments of the body
- Binding of the drug to proteins in the plasma and target tissues
- Capillary permeability and tissue volume
- Concentration of the drug between the central compartment (plasma) and the peripheral compartment (extravascular cells and tissues)

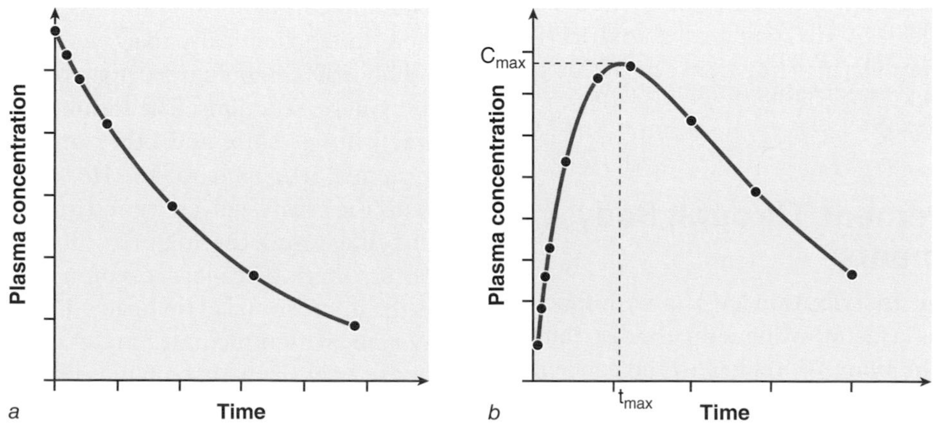

FIGURE 4.7 Typical plasma level curve after an IV bolus and oral drug administration. *(a)* Plasma level after administration of an IV bolus dose. *(b)* Plasma level after oral dosing of a drug product. C_{max} = maximum plasma concentration; t_{max} = time it takes to reach maximum plasma concentration.

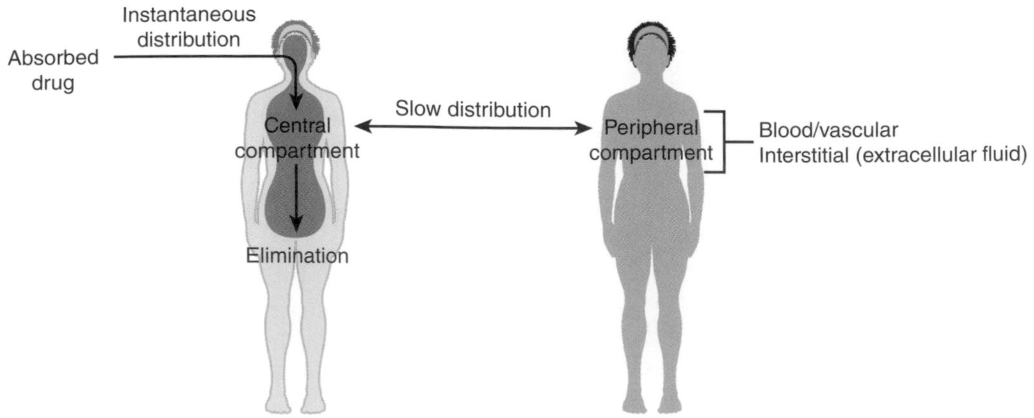

FIGURE 4.8 Distribution process of a drug reversibly leaving the bloodstream and entering and remaining in the central compartment or moving to peripheral compartment.

RED FLAG

Concerns With Prophylactic Hyperhydration

Head athletic trainers from 27 teams in the National Football League (NFL) acknowledged having given a pregame IV infusion of 1.5 L saline to select players. The intent was to minimize risk of muscle cramps, although some players admitted a psychological dependence to receiving the IV fluid. Critics noted that pregame IV fluid administration may not be medically indicated and that oral prehydration may be as effective as the IV practice and less risky. NFL athletic trainers acknowledged the occurrence of adverse events secondary to IV fluid administration, such as superficial venous thrombosis.[5] Preevent IV fluid administration is banned by the World Anti-Doping Agency (WADA) as a performance-enhancing practice during international competition unless it is medically indicated.[3,5] However, some literature critical of the NFL approach acknowledged the presence of limits and flaws in its research design.[5]

Drug Movement Through Body Compartments

The **volume of distribution** (V_d) is an important pharmacokinetic factor influencing the distribution of a drug in the body. V_d relates to the concentration of a drug in the peripheral tissue compartment compared to its concentration in the plasma in the central compartment.[6,9] Distribution of the drug to well-perfused tissues (i.e., heart, liver, kidney, and brain) is rapid, assuming that the drug is distributed in the plasma, or central compartment, and is in equilibrium with the drug that is distributed in the peripheral compartment.[14] Drug distribution to poorly perfused tissues (i.e., bone, muscle, fat) in the peripheral compartment is slower, and distribution equilibrium may not be reached for some time after drug administration. Drug concentration in poorly perfused peripheral compartments continues to increase for some time despite declining plasma concentrations. Once equilibrium is reached, plasma and tissue concentrations of free drug are considered equal and decline over time in a parallel manner.[9,14]

Drug Metabolism

Metabolism is the process in which drugs are broken down into smaller usable parts through a series of complex chemical reactions, or **biotransformation**, until chemically inactive.[4] Several organs are capable of metabolizing drugs to some extent using enzymatic reactions. The kidneys, gastrointestinal tract, lungs, skin, and other organs contribute to systemic drug metabolism. However, the liver contains the greatest diversity and quantity of metabolic enzymes, and the majority of drug metabolism occurs there. The most common metabolic pathway is the microsomal **cytochrome P450 (CYP) enzyme system**, which mediates many oxidative reactions in the liver. Hepatic enzymes chemically modify a variety of substituents on drug molecules, thereby either rendering the drugs inactive or facilitating their elimination.[1,9] An exception are **prodrugs**, which are inactive and must be metabolized into their active form. As previously discussed, the first-pass effect occurs in the liver and is a major contributor to medication metabolism. Regardless of where drug metabolism occurs, the general role of metabolism is to increase the hydrophilicity of a drug, making it more easily excreted in the urine.[13]

Half-Life

Some drugs enter and leave the body quickly, while other drugs remain active in the body for a long time. The standard method of describing how long it takes to metabolize and excrete a drug is the elimination **half-life** ($t_{1/2}$), or the time it takes the body to remove 50% of the remaining drug from the body.[4] Half-life is the determinant of the time required to reach steady state and the dosage interval. Once absorption and distribution are complete, the half-life is the time required for plasma concentrations to decrease by one-half (figure 4.9). Half-life depends on the values of clearance (described in the next section) and volume of distribution.[1,2,6,16] For most drugs, it takes 5 half-lives to reach steady state in the plasma. The half-life helps determine the following:

- **Dosage**—How much medicine needs to be administered
- **Frequency**—How often the drug should be taken
- **Duration**—How long the drug will remain in the body in significant amounts

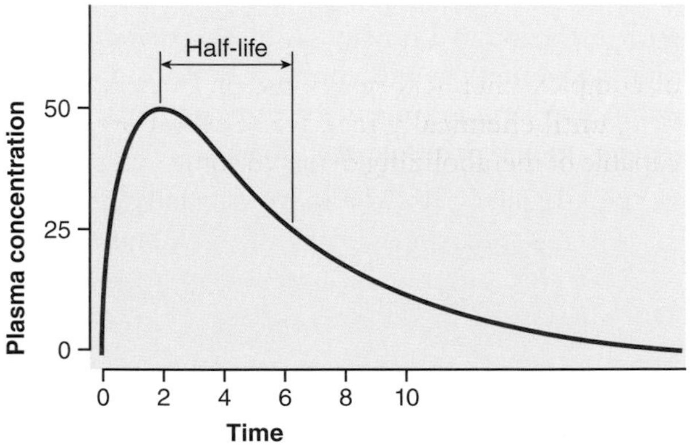

FIGURE 4.9 Elimination half-life ($t_{1/2}$) of a hypothetical drug is the time required for the concentration of the drug to reach half of its original concentration.

RED FLAG

Medication Half-Life and Dosing Frequency

If a medication with a long half-life (i.e., requires a long time for elimination) is taken too frequently, the patient may experience toxicity from the drug due to high drug concentrations in the blood. On the other hand, a drug with a long half-life may need to be taken less frequently, such as once per day. For a drug with a short half-life, such as many antibiotics, the patient must take frequent doses to maintain the correct level of the drug in the blood (dosages are detailed in chapter 6). A patient with liver or kidney dysfunction may not properly metabolize or excrete a drug, resulting in higher doses circulating for a longer time and producing symptoms of an overdose.[1,6,16,19]

Drug Elimination

Inactive chemicals, chemical by-products, and waste (**metabolites**) broken down through the process of metabolism are removed from the body through the process of **excretion**.[4] The kidney is the most important organ for excreting water-soluble drugs and their metabolites into the urine.[4] Many orally administered drugs are incompletely absorbed from the upper GI tract, and the residual drug is eliminated by fecal excretion.[1,6,13,16] Some chemicals are excreted from the lungs through breathing or lost through evaporation from the skin during sweating. Very small amounts of medication may also be excreted in tears, saliva, or the milk when breastfeeding. A patient who has poorly functioning kidneys may be unable to excrete metabolites in the urine; thus, they may accumulate in the body and become toxic.[4] For example, people with a predisposition for kidney dysfunction should avoid nonsteroidal anti-inflammatory drugs (NSAIDs), even for short-term use, due to NSAID-induced constriction of the afferent arteriole that further diminishes kidney function.

Clearance (CL) is the most important pharmacokinetic concept because it determines the steady-state concentration for a given dosage rate. Physiologically, clearance is determined by blood flow to the organ that metabolizes or eliminates the drug and the efficiency of that organ in extracting the drug from the bloodstream.[2,19,20] Clearance is defined as the volume of plasma that is cleared or removed of the drug per unit time. This quantity reflects the rate of drug elimination divided by plasma concentration. For most people, the rates of metabolism and excretion are the same.

Pharmacokinetics and Exercise

ATs must understand potential complications of medication use secondary to exercise. Little research exists on the effect of exercise on medications; however, studies indicate that there is no substantial effect of exercise on medications administered orally.[10] Exceptions to this are the antibiotic *doxycycline* and certain beta-blockers, such as *atenolol* and *propranolol*, that have demonstrated an increase in serum concentration after exercise. *Digoxin* and *warfarin* are also affected by exercise, but they are not generally used by competitive athletes.

The more common administration route for drugs used in sports medicine is the enteral oral route. Of these, medications to manage inflammation (i.e., NSAIDs) and pain (e.g., *acetaminophen*) are among the most frequently used by competitive athletes.

Evidence in Pharmacology

How Exercise Affects Plasma Concentration

Exercise reduces renal blood flow; therefore, plasma concentrations of medications eliminated by the kidneys may increase.[10] For example, an athlete with type I diabetes should be aware that there is a risk of hypoglycemia if *insulin* is injected intramuscularly immediately prior to exercise since *insulin* is metabolized in the kidney.[12]

Parenteral medications (those administered by routes other than the GI tract) have differing routes of administration that can affect their absorption and metabolism. In sports medicine clinical settings, parenteral administration routes include intramuscular injections of anti-inflammatories, certain antibiotics and corticosteroids, inhaled medications, and topical preparations.

Summary

Pharmacokinetics is a complicated concept; however, ATs need to have a working comprehension of how medications are absorbed, distributed, metabolized, and excreted. Using this knowledge will help the AT minimize the possibility of inadvertent or excessive dosing when drugs are used for multiple conditions or different drugs are taken for the same condition. This understanding of basic pharmacokinetics will help the AT enhance patient care while staying prepared to avoid unintended consequences.

This chapter provides an overview of the pharmacokinetic processes of absorption, distribution, metabolism, and excretion (ADME). An understanding of the factors that determine a drug's ability to act in an individual patient and of the changing nature of these factors over time is vitally important to the safe and efficacious use of drug therapy. The key concepts relating to the relationships among dosing, clearance, and plasma drug concentration are important to consider when making therapeutic decisions about drug regimens.[1,19,21]

This chapter also discusses many of the important biopharmaceutical factors that determine a drug's fate after the administration of a drug product to a patient. Understanding these factors, integrated with a thorough knowledge of the principles of pharmacokinetics, will enable ATs to competently monitor dosing regimens for their patients[13,21] and discuss them with the prescriber.

Case Studies

Case Study 1

Ed strained his middle and upper trapezius muscles when he was replacing a pipe underneath a sink. He tried to self-treat his pain with an over-the-counter (OTC) NSAID, but ended up seeking treatment from his physician 1 week after the injury because the condition was still hampering him at work. The physician administered a prescription medication 30 mg *ketorolac* injection in Ed's nondominant middle deltoid muscle. Ed felt less spasm and overall pain the next day at work and was able to complete his workload with much less discomfort.

Questions for Analysis

1. Why did the *ketorolac* work better than the OTC NSAID?
2. Why was the medication injected in the arm rather than directly into the spasming area?

Case Study 2

Max is a middle-aged sales representative with a history of kidney dysfunction. He sprained his ankle when he stepped off a curb. Instead of seeking a medical opinion, Max self-medicated with an OTC NSAID, doubling the recommended dosage with the hope of accelerating his recovery. After 3 days of this regimen, Max noticed blood in his urine. He then consulted his physician.

Questions for Analysis

1. With kidney dysfunction, should Max be conscientious about taking medication?
2. Why would doubling the NSAID dose be unwise for Max, considering his kidney dysfunction?

5

Pharmacodynamics

OBJECTIVES

After reading this chapter, you will be able to do the following:

- Define *pharmacodynamics* and describe how it is related to drug dosing
- Describe the lock-and-key mechanism of drug-receptor binding
- Differentiate between drug potency and efficacy in terms of dose response
- Explain common drug–receptor interactions
- Describe considerations for drug dosing

Chapter 4 discusses the concept of pharmacokinetics—what the body does to a drug through the processes of absorption, distribution, metabolism, and excretion. This chapter discusses **pharmacodynamics**, or what the drug does to the body through molecular, biochemical, and physiological effects or actions.[10,14] Understanding the basic concepts of pharmacodynamics gives the athletic trainer (AT) an awareness of the drug's effect, side effects, and interactions. During the pharmacodynamic processes, the pharmacological action of a drug takes place when the drug molecule reaches its receptor site.[3] The overall pharmacological response of a drug is predicated on 2 major factors:

1. The drug's ability to bind to the target
2. The drug's concentration at the receptor site

A general understanding of pharmacodynamics helps the AT appreciate the relationships between drug–receptor interactions and the pharmacologic effects of therapeutic medications.

Mechanism of Action

The way a drug works at the target tissue is its **mechanism of action**.[8] Most drugs exert their effects, both beneficial and harmful, by interacting with specialized target macromolecules called drug receptors that are present on or embedded in the cell membrane.[1] Reaching a drug's intended effect involves a complex interaction of the drug binding to a receptor and the chemical interactions between the drug and its target.[7] These interactions affect how a drug binds to its receptor on the cell's surface, which affects the signaling of subsequent processes in the biochemical process.[4,14]

Drug Receptors

A **drug receptor** is a specialized target macromolecule situated on the outside of the cell membrane, embedded in the cell surface or within the cell membrane, or located in the cellular cytoplasm (figure

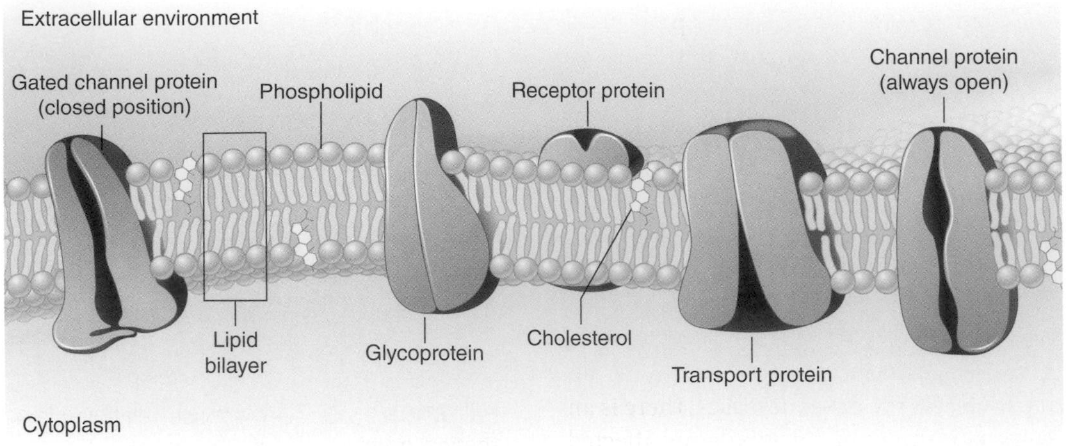

FIGURE 5.1 Various drug receptors on the cell membrane.

Evidence in Pharmacology

Direct Action of Some Drugs

Although much of this chapter focuses on the interaction of drugs with specific receptors, it is important to appreciate that not all drugs exert effects by interacting with a receptor. For example, antacids function locally by chemically neutralizing excess gastric acid, thereby reducing stomach upset.[15]

5.1). The receptor binds to a drug and mediates its mechanism of action. These drug receptors may be enzymes, nucleic acids, or specialized membrane-bound proteins. Cells have many different types of receptors that can bind with 1 or more drugs, producing a specific intracellular response.[15]

The ability of a drug to bind to a receptor is determined by the chemical structure of the drug. This drug–receptor interaction is key to the ability of the drug to facilitate its physiological effect. Most drugs achieve their desired (therapeutic) effects by interacting selectively with target molecules that play important physiologic or pathophysiologic roles.[1]

Drug–Receptor Binding

The site on the receptor where the drug binds is called its **binding site**. Drug–receptor binding is related to the 3-dimensional structure, shape, and reactivity of the binding site and the inherent structure, shape, and reactivity of the drug. Although the molecular shape of the receptor is important to its interaction with a drug, the following sections focus on the clinically important aspects of drug–receptor binding, specifically the lock-and-key mechanism.[17]

Lock-and-Key Mechanism of Drug–Receptor Interactions

Most drugs work much like a key opening a lock (figure 5.2). A drug, like a key, has a complex shape that determines its function. The drug binds to a receptor, as with a key entering a lock, and creates a response, as in opening the lock.[8] Molecules (e.g., drugs, hormones, neurotransmitters) that bind to a receptor are called **ligands**. These molecules activate or inactivate a receptor and increase or decrease the function of a particular cell. Ligands may interact with multiple receptor types; however, most drugs have relative selectivity.[3]

The combined **drug–receptor complex** unlocks the drug to act on the target tissue. Once the drug–receptor complex is created, it produces alterations in biochemical or molecular activity of a cell by a process called **signal transduction**.[15] The binding of a drug to its receptor can be reversible or irreversible.

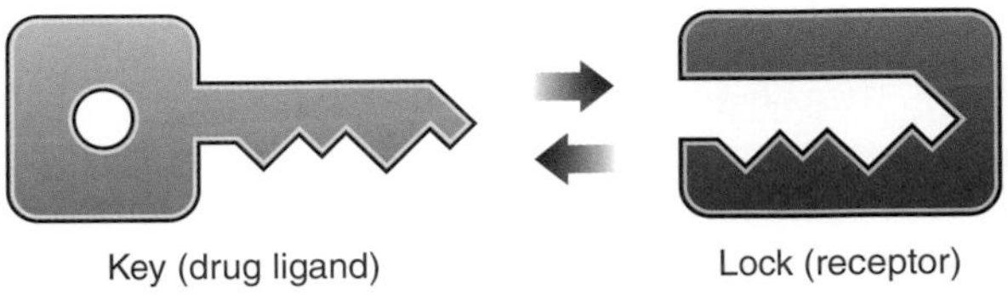

FIGURE 5.2 Lock-and-key mechanism of drug and receptor.

- **Reversible binding**—Occurs when the drug can separate from the cell's receptor, as in removing a key from a lock. When the drug is removed from the receptor, the effect of the drug stops.
- **Irreversible binding**—Occurs when the drug is not able to separate from the receptor, prolonging the drug's effect.[8]

Dose–Response Relationships

With gradually increasing (or graded) doses, there are generally greater magnitudes of response in an individual patient. As the dose increases, there is an increase in the percentage of the population affected by the drug. The lethal dose (LD) of a compound is determined experimentally, usually by administering the chemical to mice or rats. The **LD_{50}** is the dose of drug that is lethal in 50% of the population.[6] The **effective dose (ED_{50})** of a drug is the concentration of drug at which 50% of the population will have the desired therapeutic response. The **therapeutic index (TI)** or therapeutic ratio quantifies the relative safety of a drug. The TI is the **therapeutic window** calculated with this equation:

$$TI = \frac{LD_{50}}{ED_{50}}$$

Clearly, the higher the TI ratio, the safer the drug (figure 5.3).[4,6,17]

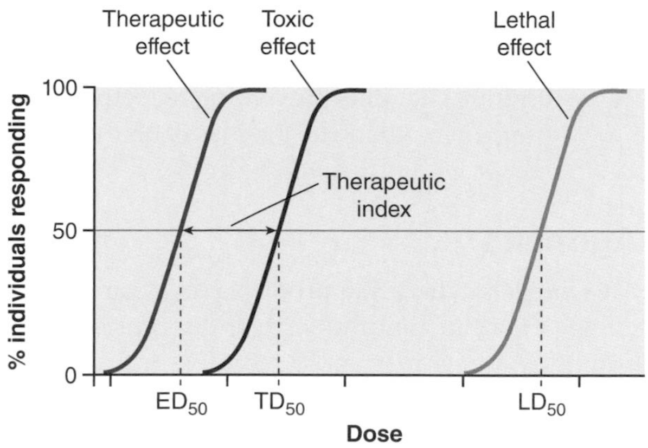

FIGURE 5.3 Dose–response relationship for a hypothetical drug.

Drug–Receptor Interactions

Many receptors for drugs can be modeled as having 2 **conformational** states (shapes) that are in reversible equilibrium with one another. These are called the *active state* and the *inactive state*. The pharmacologic properties of drugs are often based on their effects on the state of their receptors. A drug that, in binding to its receptor, favors the active receptor conformation and facilitates a receptor response is an **agonist**. A drug that inhibits the receptor response by blocking agonist-induced activation of the receptor is an **antagonist**. For the purposes of this discussion, the following pharmacologic classifications are described in more detail in the following sections.[4,8]

- **Receptor**—Unbound and available for binding (figure 5.4*a*).
- **Agonist**—Activates the receptor by inducing a conformational change in the receptor—for example, the opening of a transmembrane ion channel (figure 5.4*b*). Agonists can also function as inverse or partial agonists.
- **Competitive antagonist**—Blocks the agonist from binding to the receptor by binding to the receptor's agonist site without activating the receptor (figure 5.4*c*).

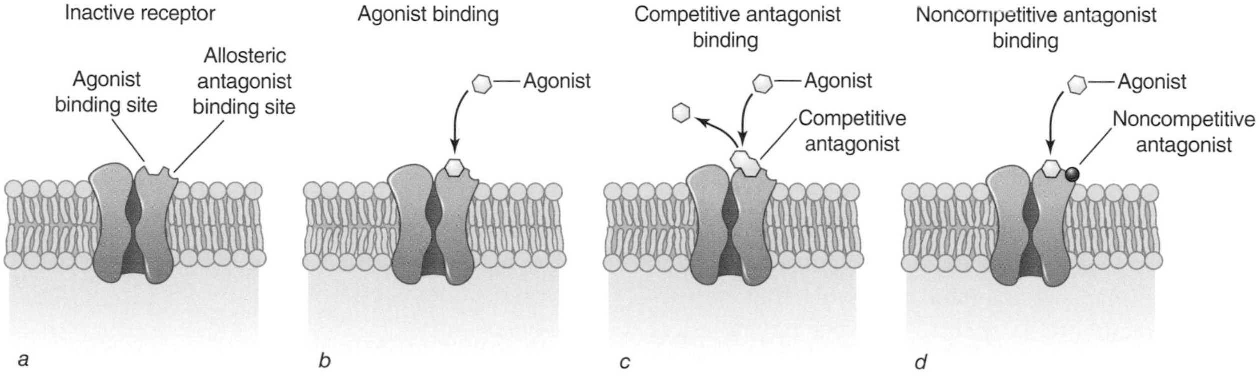

FIGURE 5.4 Agonist and antagonist receptor binding.

- **Noncompetitive antagonist**—Binds to a site different from the agonist site, the **allosteric** binding site, thus preventing receptor activation, even when the agonist is bound to the receptor (figure 5.4*d*).[7,8,17]

Agonists

An agonist is a drug that produces the desired physiologic effect in binding with the receptor. When bound by an agonist, most receptors are activated by stabilizing the receptor in a specific shape or conformation (usually, the active conformation).[4,7] For example, many hormones, neurotransmitters (e.g., acetylcholine, histamine, norepinephrine), and drugs (e.g., *morphine*, *phenylephrine*, benzodiazepines, barbiturates) act as agonists.[7] On a dose–response curve, E_{max} is the maximal response produced by the drug when all receptors are occupied by the agonist and no additional drug will produce an additional response.

- **Inverse agonists**—Bind to the same receptor as an agonist, but induce a pharmacological response opposite to that agonist.
- **Partial agonists**—Bind to and activate a receptor, but have only partial efficacy relative to a full agonist.

Antagonists

An antagonist is a drug that either diminishes or prevents the physiologic effect of the agonist[8] but has no effect in the absence of the agonist.[4] Pharmacologic antagonism occurs when an antagonist binds to a receptor and prevents the biologic effect of an agonist. Antagonists can be either competitive or noncompetitive and can bind reversibly or irreversibly.

- **Reversible antagonists**—Readily dissociate from their receptor.
- **Irreversible antagonists**—Form a stable, permanent, or nearly permanent chemical bond with their receptor.[7]

Binding of an antagonist to a receptor prevents receptor activation from producing a biological effect. The antagonist can either block or reverse the effect of an agonist. An example of an antagonist is *naloxone* (Narcan), an opioid antagonist that is structurally related to *morphine*. *Naloxone* has no effect of its own, but will reverse the effects of any opioid agonist that has been administered. Sometimes the antagonist can also reverse or block the effect of **endogenously** produced compounds. For example, beta-blockers can block the effects of endogenously produced epinephrine and norepinephrine.[7,17]

Evidence in Pharmacology

Direct and Indirect Responses

Models that study an analgesic's pharmacokinetics and pharmacodynamics in tandem try to predict the effect of the drug's concentration based on its activity in the steady state. Pharmacokinetic and pharmacodynamic models relate to the overall pharmacological effect of a drug. For example, analgesics may have a direct or indirect response. For a direct response, the plasma concentration of the drug is directly linked to the body's response to the drug. A drug that moves quickly to reach its target has a rapid response. Conversely, an indirect response is when the drug's effect increases slowly by the processes of building up or breaking down the drug.[12]

Drug Dosing

This section describes drug dosing in the context of drug efficacy versus effectiveness and introduces concepts related to dose–response relationships. Medical prescriptions are based on characteristics of the drug (e.g., indication, efficacy, safety profile, route of administration, route of elimination, dosing frequency, cost) and of the patient (e.g., age, sex, other medical problems, likelihood of pregnancy, ethnicity, other genetic determinants). Risks and benefits of the drug are also assessed; every drug poses some risk.[9]

Whether a drug is indicated for an individual patient depends on the balance of its therapeutic benefits and adverse effects. In making such judgments, prescribers consider factors that are somewhat subjective, such as personal experience, anecdotes, peer practices, and expert opinions.[13] Prescribers may use several methods to design a dosage regimen. Generally, the initial dosage of the drug is selected based on the following patient factors:

- Known diagnosis
- Pathophysiology

- Demographic
- Allergy
- Any known factor that might affect the patient's response to the dosage regimen

The starting dose of a drug and dosing interval are based on the objective of delivering a desirable (target) **therapeutic level** of the drug in the body. The drug dosage or concentration must provide safe effective therapy and work within its **therapeutic range**. After initiation of drug therapy, the patient is monitored for the **therapeutic response** by clinical and physical assessment. After evaluating the patient, the prescriber may determine that adjustments to the dosage regimen are needed.[6,18]

RED FLAG

Therapeutic Drug Monitoring

Vancomycin is a common medication of choice for the treatment of *Methicillin*-resistant *staphylococcus aureus* (MRSA). Therapeutic drug monitoring (TDM) is critical for ensuring this drug's efficiency and safety.[14] Excessive use of *vancomycin* can result in hearing loss or acute kidney damage[16] necessitating regular monitoring starting within the first 48 hours of administration.[11] The concept of TDM is important for the AT caring for competitive athletes with MRSA because highly motivated athletes sometimes opt to self-medicate under the false impression that this can accelerate their healing (i.e., more is better).

Dose Responses

A drug's **affinity** is the measure of how tightly the drug binds to the receptor. Likewise, the drug's **intrinsic activity** is a measure of its effectiveness in generating the intended change of cellular activity.[3] **Selectivity** is the degree to which a drug acts on a given receptor relative to other available cellular receptors.[7] Both the affinity of a drug for its receptor and its activity are determined by its chemical structure. The chemical structure of a drug also contributes to the drug's **specificity**. A drug that interacts with a single type of receptor on a limited number of cells exhibits high specificity. Conversely, a drug acting on a receptor found ubiquitously throughout the body exhibits widespread effects. Many clinically important drugs exhibit a broad (low) specificity because they interact with multiple receptors in different tissues. Such broad specificity might not only enhance the clinical utility of a drug but also contribute to a spectrum of adverse side effects because of off-target interactions. One example of a drug that interacts with multiple receptors is *amiodarone*, an agent used to treat cardiac arrhythmias.[5]

Potency and efficacy are often confused. **Potency** is the term used to compare the different doses of 2 medications in producing the same effect. On the other hand, efficacy is the strongest effect a drug can produce.[8] Drug responses are quantified by determining the **half-maximal effective concentration** (**EC_{50}**) for producing a given effect. For example, the relative potency of 2 hypothetical drugs (figure 5.5*a*) is a function of their relative affinities and efficacies. The EC_{50} of drug X occurs at a lower concentration than the EC_{50} of drug Y. Thus, drug X is more potent than drug Y. In the hypothetical example of drug efficacy (figure 5.5*b*), the responses are 100% for drug X and 50% for drug Y. Drug X is more efficacious than drug Y.[5]

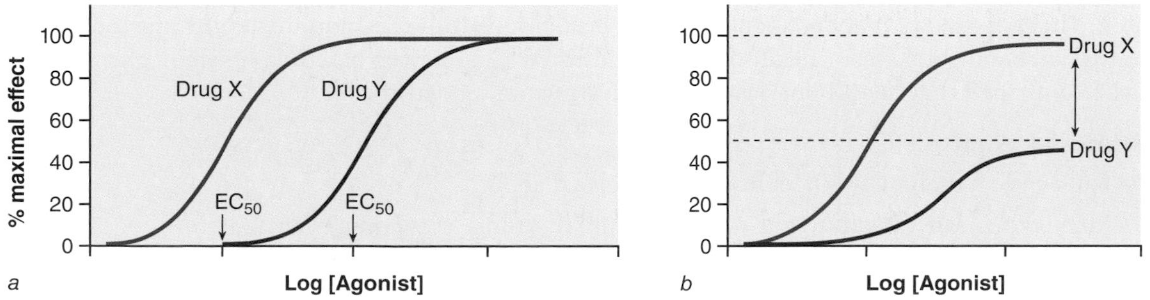

FIGURE 5.5 Relative *(a)* potency and *(b)* efficacy of 2 hypothetical drugs.

Clinical Application

Pharmacodynamics of Opioids

Pain is a complex condition to treat pharmacologically with opioids. Some opioids transfer rapidly or slowly between the plasma and its target site; their strength is classified as high or low potency. The analgesic effect of *codeine*, a low-potency opioid, is predicated on its biotransformation to *morphine* in the central nervous system. Approximately 10% of oral *codeine* is converted to *morphine* by the cytochrome P450 enzyme system. *Oxycodone* is high potency and works peripherally with the μ-opioid receptor; it is effective when there is no delay at the site of action. Metabolites of these medications, such as oxymorphone and noroxymorphone, also contribute to the analgesic effect of opioids.[12]

RED FLAG

Drug Potentiation

Drug potentiation results when one drug interacts with another, causing a greater pharmacologic response than the drugs would have independently. Warning labels associated with prescription drugs are intended to alert clinicians and patients to the prospect of inadvertent interaction. For example, it is commonly known that alcohol magnifies the sedating effects of medications. Less common, but still a significant concern, is the potential of increased bleeding risk associated when a nonsteroidal anti-inflammatory drug (NSAID) is combined with an anticoagulant.[2] The risk of drug potentiation is an additional reason why health care providers should be familiar with the medications their patients regularly use.

Summary

This chapter on pharmacodynamics (the effects of drugs on the human body) provides the clinician with a general understanding of the relationships between drugs and their targets. It also examines the mechanisms of drug–receptor interactions. It is important for the AT to have a working understanding of whether and to what extent a drug activates or inhibits its target. This understanding provides valuable information about the function of the drug inside the cell. Although the molecular details of drug–receptor interactions vary widely among drugs of different classes and receptors of different types, the fundamental mechanisms of action described in this chapter serve as paradigms for the principles of pharmacodynamics. To simplify the study of pharmacology, the student should focus on the classifications of drugs based on their receptors and mechanisms of action.

Case Studies

Case Study 1

Tim is a newly diagnosed type 2 diabetic. The nurse in his physician's office explained that he needs *insulin* to help normalize his blood sugar. Tim's physician prescribed a low dose of a long-acting *insulin* for daily injection. The nurse recommended that he take the *insulin* at bedtime and administer the injection into a fatty abdominal subcutaneous area. The dose could be adjusted in 3 months based on his daily glucose readings. Also, she confirmed that he did not have kidney dysfunction or asthma.

Questions for Analysis

1. What should a diabetic with asthma be concerned about?
2. Which is the more effective time to take *insulin*: morning or evening? Why?

Case Study 2

Jamal is a 35-year-old knee arthroscopy patient in the local sports medicine clinic who would like to return to the body weight and fitness level he had as a sophomore college football player, the final year he was a competitive athlete. After 3 weeks of rehabilitation, Jamal's clinician, Jiawen, noticed that his skin seemed a bit yellow and that the ankle on his surgical leg was abnormally swollen. Jamal admitted that his urine was an unusually dark color. He also admitted to taking a nutritional supplement to stimulate weight loss. Jiawen recommended that Jamal consult with his orthopedic surgeon promptly.

Questions for Analysis

1. What was so concerning to the clinician that he referred the patient back to his physician?
2. Could this be linked to a drug or supplement?

6

Drug Delivery, Dosages, and Procedures

OBJECTIVES

After reading this chapter, you will be able to do the following:

- Delineate the important aspects of drug delivery systems
- Summarize the different routes of administration common in the athletic training and prehospital health care settings
- Appreciate the advantages and disadvantages of common enteral and parenteral routes of administration
- Delineate the phases and disposition of oral drug delivery technology
- Differentiate between the variables in dosing regimens
- Competently administer medications in the oral route to a patient

Pharmacotherapy is the treatment and prevention of illness and disease by means of drugs of chemical or biological origin.[17] The success of drug therapy is highly dependent on the choice of the drug, the drug product, and the design of the dosage regimen. The choice of the drug is made by the prescriber after careful patient diagnosis and physical assessment. Based on the patient's individual characteristics and known pharmacokinetics of the drug, the prescriber chooses a drug product (e.g., immediate release versus modified release) and dosage regimen.[26] In the athletic training setting, the administration of medication is a common and important clinical procedure.[16]

Depending on the clinical setting, practicing athletic trainers (ATs) encounter situations where they will need to regularly administer prescription or over-the counter (OTC) medications. Although they may not use all routes of administration, should the situation arise, ATs must be familiar with the various drug delivery systems, including drug forms, drug dosing, and administration procedures.[9] Some common routes of administration determined by the prescriber include the **enteral** (gastrointestinal tract), **parenteral** (via injections), inhalation, transdermal, and topical routes. This chapter briefly summarizes important concepts from earlier chapters that are especially relevant to drug delivery.

Drug Delivery Systems

Drug delivery refers to approaches, formulations, technologies, and systems for transporting a pharmaceutical compound in the body as needed to safely achieve its desired therapeutic effect. It is often approached via a drug's chemical formulation, but it may also involve medical devices or drug–device combination products.[16,17,26] Drug delivery is an important consideration when administering medications in the athletic training clinic, and integrates the following elements:[16,26]

- Dosage form
- Dosage regimen
- Drug release formulation
- Route of administration

Biopharmaceutics links the physical and chemical properties of the drug and the drug product to their clinical performance in vivo; thus, a primary concern in biopharmaceutics is the bioavailability of drugs.[17,30] A drug product may also be **locally acting** or **extravascular**, delivering the drug directly to the site of action before reaching the systemic circulation. Examples of locally acting drug products include gastric, ophthalmic, pulmonary, and nasal drug products. Drugs with systemic bioavailability are also strongly influenced by physicochemical properties of the drug and drug product. Regardless of the intended site of drug action, biopharmaceutics aims to balance the amount and extent of drug delivered from the drug product to safely achieve optimal therapeutic efficacy for the patient.[17,25]

Routes of Administration

Selecting the proper route of administration is an important consideration for prescribers using pharmaceutical interventions. The route of drug administration (figure 6.1) is based on several factors, including the rate of drug absorption and the duration of drug action.[17,26] As discussed in chapter 4, a drug's bioavailability is the proportion of administered drug that reaches the systemic circulation and is available for distribution to the intended site of action. Drugs that are administered by direct intravenous (IV) injection are considered to have 100% bioavailability. Some drugs that are particularly well absorbed by the gastrointestinal (GI) mucosa may have bioavailability comparable to that of an IV dose (e.g., the antibiotic *ciprofloxacin*). However, most drugs do not have complete bioavailability by the oral route, so the dose administered orally is usually higher than one given parenterally. The route of administration and its **dosage form** (tablet, capsule, liquid) can clearly influence the bioavailability of a drug.[16]

Prescribers considering certain routes of administration make clinical decisions on pharmaceutical interventions based on physiologic and safety considerations. For example, intra-arterial and intrathecal drug injections are less safe than other routes of drug administration and thus are used only when absolutely necessary.[17,26] A summary of the various routes of drug administration is presented in table 6.1.[13,17,25,26,30] Advantages and limitations of each route are addressed in the sections Enteral Drug Delivery and Parenteral Drug Delivery.

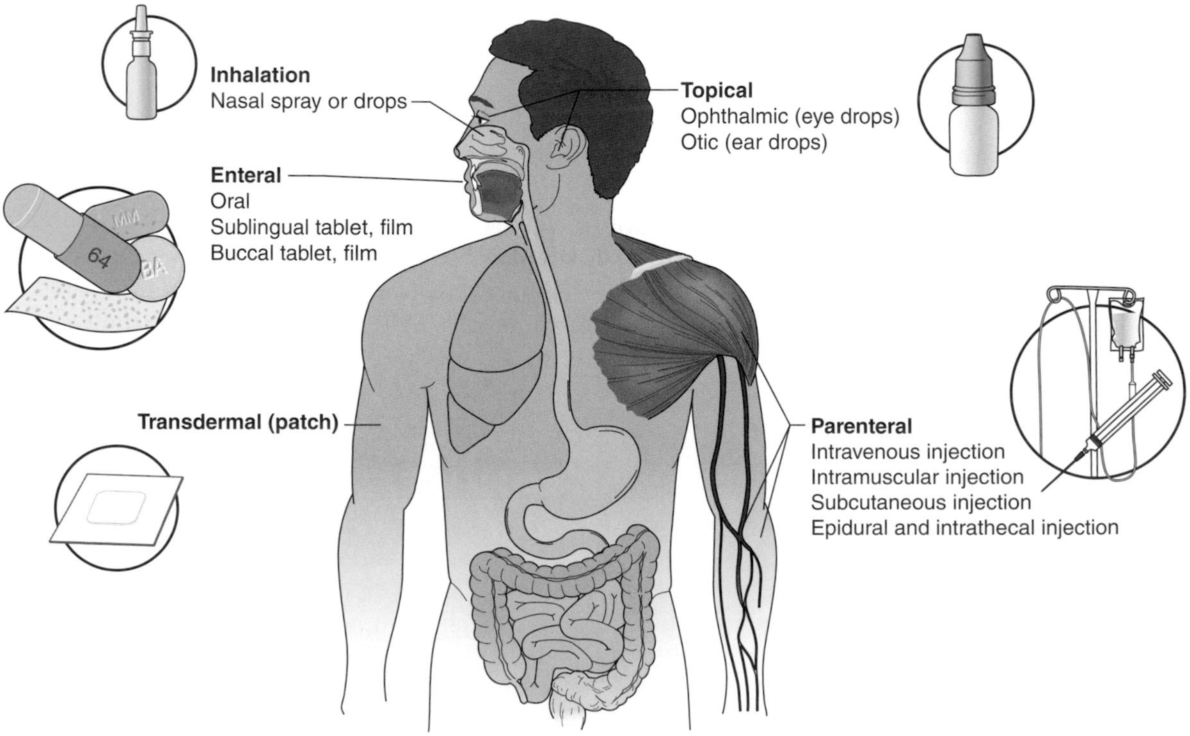

FIGURE 6.1 Common routes of extravascular and parenteral drug administration.

TABLE 6.1 Routes of Drug Administration

Route	Description
	ENTERAL: ENTRY INTO THE BODY THROUGH THE GI TRACT
Oral (swallowed)	Maximum convenience; absorption is often slower. Bioavailability is often limited by the first-pass effect, in which a significant amount of the agent is metabolized in the gut wall, portal circulation, and liver before it reaches the systemic circulation.
Rectal (through GI tract; delivered by suppository or enema)	Partial avoidance of the first-pass effect. Larger amounts of drug and drugs with unpleasant taste are better administered rectally than by the buccal or sublingual routes. Patients who lose the ability to swallow (e.g., due to hospice, stroke, diminished consciousness) may have tablets or capsules intended for oral use inserted rectally, where they are well absorbed.
	PARENTERAL: DIRECT ENTRY INTO THE BODY
Inhalation (solids, liquids, gas)	Medication is delivered to the lungs to treat respiratory diseases such as asthma. Provided in various forms (e.g., dry powder inhaler, metered dose inhaler, nebulizer, oxygen nasal cannula, anesthetic gas). Absorption usually very rapid.
Intravenous (IV)	Instantaneous and complete absorption for fastest delivery of drug throughout the body. Because of the rapid delivery mode, IV administration is frequently used in sports medicine in cases of dehydration for fluid replacement.
Intramuscular (IM)	Injection directly into a muscle that has a large blood supply, providing a faster rate of absorption than subcutaneous or intradermal injections. Large volumes may be given if the drug is not too irritating. *Lidocaine* (analgesic) is often included when the primary therapeutic agent is irritating or the dose volume is somewhat large. First-pass metabolism is avoided. The buttocks, hip, and deltoid muscles are popular sites for anti-inflammatory agents such as *ketorolac* and for vaccinations.
Subcutaneous	Bolus of drug is injected into the layer of skin directly below the dermis with few blood vessels for a slow, sustained rate of absorption. Absorption is slower than for IM injections and faster than for intradermal injections. Highly effective in administering medications such as *insulin* or *morphine*.
Intra-arterial	Specialized delivery route not commonly used in sports medicine.
Intra-articular	Drug (usually an anti-inflammatory) is injected into the affected joint. The technique may also be used to withdraw excess fluid (effusion) from a joint.
Epidural	Drug is injected into the epidural space around the spinal cord; frequently an anesthetic administered through a catheter in the epidural space. An epidural steroid injection for treating select lower back conditions is an example of this delivery route.
Intrathecal	Drugs delivered via injection into the cerebrospinal fluid (CSF) of the spinal canal or subarachnoid space, such as in spinal anesthesia, chemotherapy, pain management, or infection. Drugs may need to cross the blood-brain barrier.
	DERMAL OR MUCOUS MEMBRANE: ENTRY INTO THE BODY BY OVERCOMING THE SKIN OR MEMBRANE BARRIER
Buccal and sublingual (oral but not swallowed)	Placing the drug under the tongue (sublingual) or between the gums and cheek (buccal) allows direct absorption into the systemic venous circulation, bypassing the hepatic portal circuit and first-pass metabolism.
Topical	Application to the skin or the mucous membrane of the eye, ear, throat, or vagina for local effect. Skin topicals for musculoskeletal and dermatological conditions are commonly used in sports medicine.
Mucous membranes: ophthalmic, otologic, or nasal	Drug is introduced into the eye, ear, or nose. Nasal sprays often include locally acting (e.g., antihistamine) or systemically active drugs, such as migraine drugs, nicotine replacement, and hormone treatments.
Transdermal	Application to the skin for systemic effect. Absorption usually occurs very slowly (because of the thickness of the skin), but the first-pass effect is avoided.

Enteral Drug Delivery

Enteral administration is a method of drug delivery that involves the GI tract. Administering a drug by mouth is the most common, convenient, and economical method of drug administration and enteral delivery.[30] Oral ingestion is the safest and simplest route, with several advantages and a few disadvantages for the patient.[2,10,30]

First-Pass Effect on Enteral Drugs

Any drug that exhibits significant first-pass metabolism must be administered in a sufficient quantity to ensure that an effective concentration of active drug exits the liver into the systemic circulation, from which it can reach the target organ. Since absorption of oral drugs involves transport across membranes of the epithelial cells in the GI tract, this process is affected by the following:[15]

- Differences in luminal pH along the GI tract
- Surface area per luminal volume
- Blood perfusion
- Presence of bile and mucus
- The nature of epithelial membranes
- Inactive prodrugs that require conversion by the liver to become active

Enteral Routes of Administration

The buccal, sublingual, and rectal modes are other options for enteral administration. The oral mucosa is highly vascularized and has a thin epithelium that favors absorption. Therefore, a drug placed between the gums and cheek (buccal administration) or under the tongue (sublingual administration) is retained longer, enhancing absorption.[15] Even the rectal route has varying degrees of the first-pass effect, contrasting with other routes of administration where the drug is distributed in the body before reaching the liver.[17] Both the sublingual and buccal routes of absorption have several advantages:[2,17,30]

- Easily administered
- Rapidly absorbed
- Bypasses the harsh GI tract environment
- Avoids the first-pass effect

Rectal suppositories are viable options when oral medications are challenging—for example, for a patient who is vomiting or unconscious. In the emergency department, fast-acting antiemetic medications, analgesics, and select anti-inflammatory medications may also be administered as rectal suppositories.[2,17,30]

Oral Drug Dosage Forms

When prescribers select the oral route of administration, several factors must be considered that specifically relate to transit time in the GI tract, which may vary considerably:[17]

- Between patients and within an individual patient, with the gastric transit time being the most variable
- State of the dosage form (liquid dosage forms are emptied out of the stomach faster than solid dosage forms)
- The fasted or fed state of the patient

Refer to table 6.2 for a summary and examples of oral dosage forms.[4,17,25]

Advantages and Disadvantages of the Enteral Route of Drug Administration

Advantages

- Safest
- Most common
- Simple
- Inexpensive
- Convenient
- Painless
- No infection

Disadvantages

- Limited absorption of some drugs
- Food may affect absorption
- Drug is exposed to harsh GI environments and first-pass metabolism
- Requires GI absorption
- Slow delivery to site of pharmacologic action
- Requires patient adherence

TABLE 6.2 Oral Drug Dosage Forms

Form	Example
Tablet—Compressed powder that contains several solid phases, since drug particles are usually present together with other solid phases (e.g., filler, binder, disintegrant, glidant, and lubricant particles).	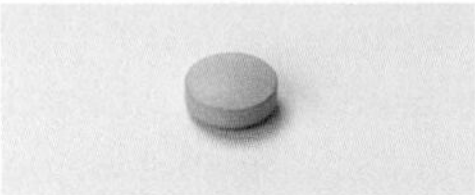
Effervescent tablet—Dissolves in water, releasing carbon dioxide. Drug product is a compression of powders into a dense tablet or granules and is packaged in a blister pack or other water-tight package. The product is dropped into water to make a solution.	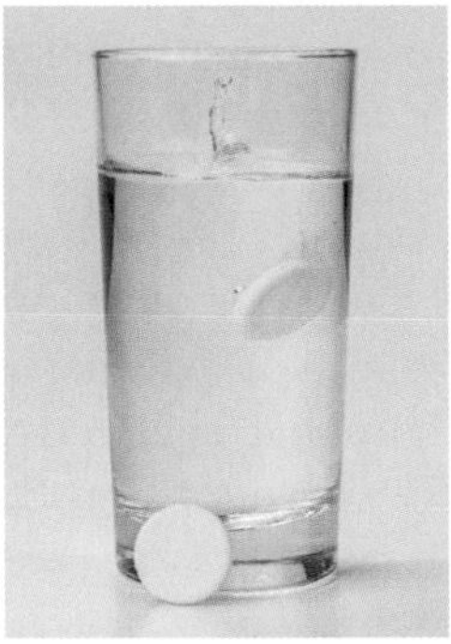
Solution—Molecularly dispersed drug that does not separate out to form larger particles if the concentration is consistent throughout.	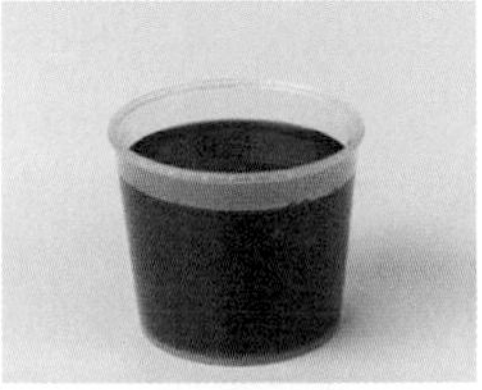
Suspension—Liquid with small pieces of drug that are not completely dissolved; must always be shaken (or stirred) before administration so that the right amount of drug is delivered.	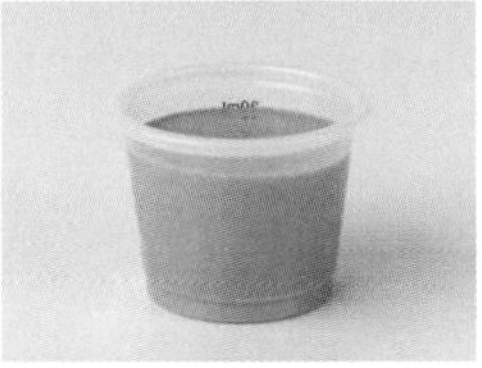
Capsule—A gelatinous envelope enclosing the active substance. Some remain intact for some hours after ingestion in order to delay absorption. Capsules may also contain a mixture of slow- and fast-release particles to produce rapid and sustained absorption in the same dose.	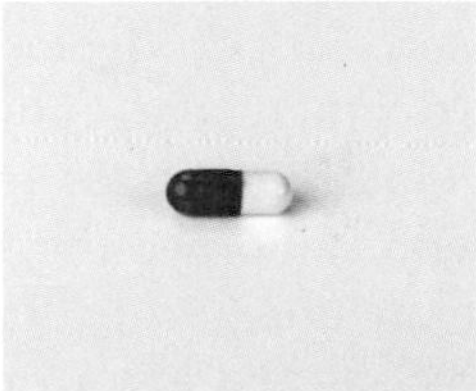
Softgels and gelcaps—Effective delivery system for oral drugs, especially poorly soluble drugs. The fill contains liquid ingredients that help increase the solubility or permeability of the drug across the membranes in the body. All softgels and gelcaps contain an aqueous solution of gelling agents, such as animal protein (mainly gelatin), plant polysaccharides, or their derivatives (e.g., carrageenan, modified forms of starch and cellulose). These dosage forms are often considered by patients to be the most efficient method of taking medication.	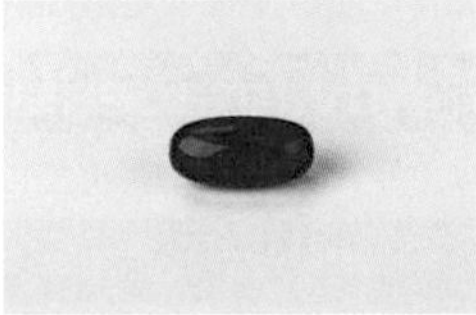
Caplet—Capsule-shaped tablet that is easier to swallow than the usual disc-shaped tablet. Caplets are prescored for splitting to provide a lower dose of the active ingredient or obtain multiple smaller doses, either to reduce cost or because the pills available provide a larger dose than required.	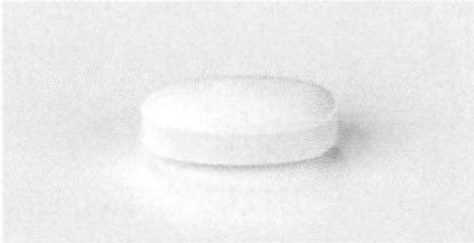

Phases of Absorption of Enteral Medications

The rate of drug release from the product and the rate and extent of drug absorption are important in determining the onset, intensity, and duration of drug action.[16,17,25,26] Systemic drug absorption from an oral drug product consists of a succession of rate processes or phases. For most orally administered drugs, the site of action is the systemic circulation, and the drug must be absorbed to achieve a pharmacological response. Absorption of oral medications involves at least 3 distinct phases:[17,25,26]

1. Disintegration (releasing the drug) or dissolution from the drug product in the body's fluids
2. Permeation of the drug across the GI linings into the systemic circulation
3. Drug disposition during GI transit (e.g., GI stability, motility, metabolism)

Modified Release of Drugs Administered Orally

Additional drug disposition may occur in the systemic circulation and thus reduce the concentration of drug available to the target tissues. By properly designing the drug product, oral drug delivery systems can vary the bioavailability of the active drug from rapid and complete absorption; slow, sustained absorption; or virtually no absorption, depending on the therapeutic objective.

Modifications in oral drug release profiles are used to improve the stability, safety, efficacy, and therapeutic profile of a drug. Drug release systems are classified according to the rate of release of a drug and the location of release. In general, drug products are either *immediate-release* or *modified-release* dosage forms. Types of modified-release form include extended-release, sustained-release, delayed-release, and controlled-release forms.

Immediate-release forms allow the drug to dissolve in the gastrointestinal contents without delaying or prolonging the dissolution or absorption of the drug. The drug is released immediately after administration.[4,15,17] However, for most oral medications, in order to achieve efficient targeted delivery, the drug release system must be designed so that the drug avoids the gastric acid mechanisms and circulates to its intended site of action.[4,25]

Modified-release oral drug systems use tablets and capsules to dissolve a drug over time; thus, the release of the drug into the bloodstream is slower and steadier. An advantage of this form is that the medication can be taken at less frequent intervals than with immediate-release formulations of the same drug. *Extended-release* is a type of modified release, and there are usually fewer side effects with extended-release formulations because the levels of the drug in the body are more consistent. Most commonly, modified-release dosage forms refer to time-dependent release in oral dose formulations. In modified-release dosage forms, the release of medication occurs after administration or to a specific target in the body. The drug release characteristics of time course and location are chosen to accomplish therapeutic or convenience objectives that are not offered by conventional dosage forms, such as a solution or an immediate-release dosage form.

Timed-release (TR) drugs have several distinct oral dosage forms:[2,4,15,17,30]

- **Sustained release (SR)**—Formulations in which there is a prolonged drug release over a period of time in a controlled manner.

Evidence in Pharmacology

Oral Drug Delivery Technology

Drug delivery technologies modify a drug's release profile, absorption, distribution, and elimination for the benefit of improving product efficacy and safety, as well as patient convenience and compliance.[16,26] Some drugs are unstable at the pH of gastric acid and need to be protected from degradation; others are irritating to the gastric lining.[17] An **enteric coating** is a chemical envelope that protects the drug from stomach acid, delivering it instead to the less acidic intestine, where the coating dissolves and releases the drug. Enteric coating is useful for certain drugs that are irritating to the stomach, such as *ibuprofen*.[2,17,30] This coating helps by protecting either the drug from the acidity of the stomach or the stomach from the detrimental effects of the drug; the coating may also help release the drug after it leaves the stomach (usually in the upper part of the small intestine).[4,15-17,26]

- **Delayed release (DR)**—Drug is released at a certain point after the initial administration.
- **Extended release (ER, XR, XL)**—Contains special coatings or ingredients that control the drug release, thereby allowing for slower absorption and prolonged duration of action to reduce dosing. ER formulations can be dosed less frequently and may improve patient compliance. ER formulations are advantageous for drugs with short half-lives.
- **Controlled release (CR)**—This form reduces dosing frequency for drugs with a short elimination half-life and duration of effect. It also limits fluctuation in plasma drug concentration, providing a more uniform therapeutic effect while minimizing adverse effects. Absorption rate is slowed by coating drug particles with wax or another water-insoluble material, embedding the drug in a matrix that releases it slowly during transit through the GI tract, or complexing the drug with ion-exchange resins. Most absorption of this form occurs in the large intestine. Crushing or otherwise disturbing a controlled-release tablet or capsule can often be dangerous.[4,15]
- **Transdermal controlled release**—Releases the drug for extended periods with consistent drug delivery over a certain length of time, sometimes for several days. Drugs for transdermal delivery must have suitable skin penetration characteristics and high potency because the penetration rate and area of application are limited.[15]

Clinical Application

Administering and Documenting Modified-Release or Timed-Release Oral Medications

Unfortunately, there is no industry standard for nomenclature or abbreviations for drug release systems. As a result, occasionally confusion and misreading occur that cause prescribing errors. When documenting drugs with multiple formulations, it is advisable to spell out the meaning in parentheses.[4,15,17]

Parenteral Drug Delivery

Parenteral administration provides the most control over the dose of drug delivered directly into the systemic circulation, cerebrospinal fluid, vascularized tissue, or some other tissue space (figure 6.2). Drugs that are administered parenterally immediately overcome barriers that can limit the effectiveness of orally administered drugs (see table 6.3).[2,30] Prescribers use parenteral administration for drugs that are poorly absorbed from the GI tract (e.g., *heparin*) or unstable in the GI tract (e.g., *insulin*). In the prehospital and emergency settings, parenteral administration is used for patients who are unable to take oral medications (e.g., unconscious patients) and in circumstances that require a rapid onset of action (i.e., emergent conditions).[6,28,30]

Parenteral administration of medications is associated with several potential disadvantages,

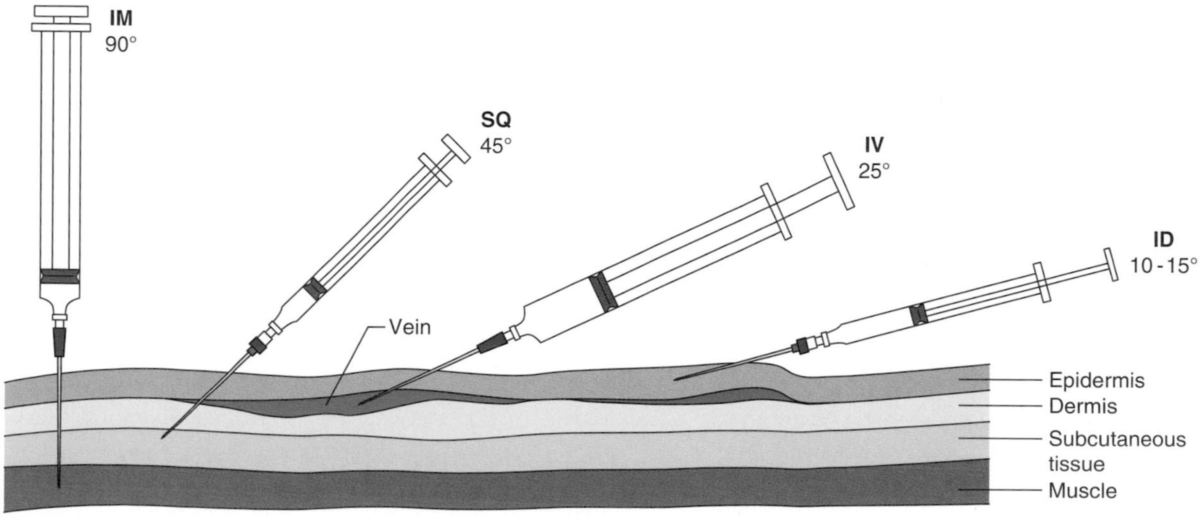

FIGURE 6.2 Most common parenteral routes of administration from deepest to most superficial. IM = intramuscular, SQ = subcutaneous, IV = intravenous, ID = intradermal.

including an increased risk of infection and the requirement for administration by a trained health care professional. The onset of action of parenterally administered drugs is often rapid, potentially resulting in increased toxicity when such drugs are administered too rapidly or in incorrect doses.[2,17]

Dosage Forms of Parenteral Drugs

Depending on the site of administration, sports medicine prescribers differentiate between intravenous (IV), intramuscular (IM), intra-articular (IART), subcutaneous (SQ), intradermal (ID), and epidural options. Other forms include intraosseous (IO), intraperitoneal, and intrathecal injection. For other routes of parenteral drug administration, the delivery systems can be aqueous, oily, or even solid (e.g., **implants**). Drugs can also be administered on the skin (transdermal) to enter the systemic circulation. Mostly, semisolid dosage forms are used for transdermal delivery, including creams, ointments, gels, and pastes. However, liquid dosage forms (e.g., emulsions) and solid dosage forms, such as transdermal controlled drug delivery systems (i.e., **patches**), are also used.[17]

Administration of medication directly into body tissue results in a rate of onset of drug action that differs among the various body tissues; absorption patterns depend on the rate of blood flow to the tissue (table 6.3).[2,10,18,30]

- Direct introduction of a drug into the venous (i.e., intravenous or, less commonly, intra-arterial) circulation or into the cerebrospinal fluid (i.e., intrathecal) results in the drug having a quicker onset of its effects.[2,30]
- Drugs administered extravascularly must be absorbed into the bloodstream and undergo first-pass metabolism. This may decrease the bioavailability, or fraction, of medication that enters the systemic circulation.

TABLE 6.3 Characteristics of Common Parenteral Routes of Administration

Route	Absorption pattern	Special utility	Limitations and precautions
Intravenous (IV)	• GI absorption circumvented • Potentially immediate effects • Suitable for large volumes, irritating substances, or complex mixtures	• Valuable for emergency use • Permits slower titration of dosage • Required for drugs with high molecular weight (e.g., peptides, proteins)	• Increased risk of adverse effects • Most solutions should be injected slowly. • Not suitable for oily solutions or poorly soluble substances
Intramuscular (IM)	• Prompt absorption from aqueous solution • Slow and sustained release from repository preparations • Depot injections are sustained release with delayed absorption.	• Suitable for moderate volumes, oily vehicles, and some irritants • Some may be appropriate for self-administration (e.g., EpiPen).	• Precautions may be needed for patients on anticoagulant medications. • May interfere with interpretation of certain diagnostic tests (e.g., creatine kinase)
Intraosseous (IO)	• Drug directly injected into bone marrow • Allows the administered medications and fluids to go directly into the vascular system • Used in life-threatening situations for quick administration access	• Provides a noncollapsible entry point into the systemic venous system • Used to provide fluids and medication when intravenous access is not available or not feasible	• Awake patients may require analgesia for IO placement by local infiltration of anesthetic at the IO site. • IO needle should be replaced with a venous line as soon as possible.
Subcutaneous (SQ)	• Prompt absorption from aqueous solution • Slow and sustained release from repository preparations (e.g., implant)	• Suitable for some poorly soluble suspensions and slow-release implants • Appropriate for self-administration or pump administration (e.g., *insulin*)	• Not suitable for large volumes • Irritants may cause pain or necrosis.

The frequency of administration can be reduced by using routes of administration that give a sustained rate of drug absorption. With drugs that are not very soluble, intramuscular injection generally provides more rapid systemic absorption than oral administration does.[26] Subcutaneous administration of a drug into poorly vascularized adipose tissue results in a slower onset of action than injection into well-vascularized intramuscular spaces.

Prescribers determine the most optimal route of administration by considering the therapeutic objectives (e.g., the need for a rapid onset, the need for long-term treatment, or restriction of delivery to a local site) and patient factors that may affect their tolerability, adherence, and ability to take the medication. Epidural analgesia is the administration of analgesics into the epidural space (figure 6.3). An example of an epidural includes an **intrathecal** injection, which delivers a drug directly into the spinal canal so that it reaches the cerebrospinal fluid (CSF). This injection is useful in spinal anesthesia, chemotherapy, and pain management, such as treating a symptomatic lumbar herniated disc. Epidural analgesics can be given either as a single injection or a continuous **infusion** via an indwelling catheter.[30]

RED FLAG

Postdural Puncture Headache

The most frequently occurring adverse event of a lumbar epidural steroid injection (ESI) is a postdural puncture headache secondary to an inadvertent lumbar dural puncture.[5,7] When a spinal needle punctures the dural space, leaking CSF causes a debilitating headache; this occurs in up to 35% of ESI patients.[21] The risk ratio of a postdural puncture headache is almost doubled when a conventional needle is used rather than an atraumatic needle. The patient will have an intense headache and difficulty standing and will feel relief when lying down.[1] Postdural puncture headaches are resolved by administering autologous blood into the epidural space.[27]

Intravenous Drug Administration

Intravenous delivery permits a rapid effect and a maximum degree of control over the amount of drug delivered (figure 6.4). When injected as a bolus, the full amount of drug is delivered to the

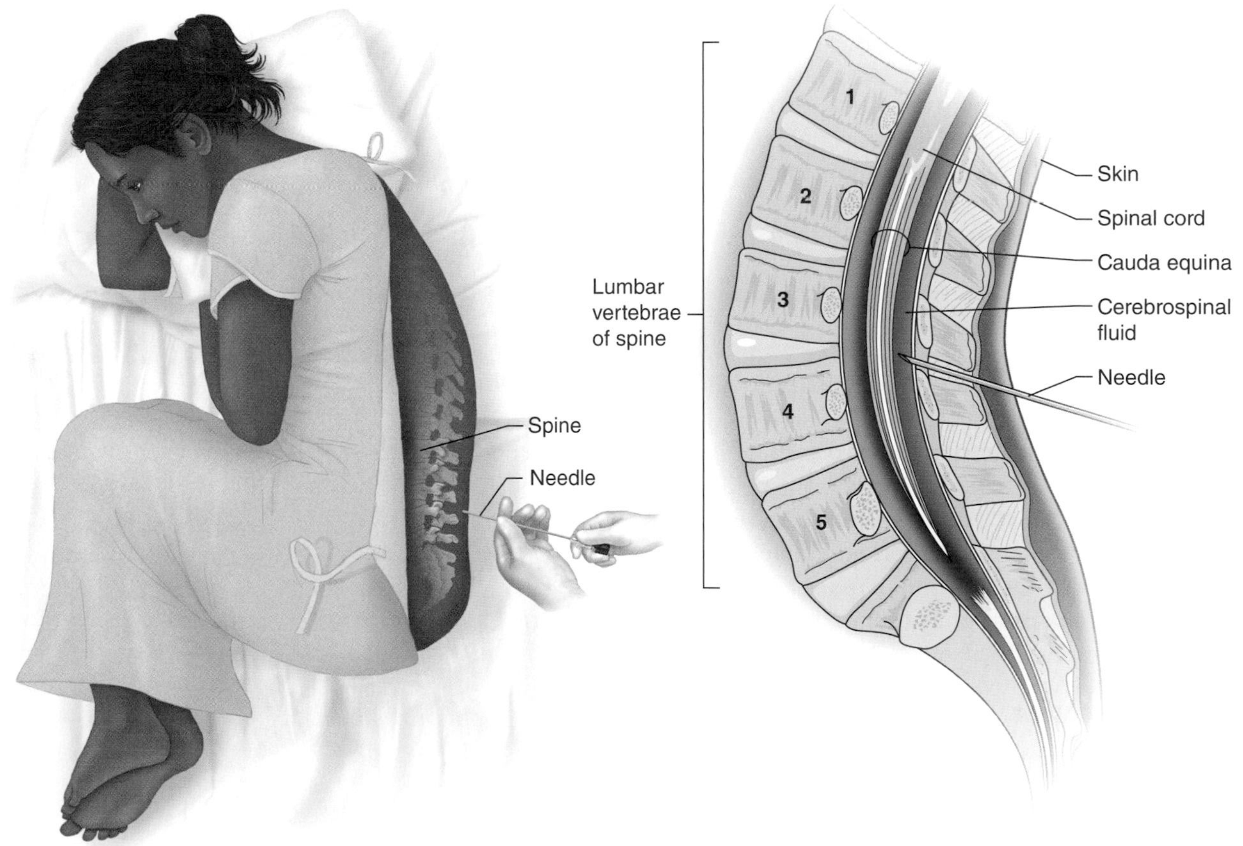

FIGURE 6.3 Epidural steroid injection is a parenteral route of administration.

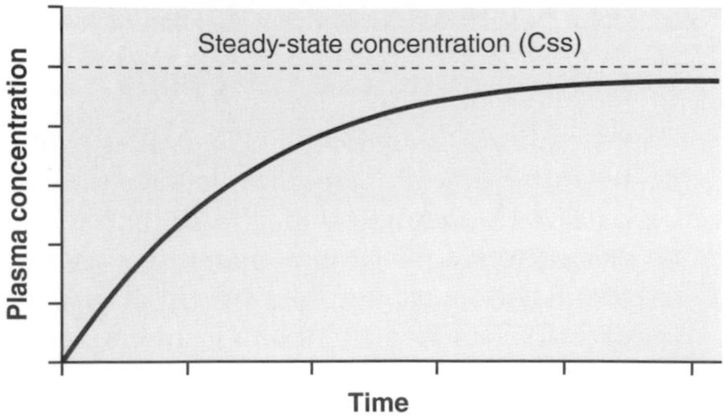

FIGURE 6.4 Continuous IV infusion of a hypothetical drug. Steady-state plasma concentration (Css) is when the amount of drug delivered in a unit of time is equal to the amount eliminated in the same unit of time.

Clinical Application

Routes of Rehydration for Heat Illness

In cases of mild dehydration, the oral route of administration is the most common option for ATs. However, for many athletes at all levels, IV administration of *normal saline* may be used to minimize the incidence of heat illness, including muscle cramping during competition. This prophylactic practice has been reported by 75% of teams in the National Football League[8] and some high school programs under appropriate medical guidance.[14] No high-level study confirms that IV prehydration prevents exercise-associated muscle cramps, and multiple studies do not support IV fluid replacement when the patient can tolerate oral fluids.[8]

systemic circulation almost immediately. If administered as an IV infusion, the drug is delivered over a longer period of time, resulting in lower peak plasma concentrations and an increased duration of circulating drug.[30] With multiple dosing, or a continuous infusion, the drug accumulates until the amount administered per unit of time is equal to the amount eliminated per unit of time (i.e., **steady-state concentration**, or **Css**).[24]

Intramuscular Drug Administration

In general, the method of drug administration that provides the most consistent and greatest bioavailability should be used to ensure maximum therapeutic effect. Certain drugs are not suitable for intramuscular administration because of erratic drug release, pain, or local irritation. Although the drug is injected into the muscle mass, it must reach the circulatory system or another body fluid in order to become bioavailable. The anatomic site of drug deposition following IM injection affects the rate of drug absorption. A drug is more rapidly absorbed when injected into the deltoid muscle than into the gluteus maximus because there is better blood flow in the deltoid muscle.[26] As the vehicle diffuses out of the muscle, the drug precipitates at the site of injection. The drug then dissolves slowly, providing a sustained dose over an extended interval of time (figure 6.5).[30]

Subcutaneous Drug Administration

Like with IM injection, subcutaneous injection provides absorption via simple diffusion and is slower than with the IV route. Subcutaneous injection minimizes the risks of hemolysis and thrombosis associated with IV injection and may provide constant, slow, and sustained effects.[30]

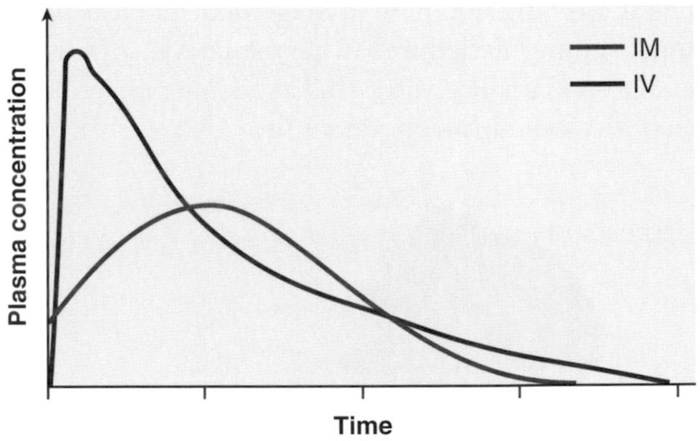

FIGURE 6.5 Plasma concentrations of a hypothetical drug after intravenous and intramuscular injection.

RED FLAG

Adverse Events Associated With Injections

Incidence of adverse events secondary to injections of corticosteroids ranges from 2% to 10%; these events can result in skin or fat atrophy at the injection site.[29] The risk of tendon rupture secondary to corticosteroid injection in the soft tissue around the Achilles tendon or plantar fascia is <1%.[23] Improper injection preparation can lead to infection, which in turn can lead to septic arthritis. However, careful sterile techniques and proper staff hygiene can reduce this risk.[19] In addition, ultrasound guidance imaging enhances the accuracy of the exact injection site.[23] Even without diagnostic imaging, 69% to 76% of the subacromial bursa injections are correctly injected, avoiding unintended injection in the surrounding structures.[19]

Mucous Membrane Drug Administration

The mucous membranes are highly vascular, permitting a drug to enter the systemic circulation rapidly and reach its target organ with minimal delay.[2] Mucous membranes are much less of a barrier to drug uptake than the skin. Some mucous membranes (e.g., small intestine) are specialized sites for absorption. Many can act as absorption sites, including the buccal, sublingual, ocular, pulmonary, nasal, rectal, and vaginal mucosa. Drugs may also be administered directly into the target organ, resulting in a virtually instantaneous onset of action. This rapid delivery is advantageous in critical conditions; for example, for acute asthma, drugs such as beta-adrenergic agonists can be administered via aerosol directly into the airways.[2] Drug delivery systems designed to give a local drug effect are considered **topical delivery systems**, and drugs providing systemic activity include many transdermal dosage forms.[2,9,17]

Topical Drug Administration

Some drugs are intended for topical or local therapeutic action at the site of administration (table 6.4). Drugs intended for local activity are designed

TABLE 6.4 Topical Drug Dosage Forms

Forms	Example
Gel—Jellylike, soft semisolid material with a 3-dimensional network that spans the volume of a liquid medium	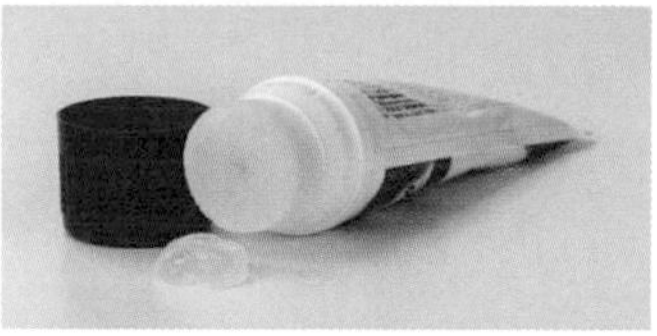
Ointment—Homogeneous, viscous semisolid preparation; most commonly a greasy, thick oil (composition 80% oil, 20% water) with a high viscosity	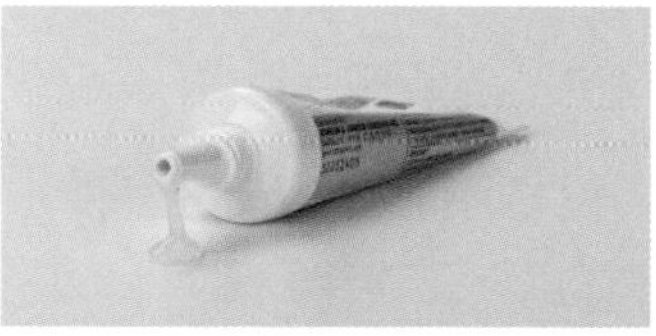
Cream—Semisolid emulsion of oil and water that may be either dispersed (water-in-oil cream) or continuous (oil-in-water cream)	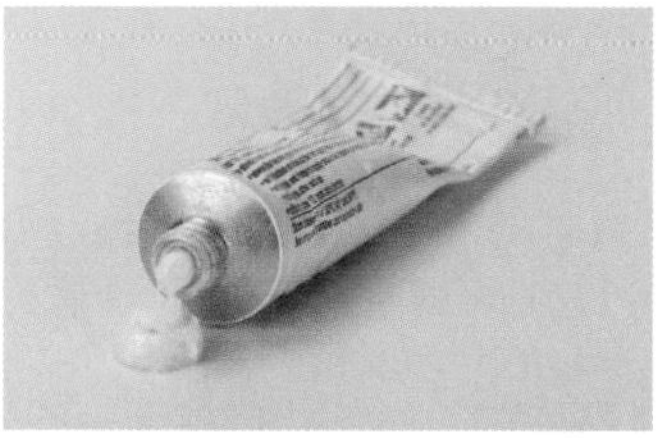
Lotion—Drug delivery system with low viscosity	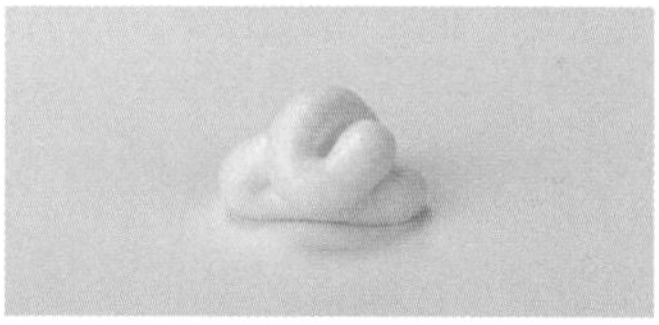
Solution—Drops, rinses, or sprays that generally have low viscosity; usually a powder dissolved in alcohol, water, and sometimes oil	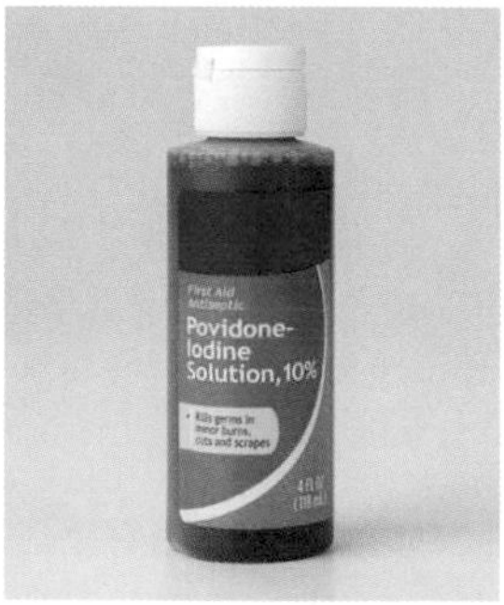

to have a direct pharmacodynamic action without affecting other body organs. For local activity, systemic drug absorption is often undesirable. Forms of drugs delivered include gels, ointments, creams, and lotions. Examples of drugs used for local action include anti-infectives, antifungals, local anesthetics, antacids, astringents, vasoconstrictors, antihistamines, bronchodilators, and corticosteroids. Although systemic absorption is undesired, it may occur with locally acting drugs; modifying the drug product design may help to mitigate systemic effects.[25]

Transdermal Drug Administration

Transdermally administered drugs are absorbed from the skin and subcutaneous tissues directly into the blood. This route of administration is ideal for a drug that must be slowly and continuously administered over extended periods of time. There is no associated risk of infection, and drug administration is simple and convenient.[2] In general, semisolid dosage forms are used for this delivery system, including creams, ointments, gels, pastes, and patches. Absorption through the skin is a special challenge since one of the main functions of the skin is to prevent particles or compounds from entering the body. The stratum corneum of the skin forms a formidable barrier against uptake; thus, transdermal delivery is difficult to achieve. Penetration enhancers are added to the delivery system to improve delivery into or through the skin. In transdermal drug delivery systems, the dosage form controls the uptake into the skin (rather than the uptake being controlled by the stratum corneum).[17] A limited number of drugs have sufficiently high lipophilicity that passive diffusion across the skin is a viable route of administration. The success of transdermal nicotine, estrogen, and *fentanyl* patches demonstrates the utility of this route of administration.[2] An example commonly used in the AT setting is the Lidoderm transdermal analgesic patch.

Medication Dosing

Optimal medication dosing ensures that the active drug is available at the site of action for the correct time and duration.[30] As noted in chapter 5, the ideal drug concentration level is in the therapeutic range (figure 6.6). In clinical practice, achieving

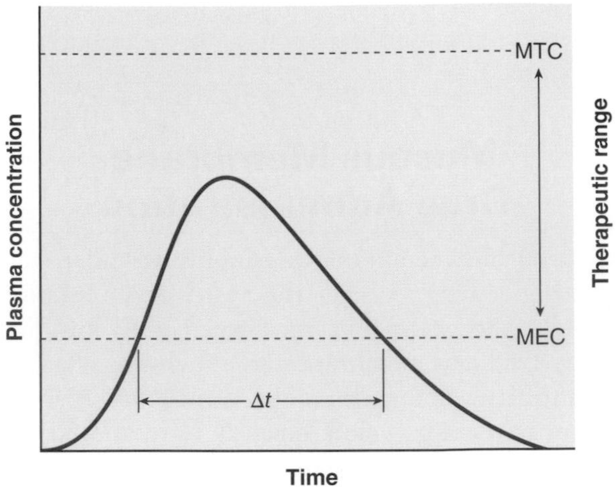

FIGURE 6.6 Drug plasma levels after oral administration of a drug in an immediate-release dosage form. *Note:* The therapeutic range is the concentration interval between the minimal effective concentration (MEC) and the minimal toxic concentration (MTC). Δt is the time interval that the drug is in the therapeutic range.

the desired concentration of a drug is dependent on a dosing regimen that is based on the following:[17]

- Drug delivery system used
- Route of administration
- Frequency of dosing
- Drug clearance rate

The goal is for the drug plasma concentration to remain within the therapeutic window, where it is effective but not toxic. Occasionally a dosing schedule can result in either the peak reaching into the toxic range, in which case the patient experiences side effects, or the trough dropping too low, which leads to the drug no longer being effective. Both of these problems can be solved by adjusting the dose and dosing schedule.[24]

Oral medications are available in different forms, and a single medication is commonly prescribed in a variety of forms.[3] The prescriber determines the appropriate form of a medication based on the nature and urgency of the medical problem that the drug is being used to treat.[9] Factors that prescribers consider with medication dosing regimens include the following:

- **Loading dose**—Once a drug is administered, the plasma concentration of the drug initially increases (figure 6.7). Distribution of the drug from the vascular (blood) compartment to body tissues causes the plasma drug con-

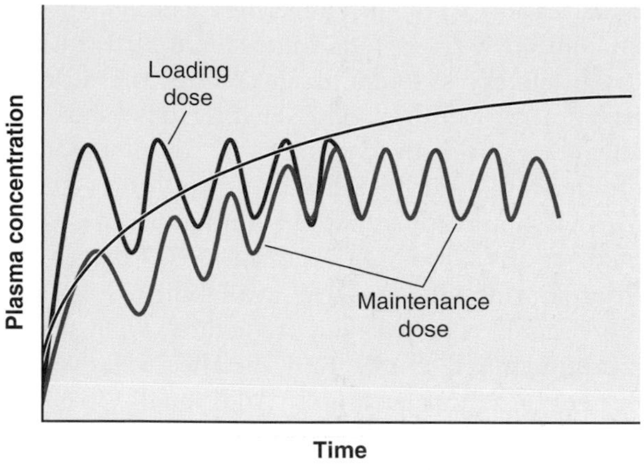

FIGURE 6.7 Dosing regimens that lead to a therapeutic dose.

centration to decrease. The rate and extent of this decrease are significant for a drug with a high volume of distribution. When the time to reach steady state is appreciable, as it is for a drug with a long half-life, it is desirable to administer a loading dose that promptly raises the concentration of drug in plasma to the target concentration.[2,11] In the absence of a loading dose, 5 half-lives must pass to achieve a steady state of the drug concentration.[9]

- **Maintenance dose**—Once steady-state drug concentration is achieved in the plasma and the tissues, subsequent doses need to replace only the amount of drug that is lost through metabolism and excretion. The maintenance dose rate of a drug is dependent on the drug clearance.[2] In most clinical situations, drugs are administered in such a way as to maintain a steady state of drug in the body—that is, just enough drug is given in each dose to replace the amount eliminated since the preceding dose. At steady state, the dosing rate (rate in) must equal the rate of elimination (rate out).[11]
- **Duration of action**—Time for a single dose of a medication to produce the desired effect.
- **Dosing frequency**—The drug dose is related to the frequency of drug administration. The more frequently a drug is administered, the smaller the amount needed to obtain the same effect. Thus, rather than a dosage of 250 mg every 3 hours (i.e., 8 times per day for 2,000 mg total), a prescriber may change the dosage to 500 mg every 6 hours (i.e., 4 times per day for 2,000 mg total) without affecting the average steady-state plasma concentration of the drug;[11,26] this choice depends on the elimination half-life of the drug and optimal liver and renal function of the patient.
- **Dosing interval**—This is determined by the elimination half-life. The longer the time between doses, the larger the amount of a drug required to maintain the average plasma drug concentration.[11,26]
- **Steady state**—Concentration eventually will be achieved when a drug is administered at a constant rate. At this point, drug elimination (the product of clearance and concentration) is equal to the rate of drug availability. This concept also extends to regular intermittent dosage (e.g., 250 mg of a drug every 8 hours). During each interdose interval, the concentration of a drug rises with absorption and falls by elimination. At steady state, the entire cycle is repeated during each interval.[10]

Clinically, drug concentrations in plasma are therapeutic, subtherapeutic, toxic, and supratherapeutic. The goal of most drug-dosing regimens is to maintain the drug at concentrations within the therapeutic range (also called the therapeutic window). If the initial (loading) dose is larger than the maintenance dose, the drug reaches its therapeutic concentration more rapidly. An excessive maintenance dose or dosing frequency could result in toxicity, while insufficient dosing will cause a subtherapeutic steady-state drug concentration.

Clinical Procedures for Enteral Drug Administration

Most oral preparations are taken by mouth, swallowed with fluid, and absorbed via the GI tract. Oral medications are available in solid forms (e.g., tablets, capsules, caplets, and enteric-coated tablets) and liquids forms (e.g., syrups, elixirs, spirits, and suspensions). For oral medication administration, the AT must be knowledgeable about the medication's purpose and adverse effects, as well as patient preferences. In addition to the patients' rights of drug administration, when administering oral medications, the AT must consider the following:[6,12,20,22,28]

- Does the patient have any medication allergies?
- Enteric-coated medication and extended- or sustained-release medications should never be chewed, broken, or crushed.
- Patients with altered GI function (e.g., vomiting and nausea) should not be administered oral medications since they would not be able to retain them.
- Oral medications are contraindicated in patients who are unconscious, uncooperative, or unable to swallow due to a medical problem.

Should any concerns arise, the AT must consult with the prescriber or a pharmacist to determine the best course of treatment for the patient.

Summary

In the prehospital clinical setting, the practicing AT must be prepared to administer medication on direction from the prescriber. The AT should be familiar with various routes of administration, drug delivery systems, drug dosing, and administration procedures. This chapter describes the advantages and disadvantages of common routes of administration in the athletic training setting. The AT should appreciate the limitations of enteral medications as well as the advantages of parenteral drug administration. Drug availability is usually more rapid, extensive, and predictable when a drug is administered by injection; the effective dose can be delivered more accurately. Additionally, in emergency situations and when a patient is unconscious, uncooperative, or unable to retain anything given by mouth, parenteral therapy may be necessary. Parenteral administration also has its disadvantages: asepsis must be maintained (e.g., injection, infusion), pain and anxiety may accompany the injection, and it is sometimes difficult for patients to perform the injections themselves if self-medication is necessary.[10]

Case Studies

Case Study 1

Alex is a professional basketball player with a history of lower back pain. To the best of his recollection, his original diagnosis was nonspecific mechanical lumbosacral dysfunction with minimal diagnostics. He thinks that he had an MRI 2 years earlier as a college senior but does not recall the findings. He has occasional right leg discomfort when he sits for extended periods of time, such as when sitting in stop-and-go traffic. Earlier this week, he reported a new popping sensation in his lower back after doing an overhead military press with a 20-kg medicine ball. He said that subsequent to this exercise, his back felt funny and he self-medicated with an over-the-counter NSAID. Evaluation indicated palpable tenderness with mild swelling along the right L3-S1 paraspinals, limited trunk flexion with a painful end point, incomplete straight leg raise due to pain from the sacrum to mid-calf, and a questionably positive sit-and-slump test for the right leg. During the exam, Alex happened to cough, which exacerbated his pain. He was referred to the orthopedic team physician, who ordered an MRI. The MRI identified a mild L5-S1 disc herniation. The initial course of action was a tapered dose of oral *prednisone* for 6 days with the customary athletic training rehabilitation protocol. At follow-up 14 days later, Alex acknowledged that his pain had improved, but he was still symptomatic; his outcome scale indicated he was at a 62% level of athletic function. An ESI was administered. After a short period of recovery from the injection, Alex resumed his rehabilitation and returned to play approximately 1 month after the strength training injury.

Questions for Analysis

1. Which administration routes were employed for the corticosteroids?
2. How does the concept of first-pass metabolism affect each of these routes?

Case Study 2

Bernie is a successful and avid golfer. She is the defending office tournament long drive champion, closest to the hole, and member of the best ball group who won the tournament. Just prior to this year's tournament, she mis-hit a shot in the sand trap and strained the flexor-pronator mass of her dominant forearm. Two days before the tournament, she saw the nurse practitioner at her local clinic for a prescription. Bernie acknowledged that she preferred not to take an oral NSAID out of concern for GI distress; therefore, the provider prescribed a Flector Patch, which is a transdermal application of the medication Voltaren (*diclofenac*). Bernie was instructed to use the patch on and off for 12-hour cycles prior to playing in the tournament. Bernie used the patch while playing and secured it with a light gauze tube around her forearm. During the tournament, she did not experience the stiffness that she had felt prior to using the patch and the patch did not affect her function as a golfer.

Questions for Analysis

1. When considering the patients' rights of drug administration, how does this choice of a patch compare to oral tablets?
2. How does the skin affect a transdermal patch?

PART II

Classes of Therapeutic Medications

Part I of this text introduced foundational concepts relating to the clinical use of medicines or drugs in the physically active population. Part II describes large classes of medications commonly used in the sports medicine setting. Chapter 7 describes types of pain and nociceptive pathways. Nonopioid analgesics and anesthetics are delineated as well as the role of the athletic trainer in the use of these medications. Chapter 8 outlines concerns about opioid medications as well as guidelines for using opioid antagonists for opioid overdose. One of the most largely used classes of drugs in sports medicine is the anti-inflammatories. Chapter 9 describes the various pathways used for the anti-inflammatory effects for steroidal and nonsteroidal medications. Finally, chapter 10 breaks down the large class of drugs used to treat infection into families of antibiotics. It discusses concerns about antibiotic resistance and responsible stewardship of antibiotics in the context of the human microbiome. These 4 chapters collectively set the stage for further study of the drugs used to treat the conditions commonly encountered in the athletic patient.

7

Drugs to Treat Pain: Nonopioid Analgesics and Anesthetics

OBJECTIVES

After reading this chapter, you will be able to do the following:

- Differentiate between the types of pain classifications
- List the therapeutic effects of each of the drug classes: nonopioid analgesics, topical analgesics, and topical and local anesthetics
- Determine the indications, contraindications, and precautions to follow for each of the drug classes discussed in this chapter
- Educate the patient on dosing schedules
- Describe the AT's role in the clinical management of acute and chronic pain

Pain is well defined as a subjective, unpleasant, sensory, and emotional experience associated with actual or potential tissue damage or abnormal functioning of nerves.[27,38] Ranging in etiology from headaches to a sprained ankle, pain is a component of virtually all clinical pathologies, and management of pain is a primary clinical imperative.[43] Just about everybody experiences pain. Approximately 100 million adults in the United States—more than the number affected by heart disease, diabetes, and cancer combined—suffer from common chronic pain conditions. Pain is one of the most frequent reasons for visiting a health care provider (HCP) and among the most common reasons for taking medication.[27] It is a complex phenomenon, and each person perceives pain differently. The effectiveness of treatment for pain often depends on a constellation of biological, psychological, and social factors. This chapter discusses pain classifications and the drugs commonly encountered by the AT in the treatment of acute and chronic pain. Opioid analgesics and antagonists are discussed in chapter 8 and nonsteroidal anti-inflammatory drugs (NSAIDs) are discussed in chapter 9.

Select Drugs Mentioned in This Chapter

Drug class	Generic name	Trade name
Analgesics		
Nonopioid oral	*acetaminophen* (sometimes *APAP* for N-acetyl-para-aminophenol)	Tylenol
	paracetamol (international)	Panadol
Topical counterirritants	*camphor*	Generic only
	capsaicin	Generic only
	menthol	Salonpas, IcyHot
Anesthetics		
Local injectable	*bupivacaine*	Marcaine
	lidocaine	Xylocaine
	procaine	Novocain
Topical cream	*lidocaine*	Lidoderm, Aspercreme
Transdermal patch	*lidocaine*	Lidocaine Patch
Various routes	*cocaine*	Illicit drug
Ophthalmic	*tetracaine*	Pontocaine eye drops

This list is not exhaustive, but rather contains drugs commonly encountered in the athletic training setting. Always consult up-to-date information, confirm with a pharmacist, or discuss the use of therapeutic medications with the prescriber of the medication.

Biopsychosocial Model

The **biopsychosocial model** is helpful for understanding health and illness. The model reflects the development of illness through the complex interaction of biological, psychological, and social factors:[14,38]

- **Biological factors (e.g., genetic, biochemical)**—The extent of an illness or injury and whether the person has other illnesses, is under stress, or has specific genes or predisposing factors that affect pain tolerance or thresholds.
- **Psychological factors (e.g., mood, personality, behavior)**—Emotions such as anxiety, fear, guilt, anger, or depression; thinking that the pain represents something worse than it does and that the person is helpless to manage it.
- **Social factors (e.g., cultural, familial, socioeconomic, medical)**—The response of significant others, friends, or teammates to the patient's response to pain.

Differentiation of Pain

When assessing and treating pain, it is helpful to classify or subdivide the presenting symptoms into types of pain.[14,38] A consensus panel commissioned by the National Institutes of Health (NIH) uses duration as the basis for categorizing pain into acute and chronic presentations.[27] Pain comes in many forms. Although acute and chronic pain are considered separately in the following sections, a person can experience both simultaneously.[38]

Acute Pain

Acute pain is of sudden onset and is expected to last a short time (i.e., <6 months).[14,27,38] Acute pain can be a useful physiologic process; its adaptive purpose is to warn a person of a disease state or a potentially harmful situation. It usually can be linked clearly to a specific event, injury, or illness—a muscle strain, a severe sunburn, a kidney contusion, or heartburn, for example. Most people can control many types of acute pain on their own with over-the-counter (OTC) medications or a short course of more potent **analgesics** and rest. Within a relatively short time, acute pain usually subsides when the underlying cause resolves, such as when the muscle strain heals. Acute pain also can be a recurrent problem, with episodes interspersed with pain-free periods,[14] as in the examples of tenosynovitis, acid indigestion (dyspepsia), and migraine headache.

Acute pain can be sharp or dull, burning, shock-like, tingling, shooting, radiating, fluctuating in intensity, varying in location, and occurring in a temporal relationship with an obvious **noxious stimulus**. Under normal conditions, acute pain subsides quickly as the healing process decreases the pain-producing stimuli; however, in some instances, pain persists for months to years, leading to a chronic pathophysiologic pain state with features quite different from those of acute pain. In many cases, the exact etiology of prolonged pain may not always be identifiable.[14,27,38]

Chronic Pain

Chronic pain is prolonged, lasting more than several months (variously defined as 3 to 6 months, but certainly longer than typical healing), and can be frustratingly difficult to treat.[14] This type of pain typically does not have any useful biologic value to patients or clinicians. Although improvement may be possible, for many patients suffering from chronic pain, a cure may be unlikely.[27] Chronic pain can become so debilitating that it affects every aspect of a person's life—the ability to attend school, practice, or work; perform activities of daily living (ADLs); or maintain friendships and family relationships. Essentially, it impedes the person's ability to participate in the fundamental tasks of daily living and appreciate the basic pleasures in life.[14]

Pathophysiology of Pain

The pathophysiology of pain involves complex interactions between neural and immune networks within the peripheral and central nervous systems (CNS) in response to afferent sensory stimuli that produce the conscious experience we know as pain. Pain can be broadly divided into 3 classes: nociceptive pain, inflammatory pain, and pathological pain.[14,27,38,39]

Nociceptive (Physiologic or Protective) Pain

Acute nociceptive pain is a physiologic, adaptive sensation elicited only by noxious stimuli that act as a warning or protective signal. In some clinical situations, such as acute trauma or surgery, it is necessary to control nociceptive pain. In these cases, the pain pathway can be interrupted by blocking transmission with local anesthetics (see the section Local Anesthetics). Alternatively, nociceptive pain may be controlled by administering opioids, such as *morphine* for postoperative pain control or *tramadol*, an opioid widely used to treat mild pain. Nociceptive pain can also be described as **somatic** (musculoskeletal) or **visceral pain**. Pain may be described as sharp, aching, or throbbing. With visceral (organ) pain, the patient often has difficulty localizing the pain or describing it in relation to a specific location, as in spleen or liver injury with **referred pain**.

Inflammatory Pain

Inflammatory pain, often considered one of the cardinal features of inflammation, is caused by activation of the immune system by tissue injury or infection. It is adaptive and protective by heightening sensory sensitivity after unavoidable tissue damage. Inflammatory pain assists in the healing of the injured body part by creating a situation that discourages physical contact and movement. Pain hypersensitivity, or tenderness, reduces further risk of damage and promotes recovery, as after a surgical wound or in an inflamed joint, where normally innocuous stimuli now elicit pain. Although this type of pain is adaptive, it still needs to be reduced in patients with ongoing inflammation, as with rheumatoid arthritis or in cases of severe or extensive injury.[39]

Pathological (Harmful or Maladaptive) Pain

Some pain is not protective but rather harmful or maladaptive. This pathological pain is not a symptom of some disorder, but rather a disease state of the nervous system. It can occur after damage to the nervous system (**neuropathic pain**), but also in conditions in which there is no such damage or inflammation (**dysfunctional pain**). Injury to a peripheral nerve yields complex anatomical and biochemical changes in the nerve and spinal cord that induce spontaneous **dysesthesia** (shooting, burning pain) and **allodynia** (hurting pain from a light touch).[38,43]

Dysfunctional pain is commonly associated with other syndromes in which there exist substantial pain but no noxious stimulus and no, or minimal, peripheral inflammatory pathology. Dysfunctional pain arises without a defined cause or injury. Conditions that evoke dysfunctional pain include the following:[27]

- Fibromyalgia
- Irritable bowel syndrome
- Tension-type or chronic headache
- Temporomandibular joint (TMJ) disease
- Complex regional pain syndrome

Many clinical pain syndromes, such as TMJ pain, typically represent a combination of inflammatory and neuropathic mechanisms. Although nociceptive pain is usually responsive to opioid analgesics, neuropathic pain typically responds less well to opioid analgesics. There is a growing perception that, in the face of chronic tissue injury or inflammation (e.g., arthritis), there can be a transition from inflammatory to neuropathic pain. Such a transition has important implications for analgesic drug efficacy.[38,43]

Analgesics

Analgesics act in various ways on the peripheral and central nervous systems to achieve analgesia, or relief from pain. The broad categories of analgesics are as follows:

- **Nonopioid analgesic drugs**—Such as *acetaminophen* (also called *APAP* for N-acetyl-para-aminophenol)
- **Nonsteroidal anti-inflammatory drugs (NSAIDs)**—Such as the propionic acid derivatives (e.g., *ibuprofen*)
- **Opioid drugs**—Such as *morphine* and *oxycodone*

These drugs are distinct from **anesthetics**, which temporarily affect or, in some instances, eliminate sensation. Anesthetics are available in 2 broad classes: general anesthetics used in surgery (discussed in chapter 22), which cause a reversible loss of consciousness, and local anesthetics, which cause a reversible loss of sensation for a limited region of the body without necessarily affecting consciousness.

Nonopioid Analgesic Agents

Analgesia should be initiated with the most effective analgesic agent that has the fewest side effects. In the treatment of mild to moderate pain, nonopioid analgesics are the preferred first-line therapies. *Acetaminophen*, the prototypical analgesic, is generally indicated as a first-line therapy in many pain-related disease states, such as osteoarthritis, although prompt reassessment should occur to evaluate effectiveness.[14,38]

The World Health Organization Guidelines for Pain Management

The World Health Organization (WHO) provides a 3-step analgesic, or pain relief, ladder as a guideline for the use of drugs in the management of pain.[42] Originally published in 1986 for the management of cancer pain, it is now widely used by medical professionals for the management of all types of pain. The 3-step pain relief ladder (figure 7.1) encourages prescribers to use more conservative therapies before initiating opioid therapy. However, in response to the current opioid epidemic, the Centers for Disease Control and Prevention (CDC) released the publication *CDC Guideline for Prescribing Opioids for Chronic Pain*.[5] The original WHO analgesic ladder indicates prompt oral administration of drugs in the following order:[42,43]

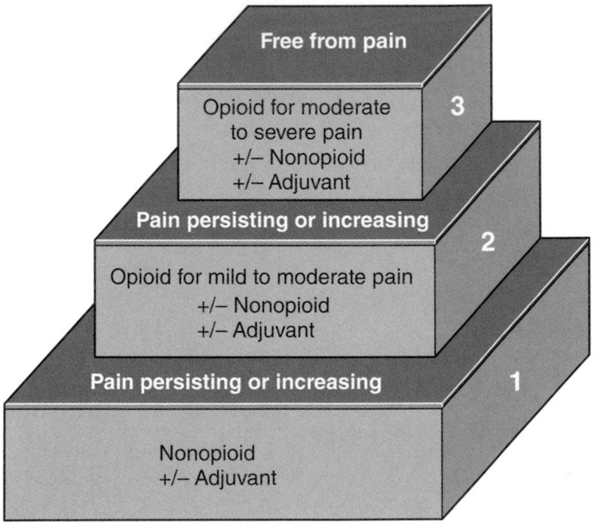

FIGURE 7.1 WHO's pain relief ladder.

Step 1—Nonopioids (*acetaminophen*, NSAIDs); if pain persists or increases, move to step 2 as necessary.

Step 2—Low-potency opioids (*codeine* or *hydrocodone* with *APAP*); if pain persists or increases, move to step 3 as necessary.

Step 3—High-potency opioids (*morphine*) until the patient is free of pain.

In addition to analgesics, the WHO recommends **adjuvants**, or additional drugs used to calm fears and anxiety; however, whenever possible, prescribers should avoid benzodiazepines (further discussed in chapter 18) when prescribing opioid pain medication.[42]

Acetaminophen (Paracetamol)

Acetaminophen or *APAP* (N-acetyl-para-aminophenol) is one of the most popular analgesic and antipyretic medications in the world;[6] >29 billion doses of the drug were sold globally in 2009.[7] *Acetaminophen* is known as *paracetamol* internationally. It became popular in the United States in the early 1980s as an option for treating fever in children without the risk of Reye's Syndrome, which is associated with use of *aspirin*.[22] In the United States, about 50 million Americans use *acetaminophen* weekly for various conditions.[16] *APAP* is available as a generic medication, with trade names including Tylenol, among others. Common conditions that *acetaminophen* treats include headache, muscle aches, arthritis, backache, toothaches, colds, and fevers.[9]

Therapeutic Effects

Acetaminophen has a role in treating mild to moderate pain and moderate to severe pain in conjunction with opiates and in reducing fever (**antipyretic**). *Acetaminophen* is widely used for reducing fever in people of all ages with minimal risk. The WHO recommends that *acetaminophen* be used to treat fever in children with a temperature >38.5°C (101.3°F).[41] *Acetaminophen* has relatively little anti-inflammatory activity, unlike other common analgesics, such as the NSAIDs (e.g., *aspirin*, *ibuprofen*). However, in the treatment of headache, *ibuprofen* and *acetaminophen* have similar effects.[23,40] *Acetaminophen* is helpful in relieving pain in mild arthritis, but has no effect on the underlying inflammation, redness, and swelling of the joint. It is better tolerated than *aspirin* due to anticoagulant (bleeding) concerns with use of *aspirin*. The American College of Rheumatology recommends *acetaminophen* as one of several treatment options for people with arthritis pain of the hip, hand, or knee that does not improve with exercise and weight loss.[21]

Mechanism of Action

The pain-relieving aspects of *acetaminophen* are facilitated through inhibiting neurotransmitters in the CNS.[1,6] Although not fully elucidated, the analgesic effects are believed to be due to activation of descending serotonergic inhibitory pathways in the CNS. Interactions with other nociceptive systems may be involved as well. Antipyresis is produced from inhibition of the hypothalamic heat-regulating center. *Acetaminophen* has some characteristics similar to NSAIDs; however, unlike NSAIDs, it is not considered an anti-inflammatory medication.[28]

Routes of Administration

As an OTC product available in a convenient tablet or caplet form, *acetaminophen* is a popular choice for ATs treating pain secondary to injuries such as sprains, strains, contusions, fever, and headache. In the sports medicine setting, the primary route of *acetaminophen* administration is oral.

Pharmacodynamics and Pharmacokinetics

Acetaminophen is absorbed primarily in the small intestine, metabolized in the liver, transported through the circulatory system, and excreted via the kidney (table 7.1). Caffeine accelerates the absorption of *acetaminophen* and slows its excretion; thus, the analgesic effect may be enhanced when combined with caffeine,[1] such as in a combination product like Excedrin. In general, *acetaminophen* can be taken without regard to meals. The rate of

TABLE 7.1 Pharmacodynamics and Pharmacokinetics of an Analgesic

Generic	*acetaminophen* (U.S.) or *paracetamol* (international)
Trade name	Tylenol (U.S.) and Panadol (international)
Category	Analgesic and antipyretic
Route	Oral, OTC or Rx; IR or ER tablet; rectal, buccal, and IV also available
Onset of action	<1 hr
Peak effect	1 hr
Duration	4-6 hr
Clinical note	When calculating the maximum daily dose, consider all sources of *acetaminophen* (prescription and OTC) and all routes of administration. Do not crush ER tablets.

Note: For oral immediate-release dosage, unless otherwise noted.
IR = immediate release; ER = extended release; IV = intravenous; OTC = over the counter; Rx = by prescription

its absorption among adults 22 to 78 years old is not significantly affected by either fasting or having eaten a light meal.

Dosing Guidelines

APAP is available in the United States in 325 mg and 500 mg strengths and has a half-life of 1.5 to 3 hours.[25] The recommended maximum daily dose for *acetaminophen* is 4,000 mg and the recommended safe dose is 3,250 mg/day (10 tablets containing 325 mg).[32] *Acetaminophen* overdose is linked to hepatotoxicity and liver failure.[25]

Indications and Precautions

Acetaminophen is a popular adjunct taken with other medications used by the sports medicine staff. Because many medications used in sports medicine contain *acetaminophen*, ATs must be cognizant of dosage amounts when overlapping drug products that include the drug to prevent inadvertent *acetaminophen* toxicity or overdoses, which have deleterious consequences. For example, OTC medicines for cold symptoms, cough, congestion symptoms, and headaches have *acetaminophen* as an active ingredient. An example is Theraflu Multi-Symptom Severe Cold—a combination of an analgesic *acetaminophen*, nonopiate antitussive *dextromethorphan*, and sympathomimetic decongestant *phenylephrine*—that is used for symptomatic relief of mild pain, fever, cough, nasal congestion, headache, and sore throat due to a common cold or influenza. This combination medication has a recommended adult dose of 650 mg *acetaminophen* per dose 4 times per day for a total of 2,600 mg, which is well within the safe level of 3,250 mg daily.[32] However, if an athlete taking the cold and flu medication sustained an injury, taking another medication containing *acetaminophen* for pain could be dangerous due to the **additive effect**. If the athlete consumed 1,000 mg of *acetaminophen* 4 times daily for the pain of the injury plus the 2,600 mg in the cold and flu medication, the total of 6,600 mg of *acetaminophen* would appreciably exceed the recommended maximum of 4,000 mg/day (or as directed by prescriber). The same concern applies to many prescription analgesics that contain *acetaminophen*, such as Norco (*acetaminophen* and *hydrocodone*).

Adverse Effects

Acetaminophen is considered a safe and efficacious medication; however, there are concerns regarding adverse effects. This medication is the leading cause of liver failure in the United States. Unintended overdose represents 50% of all *acetaminophen*-related liver failure[1] and can result after ingesting more than 4 to 10 g over a period of >24 hours.[33] Since the liver plays a central role in transforming and clearing chemicals and is susceptible to the toxicity from first-pass medications, caution is needed to not exceed a dosage of 4 g in 24 hours (4,000 mg/day); dosage at this level may lead to **hepatotoxicity**.[32] Hepatotoxicity appears to be more problematic for patients with prior hepatic disease or poor nutritional status or who have heavy alcohol use. Initially, hepatotoxicity presents with nausea, vomiting, and diarrhea within a short time, followed by liver damage 3 days after ingestion. Despite this link to liver damage, *acetaminophen* at recommended dosages is a better analgesic choice than NSAIDs for musculoskeletal pain.[1] For the AT, this condition could be a consideration for the athlete who sustains a potential liver injury.

RED FLAG

Complications Associated With *Acetaminophen*

Other concerns for *acetaminophen* complications involve asthma and pregnancy. Reports of asthma sensitivity to *acetaminophen* occurred in 34% of people who are *aspirin*-sensitive asthmatics. Complications secondary to *acetaminophen* use during pregnancy include preterm birth, low birth weight, and poor gross motor development and communication skills.[1]

Local Anesthetics

The first local anesthetic, *cocaine*, was serendipitously discovered to have anesthetic properties in the late 19th century. *Cocaine* occurs in abundance in the leaves of the coca shrub. For centuries, Andean natives have chewed these leaves for their stimulatory and euphoric effects. Because of the drug's toxicity, abuse, misuse, and addictive properties,[2] synthetic substitutes for *cocaine* led to the synthesis of *procaine*, which became the prototype for local anesthetics for nearly half a century.[30] The most widely used agents today are *lidocaine*, *bupivacaine*, and *tetracaine*,[4] otherwise known as the *-caines*. This section focuses on the local anesthetics that are commonly used in the sports medicine setting.

Therapeutic Effects

Local anesthetics provide short-term pain relief when applied to mucous membranes or skin. For most patients, treatment with local anesthetics causes the sensation of pain to disappear first, fol-

Evidence in Pharmacology

Pregame Pain-Relieving Injections

Selective use of local anesthetics prior to athletic participation may accelerate return to play without deleterious consequences.[8] However, this procedure is not without controversy in regard to sport ethics and athlete safety.[34] In a study of professional football players,[8] a pregame local anesthetic was administered under sterile technique through a peri-ligament injection for select injuries that had no risk of long-term adverse effects. Additionally, a retrospective study of professional rugby players[34] who received local anesthetics prior to participation indicated that the primary reasons for injection were a desire to prevent either missing a game (65%) or playing in pain (31%).

lowed by the loss of the sensations of temperature, touch, deep pressure, and, finally, motor function. The drug must cross the epidermal barrier, with the stratum corneum (outermost layer of the epidermis) presenting the major obstacle, to reach the Aβ-fibers and C-fibers (sensory neurons) in the epidermis. Once they have crossed the epidermis, local anesthetics are absorbed rapidly into the circulation, increasing the risk of systemic toxicity. A mixture of *tetracaine*, *epinephrine*, and *cocaine* (TAC) is a common anesthetic that has been historically used before suturing small cuts in the sports medicine setting. However, because of concern about *cocaine* toxicity, banned substances, and addiction from this formulation, alternatives that contain *lidocaine* and *prilocaine*, such as Emla cream (from EMLA, or eutectic mixture of local anesthetics), are now used (table 7.2).[2,4,14,19] Furthermore, concerns exist over **local anesthetic systemic toxicity (LAST)**, a life-threatening adverse event that may occur after the administration of local anesthetic drugs through a variety of routes.[10] The typical presentation of LAST usually begins with prodromal symptoms and signs, such as perioral numbness, tinnitus, agitation, dysarthria, and confusion.[36]

Mechanism of Action

Local anesthetics act at the cell membrane to prevent the generation and conduction of nerve impulses.

Clinical Application

Anesthetic Injection to Assist in Making the Diagnosis

An indication for administration of local anesthetic is to confirm the diagnosis of the painful os trigonum syndrome, where an extra small bone (the *os trigonum*) develops in the posterolateral aspect of the ankle. In this condition, the athlete reports a hyperplantarflexion ankle sprain and presents with inflammation in the posterior medial ankle region, incomplete range of motion, weakness, and compromised balance. Plain X-rays identify the presence of the *os trigonum*, which is revealed as a nonfracture. However, the condition is slow to respond to therapeutic treatments and rehabilitation, and an MRI does not identify soft-tissue inflammation consistent with the pain. To confirm the diagnosis of *os trigonum* syndrome, a controlled injection of 1% *lidocaine* is administered via **fluoroscopy** to anesthetize the area.[17] After the injection, the patient is asked to complete a functional task such as stair walking. If this activity is painless, the syndrome is confirmed and the *os trigonum* may be surgically excised. In a small series of soccer players and dancers,[17] this treatment was 80% to 100% successful relative to pain relief.

TABLE 7.2 Local Anesthetics Onset and Duration of Action

generic (Brand name)	Onset (min)	Duration (hr)
Esters—shorter duration		
tetracaine (Pontocaine eye drops)	≤15	2-3
Amides—longer duration		
bupivacaine (Marcaine injectable)	5	2-4
lidocaine (Xylocaine injectable)	<2	0.5-1
lidocaine and *prilocaine* topical (Emla cream)	60	1-2 hr after removal

These medications function by binding reversibly to a specific receptor site in nerve cell membranes where the pore of the sodium channels is blocked. When applied locally to nerve tissue in appropriate concentrations, local anesthetics can act on any part of the nervous system and on every type of nerve fiber, reversibly blocking the action potentials responsible for nerve conduction. Thus, a local anesthetic in contact with a peripheral nerve causes both sensory and motor paralysis in the innervated area. These effects of clinically relevant concentrations of local anesthetics are reversible with recovery of nerve function and no evidence of damage to nerve fibers or cells in most clinical applications.[24]

The chemical structure of common local anesthetics is similar among the *-caines*, and drugs in this class have a similar function within the body. *Procaine* is a prototypical local anesthetic of the ester-type group; esters generally are rapidly hydrolyzed by plasma esterases that quickly metabolize the molecule in the bloodstream, contributing to the relatively short duration of action of drugs in this group. *Lidocaine* is a prototypical local anesthetic of the amide-type group; these molecules are generally more resistant to clearance and have longer durations of action. There are exceptions—for example, *benzocaine*, which is poorly water soluble and only used topically.

Routes of Administration

Local anesthetics are commonly delivered subcutaneously by injection, transdermally by patch, and topically in creams, gels, and ointments or via ophthalmic drops. Topical administration of local anesthetics can determine both the therapeutic effect and the extent of systemic toxicity. Use of topical anesthesia makes injection unnecessary and is completely painless—factors that are particularly desirable in the sports medicine setting. Directions for use are usually given by the prescribing provider.

Recent formulations of local anesthetics for transdermal patch administration include *lidocaine* patches that deliver medication over 12 hours (figure 7.2). The 5% *lidocaine* transdermal patch was approved by the U.S. Food and Drug Administration (FDA) for treating neuropathic pain and post-herpetic **neuralgia**; however, it has successfully treated moderate to severe pain secondary to acute, soft-tissue, and connective-tissue injuries in a cohort of professional football and basketball players.[3,29] The patch was intended to reduce the need for systemic medications and complement oral medications as part of a multimodal approach for providing analgesia without anesthesia.[15,29]

Clinical Application

Ophthalmic Application of Pontocaine (*tetracaine*)

Pontocaine (*tetracaine*) is an excellent medication for mild to moderate eye pain. The AT would need standing orders to use this prescription medication. Indications include pain secondary to a direct impact to the eye that may inflame the cornea, typically from a finger poke to the eye. The patient might report transient painful and blurry (not double) vision. Pontocaine gives virtually immediate pain relief with 1 or 2 drops to the eye; return to play is likely if there are no vision concerns or other secondary injuries to the eye, such as a concussion. The patient should be examined by the team physician at an appropriate time to rule out a corneal abrasion or other serious injury.

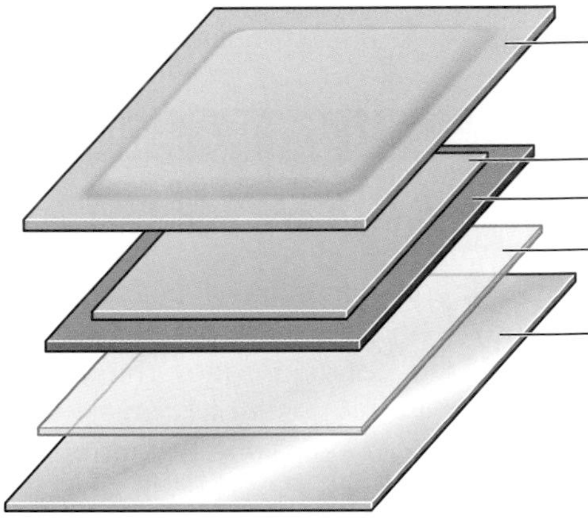

FIGURE 7.2 Transdermal drug delivery patch.

The systemic absorption of the *lidocaine* patch is minimal; however, the overall understanding of its effectiveness as an analgesic is less understood.[12] The *lidocaine* patch reduces ectopic transmission of pain signals to the dorsal horn of the spinal cord to interrupt pain signals from sodium channels in peripheral nociceptors in a localized area.[20,35] Additionally, the patch may serve as a mechanical barrier in the area of allodynia, thus preventing painful stimulation.[15] The lidocaine patch should be used for 12 hours on and 12 hours off; it initiates local analgesia within 30 minutes of application and has few associated adverse events.[20,26,29] The AT should be mindful that application instructions may vary between the transdermal medications. Long-term use of the *lidocaine* patch should occur only if there is a therapeutic benefit from its use, and caution should be recommended to patients with liver or kidney impairments.[29] Transdermal patches for pain management are also used to deliver opioids, such as *fentanyl* or other opioids (see chapter 8).

Clinical Skill

Applying and Caring for the *Lidocaine* Patch

Equipment: soap and water, shaver or scissors, clean towel or paper towel

APPLYING THE *LIDOCAINE* PATCH

1. Read the instructions that come with the patch.
   - The prescription and instructions should indicate where to place the patch, how long the patient should wear it, and when to remove and replace it.
   - The *lidocaine* patch can be cut to fit the treatment area; however, other medication patches cannot be cut.
2. When placing a patch, choose a spot where it will attach well. Choose an area of skin that is flat and hairless (if needed, trim the hair in that area with shaver or scissors). Avoid skin that has been recently shaved (wait 3 days after shaving before applying a patch to an area). Prepare and clean the skin to remove any dirt, lotions, oils, or powders. Clean the skin using warm water alone or water and a clear soap. Avoid using scented soaps or soaps that contain lotion. Dry the skin with a clean towel or paper towel.
   - Do not place the patch on skin that is too thin or thick; this could cause the body to absorb too much or too little of the drug, which could lead to increased side effects or prevent the drug from working well.
   - Do not apply the patch to skin that has been exposed to radiation (e.g., sunburned) or that is sensitive, very oily, broken out, irritated, broken, cut, or damaged (e.g., abrasions).
   - Do not apply the patch to parts of the body that move a lot or will be covered by a belt or clothing seam.

GENERAL RECOMMENDATIONS FOR CARING FOR THE *LIDOCAINE* PATCH

- It is generally recommended to rotate the locations where the patch is applied to avoid skin irritation. If instructed, keep the patch in the same area of the body; for example, if the instructions are to use the patch only on the hips and lower abdomen, rotate the patch locations within those areas.
- Do not use more than 1 patch at a time. Don't overlap patches or place 1 patch on top of another. The entire sticky side needs to be in direct contact with the skin.
- For a loose patch or one that falls off, refer to the label instructions. In general, for a loose patch, use the palm of the hand to press the patch back onto the skin. If the patch falls off completely, don't reapply it. Throw it away and apply a new patch at the next scheduled time.
- It is important to make sure the patch remains secure. A loose patch can adhere to animals and people in direct skin contact with the patient, such as teammates or children.
- The patient should shower as usual. It is OK to get the patch wet. However, the *lidocaine* patch should not be soaked or submerged under water for long periods of time. This can cause it to loosen or fall off.
- Do not use a heating pad, apply moist heat, or use another thermotherapy (e.g., hot tub) while wearing a patch. The heat can cause the patch to release its drug faster, which could cause an overdose.
- Carefully store unused patches and dispose of used ones. Both used and unused patches contain an active drug, so keep them away from children and pets.
- After removing the used *lidocaine* patch, fold it on itself and dispose it in a closed trash can.

Based on Healthline website (2019); Mayo Clinic website (2019).

Indications and Precautions

The FDA has approved *lidocaine* transdermal patches for treating neuropathic pain and post-herpetic neuralgia, however, it has also successfully treated moderate to severe pain secondary to acute, soft-tissue, and connective-tissue injuries. Clinicians should advise patients to use reasonable precautions while using topical anesthetic creams, gels, or ointments and transdermal patches.

RED FLAG

Precautions for Transdermal Anesthetics or Topical Analgesics

For all topical analgesics, these precautions should be followed:

- Do not apply to skin abrasions, burns, or open wounds. Skin that is cut or irritated may absorb more topical medication than healthy skin.
- Do not apply to swollen skin areas or deep puncture wounds.
- Avoid using the medicine on skin that is raw or blistered, such as with a severe burn or abrasions.
- Do not use in patients with sensitivity to *aspirin* (applies only to agents containing salicylates).
- Do not apply near eyes or mucous membranes.
- Do not apply over large skin areas.
- Do not apply heat to treated skin areas.
- Use the smallest amount of medication needed to numb the skin or relieve pain.
- Do not cover treated skin areas with a bandage or plastic wrap.

Adverse Effects

The most common adverse events associated with topical anesthetics are administration-site reactions, such as burning, dermatitis, erythema, pruritus, rash, skin irritation, and vesicles. In ≥10% patients, dermatologic effects are very common and include erythema and **petechiae**. Less common side effects are pruritus and rash; effects with no frequency reported include flushing, cutaneous lesions, urticaria, and dermatitis.[18]

Over-the-Counter Transdermal Analgesic Patches

OTC versions of the *lidocaine* patch (Aspercreme, Salonpas) have been developed with 1.25% *menthol* and 3.6% *lidocaine* and as a 4% *lidocaine* patch (rather than the 5% in the prescription version Lidoderm). A cohort of patients randomly treated with either patch found the OTC patch to be comparable to the prescription patch relative to safety, efficacy, and quality of life. The OTC version offers consumers a convenient option for this type of treatment. It seems to be a more successful application to superficial areas of the body, such as the wrist, thorax or ribs, acromioclavicular joint, and patellar tendon; it may also be useful in treating some foot and ankle conditions and superficial muscle strain.[20]

Topical Analgesics: Creams, Gels, and Ointments

Topical analgesics are medicines that numb and reduce the sensation of pain in the area to which they are applied. They are available as creams, ointments, solutions, eye drops, gels, or sprays. Topical analgesics may be applied to areas such as the skin, inside the mouth or throat, in the nose, or in the eyes. **Topical delivery systems** (or **vehicles**) come in both prescription and OTC strength preparations (table 7.3). Although the

TABLE 7.3 Common OTC Transdermal and Topical Analgesic Clinical Applications

Commercial product	Form	Active ingredient
Salonpas	Transdermal patch, gel, cream	*methyl salicylate, menthol*
Aspercreme	Transdermal patch, cream, topical liquid solution	*lidocaine* 4%, *trolamine salicylate,* or *menthol* 10%
IcyHot	Cream, balm, gel, spray, topical liquid solution, transdermal patch	*methyl salicylate, menthol, camphor, lidocaine* 4%
Flexall 454	Cream, gel	*methyl salicylate, menthol, camphor*
Biofreeze	Counterirritant gel	*menthol, camphor*
Salonpas Jet Spray	Spray	*methyl salicylate, menthol*
Tiger Balm	Counterirritant gel, cream, patch, ointment	*capsaicin, camphor, menthol*

terms are similar, topical preparations are not to be confused with transdermal medications. Both agents cross the stratum corneum to access C-fibers and possible nociceptor fibers in the dermal level. In contrast, transdermal medications have a slower onset and are used for more extensive analgesic for treatment times of 48 to 72 hours. Topical agents do not penetrate as deeply as transdermal medication and their serum levels are generally low.[35] The topical agent is intended to dampen pain in the peripheral nervous system through **targeted peripheral analgesia**.[29]

Over-the-Counter Topical Analgesic: Counterirritants

Menthol and *capsaicin* are popular active ingredients in many OTC pain-relieving creams, gels, sprays, and ointments. The use of *menthol* is well established and has been deemed safe by the FDA.[30,31] *Menthol* is fast acting and facilitates a reduction in blood flow. The mechanism by which *menthol* produces analgesia is unknown; however, it has been postulated that it desensitizes nociceptive C-fibers, reducing pain.[30] *Menthol* causes a tingling sensation when applied to the skin by inhibiting the calcium channel involved in regulating the pain threshold.[11] At very low concentrations, <1% *menthol* depresses sensory receptors; with concentrations between 1.25% and 16%, it stimulates sensory receptors.[30] *Capsaicin* is the active ingredient in chili peppers that makes them hot. *Capsaicin* is used in medicated creams and lotions to relieve muscle or joint pain and causes a sensation of heat that activates certain nerve cells. With regular use of *capsaicin*, this heating effect reduces the amount of substance P, a chemical that acts as a pain messenger in the body. In the clinical setting, these topical agents are used for temporary relief of muscle or joint pain caused by strains, sprains, arthritis, bruising, or backaches.

The AT's Role in the Clinical Management of Pain

Pharmacologic treatment is often considered the cornerstone of pain management. For prescribers, it is crucial to determine the optimal pain management plan for an individual patient using a benefit-to-risk assessment to select the proper therapeutic agent. The prescriber must evaluate the potential for benefit with each pharmacologic option and assess the risk of adverse effects. ATs and other HCPs treating the patient at regular intervals must frequently monitor the patient's pain and response to the medication plan.

When implementing the prescriber's pain management plan, the AT should do the following:

- Inform the patient of any modifications to therapy.
- Educate the patient and any caregivers regarding the prescriber's treatment plan, ensuring that they understand all instructions.
- Complete validated **patient-reported outcome (PRO)** scales.
- Discuss symptom-specific lifestyle modification (e.g., pain-trigger avoidance); this should include diligently complying with treatment plan to avoid exacerbating the original injury.
- Perform nonpharmacologic treatment modalities.
- Review the patient's drug therapy regimen, including dose, route, frequency, and duration.
- Monitor the drug therapy regimen with the patient, including efficacy, toxicity, misuse, and adverse effects.
- Educate the patient on safe use, storage, and disposal of medications.
- Schedule follow-up appointments.

Monitoring the Patient's Pain and Response to the Medication Plan

For the AT in the clinical setting, tracking function as well as pain is critical in determining the patient's ongoing response to opioids and allowing the prescriber to determine whether any potential changes in opioid dosing are needed. Because of the well-documented evidence of overdose risk and the limited evidence of opioid effectiveness beyond the period of acute pain, the use of opioids should result in clinically meaningful improvement in function and pain and, therefore, **health-related quality of life (HRQOL)**. For there to be considered **clinically meaningful improvement**, there must be documented improvement in pain and function of at least 30% compared to the start of treatment or in response to a dose change. A decrease in pain intensity in the absence of improved function is not considered meaningful improvement except in very limited circumstances, such as catastrophic injuries (e.g., multiple traumas, spinal cord injury).[37]

Clinical recommendations for patient monitoring involve regularly assessing and documenting function and pain using only validated instruments to measure clinically meaningful improvement (30% from baseline) in function and pain.[37]

Additionally, the AT plays an essential role in monitoring and evaluating the patient's response to the pain management plan. When monitoring the patient's response to the plan, the AT should do the following:

- Assess attainment of treatment goals (e.g., improved activity, improved sleep, improved sport participation).
- Identify the presence of adverse effects or aberrant drug-taking behaviors.
- Complete PRO scales.
- Frequently review the pain management plan and PROs.
- Discuss patient adherence to all facets of treatment plan, including nonpharmacologic modalities.

Summary

Given its profound effect on patient physiology and quality of life, the management of pain must be an important element in any therapeutic intervention. Appropriate pain assessment and adequate pain management are considered the standard of care, and some people consider pain to be the fifth vital sign.[43] The AT plays a critical role in the clinical management of the patient's pain. Often, the AT is the only clinician interacting with the patient on a regular basis. This frequent interaction provides an opportunity for the AT to engage with the patient that few other HCPs have. The period of discomfort and uncertainty for the patient when healing from pain allows a special therapeutic relationship to develop between the AT and the patient. ATs administer medications under the direction of a licensed physician. Therefore, they must have a working knowledge of analgesics, one of the most important drug classes in sports medicine. This chapter discusses analgesics and their critical role in the WHO pain relief ladder. Treatment of pain should follow a progressive approach, beginning with mild pain relievers that are commonly used in the AT setting, the nonopioid analgesics. Specifically, treatment should begin with *acetaminophen* (Tylenol), local anesthetics, and topical analgesics. Finally, this chapter discusses the AT's role in monitoring the patient's pain and response to treatment using patient-reported outcomes to improve patient care.

Case Studies

Case Study 1

Paul was an elite professional basketball player who sustained a laceration to his right eyebrow. Evaluation showed no indication of concussion or eye damage; thus, he was referred to the team physician for suturing. Because Paul was eager to return to the game, the physician asked, "Do you want to be sutured like a basketball player or a hockey player?" Paul asked about the difference, and the physician noted that the technique was identical, but that hockey players do not use numbing medicine. Paul received 4 sutures without *lidocaine* and was able to finish the game without sequelae.

Questions for Analysis

1. How much longer would the process have taken if the laceration were infiltrated with *lidocaine*?
2. Did there seem to be any unusual risks associated with not using lidocaine to anesthetize the area?

Case Study 2

Clifford was a postal service letter carrier. While delivering mail in the winter, he sprained his left ankle while stepping incorrectly off an icy curb. He was diagnosed with a mild ankle sprain, and his physician prescribed analgesic tablets for 7 days. A friend of Clifford's mentioned that this medication was contraindicated for the driving that was required on the postal route. Clifford's physician agreed and prescribed a 1-week dose of Lidoderm patches to be used in conjunction with an ankle brace while Clifford was out delivering mail but removed when he returned home. Clifford also appreciated the prescription of the Lidoderm patch rather than an oral medication since he had experienced nausea while taking pain medication in the past.

Questions for Analysis

1. What is an advantage of the Lidoderm patch?
2. Why did Clifford need to remove the patch when he returned home?

Drugs Described in This Chapter

generic (pronunciation) Trade name	Therapeutic uses	Clinical concerns
acetaminophen (a seet a MIN oh fen) or the abbreviation *APAP* (N-acetyl-para-aminophenol) Tylenol (in the United States) *paracetamol* (par RA cet a MOL) Panadol (international)	Fever reducer, mild pain, and severe pain when combined with opiates Oral: 325-650 mg every 4-6 hr Maximum dose: 1 g (1,000 mg) per dose and 3.5 g (3,500 mg) per day, unless otherwise directed by prescriber	Hepatotoxicity, acute liver failure, sometimes resulting in liver transplantation and death; usually associated with doses that exceed the maximum. Consuming *APAP* products together may lead to fatal overdose. Regular alcohol use and *APAP* may result in liver toxicity. Does not cause stomach upset; thus can be taken on an empty stomach.
lidocaine (LYE doe kane) Lidoderm, Aspercreme Lidocaine Patch	Apply the prescribed number of patches (maximum of 3) to painful area once for ≤12 hr within a 24-hr period. Each adhesive patch contains 700 mg of *lidocaine* (50 mg medication per g of adhesive) in an aqueous base with other inactive ingredients.	Excessive dosing by applying the *lidocaine* patch to larger areas or using for longer than the recommended wearing time could result in increased absorption of *lidocaine* and high blood concentrations, leading to serious adverse effects. If irritation or a burning sensation occurs during application, remove the patch and do not reapply until the irritation subsides.

8

Drugs to Treat Pain: Opioid Analgesics

OBJECTIVES

After reading this chapter, you will be able to do the following:

- Differentiate between endogenous and exogenous opioids
- Discuss the various routes of administration of opioid medications
- Summarize the classes of opioids
- Recognize the signs of opioid misuse, abuse, and overdose
- Administer emergency Narcan nasal spray in cases of known or suspected opioid overdose

Select Drugs Mentioned in This Chapter

Drug class	Generic name	Trade name
Opioid, low potency	*codeine*	Many
Opioid, medium potency	*morphine*	MS Contin
Opioid	*hydrocodone*	Zohydro
Opioid	*oxycodone*	OxyContin
Opioid, extremely high potency	*fentanyl*	Many
Opioid, illegal	*heroin*	Illegal drug
Opioid antagonist	*naloxone*	Narcan

This list is not exhaustive, but rather contains drugs commonly encountered in the athletic training setting. Always consult up-to-date information, confirm with a pharmacist, or discuss the use of therapeutic medications with the prescriber of the medication.

After nonopioids, therapeutic medications used on the next steps of the World Health Organization's (WHO) 3-step analgesic (pain relief) ladder[20] are the low-potency **opioids** followed by the high-potency opioids. The term *opioid* is generally used to refer to drugs or chemicals that interact with opioid receptors in the body. In contrast, the term *opiate* refers to compounds structurally related to products found in opium, a word derived from *opos*, the Greek word for "juice." Natural opiates are derived from the resin (milk or juice) of the opium poppy (figure 8.1). Opioids include analgesic drugs, such as *codeine* and *morphine*, as well as many semisynthetic and synthetic derivatives. Endogenous opioids are naturally occurring peptide ligands for opioid receptors found in the human brain. The term **endorphin** is not only used synonymously with the term *endogenous opioid peptides*, but also refers to a specific endogenous opioid, **beta-endorphin** (or **β-endorphin**). The term **narcotic** was derived from the Greek word *narkotikos*, for "numbing" or "stupor." Although the term *narcotic* originally referred to any drug that induced narcosis (i.e., sleep), the word has become associated with opioids and is often used in a legal context to refer to substances with potential for abuse or addiction.[13,21]

Use of the opioid medication class of analgesics may be an effective treatment option in the management of chronic (noncancer) pain; however, this practice continues to be increasingly controversial.[6] Data indicate that >700,000 people died in the United States from drug overdoses between 1999 and 2017, with 70,237 deaths in 2017 alone. Of these 70,237 deaths, 67.8% involved an opioid.[12] The age-adjusted drug overdose death rate significantly increased from 6.0 (1999) to 21.7 (2017) deaths per 100,000 people.[17] Prescription or illicit opioids were involved in 67.8% (47,600) of these deaths. Among opioid-involved deaths, the category of synthetic opioids other than *methadone* (a category that includes the illicitly manufactured *fentanyl*) was the most common (28,466 deaths). The prescription opioids category, which includes natural and semisynthetic opioids (e.g., *oxycodone* and *hydrocodone*) and *methadone*, was the second most common, with 17,029 deaths.[12] In the treatment of chronic pain, nonpharmacologic therapy and nonopioid pharmacologic therapy are preferred. Prescribers should consider opioid therapy only if the expected benefits for both pain and function are anticipated to outweigh the risks to the patient. If opioids are used, they should be combined with nonpharmacologic therapy and nonopioid pharmacologic therapy, as appropriate.[11]

Appropriate Use of Opioid Analgesics

In response to the opioid epidemic, the Centers for Disease Control and Prevention (CDC) has released guidelines for prescribers on the appropriate use of opioids for chronic pain. The CDC guidelines provide prescribers with recommendations for safer care for all patients. These guidelines focus on more specific recommendations compared to previous guidelines on monitoring and discontinuing opioids when risks and harms outweigh benefits. Recommendations for prescribers are as follows:[1]

- Opioids should not be first-line or routine therapy for chronic pain.
- Clinicians should establish and measure goals for pain and function.

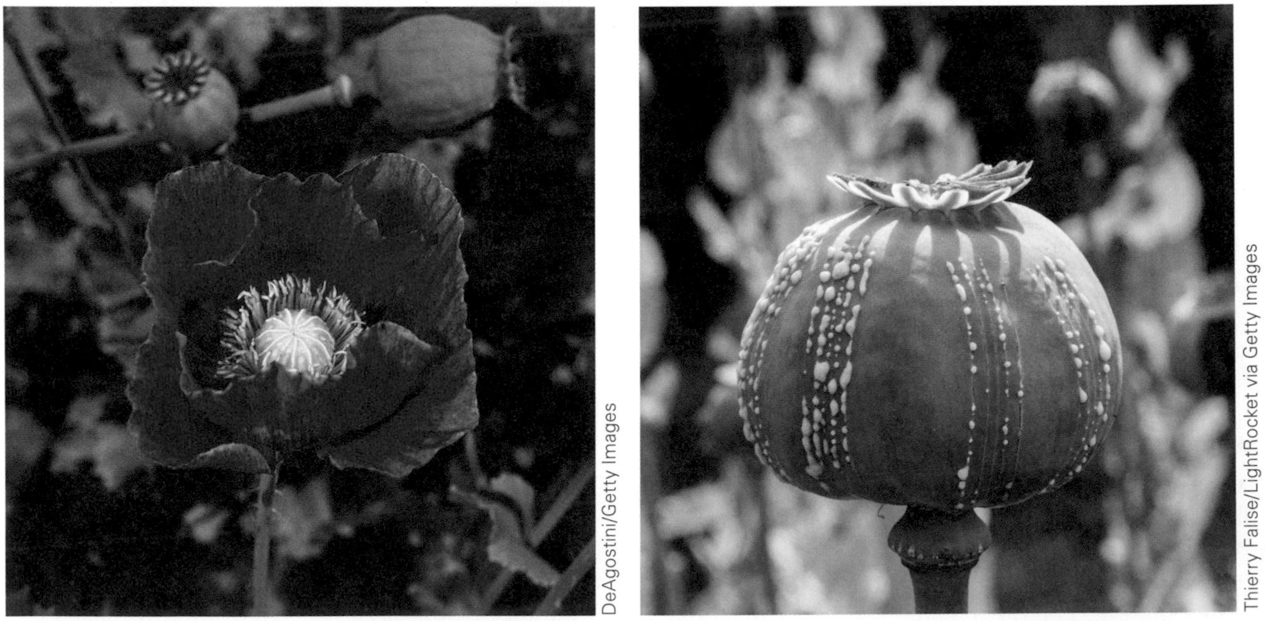
DeAgostini/Getty Images
Thierry Falise/LightRocket via Getty Images

a b

FIGURE 8.1 *(a)* Flower and *(b)* milk of the opium poppy.

- Clinicians should discuss the benefits and risks of opioid treatment and the availability of nonopioid therapies with patients.
- Prescribe immediate-release opioids only when treating acute pain.
- Start low and go slow—prescribe only the lowest effective dosage and carefully determine the need for increased dosage.
- When opioids are needed for acute pain, prescribe no more than needed.
- Do not prescribe extended-release or long-acting opioids for acute pain.
- Follow up with patients and reevaluate the risk of harm; reduce the dose or taper and discontinue if needed.

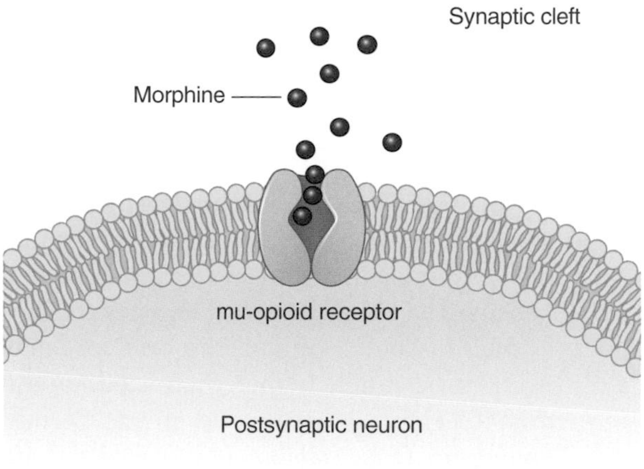

FIGURE 8.2 Opioid agonist ligand binding with the mu-opioid receptor (MOR) on the postsynaptic neuron.

Therapeutic Effects

Opioid analgesics produce effects primarily on the central nervous system (CNS); the important among these are analgesia, **euphoria**, sedation, and respiratory depression. When therapeutic doses of opioids are administered for pain, patients report that the pain becomes less intense or disappears entirely. In addition to relieving distress, opioid analgesics may cause some patients to experience euphoria. Analgesia often occurs without loss of consciousness, although drowsiness commonly occurs, and usually does not cause slurred speech, emotional lability, or significant impairment of motor coordination. Opioid analgesics relieve continuous dull pain (as generated by tissue injury and inflammation) more effectively than sharp intermittent (incident) pain, such as that associated with the movement of an inflamed joint. With sufficient amounts of opioid medication, it is possible to relieve even the severe piercing pain associated with an acute bone fracture or a kidney stone, for example.[21]

When an analgesic dose of opioid medication is administered to pain-free patients, the recipient may report the drug experience to be unpleasant (side and adverse effects are described later in this chapter). The healthy patient dosed with an opioid may also experience drowsiness, difficulty in **mentation**, **apathy**, and reduced physical activity. As the dose is increased, the subjective, analgesic, and toxic effects, including respiratory depression, become more pronounced[21] and the risk of fatal overdose increases.

Mechanism of Action

Opioid drugs act by binding to **opioid receptors**, primarily located in the CNS, the peripheral nervous system, and the gastrointestinal tract. The binding of opioids with these receptors mediates both the psychoactive and the somatic effects of these drugs.[5] Opioids, such as *morphine* and *heroin*, are considered **mu-opioid receptor** (**MOR**; also **μ-opioid receptor**) agonists, since they bind specifically with the MOR, the major analgesic opioid receptor (figure 8.2). It is the activation of the MOR that produces the analgesic, euphoric, and sedative effects involved in the addictive qualities of opioid drugs.[18] Since MOR activation is the most common mechanism of action for opioids, it serves as the focus of this discussion.

Routes of Administration

The route of administration of opioid medications depends on individual patient needs. Although the oral route is preferred, intravenous (IV), intranasal (IN), subcutaneous (SQ), intraspinal (epidural or intrathecal), and intramuscular (IM) options may be indicated. The onset of analgesic effect for oral medications is approximately 45 minutes and the peak effect usually occurs 1 to 2 hours after administration. This delay must be considered when immediate relief is needed in the management of acute pain (i.e., postsurgical or breakthrough pain). When the patient is unable to take oral medications, alternative routes of therapy, such as IV administration, may be preferred.[6]

Pharmacodynamics and Pharmacokinetics

Although they are administered in various forms, the drugs in the opioid class of medications generally have similar pharmacokinetics. The sections that follow include pharmacodynamic and pharmacokinetic tables for the most common opioids encountered in the sports medicine setting. Major differences among this class of drugs are discussed in subsections for each specific drug.

- **Absorption**—Most opioid analgesics are well absorbed when administered by subcutaneous, intramuscular, and oral routes. However, because the first-pass effect reduces the bioavailability of the opioid,[15] an oral dose may need to be much higher than a parenteral dose to elicit a therapeutic effect. Certain analgesics (e.g., *codeine* and *oxycodone*) are effective orally because they have reduced first-pass metabolism. By avoiding first-pass metabolism, **nasal insufflation** of certain opioids can rapidly result in therapeutic blood levels.
- **Distribution**—The uptake of opioids by various organs and tissues is a function of both physiologic and chemical factors. For distribution of opioids through the bloodstream, the molecules bind to plasma proteins and the drugs rapidly leave the blood compartment. Once the drug has left the circulatory system, the molecules concentrate most densely in highly perfused tissues, such as the brain, lungs, liver, kidneys, and spleen. Drug concentrations in skeletal muscle may be much lower, but this tissue serves as the main reservoir because of its greater bulk. Even though blood flow to fatty tissue is lower than to highly perfused tissues, accumulation in adipose tissue can be very important, particularly after frequent high-dose drug administration or continuous infusion of opioids that are slowly metabolized.
- **Metabolism**—Most opioids undergo extensive first-pass metabolism in the liver before entering the systemic circulation. Opioid metabolism in the liver requires that the cytochrome P450 enzymes facilitate metabolic reactions. Opioids are typically lipophilic, which allows them to cross cell membranes to reach target tissues.
- **Excretion**—Polar metabolites of opioid analgesics are excreted mainly in the urine. Small amounts of unchanged drug may also be found in the urine. Although small molecules are found in the bile, enterohepatic circulation represents only a small portion of the excretory process of these polar metabolites. Patients with potential renal insufficiency (e.g., due to shock, heatstroke, or rhabdomyolysis) should be carefully evaluated before receiving high-potency opioids—especially when administered at high doses—due to the risk of sedation and respiratory depression.[13]

Dosing Guidelines

Individual patient factors (e.g., renal or liver dysfunction) may lead prescribers to initiate therapy with an opioid to optimize pain relief while minimizing adverse effects.[6] The WHO 3-step pain relief ladder encourages using more conservative therapies before initiating opioid therapy. Weaker opioids can be supplanted by stronger opioids in cases of moderate and severe pain. Antidepressants such as *amitriptyline* and *duloxetine* that are used as adjuncts in the treatment of chronic neuropathic pain have limited intrinsic analgesic actions in acute pain; however, antidepressants may enhance *morphine*-induced analgesia. In the presence of

RED FLAG

Characteristics of Opioid Addiction

Opioid addiction or opioid use disorder (OUD) can affect one's health and relationships to the point that the person's life becomes organized around using the drug.[7] Opioid addiction can present over the span of a few weeks or much earlier, depending on each individual patient, and can worsen over time.[7] The diagnosis for OUD requires presentation of at least 2 of 11 criteria over a 1-year period of time. The following are examples of symptoms of OUD:[8,9]

- Inability to control opioid use
- Uncontrollable cravings
- Drowsiness
- Changes in sleep habits
- Weight loss
- Frequent flulike symptoms
- Decreased libido
- Lack of hygiene
- Changes in exercise habits
- Isolation from family and friends
- Stealing from family, friends, or businesses
- New financial difficulties

severe pain, opioids should be considered sooner rather than later.[21]

The opioid dosing schedule typically begins with administration of a starting dose and then titrates the dose up or down, depending on the patient's degree of pain and demonstrated side effects (e.g., sedation). As-needed dosing schedules may produce wide swings in analgesic plasma concentrations, resulting in alternating states of uncontrolled pain and sedation. This, in turn, may initiate a vicious cycle where increasing amounts of pain medications are needed for relief. As the painful state subsides and the need for medication decreases, PRN (as needed) schedules may be appropriate, which may also be useful in patients who present with pain that is intermittent or sporadic in nature. Patients with high pain tolerance may be able to transition from opioid treatment following orthopedic surgery to an anti-inflammatory medication and over-the-counter (OTC) pain reliever.

Combination Therapy

In general, the use of combinations of drugs (table 8.1) that have the same mechanism of action is not warranted (e.g., *morphine* plus *methadone*). The same principle holds if the drugs have overlapping targets and opposing effects. On the other hand, certain opioid combinations are useful. For example, in a chronic pain state with periodic incident or breakthrough pain, the patient might receive a slow-release formulation of *morphine* for baseline pain relief, and the acute incident (breakthrough) pain may be managed with a rapid-onset and short-lasting formulation. For inflammatory or nociceptive pain, opioids may be usefully combined with other analgesic agents, such as *acetaminophen* (table 8.2) or other NSAIDs (refer to chapter 9). For example, antidepressants that block amine reuptake, such as *amitriptyline* or *duloxetine*, and anticonvulsants, such as *gabapentin*, may enhance the analgesic effect and may be synergistic in some pain states.[21]

TABLE 8.1 Combinations of Analgesics, Opioids, and NSAIDs Commonly Prescribed in Sports Medicine

Trade name	Generic name
Demerol	*meperidine*
Dilaudid*	*hydromorphone**
Norco, Lortab, Vicodin	Multiple options of these medications are available with different strengths of a combination of *hydrocodone* and *acetaminophen*
OxyContin*	*oxycodone**
Percocet	*oxycodone** and *acetaminophen*
Tylenol with Codeine	*codeine* and *acetaminophen*
Ultram	*tramadol*
Vicoprofen	*hydrocodone* and *ibuprofen*

*Medication banned for international competition by the World Anti-Doping Association (WADA); further discussed in chapter 21.

TABLE 8.2 Example Dosing Guidelines for a Combination Opioid and Analgesic (Norco)

Product strength	Usual adult dosage PRN	Total daily dosage should not exceed
5 mg *hydrocodone* and 325 mg *acetaminophen*	1 or 2 tablets every 4-6 hr	8 tablets
7.5 mg *hydrocodone* and 325 mg *acetaminophen*	1 tablet every 4-6 hr	6 tablets
10 mg *hydrocodone* and 325 mg *acetaminophen*	1 tablet every 4-6 hr	6 tablets

In the management of persistent chronic pain or following surgical procedures, physicians may prescribe opioids on an around-the-clock dosing schedule, such as every 3 to 6 hours. While on around-the-clock dosing, patients may experience **breakthrough pain** during acute situations, such as rehabilitation sessions, movement, or wound cleaning of the affected area, or if the underlying persistent pain is not otherwise controlled. For example, *tramadol* (Ultram, Ultram ER), a narcotic pain reliever, is used to treat moderate to severe pain in adults. The extended-release (ER) form of all opioids should be used only for chronic pain and is dosed around the clock, rather than on an as-needed basis.[3] Physical dependence can occur even with appropriate opioid use. See the Red Flag sidebar for characteristics of opioid addiction.

Indications and Precautions

Opioids are often used in the second step on the WHO pain ladder in the management of acute pain and some types of chronic pain. Although they are controversial and potentially addictive and abused, drugs in this medication class may be an effective treatment option in the management of chronic noncancer pain. When a trial of opioids is warranted, it should follow a complete assessment of the pain complaint and an assessment of the patient's functionality goals and risk factors for opioid misuse, abuse, diversion, or overdose. Opioid choice should be based on patient acceptance, analgesic effectiveness, and pharmacokinetic, pharmacodynamic, and side-effect profiles.[6,21] Similarly, since use of opioids often leads to **opioid-induced constipation** (OIC), patients taking opioids should be counseled on proper intake of fluids and fiber, and a stimulant laxative or stool softener may be added to the dosing schedule.[6]

Adverse Effects

Opioids share related pharmacologic attributes and exert a profound effect on the CNS and gastrointestinal (GI) tract. Mood changes, sedation, nausea, vomiting, decreased GI motility, constipation, respiratory depression, dependence, pruritus, and tolerance are evident in varying degrees with all opioid agents. Tolerance to side effects (except to constipation) often develops over time. Some differences exist among the opioids in regard to incidence of side effects, which may assist in selection of the most appropriate agent.[6,21] Side effects can be numerous—for example, when *morphine* is first initiated or when doses are significantly increased. Many patients can experience nausea and vomiting through direct stimulation of the chemoreceptor trigger zone, decreased peristalsis, and a vestibular mechanism. Opioid-induced nausea may be incredibly troublesome to patients, especially following surgery.

As doses of opioids are increased, the respiratory center becomes less responsive to carbon dioxide, causing progressive respiratory depression. Res-

Evidence in Pharmacology

Opioid-Induced Constipation

Opioid-induced constipation is a reduction of spontaneous bowel movement from baseline to typically <3 bowel movements per week after commencing opioid therapy.[14,16] In some cases, OIC may not respond well to laxatives; therefore, prescription medications have been tailored for this condition. Peripherally acting mu-opioid receptor agonists (PAMORA) are intended to reverse the constipation associated with opioids.[16] Examples of these medications are Relistor (*methylnaltrexone*), Amitiza (*lubiprostone*), and Movantik (*naloxegol*). These medications should be administered precisely according to dosage instructions and ceased when opioid use ends. They are contraindicated for patients with a GI tract obstruction or hepatic impairment.[14]

RED FLAG

Concerns With Combining Opioids and Benzodiazepines

Well-known adverse outcomes of concomitant use of opioids with benzodiazepines include significant sedation, respiratory depression, coma, and death. Alcohol should also be avoided when using opioids because of the concern of potentiation of the sedative effect. At a minimum, these concerns validate the medication warning that combining these medications should be avoided, especially while driving, until the effect of the medication is understood. Doses should always be the minimum necessary for accomplishing therapeutic goals.

piratory depression often manifests as a decrease in respiratory rate. Caution is also urged when combining opioid analgesics with alcohol or other CNS depressants (i.e., benzodiazepines and sleep hypnotics), because this combination can result in potentially lethal respiratory depression.[6]

Opioid Warnings

Narcotic (opioid) analgesics are one of the most widely used analgesics for pain relief; however, they have been overused, overprescribed, and misused, resulting in >2 million people in the United States having a substance misuse disorder connected with prescription narcotic analgesics. These medications are among the drug classes that have a heightened risk of causing significant harm when used in error. Black box warnings are listed for virtually all opioid medications. The U.S. Food and Drug Administration (FDA) guidelines for use recommend that opioids should be reserved for patients for whom alternative treatment options (e.g., nonopioid analgesics, opioid combination products) are ineffective, not tolerated, or would be otherwise inadequate to provide sufficient management of pain. Considering the severity of pain response, prescribers must individualize opioid doses based on the patient's prior analgesic treatment experience and risk factors for addiction, abuse, and misuse. The lowest effective dose for the shortest duration consistent with individual patient treatment goals should be used. The 3 primary FDA opioid warnings are as follows:[4,6,10,19]

1. **Risk of addiction, abuse, and misuse.** Opioids expose patients and other users to the risks of opioid addiction, abuse, and misuse, which can lead to overdose and death. Each patient's risk should be assessed prior to prescribing these drugs and all patients should be monitored regularly for the development of these behaviors and conditions.
2. **Life-threatening respiratory depression.** Serious, life-threatening, or fatal respiratory depression may occur with the use of opioids. Patients should be monitored for respiratory depression, especially during initiation of drug or following a dose increase.
3. **Risks from concomitant use with benzodiazepines or other CNS depressants.** Concomitant use of opioids with benzodiazepines or other CNS depressants, including alcohol, may result in profound sedation, respiratory depression, coma, and death. Physicians should reserve concomitant prescribing of opioids and benzodiazepines or other CNS depressants for use in patients for whom alternative treatment options are inadequate. Dosages and durations should be limited to the minimum required. Patients should be monitored for signs and symptoms of respiratory depression and sedation.

Narcotic analgesics are potentially addictive, and the risk of becoming emotionally and physically dependent on these drugs increases as the patient takes higher dosages for longer durations of time. When prescribed by a physician and used for short periods of time (e.g., <5 days) for pain relief after surgery, the risk of becoming addicted to narcotic analgesics is relatively low. HCPs must understand that with chronic opioid use, physical dependence is to be expected. A baseline assessment and ongoing evaluation of these behaviors and the patient's risk of misuse, abuse, and addiction are critical for mitigating risks of chronic opioid therapy and ensuring patient safety. The mechanisms underlying abuse, misuse, addiction, chronic tolerance, and dependence and withdrawal are further discussed in chapter 18.

Classes of Opioid Analgesics

The common opioids that an AT is likely to encounter while providing medical care to healthy, physically active people are listed in table 8.3. Following the WHO pain ladder, this section begins by describing a common example of a low-potency opioid analgesic, *codeine*, followed by the prototypical medium-potency opioid, *morphine*. Most all other opioids are compared to *morphine* for **therapeutic equivalence**. Other medium-potency opioids the AT may encounter in the sports medicine setting include the semisynthetic derivatives of *morphine*, *oxycodone* and *hydrocodone*. Extremely high-potency opioids, such as *fentanyl*, are discussed in relation to their prominent use in the treatment of severe pain and the management of chronic pain.

Low-Potency Analgesic: *Codeine*

Codeine (no trade name) is a low-potency opioid used for treating mild to moderate pain, as well as for its antitussive and antidiarrheal effects. Since its abuse potential is highest when used as a single entity, it is often combined with other analgesic products (e.g., *acetaminophen*).[6,21] Because *codeine*

TABLE 8.3 Classes of Opioids

Opioid class	Example generic drug
Low-potency opioids	*codeine*
Medium-potency opioids	*morphine, oxycodone, hydrocodone*
Extremely high-potency opioids	*fentanyl*
Schedule I illicit drug	*heroin*
Opioid antagonists	*naloxone*

has considerably higher oral bioavailability than *morphine*, it is also used in conditions for which a low-potency oral opioid analgesic is preferred, such as combined with *acetaminophen* or *aspirin*.[21]

Like other opioids, the mechanism of action for *codeine* is as an MOR agonist. The drug binds to mu-opioid receptors in the CNS, causing inhibition of ascending pain pathways and thereby altering the perception of and response to pain. *Codeine* also has antitussive (cough suppression) effects by direct central action in the medulla and can produce generalized CNS depression, leading to lethargy and drowsiness. *Codeine* is about 60% as effective as an analgesic and a respiratory depressant when taken orally compared to parenterally.[21] The pharmacodynamics and pharmacokinetics of *codeine* as a prototypical low-potency opioid are presented in table 8.4.

Medium-Potency Opioid Analgesics: *Morphine* and Its Derivatives

Morphine (MS Contin) is considered the prototypical medium-potency opioid drug, and its semisynthetic derivatives are the most widely used opioids for control of pain outside of the context of anesthesia or procedural sedation.[5] Despite the availability of several newer therapeutic medications, *morphine* remains the standard (**equianalgesic**) against which new analgesics are measured.[6] The pharmacodynamics and pharmacokinetics of *morphine*, a prototypical medium-potency opioid, are provided in table 8.5.

Many semisynthetic derivatives, or **congeners**, of *morphine* are produced by making relatively simple modifications to the molecular structure;

TABLE 8.4 Pharmacodynamics and Pharmacokinetics of a Prototypical Low-Potency Opioid

Generic name	*codeine*
Trade name	Generic only
Category	Low-potency opioid analgesic, antitussive
Route	Immediate-release (IR) oral tablet, 15 mg (other preparations available)
Onset of action	0.5-1 hr
Peak effect	1-1.5 hr
Duration	4-6 hr
Bioavailability	53%
Half-life	3 hr
Absorption	Adequate
Distribution	3-6 L/kg
Metabolism	Hepatic
Excretion	Urine, feces
Clinical note	Reserve *codeine* for use in patients for whom alternative treatment options (e.g., nonopioid analgesics, opioid combination products) are ineffective, not tolerated, or would be otherwise inadequate.

TABLE 8.5 Pharmacodynamics and Pharmacokinetics of a Prototypical Medium-Potency Opioid

Generic name	*morphine*
Trade name	MS Contin
Category	Medium-potency opioid analgesic
Route	Oral (IR, ER), rectal, IV, IM, and SQ
Onset of action	~30 min Patient dependent; dosing must be individualized.
Peak effect	1 hr
Duration	Pain relief is patient dependent; dosing must be individualized.
Bioavailability	17% to 33% (First-pass effect limits oral bioavailability.)
Half-life	2-4 hr
Absorption	Variable
Distribution	Skeletal muscle, liver, kidneys, lungs, intestinal tract, spleen, and brain 1-6 L/kg Binds to opioid receptors in the CNS and periphery (e.g., GI tract)
Metabolism	Hepatic
Excretion	Urine and feces
Clinical note	Use *morphine* for management of pain severe enough to require daily, around-the-clock, long-term opioid treatment and for which alternative treatment options are inadequate.

Note: For oral immediate-release dosage, unless otherwise noted.

some derivatives have >1,000 times the potency of *morphine*.[6,21]

Synthetic Derivatives of *Morphine*: *Oxycodone* and *Hydrocodone*

The semisynthetic compounds *oxycodone* (OxyContin) and *hydrocodone* (Zohydro) are potent analogues of *codeine* that are also orally available and are widely used, often in combination with *acetaminophen*. At present, *oxycodone* is one of the most commonly abused pharmaceutical drugs in the United States.[21] *Oxycodone* and *hydrocodone* are metabolized in the liver through the cytochrome P450 system to a highly potent opioid agonist.[5] *Oxycodone* is a useful oral analgesic for moderate to severe pain, which is especially true when the product is used in combination with nonopioids. Although *oxycodone* shares basic characteristics with *morphine*, the availability of both immediate-release and controlled-release oral dosage forms also makes it very useful in treating both chronic pain and acute pain.[6] *Oxycodone* is available as single-ingredient medication in immediate-release and controlled-release formulations. *Hydrocodone* is a commonly prescribed strong opioid and is available orally in immediate-release form combined with nonopioid analgesics, as well as in extended-release formulations. *Hydrocodone* is approximately equipotent to *oxycodone*, with an onset of action of 10 to 30 minutes, duration of 4 to 6 hours, and a serum half-life of about 4 hours.[21] The pharmacodynamic and pharmacokinetic properties of *oxycodone* and *hydrocodone* are similar to those of *morphine*.[6]

High-Potency Opioids: *Fentanyl*

Fentanyl is a synthetic opioid agonist used for severe pain and is 100 times more potent than *morphine*. *Fentanyl* is most widely used for intraoperative and periprocedural analgesia due to its high potency and rapid onset of action.[5] The time to peak analgesic effect after IV administration of *fentanyl* (~5 minutes) is much less than that for *morphine* (~15 minutes), and recovery from analgesic effects also occurs more quickly. However, with larger doses or prolonged infusions, the effects of *fentanyl* become more lasting, with durations of action becoming similar to those of longer-acting opioids.[21]

Fentanyl is used in the management of acute severe pain, but its use in chronic pain treatment has become more widespread.[5,6,21] Because *fentanyl* is poorly absorbed in the GI tract, the transdermal or buccal administration methods are preferred when using the drug for chronic pain management. Transdermal *fentanyl* patches (Duragesic) provide sustained release for 48 to 72 hours (figure 8.3); however, factors promoting increased absorption (e.g., fever, moist heat) can lead to overdosage and increased side effects (as discussed in chapter 7). The transdermal patch *fentanyl* is indicated only for opioid-tolerant patients (patients who have been on 60 mg of *morphine*/day or an equianalgesic dose of another opioid for at least a week). Transbuccal administration modes, such as buccal tablets, intranasal spray, soluble films, and lollipop-like lozenges or troches, permit rapid absorption. This method has found use in the management of acute incident pain and for the relief of breakthrough chronic pain. Illicit use (self-administration by chewing) of *fentanyl* patches or lollipops can be deadly, and ATs must be aware of this potential if these modes are prescribed to a patient.[21]

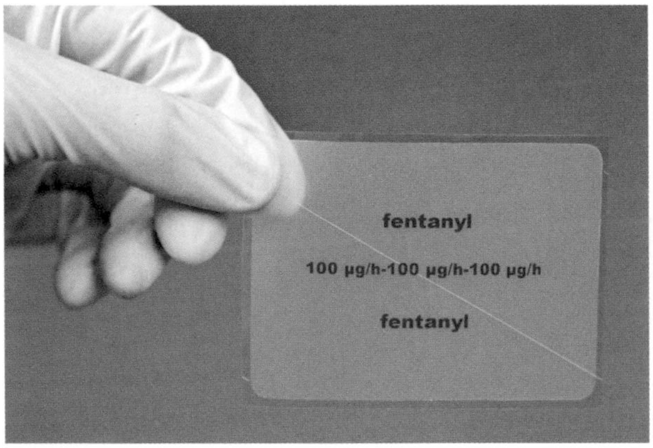

Carsten Rehder/picture alliance via Getty Images

FIGURE 8.3 Transdermal *fentanyl* patch.

Opioid Antagonists: *Naloxone*

The opioid antagonist *naloxone* (Narcan) binds competitively to opioid receptors but does not produce an analgesic or opioid side-effect response (figure 8.4). Therefore, it is used most often to reverse the toxic effects of opioid agonists.

Naloxone (Narcan) is indicated for the emergency treatment of opioid overdose as manifested by respiratory or CNS depression. Opioid antagonists, particularly *naloxone*, have an established use in the treatment of opioid-induced toxicity, especially respiratory depression leading to unconsciousness and death from overdose. *Naloxone* acts rapidly to reverse the respiratory depression associated with even high doses of opioids. Within the scope of an AT's practice, *naloxone* is administered intranasally (figure 8.5) or intramuscularly; it is intended for immediate administration as an emergency rescue drug. *Naloxone* can completely or partially reverse opioid depression (including respiratory depression) induced by natural and synthetic opioids. The duration of action of *naloxone* is relatively short, and 2 mg of *naloxone* can be administered every 2 or 3 minutes while waiting for emergency medical assistance.[21] Immediate transport to a hospital is necessary after administration of *naloxone*.

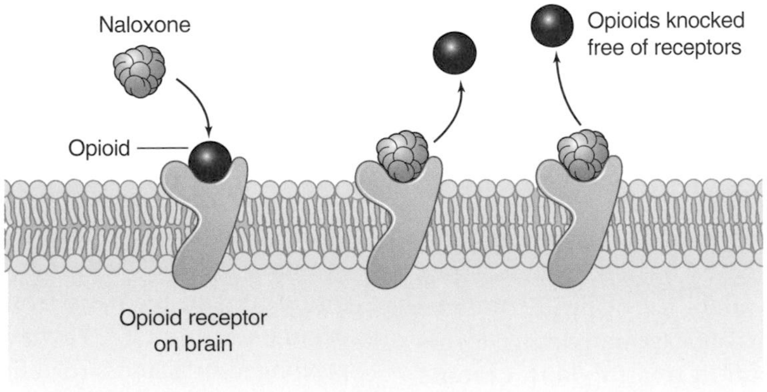

FIGURE 8.4 Reversing opioid overdose: Opioid receptor antagonists' mechanism of action.

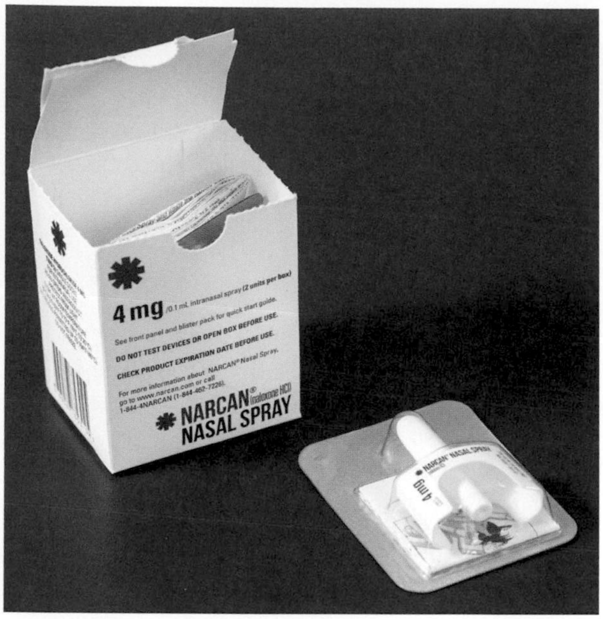

FIGURE 8.5 Narcan (*naloxone*) nasal spray for the rapid treatment of opioid overdose.

Summary

Opioid analgesics are effective treatment options in the management of acute and chronic (noncancer) pain; however, concerns exist about overdose deaths, which have been driven by dramatic increases in the prescribing of opioids for chronic pain. The AT treating chronic pain should prioritize nonpharmacologic therapy and nonopioid pharmacologic therapy. Prescribers should consider opioid therapy only if the expected benefits for both pain and function are anticipated to outweigh the risks to the patient. In the management of pain following surgical procedures, around-the-clock administration schedules should be used to maintain freedom from pain. This chapter discusses the therapeutic effects as well as the disadvantages of and concerns about the use of opioid analgesics. The AT should understand the warning signs of opioid physical dependence, misuse, and abuse. Recognizing the signs of opioid overdose and being proficient in the emergency administration of *naloxone* are essential skills for the AT in practically all practice settings.

Case Studies

Case Study 1

After ankle surgery, Miles was prescribed Vicoprofen, a combination of *hydrocodone* and *ibuprofen*. A few days after surgery, Miles noted bowel movement irregularity and started to pay closer attention to his digestion. After 6 days, he'd had only 2 bowel movements. He started OTC stool softeners and natural remedies for constipation with little success. He mentioned this concern to his physician at the 10-day post-op exam. During that exam, Miles acknowledged that his pain was more tolerable. His physician stopped the prescription for Vicoprofen and recommended *acetaminophen* and *ibuprofen* as needed.

Questions for Analysis

1. What caused his constipation?
2. Will the change of medication likely help the patient with constipation?

Case Study 2

Delores is a college athlete who recently had knee arthroscopy. As is done with many athletes at her school, she was prescribed *acetaminophen* with *codeine* following surgery. Her rehabilitation program was progressing slowly, in part due to her low pain threshold. After 3 weeks, Delores reported that she had lost her remaining supply of pain medication and asked to have it refilled since she was still in pain. The team physician acknowledged this was a bit unusual but recognized Delores' poor rehabilitation and refilled the prescription. Over the next 2 weeks, Delores was inconsistent with her rehabilitation appointments and academic work; she acknowledged that she continued to have significant pain and asked for another medication refill.

Questions for Analysis

1. What seems unusual about Delores' case?
2. What aspects of this case present a concern about the prospect of an opioid addiction? Why?

Drugs Described in This Chapter

generic (pronunciation) Trade name	Therapeutic uses Indications and dosage	Clinical concerns
codeine (KOE deen) No trade name	Management of mild to moderately severe pain and antitussive (cough suppressant) Oral: 15-60 mg every 4 hr as needed Maximum dose: 360 mg/day	Commonly reported: drowsiness lightheadedness, dizziness, sedation, shortness of breath, nausea, vomiting, sweating, and constipation. ***Opioid warnings**
morphine (MOR feen) MS Contin	Moderate to severe pain Oral: 10-30 mg every 4 hr as needed Commonly administered IM, SQ, and IV with continuous infusion or with patient-controlled analgesia (PCA)	*Risk of respiratory depression* Avoid concurrent use of benzodiazepines. Associated with addiction, abuse, and misuse. ***Opioid warnings**
naloxone (nal OKS one) Narcan intranasal spray; Evzio (auto-injector)	Acute opioid toxicity Intranasal: 2 or 4 mg sprayed into 1 nostril *Naloxone* has a short half-life. Rescue medication (nasal spray) used for opioid toxicity (overdose)	Cardiac arrhythmia, hypertension, hypotension, hepatotoxicity, pulmonary edema, opioid withdrawal (shared adverse effects), nausea, vomiting, and acute opioid withdrawal (shared adverse effects)

Notes: Unless otherwise specified, oral dosing reflects the use of immediate-release formulations. Contraindications to all medications are always hypersensitivity, allergic reaction, or anaphylaxis with symptoms such as hives, difficulty breathing, and angioedema (swelling of lips, tongue, or throat).

***Opioid warnings:** The Institute for Safe Medication Practices (ISMP) includes opioid medications among its list of drug classes that have a heightened risk of causing significant harm when used in error. These drugs expose patients and other users to the risks of opioid addiction, abuse, and misuse, which can lead to overdose and death. Assess each patient's risk prior to prescribing this drug and monitor all patients regularly for the development of these behaviors and conditions.

Limitations of use. Reserve for use in patients for whom alternative treatment options (e.g., nonopioid analgesics, opioid combination products) are ineffective, not tolerated, or would be otherwise inadequate to provide sufficient management of pain.

Black box warning: Life-threatening respiratory depression. Serious, life-threatening, or fatal respiratory depression may occur with use of opioids. Patients must be monitored for respiratory depression, especially during initiation of the drug or following a dose increase.

Black box warning: Risks from concomitant use with benzodiazepines or other CNS depressants. Concomitant use of opioids with benzodiazepines or other CNS depressants, including alcohol, may result in profound sedation, respiratory depression, coma, and death. Reserve concomitant prescribing of opioids and benzodiazepines or other CNS depressants for use in patients for whom alternative treatment options are inadequate. Limit dosages and durations to the minimum required. Patients should be followed for signs and symptoms of respiratory depression and sedation.

9

Drugs to Treat Inflammation: Steroidal and Nonsteroidal Anti-Inflammatories

OBJECTIVES

After reading this chapter, you will be able to do the following:

- Differentiate between the actions of steroidal and nonsteroidal anti-inflammatory medications on the inflammatory process
- Contrast the functions of COX-1 and COX-2 inhibitors
- Compare the adverse and toxic effects of corticosteroids, *aspirin*, nonselective COX inhibitor NSAIDs, and the COX-2-selective drug
- Describe anti-inflammatories commonly used in the athletic training setting

Select Drugs Mentioned in This Chapter

Drug class	Generic name	Trade name
Corticosteroid	*prednisone*	Generic only
Salicylate, nonselective irreversible COX-1 and COX-2 inhibitor	*aspirin* or *acetylsalicylic acid (ASA)*	Bayer, Bufferin, many others
Nonsteroidal, nonselective COX-1 and COX-2 inhibitor	*naproxen*	Aleve, Naprosyn
Propionic acid derivative, nonselective COX-1 and COX-2 inhibitor	*ibuprofen*	Motrin, Advil
Nonsteroidal, selective COX-2 inhibitor	*celecoxib*	Celebrex

This list is not exhaustive, but rather contains drugs commonly encountered in the athletic training setting. Always consult up-to-date information, confirm with a pharmacist, or discuss the use of therapeutic medications with the prescriber of the medication.

Inflammation is a complex response to cell injury that primarily occurs in vascularized connective tissue, with inflammatory mediators functioning to eliminate the cause of cell injury and clear away debris in preparation for tissue repair. The response is activated by noxious agents, infections, or physical injuries that release damage- and pathogen-associated molecules, which are then recognized by immune system cells. Although the inflammatory response is a normal protective process, its intensity and duration may become inappropriate and destructive, resulting in chronic inflammatory conditions. Drugs with anti-inflammatory actions may be indicated for these conditions.[4]

Pharmacological interventions for inflammation involve the large category of anti-inflammatory drugs, which are directed at controlling the inflammatory process and minimizing inflammatory pain. The 2 major classes of anti-inflammatory medications are the corticosteroids, specifically the **glucocorticoids**, and the **nonsteroidal anti-inflammatory drugs (NSAIDs)**. This chapter describes the use of pharmacological interventions for effectively controlling inflammatory pain and reducing inflammation.[14]

Inflammatory Process

The acute phase response, or inflammation, is a physiologic response to tissue injury and infection. (Although it is similar in its physiological responses, inflammation is not a synonym for infection.) Vascular changes account for the familiar clinical signs of inflammation: redness, heat, pain, and swelling. Vasodilation and increased blood vessel wall permeability are the most consistent vascular responses. Vasodilation accommodates an increase in blood flow, or **hyperemia**, producing redness and heat. An increase in the permeability of vascular endothelium allows exudation of plasma, producing swelling and pain. Both vascular changes are brought about by local chemical mediators, or **cytokines**. These substances are either released by damaged cells or synthesized within the injured tissue. They include **histamine**, bradykinin, **prostaglandins**, and a variety of other complex agents. Some of these substances also sensitize sensory nerve endings and enhance nociception and pain transmission.[4]

Acute Inflammation

When tissue damage occurs (regardless of mechanism), transient local vasodilation and increased capillary permeability occur. The 3 major phases (figure 9.1) of acute inflammation are as follows:[4,11,14]

- **Vascular phase**—Following tissue damage or introduction of a pathogen to the tissues, vasoactive mediators (cytokines) cause arterioles to dilate and endothelial cells to shrink, making capillaries and venules more

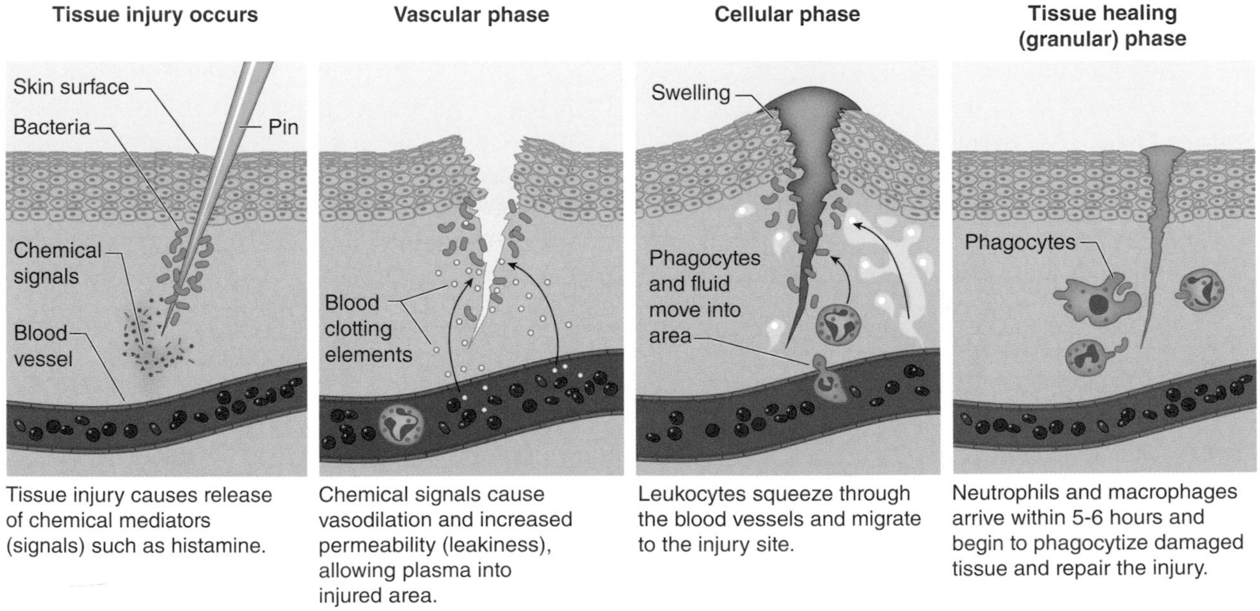
Tissue injury occurs
Vascular phase
Cellular phase
Tissue healing (granular) phase
Skin surface
Bacteria
Pin
Chemical signals
Blood vessel
Blood clotting elements
Swelling
Phagocytes and fluid move into area
Phagocytes
Tissue injury causes release of chemical mediators (signals) such as histamine.
Chemical signals cause vasodilation and increased permeability (leakiness), allowing plasma into injured area.
Leukocytes squeeze through the blood vessels and migrate to the injury site.
Neutrophils and macrophages arrive within 5-6 hours and begin to phagocytize damaged tissue and repair the injury.

FIGURE 9.1 Major events in the acute inflammatory process.

permeable. Increased intracellular permeability allows extravasation of plasma, leading to swelling and pain.

- **Cellular phase**—Within a few hours of the vascular changes, **chemotactic** mediators target leukocytes (white blood cells), which adhere to endothelium (margination), squeeze through the openings (**diapedesis**) in the capillaries, and migrate out into the tissues (emigration). Additionally, **chemokines** attract macrophages to the site of inflammation.
- **Tissue healing (granular) phase**—Within 6 hours after the onset of the inflammatory response, macrophages arrive at the damaged tissue. Activated macrophages secrete 3 major proinflammatory cytokines: **interleukin-1 (IL-1)**, **interleukin-6 (IL-6)**, and **tumor necrosis factor alpha** (TNF-α). These cytokines induce coagulation, increase vascular permeability, and promote the acute-phase response.

Acute inflammation is characterized by a rapid onset following tissue injury that resolves relatively quickly. The resulting tissue pathology is typically mild and localized.[14] Whether it occurs in response to tissue injury or due to the body's attempt to limit invading pathogens, the acute inflammatory response is similar.[11,14]

Chronic Inflammation

Chronic inflammation results from continuous or repeated exposure to the offending element or process. This physiological process can result from continued tissue damage, persistence of pathogens, autoimmune diseases, and cancers. The hallmark of chronic inflammation is the accumulation and activation of macrophages and lymphocytes, as well as fibroblasts that replace the original, damaged, or necrotic tissue. Soluble factors released by macrophages and lymphocytes play an important role in the development of chronic inflammation. Replacement of damaged tissue by fibroblasts leads to **fibrosis**, an excessive deposition of fibrous tissue that can interfere with normal tissue function due to excessive amounts of growth factors (platelet-derived growth factor, fibrogenic cytokines [IL-1 and TNF-α], and angiogenic factors (fibroblast growth factor, vascular endothelial growth factor). Chronic inflammation can also lead to the formation of **granulomas**—a mass of cells consisting of activated macrophages surrounded by activated lymphocytes.[11]

Controlling Inflammation

Many drugs are available to decrease joint pain, swelling, and inflammation and possibly prevent or minimize the progression of the inflammatory response. The 2 major categories of anti-inflammatory drugs are as follows:

1. Corticosteroids, such as *prednisone* or *hydrocortisone*
2. Nonsteroidal anti-inflammatory drugs (NSAIDs), such as *aspirin*, *ibuprofen*, or *naproxen*[11,25]

NSAIDs inhibit the vascular phase of inflammation, and corticosteroids inhibit primarily the cellular phase of inflammation.[4] Corticosteroids function to profoundly alter the immune responses of lymphocytes; this is an important aspect of the anti-inflammatory and immunosuppressive actions of these drugs. Although the use of corticosteroids as anti-inflammatory agents does not address the underlying cause of the disease or condition, the suppression of inflammation is of enormous clinical utility, which has made these drugs among the most frequently prescribed pharmacological agents.[31]

Anti-inflammatory medications function to inhibit various parts of the **arachidonic acid cascade**. Nonselective NSAIDs target cyclooxygenase (COX), the rate-limiting enzyme in the production of prostaglandins. In contrast, corticosteroids prevent the liberation of arachidonic acid from plasma-membrane phospholipids (figure 9.2) and thus reduce the synthesis of the **eicosanoids** (e.g., prostaglandins, thromboxanes, and leukotrienes).[11]

NSAIDs are widely used for their anti-inflammatory and analgesic effects. NSAIDs are a necessary choice in pain management because of the integrated role of the COX pathway in the generation of inflammation and the biochemical recognition of pain.[25]

Corticosteroids

Corticosteroids (also called *glucocorticoids* or *steroids*) are **endogenous hormones**, such as the glucocorticoid cortisol, that are secreted naturally by the zona fasciculata of the cortex of the adrenal glands (figure 9.3). **Cortisol** is released in response to stress and has numerous effects on the body that are essential for life. **Corticosteroid** medications are a synthetic version of cortisol, such as *cortisone*, *prednisone*, or *hydrocortisone*, that are very effective at reducing inflammation and suppressing the immune system.[12] Corticosteroids have historically

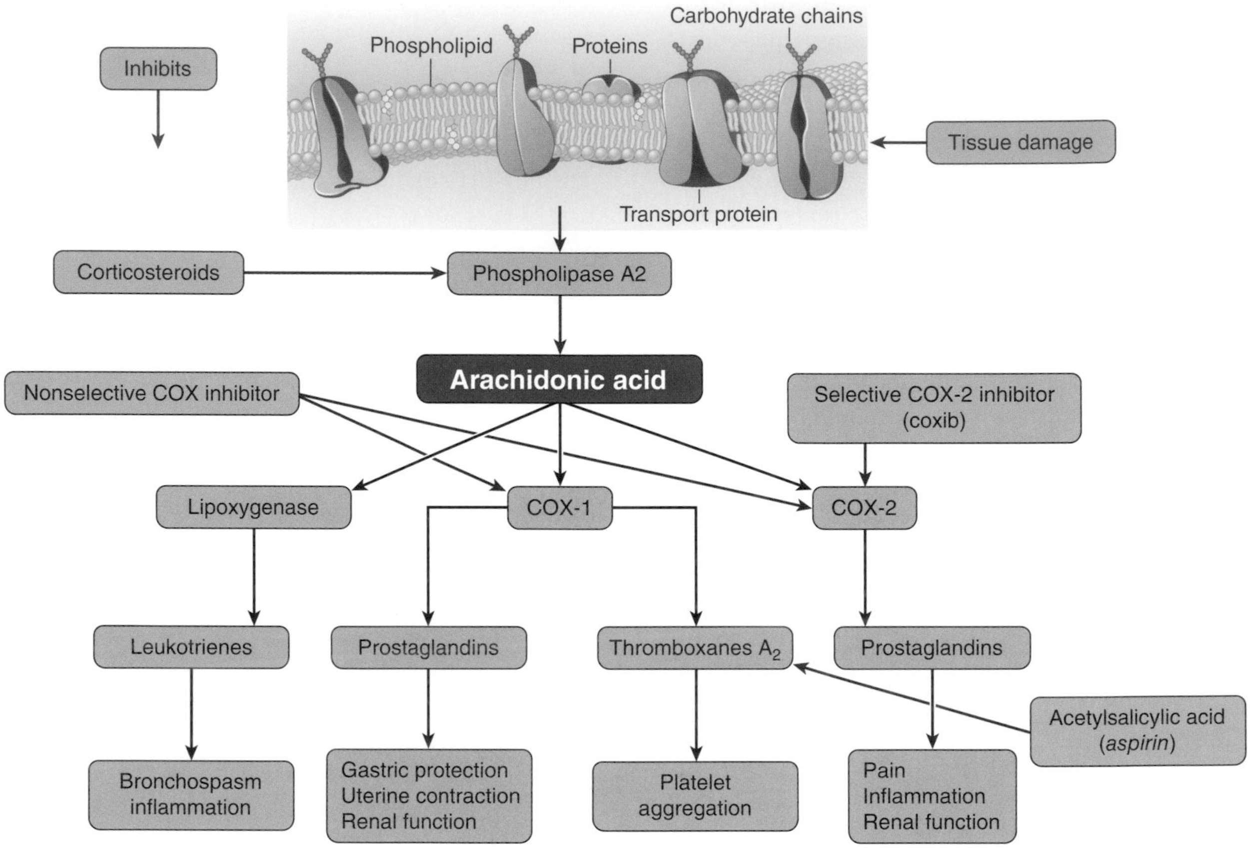

FIGURE 9.2 The arachidonic acid cascade.

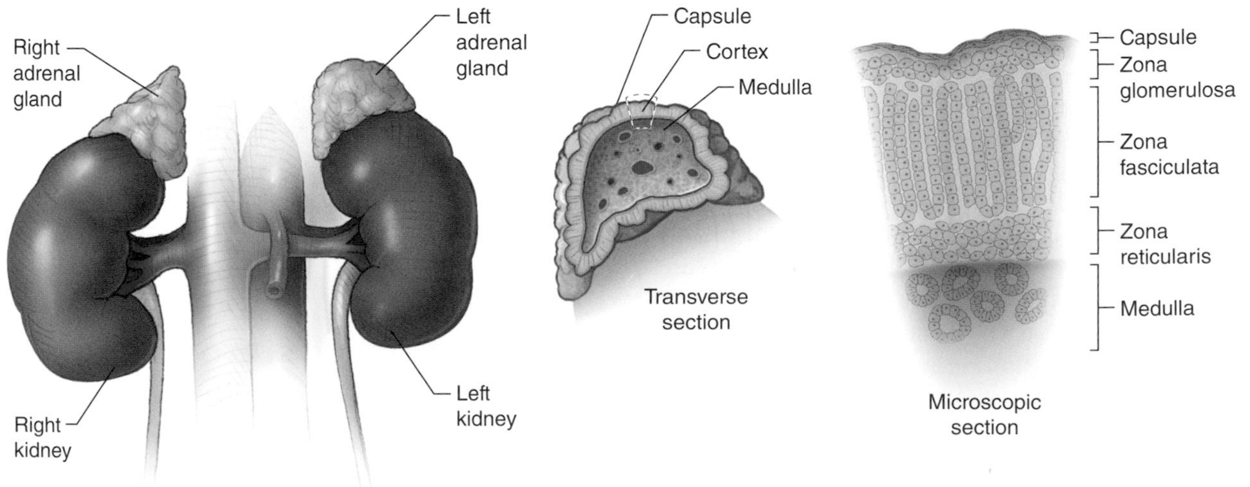

FIGURE 9.3 Location, transverse section, and microscopic section of the adrenal cortex and the zona fasciculata that produce cortisol, an endogenous corticosteroid cortisol.

TABLE 9.1 Examples of Corticosteroid Anti-Inflammatories

Generic name	Brand name
betamethasone	Celestone Soluspan
dexamethasone	Decadron, DexPak, others
hydrocortisone	Cortef, Solu-Cortef, others
methyl-prednisolone	Medrol Dosepak, Solu-Medrol, Methylpred-DP, DEPO-Medrol
prednisone	Generic only
prednisolone	Millipred, Pred Forte, Pred Mild, Orapred, Veripred 20
triamcinolone	Kenalog, Aristospan, Azmacort, others

been used for pain relief in inflammatory conditions. The use of corticosteroids to treat inflammatory and autoimmune diseases makes them among the most frequently prescribed classes of drugs. Because corticosteroids exert effects on almost every organ system, extended administration and withdrawal that is made too rapidly may be complicated by serious side effects. Therefore, the decision to institute therapy with systemic corticosteroids always requires careful consideration of the relative risks and benefits in each patient.[31] Refer to table 9.1 for examples of corticosteroid medications, called "the *-ones*" (rhymes with "zones"), since the end of each generic name ends in *-one*.

Therapeutic Effects

Corticosteroids inhibit the inflammatory response to tissue injury. Endogenous corticosteroids also suppress manifestations of allergic disease due to the release of histamine from mast cells and basophils. These anti-inflammatory effects require high levels of circulating corticosteroids and cannot be produced by administering **exogenous** corticosteroids without producing the other manifestations of corticosteroid excess (see the section Dosing Guidelines). The **hypothalamic-pituitary-adrenal (HPA) axis** (figure 9.4) can be suppressed in patients who are receiving corticosteroids for prolonged periods.[22] Large doses of exogenous corticosteroids inhibit **adrenocorticotropic hormone (ACTH)** release from the pituitary gland. ACTH stimulates the release of cortisol from the adrenal cortex. ACTH secretion to the point of severe adrenal insufficiency can be a dangerous problem when therapy is stopped abruptly. However, local administration of corticosteroids—for example, by injection into an inflamed joint or near an irritated nerve—produces a high local concentration of the steroid, often without enough systemic absorption to cause serious side effects.[4] The main differences among corticosteroids lie in their potency (dose), the time they last in the body (half-life), and their propensity for fluid retention due to effects on sodium retention.[12]

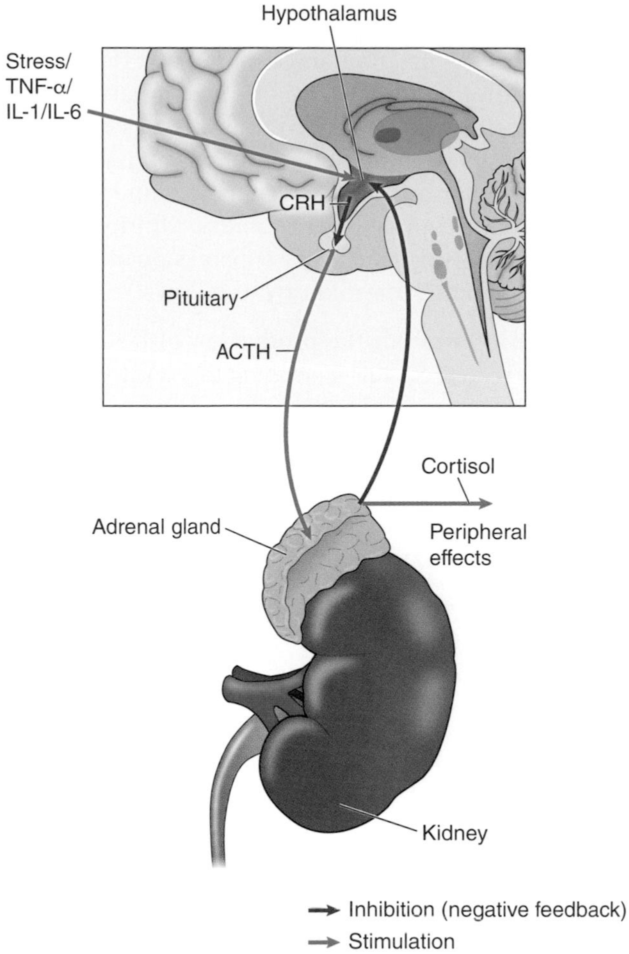

FIGURE 9.4 The hypothalamic-pituitary-adrenal (HPA) axis. CRH = corticotropin-releasing hormone; AVP = arginine vasopressin; ACTH = adrenocorticotropic hormone; IL-1 = interleukin-1; IL-6 = interleukin-6; TNF-α = tumor necrosis factor alpha.

Steroid Hormones

The word *steroid* may sound concerning because of the media attention given to the anabolic steroids that some athletes use to gain muscle. However, steroids are a large group with many different functions, and those used to treat inflammation—specifically, corticosteroids—are different than the steroids you may hear about athletes using on the news.[16]

Mechanism of Action

The primary mechanism of action of the corticosteroids includes both anti-inflammatory and immunosuppressive actions. These drugs function to decrease inflammation by suppression of migration of polymorphonuclear leukocytes and reversal of increased capillary permeability. Multiple other mechanisms involved in the suppression of inflammation by corticosteroids are as follows:[31]

- Inhibition of the production of factors that are critical for generating the inflammatory response
- Decreased release of vasoactive and chemoattractive factors
- Diminished secretion of lipolytic and proteolytic enzymes
- Decreased extravasation of leukocytes to areas of injury
- Decreased fibroblast activity at the site of injury

The anti-inflammatory effects of corticosteroids are largely due to a reduction in the synthesis or release of a variety of inflammatory mediators, including the prostaglandins, which are also inhibited by NSAIDs. The sum of these actions results in suppression of the vascular changes responsible for the cardinal signs of inflammation. Corticosteroids also inhibit certain aspects of leukocyte function, which accounts largely for their immunosuppressant effect.[4,31]

Routes of Administration

Corticosteroids are used to treat a variety of inflammatory conditions and can be administered intravenously, orally, intra-articularly, topically, intralesionally, or transcutaneously. Corticosteroids marketed as anti-inflammatories are often topical formulations, such as nasal sprays for rhinitis or inhalers for asthma. Generic oral formulations of *prednisone*, *methylprednisolone*, and *triamcinolone* typically last for 12 to 36 hours in the body, whereas *dexamethasone* and *betamethasone* last for 32 to 72 hours. *Prednisone* is one of the most commonly used corticosteroids because of its low cost and is available only in oral form. These medications should be administered with food to decrease GI upset. Some corticosteroids are formulated in a way that extends their duration of action; for example, depot preparations of *methylprednisolone* provide anti-inflammatory effects for 1 to 4 weeks. The long-acting repository (depot) formulations are intended for intramuscular or intra-articular injection.[4]

Pharmacodynamics and Pharmacokinetics

Corticosteroids are strikingly similar in their molecular structures and clinical effects. All oral corticosteroids undergo first-pass metabolism during absorption. When dosed equivalently, the various corticosteroids are equivalent in anti-inflammatory efficacy and have similar side-effect profiles, except for fluid retention. For these reasons, preparations are readily interchangeable, provided that equipotent doses are prescribed.[4] The pharmacodynamics and pharmacokinetics of the prototypical corticosteroid drug *prednisone* are described in table 9.2.

Dosing Guidelines

Dosing of corticosteroids depends on the condition being treated and the response of the patient. For people who are taking corticosteroids long term, the provider may prescribe extra doses during times of acute stress, such as severe infection or surgery. Corticosteroids mimic the cortisol surge that is normally produced by the body, particularly during stressful events, so that healing is not delayed or incomplete. Discontinuation of therapy that has lasted longer than 7 days may require tapering of the drug to prevent **adrenal crisis**. Standard formulations of *prednisone*, *methylprednisolone*, and *triamcinolone* last for around 12 to 36 hours in the body, whereas *dexamethasone* and *betamethasone* last for 32 to 72 hours.[12] Dose requirements are variable; individualized doses are based on disease and patient response. For example, a *methylprednisolone* (Medrol Dosepak) is a low-dose oral corticosteroid treatment course used in sports medicine to treat lower back injuries and other musculoskeletal conditions. This pack contains 21 tablets of *methylprednisolone* 4 mg that are taken over a 6-day period.[4,9]

When corticosteroids are administered at recommended dosages for short durations of time, these potent anti-inflammatories are considered safe. More regular or extended dosing has been associated with several severe adverse effects.[12] Use of high-dose corticosteroids, particularly long term, can cause **avascular necrosis**, especially of the head of the femur and humerus. The reason is unknown, but one hypothesis is that corticosteroids can increase lipid levels in the blood, thereby reducing blood

TABLE 9.2 Pharmacodynamics and Pharmacokinetics of a Prototypical Corticosteroid Drug

Generic	*prednisone*
Trade name	Tablet (generic only), oral solution (Prednisone Intensol), delayed-release tablet (Rayos)
Category	Anti-inflammatories: corticosteroids
Route	Oral tablet
Onset of action	Depends on drug formulation
Peak effect	Oral: Immediate-release tablet: 2 hr Delayed-release tablet: 6-6.5 hr
Duration	12-36 hr
Bioavailability	Interindividual variability: 44% (reported range: 20% to 95%)
Half-life	2-3 hr
Absorption	50% to 90% (may be altered in hepatic failure, chronic renal failure, inflammatory bowel disease, or hyperthyroidism, and in the elderly)
Distribution	Protein bound (concentration dependent): 70%
Metabolism	Hepatic to metabolite *prednisolone* (active)
Excretion	Urine
Clinical note	**Anaphylactoid reactions:** Rare cases of anaphylactoid reactions have been observed in patients receiving corticosteroids. **Immunosuppression:** Prolonged use of corticosteroids may increase the incidence of secondary infection, mask acute infection (including fungal infections), prolong or exacerbate viral infections, or limit response to killed or inactivated vaccines. **Musculoskeletal adverse effects:** These include arthralgia, osteonecrosis of femoral and humeral heads, increased risk of fracture, loss of muscle mass, muscle weakness, myalgias, osteopenia, osteoporosis, pathologic fracture of long bones, steroid myopathy, tendon rupture (particularly of the Achilles tendon), and vertebral compression fractures.

flow. If untreated, avascular necrosis worsens with time, and eventually the bone can collapse. Avascular necrosis also causes bone to lose its smooth shape, potentially leading to severe arthritis.[10]

RED FLAG

Potential Consequences of Corticosteroid Use

Corticosteroids are used to treat spinal disc herniation, chronic tendinopathy, and autoimmune or inflammatory diseases, such as systemic lupus erythematosus.[19] Multiple studies have linked **osteonecrosis** of the hip to corticosteroid use. High-dose corticosteroid use is the independent factor most frequently associated with the development of osteonecrosis, particularly of the femoral head.[19,20] A *methylprednisolone* (Medrol) taper pack (MTP) is a low-dose oral corticosteroid treatment. Little evidence exists linking a single course of MTP to osteonecrosis.[8] The AT should be aware that osteonecrosis is responsible for >10% of all hip arthroplasties in the United States and Europe and is the most common reason that many physicians do not routinely prescribe corticosteroids.

Indications and Precautions

Short-term administration (for acute episodes or exacerbations) of corticosteroids may be prescribed for patients with acute and subacute bursitis, acute nonspecific tenosynovitis, ankylosing spondylitis, epicondylitis, posttraumatic osteoarthritis, and several types of arthritis (e.g., acute gouty arthritis, psoriatic arthritis, rheumatoid arthritis, and synovitis of osteoarthritis). During an exacerbation or as maintenance therapy, the prescriber may consider corticosteroids for select cases of acute rheumatic carditis, systemic dermatomyositis (polymyositis), and systemic lupus erythematosus.[16] Prolonged use of corticosteroids may result in **immunosuppression** that increases the incidence of secondary infection, mask acute infection (including fungal infections), prolong or exacerbate viral infections, or limit response to certain vaccines. Because corticosteroids suppress the immune system, they increase the risk of infection. Certain viral infections, such as chicken pox or measles, may have a more severe course in people taking corticosteroids.[12] Other precautions for patients prescribed corticosteroid therapy are discussed in the Evidence in Pharmacology sidebar.

Prescription doses of exogenous corticosteroids can cause higher than normal levels of cortisol in the blood. High levels of exogenous corticosteroids for a prolonged time cause the hypothalamus to secrete less **corticotropin-releasing hormone (CRH)**, which reduces ACTH, thereby causing the adrenal glands to stop making cortisol.[22,35] This condition is of concern if the medication is suddenly stopped because the adrenal cortex will not immediately begin producing corticosteroids again. This is called **acute adrenal insufficiency** (also Addison's disease), and symptoms include irritability, nausea, joint pain, dizziness, and low blood pressure.[35] To avoid this condition, steroid medication should be withdrawn slowly over several days or weeks to allow the adrenal cortex to fully resume its functioning capacity again.[12,22,35]

Evidence in Pharmacology

Corticosteroid Injections and Pregnancy

Corticosteroid use is preferred for pregnant women with musculoskeletal inflammation late in pregnancy because NSAIDs are contraindicated during the third trimester.[21] Additionally, corticosteroids are used during pregnancy to treat an autoimmune disorder of the mother that could be more harmful to fetal health than high doses of the medication.[3] A historical link was found between corticosteroids and cleft lip births; however, contemporary evidence indicates this incidence is modest.[37] Other corticosteroid risks during pregnancy include preeclampsia, low birth weight, preterm birth, and potential hyperglycemia and ketoacidosis for the patient with gestational diabetes.[3,21] Corticosteroid use following birth can disturb normal lactation, but this is reversible after stopping use of the medication.

Adverse Effects

In cases of adrenal insufficiency, there is suppression of the HPA axis in patients receiving high doses of corticosteroids for prolonged periods of time. With prolonged suppression, the adrenal glands atrophy and can take months to recover full function after discontinuation of the exogenous corticosteroid. Overuse of steroid joint injections may also result in adrenal suppression after their discontinuation.[22] HPA axis suppression may lead to acute adrenal crisis, a potentially life-threatening medical condition requiring immediate emergency treatment. Withdrawal and discontinuation of a corticosteroid should be conducted slowly and carefully. Adult patients receiving >20 mg per day of *prednisone* (or equivalent) may be most susceptible. Thus, it is critical for any patient prescribed corticosteroids to follow precise instructions of the daily schedule without deviation. Anaphylactoid reactions are rare but have been observed in patients receiving corticosteroids. Corticosteroids have been associated with many side effects:

- Agitation and irritability
- Blurred vision
- Difficulty concentrating
- Dizziness
- Facial hair growth in female patients
- Fast or irregular heartbeat
- Fluid retention
- Headache
- High blood pressure
- Increased blood sugar, cholesterol, or triglycerides
- Increased risk of gastric ulcers or gastritis
- Loss of potassium
- Shortness of breath
- Sleeplessness
- Weight gain

This is not a comprehensive list of all side effects. The AT should consult the prescriber with any additional questions or concerns.

Long-term use of exogenous corticosteroid therapy may cause abnormally high cortisol levels and lead to **Cushing's syndrome** (hypercortisolism). Typical undesired effects of corticosteroids present quite uniformly as drug-induced Cushing's syndrome, caused by long-term exposure to an excess of cortisol. Symptoms include a fatty (buffalo) hump between the shoulders, a round face, weight gain, irregular menstrual cycles, fatigue, and depression.

Nonsteroidal Anti-Inflammatory Drugs

Nonsteroidal anti-inflammatory drugs (NSAIDs) are among the most commonly used groups of drugs.[15] More than 20 different NSAIDs are available commercially, and these agents are used worldwide. All the NSAIDs (including *aspirin*) have analgesic, antipyretic, and anti-inflammatory effects. The traditional (nonselective) NSAIDs also have **antithrombotic** effects.[33] These medications relieve pain by blocking the production of pain-signaling molecules. One of the steps in this pathway involves certain types of **cyclooxygenase** (COX-1 and COX-2) enzymes. By inhibiting the COX enzymes, NSAIDs relieve pain in joints, muscles, and other soft tissues.[7]

NSAIDs are a choice in pain management because of the integral role of the COX pathway in the generation of inflammation and the biochemical recognition of pain. The agents differ with respect to their side effects, duration of action, degree of platelet antagonism (bleeding), and gastrointestinal (GI) toxicity.[33] Both traditional nonselective COX inhibitor NSAIDs and the selective cyclooxygenase COX-2 inhibitors are widely used for their anti-inflammatory and analgesic effects (figure 9.5).[17,23,25,33] The NSAIDs are grouped by their chemical similarity, which leads to functional similarity. This chemical diversity yields a broad range of pharmacokinetic characteristics. Although there are many differences in the kinetics of NSAIDs, the drugs have many general properties in common.[13,15,23] There are 2 major categories of NSAIDs (see table 9.3 for examples of medications):

1. **Nonselective (traditional, classic, older) COX inhibitor NSAIDs**—Vary primarily in their potency, analgesic and anti-inflammatory effectiveness, and duration of action. Some have better anti-inflammatory effectiveness and others have better analgesic effectiveness.
2. **Selective (newer) cyclooxygenase-2 (COX-2) inhibitor NSAIDs**—All named with the ending *-coxib*, these medications produce analgesia equivalent to that of the nonselective NSAIDs while decreasing the adverse effects, specifically the GI toxicity associated with chronic NSAID use. Unfortunately, postclinical experience involving some of the highly selective COX-2 inhibitors has shown a higher incidence of cardiovascular

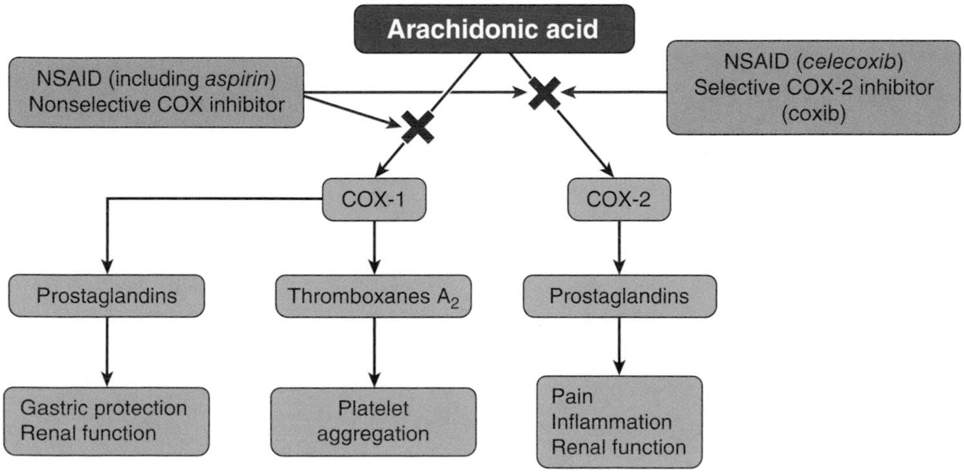

FIGURE 9.5 Role of NSAIDs in inhibiting the cyclooxygenase enzymes.

TABLE 9.3 Examples of Nonselective COX Inhibitors and Selective COX-2 Inhibitors

Generic name	Brand name
NONSELECTIVE COX INHIBITORS	
aspirin, acetylsalicylic acid (ASA)	Bayer, Bufferin, many others
diclofenac	Voltaren
ibuprofen	Motrin, Advil
indomethacin	Indocin
ketoprofen	Orudis
ketorolac	Toradol
naproxen	Aleve, Naprosyn
SELECTIVE COX-2 INHIBITOR	
celecoxib	Celebrex

thrombotic events than with the nonselective drugs.[17] Since then, both *rofecoxib* (Vioxx) and *valdecoxib* (Bextra) have been withdrawn from the market because of an increased risk of adverse cardiovascular events at high doses in the elderly (heart attack, stroke) and skin reactions.[14] Only *celecoxib* (Celebrex) is currently available for use in the United States despite having similar risks.

Evidence in Pharmacology

Cardiovascular Risk Associated With NSAIDs

Some drugs used to treat noncardiovascular conditions may adversely affect the cardiovascular status of patients both with and without known cardiovascular disease. Findings from the Coxib and traditional NSAID Trialists' (CNT) Collaboration—which evaluated the cardiovascular safety of NSAIDs, including *celecoxib, valdecoxib* (withdrawn), and *rofecoxib* (withdrawn)—revealed an increase in the incidence of myocardial infarction, stroke, and vascular death. Major vascular events were increased by about a third by a coxib (rate ratio [RR] 1.37, 95% confidence interval [CI] 1.14-1.66; $p = 0.0009$). The nonselective COX inhibitor, *diclofenac* (RR 1.41, CI 1.12-1.78; $p = 0.0036$), is primarily prescribed topically chiefly due to an increase in major coronary events (*diclofenac* RR 1.70, CI 1.19-2.41; $p = 0.0032$).[2,5]

Therapeutic Effects

The NSAIDs are antipyretic, analgesic, and anti-inflammatory medications. NSAIDs provide mostly symptomatic relief from pain and inflammation associated with musculoskeletal disorders, such as strains, sprains, and various symptoms associated with rheumatoid arthritis and osteoarthritis. Patients with more debilitating disease may not respond adequately to full therapeutic doses of NSAIDs and may require aggressive therapy with second-line agents such as analgesics or corticosteroids.[14,15] Genomic variation may also affect a person's success rate with a particular NSAID; thus, there are >20 treatment options.

The NSAIDs are effective against inflammatory pain of low to moderate intensity. Although their maximal efficacy is generally less than that of opioids, NSAIDs lack the unwanted adverse effects of opiates in the central nervous system (CNS), including respiratory depression and the potential for the development of physical dependence. Coadministration of NSAIDs can reduce the opioid dose needed for sufficient pain control and thus, reduce the likelihood of adverse opioid effects. For example, *ibuprofen* can be prescribed in combination with *hydrocodone*. Although NSAIDs do not change the perception of sensory modalities other than pain, NSAIDs are particularly effective when inflammation has caused sensitization of pain perception. Thus, postoperative pain or pain arising from inflammation, such as arthritic pain, is controlled well by NSAIDs, whereas pain arising from the hollow viscera usually is not relieved. An exception to this is menstrual pain; treatment of menstrual pain with NSAIDs is often useful. NSAIDs are commonly used to treat migraine attacks and can be combined with **antiemetics** to aid relief of the associated nausea. NSAIDs (and opioids) generally lack efficacy in neuropathic pain, such as diabetic neuralgia or pain associated with shingles (postherpetic neuralgia). However, *ketorolac* (Toradol) 60 mg administered intramuscularly (IM) has been shown to produce analgesia equivalent to *morphine* 10 mg IM for this type of pain.[14]

Mechanisms of Action

The classic COX inhibitors are not selective and inhibit all types of COX enzyme activity, thus impairing the ultimate transformation of arachidonic acid to prostaglandins, prostacyclin, and thromboxanes (recall the depiction from figure 9.2). The resulting inhibition of prostaglandin and thromboxane synthesis has the effect of reduced inflammation, as well as antipyretic, antithrombotic, and analgesic effects. NSAIDs affect pain pathways in at least 3 ways:[13,14,33]

1. Prostaglandins reduce the activation threshold at the peripheral terminals of primary afferent nociceptor neurons. By reducing prostaglandin synthesis, NSAIDs decrease inflammatory hyperalgesia and allodynia.
2. NSAIDs decrease the recruitment of leukocytes and, thereby, the production of leukocyte-derived inflammatory mediators.
3. NSAIDs that cross the blood-brain barrier prevent the generation of prostaglandins that act as pain-producing neuromodulators in the spinal cord dorsal horn.

Route of Administration

NSAIDs are used for the treatment of mild to moderate pain, especially the pain associated with musculoskeletal inflammation, such as in arthritis and gout. The primary route of NSAID administration is oral for both prescription and over-the-counter (OTC) medicines. *Ketorolac* (Toradol) is the only NSAID routinely administered via the parenteral route.

Topical NSAIDs have decreased systemic exposure (i.e., lower absorption into the systemic circulation) compared to the oral and intravenous formulations; therefore, they are expected to cause less serious side effects. According to a recent Cochrane systematic review, *diclofenac* gel, *ketoprofen* gel, *piroxicam* gel, and *diclofenac* plaster work reasonably well for strains and sprains. For hand and knee osteoarthritis, topical *diclofenac* and topical *ketoprofen* rubbed on the skin for ≥6 weeks helped reduce pain by at least half in a modest number of people.[34] Methods that enhance transdermal delivery, such as iontophoresis or chemical penetration enhancers, continue to be investigated.[14]

Although topical and oral NSAIDs may produce similar efficacy, patients receiving topical NSAIDs reported fewer GI side effects compared with those using oral formulations.[15] The cardiovascular and renal safety profile of topical NSAIDs (see Adverse Effects section that follows) remains to be assessed, and the possibility of skin rashes due to topical application of NSAIDs should be kept in mind. However, the lower systemic exposure that is expected from topical usage may result in a better overall safety profile for these routes of administration.[15]

Pharmacokinetics

The major differences between NSAIDs are their therapeutic half-lives and safety profiles. NSAIDs are systemic drugs that are distributed throughout the body and readily penetrate synovial joints, which makes these drugs ideal for reducing musculoskeletal inflammation.

Absorption and Distribution

Most NSAIDs are acidic compounds with a relatively high bioavailability. After oral administration, the absorption of NSAIDs is generally rapid, and peak plasma concentrations are reached within 3 hours. Oral NSAIDs undergo hepatic first-pass metabolism, resulting in reduced bioavailability. Food intake may delay absorption and systemic availability. Antacids, commonly prescribed to patients on NSAID therapy, variably delay absorption. *Aspirin* begins to acetylate platelets within minutes of reaching the presystemic circulation.[14]

For distribution, NSAIDs bind to plasma proteins; they are usually metabolized in the liver and excreted in the urine.[15,36] Most NSAIDs are extensively bound (95% to 99%) to plasma proteins, usually albumin,[6,14] and achieve sufficient concentrations in the CNS to have a central analgesic effect.[14] Most NSAIDs are distributed widely throughout the body and readily penetrate synovial joints, yielding synovial fluid concentrations in the range of half the plasma concentration.[14] The volume of distribution of NSAIDs is low, ranging from 0.1 to 0.3 L/kg, suggesting minimal tissue binding. NSAID binding in plasma can be saturated when the concentration of the NSAID exceeds that of albumin.[6,14]

Metabolism and Excretion

Hepatic biotransformation and renal excretion are the principal routes of metabolism and elimination of the majority of NSAIDs. Common NSAIDs have a variable half-life ($t_{1/2}$). *Aspirin* has a $t_{1/2}$ of 0.25 to 0.3 hours. *Ibuprofen* has a $t_{1/2}$ of about 2 hours, is relatively safe, and is the least expensive of the traditional nonselective NSAIDs.[17] *Naproxen* has a comparatively long but highly variable $t_{1/2}$ ranging from 12 to 17 hours. Genetic variation in the major metabolizing enzymes and variation in the composition of the intestinal microbiome may contribute to variability in metabolism and elimination. In general, NSAIDs are not recommended in patients with advanced hepatic or renal disease due to the drugs' potential altered pharmacokinetic effects, which can potentiate increased adverse pharmacodynamic effects, including risk of bleeding and acute kidney injury.[6,14] NSAID elimination is dependent on the free (unbound) fraction of the drug within the plasma and the intrinsic enzyme activities of the liver to metabolize the drug to an excretable metabolite.

Dosing Guidelines

Most patients take therapeutic doses of NSAIDs for short durations of time and usually tolerate them well. NSAIDs have a dose-dependent relationship between concentration and therapeutic effects. All NSAIDs pose dose- and age-related risks of gastropathy and renal impairment. The enzyme COX-1 plays a role in protecting the stomach lining. Because most NSAIDs block COX-1, they all increase the risk of stomach ulcers and GI bleeding. *Naproxen* is the only NSAID with a neutral-positive cardiac profile. Some selective NSAIDs, along with some of the nonselective COX-inhibitor NSAIDs, were found to increase the risk of heart attacks (see Cardiovascular Effects section).

Precautions

Safety concerns exist for NSAID use in patients with, or at elevated risk for, cardiovascular disease, diabetes, or thrombotic events. NSAIDs should be avoided in patients with renal insufficiency (creatinine clearance <60 mL/min), GI bleeding, platelet dysfunction, reduced cardiac output, difficult-to-control hypertension, hypovolemia, hyponatremia, aspirin-sensitive asthma, or cirrhosis. NSAIDs may have a drug–drug interaction that induces hypoglycemia among diabetic patients prescribed other drugs.[18] Prescribers must use with caution or avoid NSAIDs in patients receiving anticoagulants, systemic corticosteroids, lithium, loop diuretics, and other interacting drugs.[29]

Drug–Drug Interactions

All the nonsalicylate, nonselective NSAIDs and acetylsalicylic acid (*aspirin*) inhibit platelet aggregation via inhibition of platelet COX-1 activity. NSAIDs may augment the risk of bleeding in patients receiving *warfarin* (Coumadin) and other blood thinner medications. The **anticoagulant** effects occur because almost all NSAIDs temporarily suppress normal platelet function during the dosing interval and because some NSAIDs also increase *warfarin* levels by interfering with its metabolism. Thus, concurrent administration of these medications should be avoided.[14,32] Low-dose *aspirin* is a special case relating to reducing risk of cardiovascular events, with the benefit of reducing the risk of secondary thrombotic cardiovascular events. These properties may be important enough to warrant its continued use in the patient who also needs a typical NSAID.[32]

Adverse Effects

The AT must realize that all NSAIDs may cause GI damage, although with varying intensity. Of note is the risk of distal GI toxicity of NSAIDs, which appears to increase with formulations that release drugs in the intestine (e.g., enteric-coated and sustained-release formulations).[15]

Gastrointestinal Toxicity

Many patients who develop a serious upper GI adverse event while receiving NSAID therapy are asymptomatic prior to diagnosis. The most common adverse effect of NSAIDs is GI injury,[15,32,33] which is often asymptomatic and may heal spontaneously.[14,15] The mechanism underlying NSAID-induced GI adverse effects is inhibition of prostaglandin synthesis, which causes weakening of the protective GI mucosal barrier, predisposing the stomach to bleeding.[36] All NSAID regimens have been shown to increase risk of upper GI complications.[5] In about 40% of patients, the most common GI symptoms associated with NSAIDs were dyspepsia, abdominal pain, nausea, and diarrhea. GI inflammation secondary to NSAID use can result in a peptic ulcer or gastroesophageal reflux disease, as reported by 48% of NSAID users taking the medication for ≥6 days.[30]

Platelet inhibition by NSAIDs increases the likelihood of gastric bleeding when mucosal damage has occurred. Coadministration of proton pump inhibitors or H_2 antagonists in conjunction with NSAIDs reduces the rate of duodenal and gastric ulceration;[14] however, the long-term use of these medications has become controversial.

Cardiovascular Effects

Monitoring patients, particularly those with renal or cardiovascular comorbidities, is essential. Overall, considering the increased incidence of cardiovascular complications associated with inflammatory conditions, NSAID use where there is even a slight risk of aggravating these adverse effects may result in serious outcomes, particularly in high-risk patients. Cardiovascular adverse events such as myocardial infarction, cerebrovascular accidents (stroke), and death are associated with several NSAIDs.[15]

Nephrotoxicity

The use of all NSAIDs has been associated with dose-dependent renal side effects with various etiologies.[15] Compared with GI and cardiovascular risks, renal side effects of NSAIDs are considered uncommon at doses recommended in the manufacturer's labeling.[36] However, there is a risk of renal damage with any of the NSAIDs, especially in elderly patients or patients with preexisting renal disease. Because these drugs are cleared by the kidney, renal damage results in higher, more toxic serum concentrations.[17,36] NSAIDs cause inhibition of prostaglandin and thromboxane synthesis, leading to renal vasoconstriction and consequently reduced renal perfusion and aberrant renal function. Clinical manifestations of NSAID-induced nephrotoxicity include electrolyte abnormalities such as hyperkalemia, reduced glomerular filtration rate, nephrotic syndrome related to drug-induced minimal change disease, chronic kidney disease, acute interstitial nephritis, sodium retention, edema, and renal papillary necrosis.[36]

Genetics appears to have an influence on the effects of NSAIDS on kidney function and risk of kidney disease. A study of U.S. military members (>22 years old and <50 years old; average age 28) centered on the association of NSAIDs and acute and chronic kidney disease reported that African American soldiers had at least twice the hazard of chronic kidney disease when compared to white and Hispanic soldiers.[24] The AT caring for a patient population within this range should be cognizant of the prospect of kidney dysfunction with NSAID use.

RED FLAG

Unintended Consequences of NSAIDs on the Kidneys

With the use of NSAIDs comes the associated risk of acute kidney injury (AKI), which can lead to chronic kidney disease. AKI is the result of compromised renal hemodynamics, intravascular volume depletion, and reduction of glomerular capillary pressure.[27] Acute kidney compromise can occur with a single NSAID dose; however, an online survey of *ibuprofen* users indicated that 15% of participants admitted exceeding the recommended daily dose.[26,27] Not recognizing AKI could potentially lead to a more significant disease process that requires dialysis.[12]

Acute kidney injury results from a reduction in **glomerular filtration rate (GFR)** that causes injury to the proximal tubule and may result in chronic kidney disease.[15] Acute forms of side effects secondary to NSAID use are dependent on dose and duration, and many of the side effects are short term and reversible on NSAID withdrawal. Chronic use of NSAIDs is relatively free of renal side effects in the average patient. However, in some patients—particularly those who have other risk factors or are using other drugs that can cause kidney damage, such as diuretics and angiotensin-converting enzyme (ACE) inhibitors—chronic NSAID use may result in end-stage chronic renal disease. However, for the majority of patients, renal side effects of NSAIDs are rare, particularly if high or supratherapeutic doses are avoided.[15]

Hypersensitivity

Hypersensitivity symptoms to *aspirin* and NSAIDs range from vasomotor rhinitis, generalized urticaria, and bronchial asthma to laryngeal edema, bronchoconstriction, flushing, hypotension, and shock. *Aspirin* intolerance (including aspirin-associated asthma) is a contraindication to therapy with any

Evidence in Pharmacology

Excessive Doses of NSAIDs Can Cause Acute Kidney Injury

It is estimated that NSAID prescriptions were issued to >98 million Americans in 2012. A variety of OTC NSAIDs are available for purchase in pharmacies, grocery stores, and vending machines, and 36 million Americans have used OTC versions of these medications. With the easy access of NSAIDs comes the risk of acute kidney injury (AKI) and chronic kidney disease (CKD). Acute kidney compromise can occur with a single NSAID dose. An online survey of *ibuprofen* users indicated that 15% of participants admitted exceeding the recommended daily dose. Several diagnostic tests are available to a physician to diagnose kidney dysfunction; however, the presence of **hematuria** should be a red flag to the AT with patients who take NSAIDs.[27]

One such case of kidney disease involved a professional football player who used excessive doses of an OTC NSAID for ≥3 months, resulting in the premature end of his football career.[1] AKI results from reduced renal plasma flow due to a decrease in the renal prostaglandins that regulate vasodilation to the glomerular level.[9] Compromises of renal hemodynamics, intravascular volume depletion, and reduction of glomerular capillary pressure also contribute to AKI.[27] Another mechanism of AKI, acute interstitial nephritis (AIN), is the presence of inflammatory cells that have infiltrated the kidney's interstitium.[9] Patients with AKI are at greater risk of developing CKD, which presents as reduced kidney function or evidence of kidney damage. Adverse kidney events secondary to NSAID use occur in 1% to 5% of all patients exposed to NSAIDs, but account for 37% of all drug-reported cases of AKI.[26,27] If the AT suspects that a patient may have AKI as a result of NSAID use, it is recommended that the patient be referred and evaluated by the prescriber.[9]

---

other NSAID because of cross-sensitivity. Although less common in children, this cross-sensitivity may occur in 10% to 25% of patients with asthma, nasal polyps, or chronic urticaria and in 1% of apparently healthy people. Hypersensitivity reaction can be provoked by even low doses (<80 mg) of *aspirin* and involves COX inhibition. Treatment of hypersensitivity to *aspirin* and other NSAIDs is similar to that for other severe hypersensitivity reactions: support of vital organ function and administration of epinephrine.[14]

The following sections present a summary of the NSAID classes most commonly used in the AT setting: the salicylates and the propionic acid derivatives. These 2 medication classes have the same effects as other NSAIDs, so the discussion of each of these drug classes is limited to the differences specific to each.

Salicylates

Acetylsalicylic acid (ASA or *aspirin*), the prototypical salicylate NSAID, is a widely consumed analgesic, antipyretic, and anti-inflammatory agent (table 9.4).[13,33] Initially found in the bark of the willow tree, it is considered the original NSAID. *Aspirin* is one of the most widely used medications globally and is on the World Health Organization's (WHO's) list of essential medicines, a list of the safest and most effective medicines needed in a health system.[37]

The effects of *aspirin* are largely caused by its capacity to acetylate proteins. Other salicylates generally act by virtue of their content of salicylic acid, which is a relatively weak inhibitor of the purified COX enzymes.[14] The major difference between the mechanisms of action of *aspirin* and those of other NSAIDs is that *aspirin* irreversibly inhibits COX and platelet functioning for the life of the platelet (7 to 10 days).[32] The irreversible action of *aspirin* results in a longer duration of its antiplatelet effect and is the basis for its use as an antithrombotic drug.[17,32]

The dose of a typical *aspirin* tablet is 325 mg. In general, for fever or as an analgesic, the usual dose is 325 to 650 mg every 4 to 6 hours or 1,000 mg every 6 hours up to 3 times per day. The maximum recommended dose per day is 3,000 mg.

The beneficial effects of *aspirin* may be attenuated by prior or ongoing administration of some nonselective NSAIDs, such as *ibuprofen* or *naproxen*. Thus, regular NSAID use should be avoided, if possible, in patients taking low-dose *aspirin* for cardiovascular protection. In patients on aspirin who require NSAIDs on an occasional short-term basis, extend-

TABLE 9.4 Pharmacodynamics and Pharmacokinetics of a Prototypical Salicylate NSAID

Generic name	*acetylsalicylic acid (ASA), aspirin*
Trade name	Bayer, Bufferin, many others
Category	Nonselective COX inhibitor NSAID, nonopioid analgesic, antiplatelet agent
Route	Oral: immediate release or extended release
Onset of action	Within 1 hr (nonenteric coated); onset of enteric-coated aspirin is expected to be delayed.
Peak effect	Immediate release: ~1-2 hr (nonenteric coated), 3-4 hr (enteric coated) Extended-release capsule: 2 hr Chewing nonenteric-coated tablets results in a time to peak concentration of 20 min. Chewing enteric-coated tablets results in a time to peak concentration of 2 hr.
Duration	4-6 hr; however, platelet inhibitory effects last the lifetime of the platelet (~10 d) due to its irreversible inhibition of platelet COX-1.
Bioavailability	50% to 75% reaches the systemic circulation.
Half-life	Plasma concentration: 15-20 min Dose dependent: 3 hr at lower doses (300-600 mg), 5 to 6 hr (after 1 g), 10 hr with higher doses
Absorption	Rapidly absorbed in stomach and upper intestine
Distribution	Readily distributed into most body fluids and tissues, red blood cells, synovial fluid, and blood
Metabolism	Hydrolyzed to salicylate (active) in GI mucosa. Metabolism of salicylate occurs primarily by hepatic conjugation. Metabolic pathways are saturable.
Excretion	Urine (75% as salicyluric acid, 10% as salicylic acid, and 15% other metabolites)
Clinical note	Chewing nonenteric-coated or enteric-coated tablets results in inhibition of platelet aggregation within 20 min; therefore, nonenteric-coated tablets should be chewed in settings where a more rapid onset is required (e.g., acute MI) and enteric-coated tablets may be chewed when a rapid effect is required and immediate-release nonenteric-coated tablets are not available.

NSAID = nonsteroidal anti-inflammatory drug; COX-1 = cyclooxygenase-1; MI = myocardial infarction

ed-release *aspirin* should be taken ≥2 hours before or ≥8 hours after the NSAID.[32]

Aspirin is rapidly absorbed and distributed throughout the body, which can lead to several adverse effects. Chronic *aspirin* use can produce gastric irritation and erosion, hemorrhage, vomiting, and renal tubular necrosis. These concerns limit the usefulness of *aspirin* primarily to acute pain settings.[13] **Reye's syndrome** is a rare but serious disorder of rapid liver degeneration and brain damage.[17,33] The cause of Reye's syndrome is unknown, but many cases seem to follow infection with influenza A or B or varicella. Using *aspirin* during such illness increases the risk of Reye's syndrome by as much as 35-fold.[28] Fortunately, the incidence of Reye's syndrome has fallen dramatically as the public has been educated not to give *aspirin* to children.[14,17,33]

Propionic Acid Derivatives

Among the propionic acid derivatives, *ibuprofen* (Advil, Motrin) is the most commonly used NSAID in the United States and is available OTC or with a prescription. Used primarily for its analgesic and anti-inflammatory effects, *ibuprofen* is also an antipyretic, and it has a lower incidence of adverse effects than *aspirin*. Propionic acid derivatives are nonselective COX inhibitors with the effects and side effects common to other NSAIDs. In addition to the prototypical drug, *ibuprofen*, other propionic acids include the following:[14,17,32,33]

- *naproxen* (Aleve, Naprosyn)
- *ketoprofen* (Orudis, Oruvail, Actron)
- *fenoprofen* (Nalfon, Fenortho, ProFeno)

Ibuprofen is absorbed rapidly, binds avidly to protein, and undergoes hepatic metabolism (90% is metabolized) and renal excretion of metabolites. It is short acting, with a $t_{1/2}$ of about 2 hours (see table 9.5); however, slow equilibration with the synovial space means that its antiarthritic effects may persist after plasma levels decline. *Ibuprofen* is supplied as tablets, chewable tablets, capsules, caplets, and gel caps containing 50 to 800 mg; as oral suspension; and as an injectable. Solid oral dosage forms containing 200 mg are commonly available without a prescription. *Ibuprofen* is licensed for marketing alone and in fixed-dose combinations with antihistamines, histamine-2 blockers, decongestants, and *hydrocodone*. The usual dose for mild to moderate pain is 400 mg every 4 to 6 hours as needed.[14]

Other propionic acid derivatives, particularly *naproxen* (Aleve, Naprosyn), have inhibitory effects on leukocyte function. Some evidence suggests that compared to *ibuprofen*, *naproxen* may have slightly better efficacy with analgesia and relief of morning stiffness. This benefit accords with the longer $t_{1/2}$ of *naproxen* in comparison to other propionic acid derivatives.[13,14] The longer $t_{1/2}$ of *naproxen* allows this drug to be administered less frequently with equivalent analgesic efficacy. Its adverse effect profile is similar to *ibuprofen*, and it is generally well tolerated. As with all NSAIDs, *ibuprofen* and *naproxen* can cause GI complications ranging from dyspepsia to gastric bleeding.[13]

Summary

This chapter describes the mechanism of action of anti-inflammatory medications, including corticosteroids and NSAIDs. Anti-inflammatory medications are potent drugs with important adverse effects. Compared to NSAIDs, corticosteroids exhibit superior anti-inflammatory efficacy, particularly for the medical management of systemic inflammatory conditions. *Prednisone*, a widely used systemic preparation, is a potent anti-inflammatory and immunosuppressive drug that has serious potential adverse effects if overused. Chronic use

TABLE 9.5 Pharmacodynamics and Pharmacokinetics of a Prototypical Propionic Acid NSAID

Generic name	*ibuprofen*
Trade name	Advil, Motrin
Category	Nonselective COX inhibitor NSAID, nonopioid analgesic, antipyretic
Route	Oral, injectable
Onset of action	Analgesic: within 60 min
Peak effect	1-2 hr
Duration	6-8 hr
Bioavailability	80%
Half-life	2 hr
Absorption	Rapid (85%)
Distribution	V_d = 0.12 L/kg
Metabolism	Hepatic
Excretion	Urine (primarily as metabolites: 45-80%), some in feces
Clinical note	To avoid gastric upset, patients should be instructed to take medication after meals and educated about the signs of a significant hypersensitive reaction (e.g., wheezing; chest tightness; fever; itching; bad cough; blue skin color; seizures; or swelling of face, lips, tongue, or throat). Note: This is not a comprehensive list of all side effects. Patients should consult the prescriber with additional questions.

Evidence in Pharmacology

Adverse Cardiac Effects of NSAIDs

Ibuprofen (Advil, Motrin) has been associated with significantly increased major coronary events (RR 2.22, 99% CI 1.10-4.48; $p = 0.0253$), but not major vascular events (RR 1.44, CI 0.89-2.33).[2,5] Compared with patients who used a placebo, among the 1,000 patients allocated to a *-coxib* or *diclofenac* (Voltaren) for a year, there were more major vascular events, 1 of which was fatal. *Naproxen* (Aleve, Naprosyn) did not significantly increase major vascular events (RR 0.93, CI 0.69-1.27). Vascular death was increased significantly by *-coxibs* (RR 1.58, 99% CI 1.00-2.49; $p = 0.0103$) and *diclofenac* (RI 1.65, CI 0.95-2.85, $p = 0.0187$) and nonsignificantly by *ibuprofen* (RR 1.90, CI 0.56-6.41; $p = 0.17$), but was not increased by *naproxen* (RR 1.08, CI 0.48-2.47, $p = 0.80$). The proportional effects on major vascular events were independent of baseline characteristics, including vascular risk. Heart failure risk was roughly doubled by all NSAIDs. Additionally, all NSAID regimens increased upper GI complications.[2,5] It is best to minimize the use of NSAIDs in general and especially in patients with cardiovascular disease. If an NSAID must be used, the best advice for practice is to use the drug with the safest profile in the lowest dose for the shortest period of time.[2] The FDA has determined that the data differentiating the risk between distinct NSAIDs is not sufficient to distinguish between drugs on the regulatory level; thus, a cardiovascular risk warning is included on the label of all NSAIDs.[14]

---

of corticosteroids is associated with many adverse effects, such as Cushing's syndrome; however, a few days or even a week of corticosteroid therapy generally has minimal to no side effects. In the sports medicine setting, corticosteroids are commonly used for the reduction of inflammation and joint pain. Increasingly, topical medications are being used to locally provide anti-inflammatory effects. Some corticosteroids are formulated as a long-acting depot formulation intended for intramuscular, intralesional, or intra-articular injection, a formulation that provides an extended duration of action (for example, depot preparations of *methylprednisolone* provide anti-inflammatory effects for 1 to 4 weeks).[4,31]

This chapter also provides a detailed discussion of nonsteroidal anti-inflammatory drugs (NSAIDs), which are used to reduce chronic and acute inflammation in patients with a variety of conditions. Both therapeutic and adverse effects of NSAIDs are due to inhibition of the cyclooxygenase (COX) enzyme. NSAIDs are classified as nonselective and COX-2-selective inhibitors (*-coxibs*) based on their extent of selectivity for COX inhibition. However, regardless of their COX selectivity, common side effects of NSAIDs involve the GI tract, sometimes with serious GI complications, renal disturbances, and cardiovascular events. Indeed, several *-coxib* medications have been withdrawn due to serious cardiovascular side effects. In the sports medicine setting, there is a tendency to believe that all NSAIDs can be safely taken on a regular basis for acute and chronic pain.[15] However, solid evidence demonstrates that caution is necessary when administering these medications in the athletic training setting.

Case Studies

Case Study 1

Antoinette is a local fire fighter who recently resumed the strength training and fitness program she had participated in 10 years earlier. To complement her fitness program, she tried to lose weight by cutting back on her food intake. She strained her lower back at a fire scene and subsequently reduced her strength training and fitness work. Antoinette was prescribed an NSAID and was adherent in taking it, particularly first thing in the morning. She experienced intermittent stomach pain that increased as she continued the NSAID treatment. When she began to have a bloody stool, which concerned her, Antionette returned to her physician. The physician determined that Antoinette had been taking her morning NSAID dose without food.

Questions for Analysis

1. Why should an NSAID be taken with food?
2. How much food taken with the medication is generally enough to prevent the side effects associated with NSAID use?

Case Study 2

Karen is a skilled softball player dedicated to playing every game during her senior season. After sustaining an ankle sprain, her team physician prescribed the NSAID *naproxen* to manage inflammation. In addition, Karen self-medicated with OTC *ibuprofen*, reasoning that the medications had different names and functions. Because of this combination of drugs, Karen ran the risk of exceeding the recommended daily dose of NSAID medications, which could contribute to renal or gastrointestinal complications. Karen mentioned this to her athletic trainer, who advised her to stop the *ibuprofen* immediately and use only the medication prescribed by the team physician.

Questions for Analysis

1. A scenario like this is not unusual: A highly motivated, goal-oriented patient is trying to accelerate recovery. How could this have been prevented?
2. Is there any concern for stopping the *ibuprofen* earlier than otherwise expected?

Drugs Described in This Chapter

Drug class	*generic* (pronunciation) Trade name	Therapeutic uses	Clinical concerns
Anti-inflammatories: corticosteroids	*prednisone* (PRED ni sone) Generic only	Immediate-release only: as adjunctive therapy for short-term administration in acute and subacute bursitis, acute gout flares, acute nonspecific tenosynovitis, ankylosing spondylitis, epicondylitis, posttraumatic osteoarthritis, and synovitis of osteoarthritis. Dose depends on the condition being treated and the response of the patient.	Patient is more susceptible for infection; risk is greater with higher dosages. Some signs of an infection may be masked by *prednisone*. Side effects are more likely to be experienced at dosages >7.5 mg/d and with long-term therapy. **Neuromuscular and skeletal:** Effects include amyotrophy, aseptic necrosis of bones (femoral and humeral heads), osteoporosis, pathological fracture (long bones), rupture of tendon (particularly Achilles tendon), steroid myopathy, and vertebral compression fracture. **Endocrine and metabolic:** Long-term *prednisone* administration has been associated with the suppression of the hypothalamic-pituitary-adrenal (HPA) axis. Suppression of this axis can result in corticosteroid insufficiency. Cushing's syndrome: Consider alternate-day therapy for long-term use. Discontinuation of long-term therapy requires gradual withdrawal by tapering the dose.

Drug class	*generic* (pronunciation) Trade name	Therapeutic uses	Clinical concerns
Anti-inflammatories: nonsteroidal, nonselective COX inhibitors	*aspirin* (AS pir in) Bayer, Bufferin, many others	Inhibits platelet aggregation; has antipyretic, analgesic, and anti-inflammatory properties. **Emergency treatment of acute myocardial infarction:** Nonenteric-coated, chewable 81 to 325 mg tablets given on presentation. Analgesic and antipyretic, oral tablet 325 to 650 mg as needed every 4 hr or as directed by health care provider. Maximum daily dose: 4 g/d	Do not use extended-release capsules in situations for which a rapid onset of action is required (such as emergency treatment of acute MI); use immediate-release formulations instead. Administer medication with food or a full glass of water to minimize GI distress. Extended-release capsules: Do not cut, crush, or chew. Do not administer 2 hr before or 1 hr after alcohol consumption. Serious adverse effects include GI toxicity, nephrotoxicity, and increased bleeding time at therapeutic levels, bronchoconstrictor reaction due to increased leukotrienes, tinnitus, hyperventilation, metabolic acidosis, hyperthermia, coma in overdose.
	ibuprofen (eye byoo PROE fen) Advil, Motrin, many others	Reduction of fever, headache, migraine, sore throat, arthritis, physical or athletic overexertion (e.g., sprains and strains), menstrual pain, dental pain, backache, pain due to the common cold and flu; minor muscle, bone, or joint pain. OTC doses are 200 mg every 4-6 hr as needed; if no relief, the patient may increase the dose to 400 mg every 4-6 hr as needed (maximum: 1,200 mg/d). Duration: treatment for >10 d as an analgesic or >3 d as an antipyretic is not recommended unless directed by prescriber. Prescription doses allow for 400 to 3,200 mg daily.	**U.S. boxed warning:** Serious cardiovascular thrombotic events can occur. *Ibuprofen* causes increased risk of serious cardiovascular thrombotic events, including myocardial infarction, and stroke, which can be fatal. This risk may occur early in treatment and may increase with duration of use. **U.S. boxed warning:** NSAIDs cause an increased risk of serious GI inflammation, ulceration, bleeding, and perforation (may be fatal). These events may occur at any time during therapy and without warning. Avoid use in patients with active GI bleeding. Platelet adhesion and aggregation may be decreased. NSAID use may prolong bleeding time; patients with coagulation disorders or who are receiving anticoagulants should be monitored closely. Have the patient report immediately to the prescriber signs of aseptic meningitis, abdominal ulcers, signs of internal bleeding, shortness of breath, swelling of arms or legs, angina, tachycardia, severe headache, severe dizziness, passing out, severe loss of strength and energy, tinnitus, severe nausea, vomiting, severe abdominal pain, severe back pain, and vision changes.

This is not a comprehensive list of all side effects. Patients should consult their prescriber with additional questions.

10

Drugs to Treat Infection: Antibiotics

OBJECTIVES

After reading this chapter, you will be able to do the following:

- Describe the various types of antimicrobial medications
- Describe the mechanism of action for antibiotic medications
- List general considerations of antibiotic use and people at risk for bacterial infections
- Recognize clinical manifestations of bacterial infections
- Identify clinical scenarios in which use of antibacterial agents is inappropriate
- Collaborate with prescribers and other health care providers on antibiotic misuse and stewardship

Antimicrobial agents have had a major influence on human health. Together with vaccines, **antimicrobials** have contributed to reduced mortality, extended life span, and enhanced quality of life. However, antimicrobial drugs must be used with caution because they promote the occurrence of drug resistance in both the pathogens they are designed to treat and in other bystander organisms. Antibiotics are prescribed to approximately one-third of all hospitalized patients and account for >10% of hospital pharmacy expenditures. Up to half of antibiotic orders may be unnecessary, poorly chosen, or dosed incorrectly.[10] The overuse of antibiotics has led to a decrease in their effectiveness and the emergence of superbugs, or **multidrug-resistant organisms (MDROs)**. These are strains of bacteria that have developed resistance to many different types of antibiotics. The following bacteria are examples of MDROs:[22]

- *Methicillin*-resistant *Staphylococcus aureus* (MRSA)
- *Pseudomonas aeruginosa*
- *Vancomycin*-resistant *enterococcus* (VRE)

Of great concern is that new strains of bacteria may emerge that cannot be treated by any existing antibiotics.[22] Antibiotics are used to treat or prevent **infections** by pathogens, specifically, bacterial infections. They are not effective against viral infections, such as the common cold or influenza.[10,15,31]

In this chapter, the terms *antibacterial agents* and *antibiotic drugs* are used interchangeably. The term **antibiotic** refers to medicines that treat infections.[10] Prescribers select the **antibacterial** drug based on an understanding of each drug's mechanism of action, spectrum of activity, mechanisms of resistance, pharmacology, and adverse effect profile.[15] Since the category of antibiotics is so broad, these drugs are

Select Drugs Mentioned in This Chapter

Antibiotic types	Generic name	Trade name
β-lactam (broad-spectrum) aminopenicillins	*amoxicillin* *penicillin* *ampicillin*	Amoxil Generic only Generic only
β-lactam cephalosporins	*cephalexin* *ceftriaxone*	Keflex Rocephin
β-lactam carbapenems	*imipenem* *meropenem*	Primaxin Merrem
Macrolides	*azithromycin* *erythromycin* *clarithromycin*	Zithromax, Z-pak Ery-Tab Biaxin
Tetracyclines	*doxycycline* *tetracycline*	Vibramycin, Monodox Tetracap (many others)
Fluoroquinolones	*ciprofloxacin*	Cipro
Aminoglycosides	*gentamicin* *tobramycin*	Cidomycin, Clindacin (topical) Tobrex
Nitroimidazoles	*metronidazole*	Flagyl, MetroGel
Sulfonamides (also called sulfa drugs)	*sulfamethoxazole* and *trimethoprim**	Bactrim, Septra
Glycopeptides	*vancomycin*	Vancocin

This list is not exhaustive, but rather contains drugs commonly encountered in the athletic training setting. Always consult up-to-date information, confirm with a pharmacist, or discuss the use of therapeutic medications with the prescriber of the medication.
**Trimethoprim* is not a sulfonamide. Although it is chemically dissimilar to *sulfamethoxazole*, it has a similar mechanism of action.

Antimicrobial Medicines

Antimicrobial medicines are grouped according to the microorganisms they primarily act against. Microorganisms—also called microbes—include bacteria, viruses, fungi, and parasites. Antimicrobials are medicinal products that kill or stop the growth of living microorganisms and include the following:[9,10,15]

- **Antibacterials** (also called antibiotics)—Drugs active against bacterial infections
  - **Bactericidal**—Agents that kill bacteria
  - **Bacteriostatic**—Agents that slow down or stall the growth of bacteria
- Medications that do not treat bacterial infections but are critical to treating microorganisms
  - **Antivirals**—Drugs active against viral infections
  - **Antifungals**—Drugs active against fungal infections
  - **Antiparasitics**—Drugs active against malaria and other infections due to parasites

Many of these drugs are discussed in future chapters.

subdivided into functional drug groups or classes to facilitate understanding and prescribing practices. To assist the learning of this class of medication, this chapter describes the classes of antibacterial medications and collectively provides the therapeutic effects, mechanism of action, route of administration, pharmacodynamics, pharmacokinetics, dosing guidelines, indications and precautions, and adverse effects of these medicines. Athletic trainers (ATs) do not need to know all the available antibiotic medications; rather, a general understanding of the classes of antibiotics and representative examples will help to advise patients and discuss patient care with prescribers and other health care providers. Topical antibiotics used in the treatment of dermatological conditions are discussed in chapter 16.

Indications for Use

Manifestations of a bacterial infection may present as local (e.g., cellulitis, abscess) or systemic (e.g., most often fever). Manifestations can develop in multiple organ systems and may lead to severe, generalized infections that have life-threatening consequences (e.g., sepsis and septic shock). Most manifestations resolve with successful treatment of the underlying infection.[4] Prescribers use their findings from the physical examination along with the clinical presentation to determine the anatomic location of the infection. Often with diagnostic or laboratory testing, prescribers can discern the most probable pathogens associated with disease (figure 10.1). A common host response to bacterial toxins accompanying bacterial infection is fever, which is a rise in body temperature above the normal 98.6°F (37°C).[28]

Bacteria are classified by the following:

- **Morphology (shape)**—Classified by spheres (cocci), rods (bacilli), and spirals or helixes (spirochetes; see figure 10.2).
- **Gram staining**—A bacteriological laboratory technique used to differentiate bacterial species into **Gram-positive** and **Gram-negative** groups based on the physical properties of their cell walls.
- **Encapsulation**—Encapsulated bacteria (e.g., *Streptococcus pneumoniae, Haemophilus influenzae*) are protected from ingestion by phagocytes, thereby increasing bacterial **virulence**.
- **Oxygen requirements**—Aerobic bacteria (obligate aerobes) require oxygen to produce energy and grow in culture. Anaerobic bacteria (obligate anaerobes) do not require oxygen and do not grow in culture if air is present. Anaerobic bacteria are common in the gastrointestinal tract, vagina, dental crevices, and chronic wounds when blood supply is impaired. These bacteria occur naturally and are the most common flora in the body. In their natural state, they don't cause infection. However, they can cause infections after an injury or trauma to the body.

The following sections discuss commonalities among antibacterials as a class of medication. The use of specific medications from common groups of antibacterials used in the athletic training setting is described in the Indications and Precautions section found later in this chapter.

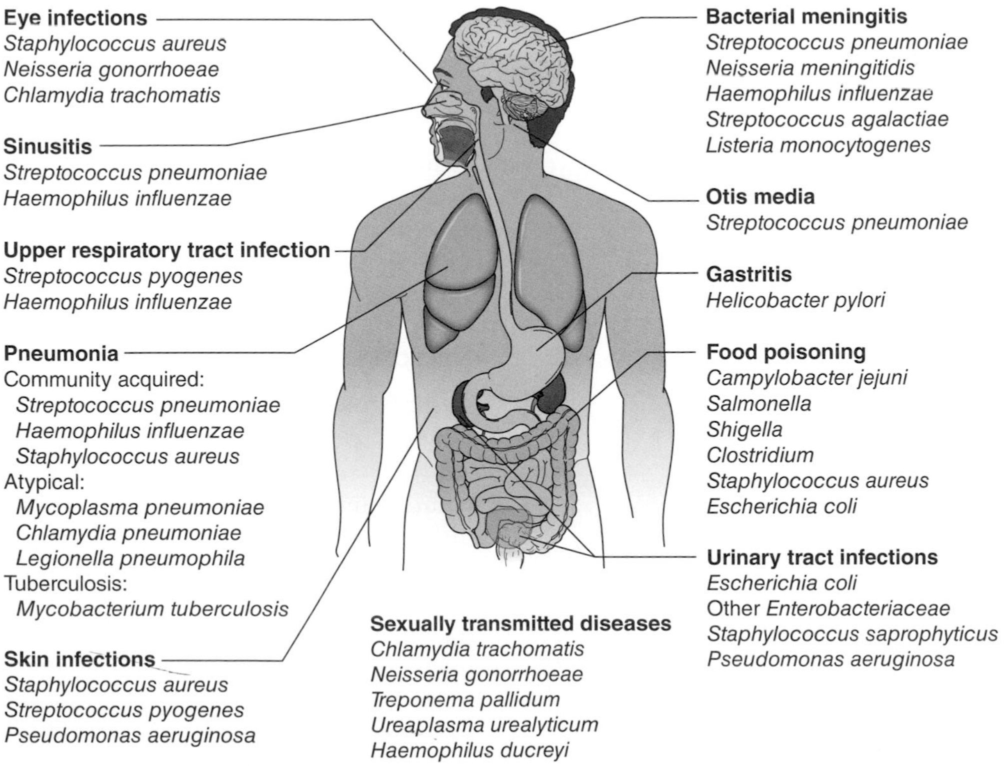

FIGURE 10.1 Common bacterial infections.

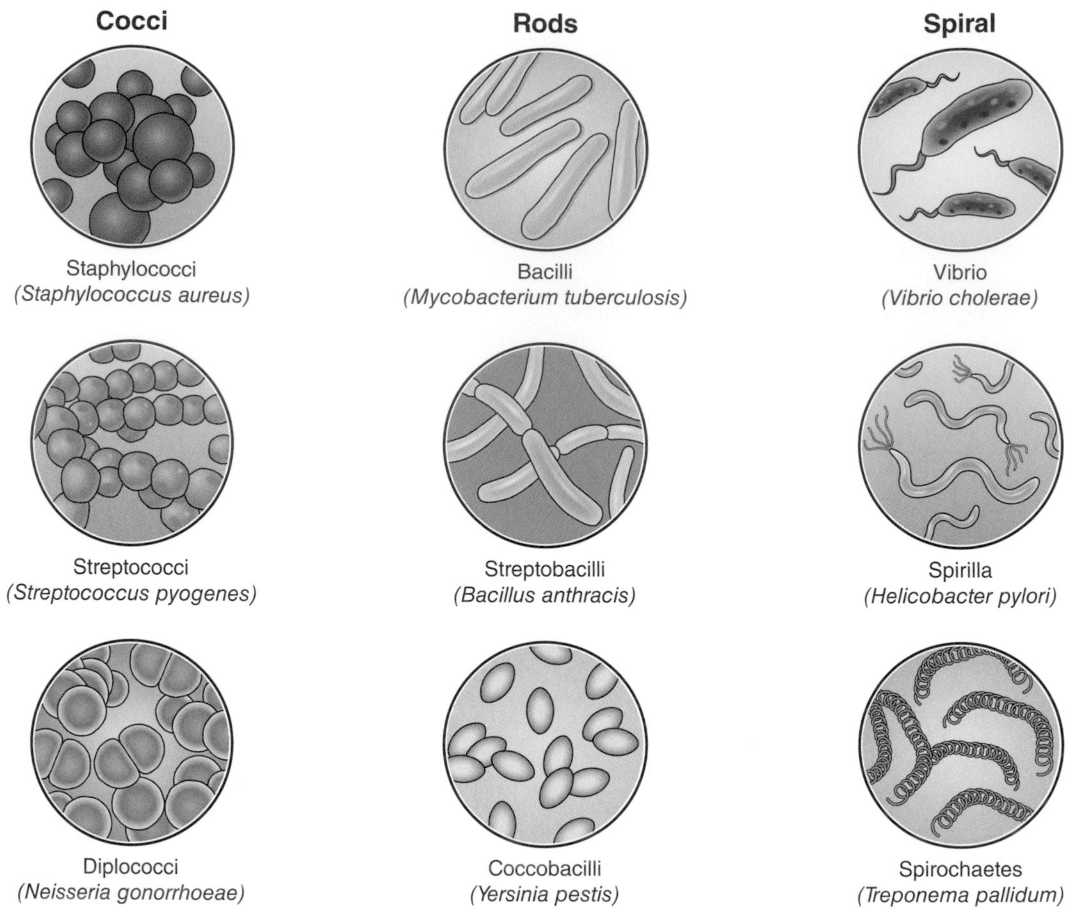

FIGURE 10.2 Shapes of bacteria.

Mechanism of Action

Antibiotics have many mechanisms of action (figure 10.3):[15,22]

- Inhibition of cell wall synthesis (most common mechanism)
- Inhibition of protein synthesis (second largest class)
- Alteration of cell membrane structure
- Inhibition of nucleic acid synthesis
- Antimetabolic activity

Human Microbiome

Some bacteria cause disease; however, others normally occupy a particular site in the body as **resident flora** (or **microbiome**) and do not usually cause disease.[4,29] Healthy people live in harmony with most of the microorganisms that establish themselves, or colonize, in nonsterile parts of the body, such as the skin, nose, mouth, throat, large intestine, and vagina. Cells of the microbiome outnumber a person's own cells 10:1.[4,30] The resident flora at each site include several different types of microorganisms, and some sites are normally colonized by several hundred different types of microorganisms. Environmental factors, such as diet, antibiotic use, sanitary conditions, air pollution, and hygienic habits, influence what species make up a person's microbiome. If disturbed (for example, by washing the skin or using antibiotics), the microbiome usually promptly reestablishes itself.

Spectrum of Activity

Antimicrobials vary in their ability to inhibit or kill different species of bacteria. Antimicrobials that kill many different species of bacteria are **broad-spectrum** antimicrobials, whereas those that kill fewer different species of bacteria are **narrow-spectrum** antimicrobials. Broad-spectrum antimicrobial coverage increases the likelihood of empirically treating a causative pathogen; unfortunately, secondary infections caused by certain antimicrobial-resistant pathogens commonly develop. In addition, adverse events may complicate up to 10% of antimicrobial therapy (adverse event rate is higher for select

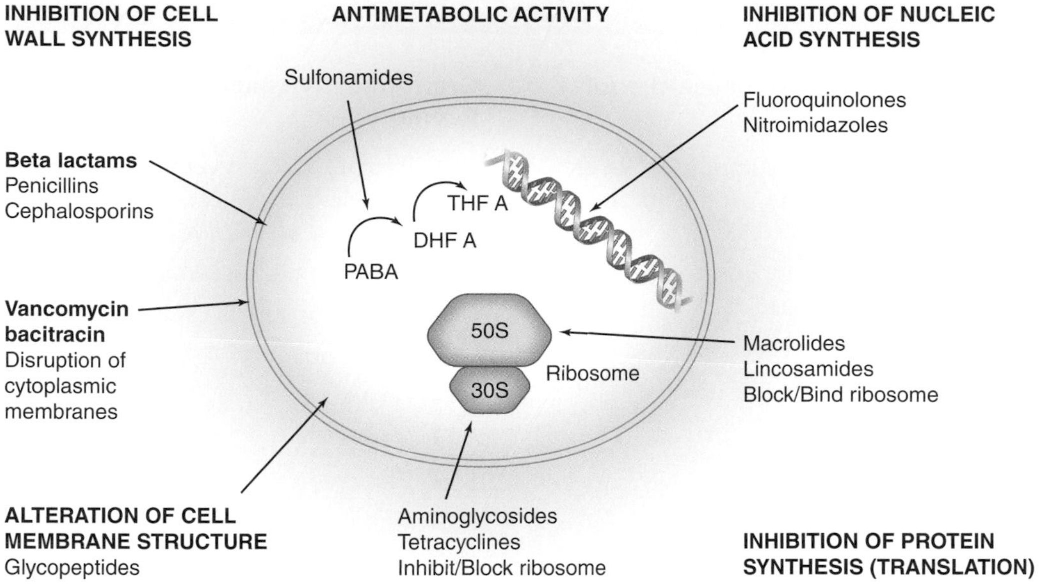

FIGURE 10.3 Mechanisms of action of antibiotics on bacterial cells.

Infections and the Human Microbiome

Rather than causing disease, the microbiome protects the body against disease-causing organisms. However, under certain conditions, microorganisms that are part of a person's microbiome may cause disease. Such conditions include the following:[4,30]

- The use of antibiotics
- Injury or surgery
- A weakened immune system (as occurs in people with AIDS, people taking corticosteroids, or those receiving cancer chemotherapy)

When antibiotics are used to treat an infection, they also kill a large proportion of certain types of bacteria of the microbiome; thus, other resident bacteria or fungi can grow unchecked. For example, if a woman takes antibiotics for a urinary tract infection, the antibiotics kill some of the resident flora, allowing yeast in the vagina to multiply and cause a vaginal yeast infection.[4,30]

agents).[22,28,31] Identifying the specific pathogen or microorganism using laboratory tests such as Gram staining (e.g., throat culture for *Streptococcus*) is important in selecting the correct antibiotic for the patient's condition.

Some Gram-positive bacteria are resident microorganisms that occupy sites in the body, such as the skin. These bacteria do not usually cause disease. However, some Gram-positive bacteria do cause disease; these are increasingly becoming resistant to antibiotics. For example, *Staphylococcus aureus*, a Gram-positive aerobic bacterium, is highly pathogenic. It commonly causes skin infections and abscess formation and sometimes pneumonia, endocarditis, and osteomyelitis. *Methicillin*-resistant *Staphylococcus aureus* (MRSA) bacteria have developed resistance to most antibiotics related to *penicillin* (*methicillin* is a type of extended-spectrum *penicillin*).[5] MRSA strains are commonly involved in infections acquired in health care facilities (health care–associated infections) as well as community-acquired infections (acquired outside of health care facilities). Among Gram-positive pathogens, *Staphylococcus aureus*, *Streptococcus pneumoniae*, and, more recently, *Enterococcus* species present global antibiotic resistance challenges that cause significant public health concerns and add to the cost of health care.[31]

Spectrum of Bacteria

Gram-positive bacteria can cause the following:

- Skin and soft-tissue infections, heart valve infections, bone infections, and septicemia (*Staphylococcus aureus*)
- Pneumonia, meningitis, and middle ear infections (*Pneumococcus*)
- Pharyngitis or strep throat, pneumonia, wound and skin infections, sepsis, and endocarditis (*Streptococcus*)
- Endocarditis, urinary tract infections, prostatitis, intra-abdominal infection, cellulitis, wound infection, and concurrent bacteremia (*Enterococcus*)
- Toxic shock syndrome
- Diphtheria
- Anthrax

Gram-negative bacteria can cause the following:

- Urinary tract infections, watery diarrhea (traveler's diarrhea), pelvic inflammatory disease (*Escherichia coli*, or *E. coli*)
- Bloodstream infections
- Wound or surgical site infections
- Meningitis
- Peritonitis
- Plague
- Cholera
- Typhoid fever

Gram-negative bacterial infections can be serious. Gram-negative bacteria are enclosed in a protective cell wall that prevents the white blood cells in the immune system from ingesting the bacteria. This outer membrane protects the bacteria against certain antibiotics, such as *penicillin*. When disrupted, this membrane releases toxic substances (endotoxins) that contribute to the severity of symptoms during infections with Gram-negative bacteria. Some Gram-negative bacterial infections are common in the United States. For example, the Gram-negative bacteria *Escherichia coli* (*E. coli*) are the most numerous aerobic **commensal** inhabitants of the large intestine. Certain strains cause diarrhea, and all can cause infection when they invade sterile sites (e.g., the urinary tract).

Therapeutic Effects

Although there are hundreds of different types of antibiotics, many are structurally related and thus grouped into classes. Drugs within each class share structural and functional similarities, although they often have different pharmacology and spectra of activity.[30] Most antibiotics can be classified into specific groups based on mechanism of action and spectrum of bactericidal activity (table 10.1).[15,19,22]

Routes of Administration

Most antibiotics prescribed to patients are delivered via the enteral (gastrointestinal) route. These are typically in the form of pills, tablets, or capsules, and are occasionally liquid. Patients with a functioning gastrointestinal (GI) tract and without hemodynamic instability may receive oral antibacterials, especially if the agent has good bioavailability. However, patients manifesting systemic signs of infection such as hypotension or hypoperfusion should receive intravenous (IV) antibacterials. Antibacterials with poor bioavailability should be administered intravenously for systemic infections (e.g., *vancomycin*, IV *vancomycin*). IV administration of orally available drugs is preferred in the following circumstances:[30]

- Oral antibiotics cannot be tolerated (e.g., because of vomiting).
- Oral antibiotics are poorly absorbed (e.g., because of malabsorption after intestinal surgery; impaired intestinal motility, such as due to opioid use).
- Patient is critically ill, requiring the most immediate medication effect or possibly having impaired GI tract perfusion.

TABLE 10.1 Mechanism of Action of Antibiotic Drugs, Spectrum of Antibacterial Activity, and Therapeutic Indications

Antibiotic category	Example drugs: *generic* and Trade names	Spectrum of antibacterial activity	Therapeutic indications
	INHIBITION OF CELL WALL SYNTHESIS		
β-lactams: broad-spectrum *penicillins*	*amoxicillin* (Amoxil) *penicillin* (generic only) *ampicillin* (generic only)	First medications to be effective against many bacterial infections caused by staphylococci and streptococci. Still widely used today, though many types of bacteria have developed resistance following extensive use.	Most commonly prescribed antibiotics. Used widely to treat a variety of infections, including skin infections, chest infections, and urinary tract infections.
β-lactams: cephalosporins	*cephalexin* (Keflex) *ceftriaxone* (Rocephin)	Variable activity against Gram-positive cocci, excellent for pneumococci.	Used to treat a wide range of infections. Some are also effective for treating more serious infections, such as septicemia and meningitis. Each successive generation possesses a different empiric activity profile (Gram positive vs. Gram negative).
β-lactams: carbapenems	*imipenem* (Primaxin) *meropenem* (Merrem)	Have the broadest spectrum of activity.	Used for severe infections or as last-line medication.
	INHIBITION OF PROTEIN SYNTHESIS		
Macrolides	*erythromycin* (Ery-Tab) *clarithromycin* (Biaxin) *azithromycin* (Zithromax)	Good against Gram-positive cocci, such as streptococci (excludes many staphylococci and most enterococci).	Useful for treating lung and chest infections and *penicillin*-resistant strains of bacteria. Good alternative for people with a *penicillin* allergy.
Tetracyclines	*doxycycline* (Vibramycin) *tetracycline* (Tetracap, many others)	Similar to macrolides, *Brucella* species, and spirochetes.	Used to treat a wide range of infections. Commonly used to treat acne and rosacea.
Aminoglycosides	*gentamicin* (Cidomycin) *tobramycin* (Tobrex)	Gram-negative bacteria, including multidrug-resistant *K. pneumoniae*, *A. baumannii*, and *P. aeruginosa*. Moderate activity against Gram-positive cocci. Poor anaerobic activity.	Used primarily in the hospital to treat very serious illnesses such as septicemia. Can cause serious side effects, including hearing loss and kidney damage. Mostly administered by injection, but may be administered as drops for some ear or eye infections.

(continued)

Table 10.1 *(continued)*

Antibiotic category	Example drugs: *generic* and Trade names	Spectrum of antibacterial activity	Therapeutic indications
INHIBITION OF NUCLEIC ACID SYNTHESIS			
Fluoroquinolones	*ciprofloxacin* (Cipro) *levofloxacin* (Levaquin) *ofloxacin* (Floxin)	Wide Gram-negative activity. Additional activity against intracellular microbes. Moderate activity against Gram-positive cocci.	Broad-spectrum antibiotics that were once used to treat a wide range of infections, including traveler's diarrhea and respiratory and urinary tract infections. These antibiotics are no longer used in the active population because of the risk of serious side effects (tendinopathy).
Nitroimidazoles	*metronidazole* (Flagyl)	Excellent antianaerobic activity.	Used to treat bacterial infections of the vagina, stomach or intestines, liver, skin, joints, brain, heart, and respiratory tract that are caused by anaerobic pathogens.
ALTERATION OF CELL MEMBRANE STRUCTURE			
Glycopeptides	*vancomycin* (Vancocin)	Excellent activity against Gram-positive cocci, including MRSA, highly resistant pneumococci, enterococci, *C. difficile*, and streptococci.	Used orally to treat an infection of the intestines caused by *C. difficile*, which can cause watery or bloody diarrhea. Used intravenously to treat serious bacterial infections of the skin and soft tissues or the blood caused by *Methicillin*-resistant *S. aureus*.
ANTIMETABOLIC ACTIVITY			
Sulfonamides (sulfa drugs)	*sulfamethoxazole* and *trimethoprim* (Bactrim, Septra)	Moderate antistaphylococcal activity. Effective against some MRSA but poor against streptococci and enterococci. Good Gram-negative activity. Poor anaerobic activity.	Used to treat ear infections, urinary tract infections, bronchitis, infections of the intestines, and some types of pneumonia.

Adapted from Falagas and Bliziotis (2016); Kapoor, Saigal, and Elongavan (2017); Hooper, Shenoy, and Varughese (2018); National Health Service website (2019).

Hospitalized patients with mild to moderate infections who have normal GI function are candidates for treatment with well-absorbed oral antibacterial agents. For many antibiotics, oral administration results in therapeutic blood levels nearly as rapidly as IV administration does. Furthermore, patients initially treated with parenteral therapy can be safely switched to oral antibiotics when they become clinically stable.[18] Oral or parenteral administration of anti-infectives depends on the severity of illness and the location of the infection.

Pharmacokinetics

Many factors can affect an antibiotic drug's absorption, including the timing of food consumption

Clinical Application

Osteomyelitis

Osteomyelitis, a bone infection, is a serious complication of a compound fracture (e.g., a football player sustained a metacarpal compound fracture that required surgery) that is viable for 2 weeks to several months.[2] When the infection is diagnosed, an early option is an IV of antibiotic. A variation of IV therapy is to use a **peripherally inserted central catheter (PICC line)** to administer antibiotics directly into the systemic circulation (figure 10.4). Although use of a PICC line has potential complications, it is useful for administering higher concentrations of medication. Measuring the **C-reactive protein (CRP)** level and repeating images are recommended as follow-up to the initial diagnosis.

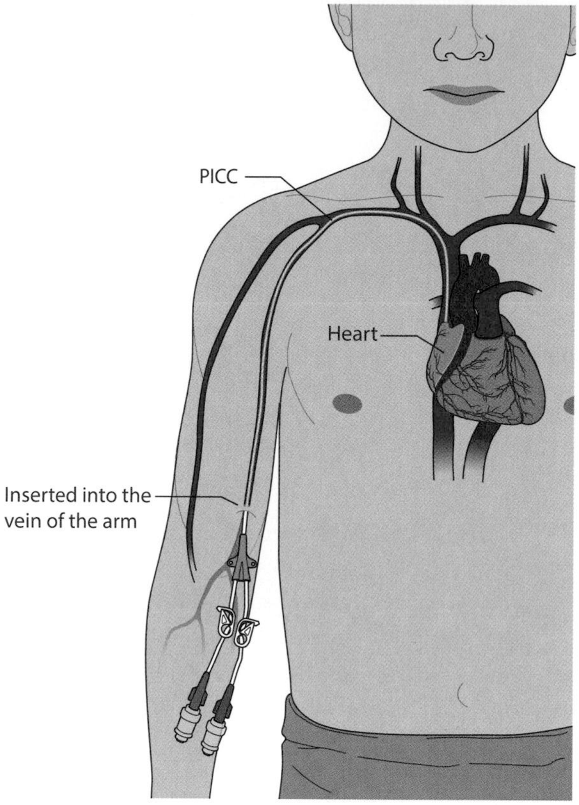

FIGURE 10.4 Peripherally inserted central catheter (PICC line).

relative to drug administration, drug-metabolizing enzymes, or underlying conditions such as diarrhea or **ileus** that can affect the site of drug absorption and thereby alter bioavailability. Certain orally administered drugs have lower bioavailability because of the first-pass effect—the process by which drugs are absorbed in the small intestine through the hepatic portal circulation and then directly transported to the liver for metabolism.[15]

Antibacterial drugs are distributed by binding to serum proteins, and a given drug is usually described as either poorly or highly protein bound. Only the unbound (free) drug is active and available to exert antibacterial effects.[15] Distribution of antibiotics within the tissues (penetration) varies with the site of infection. The central nervous system (CNS) is one body site where antibacterial penetration is defined and correlations with clinical outcomes are established. Caution must be used when selecting an antibacterial on the basis of tissue or fluid penetration. Body fluids where drug concentrations are clinically relevant include cerebrospinal fluid, urine, synovial fluid, and peritoneal fluid. Apart from these areas, more attention should be paid to clinical efficacy, antibacterial spectrum, adverse effects, and cost than to comparative data on penetration.[28]

Like many drugs, antibiotics are metabolized by the cytochrome P450 (CYP) enzyme system in the liver. The CYP3A4 enzyme is a common subfamily responsible for metabolism of the majority of antibiotic drugs. Antibacterial drugs can be substrates, inhibitors, or inducers of a particular CYP enzyme, and therefore affect the concentration of the drug.[15] For excretions, approximately 5 to 7 half-lives are required for an antibacterial drug to reach steady state when multiple doses are given in a time frame shorter than the half-life itself.[15]

Pharmacodynamics

Four important pharmacodynamic parameters (figure 10.5) are related to antibacterial efficacy:[15,30]

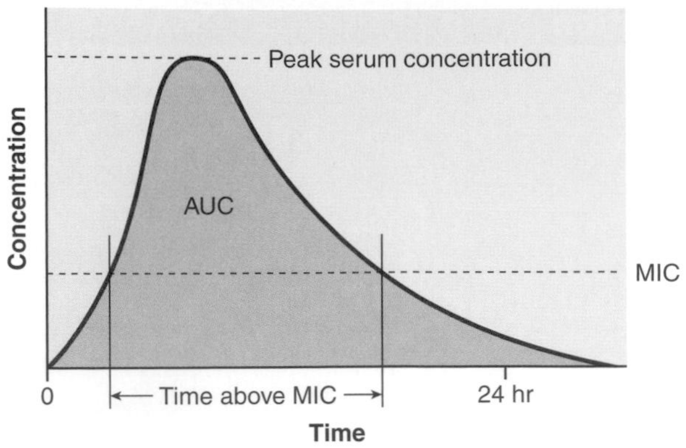

FIGURE 10.5 Time versus concentration of a single dose of a theoretical antibiotic. AUC = area under the curve (amount of drug); MIC = minimal inhibitory concentration (lowest concentration needed to achieve an effect).

1. **Minimal inhibitory concentration (MIC)**—Lowest drug concentration that inhibits the growth of a microorganism under standardized laboratory conditions.
2. **Peak-to-MIC ratio**—Best correlated with antibacterial activity, the ratio of peak serum concentration to MIC, or the magnitude by which the peak concentration exceeds the MIC.
3. **Percentage of time above MIC**—Duration of dosing interval in which the antibiotic concentration exceeds the MIC that best correlates with antibacterial activity.
4. **24-hour area under the concentration-time curve (AUC24)**—The AUC24-to-MIC ratio that best correlates with antibacterial activity.

Antibacterials are categorized based on the pharmacodynamics that optimize antibacterial activity. The general categories based on their concentration-related effects on bacteria are as follows:[3,28,30]

1. **Concentration-dependent activity**—Occurs when higher drug concentrations are associated with greater rate and extent of bacterial killing; the magnitude by which the peak concentration exceeds the MIC that best correlates with antimicrobial activity. Aminoglycosides, fluoroquinolones, and *metronidazole* are examples of antimicrobials that exhibit concentration-dependent activity.
2. **Time-dependent activity**—Duration of the dosing interval in which the antibiotic concentration exceeds the MIC and best correlates with antimicrobial activity. β-lactams, *erythromycin*, and *clarithromycin* exhibit time-dependent bactericidal activity.
3. **Exposure-dependent activity**—Amount of drug given relative to the AUC24-to-MIC ratio that best correlates with antibacterial activity. Most antibiotics have exposure-dependent antibacterial activity that is best characterized by the AUC-to-MIC ratio. *Vancomycin*, *tetracycline*, and *clindamycin* are examples.

Dosing Guidelines

The timing of initial therapy should be guided by the urgency and severity of the patient's condition. For patients with severe illness, a common approach is to use broad-spectrum antibacterial agents as initial empiric therapy; here, the intent is to cover multiple possible pathogens commonly associated with the specific clinical syndrome to ensure adequate treatment of possible pathogens while additional data are being collected.[18]

Evidence in Pharmacology

Patient Adherence

Patients should take their full course of antibiotics as prescribed, even if their symptoms have resolved. A common mistake patients make is to stop taking their antibiotic treatment once they start to feel better.[24] However, this practice can promote resistance or the development of a superinfection and increase the risk of relapse. As with any drug, patients typically have better adherence to a drug that they have to take once a day versus a drug that they have to take multiple times a day. A shorter course of medication may also be preferable. For example, patients with streptococcal tonsillopharyngitis who were prescribed a 3-day course of *azithromycin* reported a 94% to 95% adherence, whereas those who received a 10-day course of *penicillin V* reported 62% adherence.[16] The choice of medication and dosage is the prescriber's responsibility.

Adverse Effects

Antibacterial medications are among the most commonly prescribed drugs worldwide and are used for a wide range of infections. However, antibiotics also expose people to the risk of adverse effects. Some side effects are common and to be expected, such as antibiotic-induced diarrhea. Other adverse effects are uncommon. ATs should be aware of a few rare adverse effects that manifest specifically in the athletic population, such as the relationship between *ciprofloxacin* and tendon injury (described further in the sidebar Risks Associated With Fluoroquinolones).[27] Similarly, some antibiotics have specific instructions that improve the effectiveness of the medication. For example, *ciprofloxacin* should not be taken with calcium-rich foods like dairy or antacids. With some antibiotics, the AT should be aware of common special instructions that the clinical pharmacist provides to the patient, such as how *tetracycline* causes sensitivity to the sun.

Indications and Precautions

Although antibiotics are no longer routinely used to treat certain infections, antibiotic therapy is appropriate for some conditions. Prescribers should holistically assess the patient and provide antibiotics for conditions that meet the following criteria:[22]

- Not serious but unlikely to clear up without antibiotics (e.g., acne)
- Not serious but could spread to other people if not promptly treated (e.g., the common skin infection impetigo, common foodborne illnesses such as *Salmonella*)
- Supported by evidence suggesting that antibiotics could significantly speed up recovery (e.g., kidney infection)
- At high risk of more serious complications (e.g., cellulitis, pneumonia)

Antibiotic medication may be recommended for people who are more vulnerable to the harmful effects of bacterial infection, including the following:[22]

- Over 75 years old
- With heart failure
- Who have to take *insulin* for diabetes
- With a weakened immune system, either because of an underlying health condition such as HIV or as a side effect of certain treatments such as chemotherapy

Evidence in Pharmacology

Penicillin Allergy

Immunologically mediated adverse reactions to β-lactam antibiotics may occur in up to 10% of patients receiving that agent, whereas anaphylaxis occurs in approximately 0.01% of patients. Patients who claim to have a *penicillin* allergy may not really have a true *penicillin* allergy, although the cross-reactivity between a *penicillin* allergy and cephalosporins is extremely low (<1%). Infrequent adverse hypersensitivity effects include fever, vomiting, erythema, dermatitis, angioedema, and pseudomembranous colitis.[23]

β-Lactams

Broad-spectrum β-lactam antibiotics, including the *penicillins*, carbapenems, and cephalosporins, are active against various bacteria. Common adverse drug reactions for β-lactam antibiotics include diarrhea, nausea, rash, urticaria, and superinfection (including candidiasis).[6] *Penicillin* allergies are a serious concern, and all prescribers must determine the presence of allergy before prescribing this medication. Carbapenems are one of the broadest drug classes available. They are highly effective antibiotic agents that are commonly reserved for use in the treatment of severe or high-risk bacterial infections and for known or suspected multidrug-resistant bacterial infections.

Macrolides

This group of medications, which includes *erythromycin* (Ery-Tab), *clarithromycin* (Biaxin), and *azithromycin* (Zithromax), is among the most commonly prescribed class of antibiotics worldwide and is used for a wide range of infections.[7] In a systematic review from the Cochrane Library, most studies (89%) reported at least some adverse events with the use of macrolides, with GI adverse events most commonly reported. *Erythromycin* caused GI side effects in a significant proportion of patients.[13] Other macrolides have been developed that produce fewer side effects and are more easily absorbed, including *clarithromycin* and *azithromycin*.

Tetracyclines

Tetracyclines were discovered in the 1940s. They exhibit broad-spectrum activity against a wide range of microorganisms, including Gram-positive and Gram-negative bacteria. Rather than killing the infectious agent (bactericidal), tetracyclines inhibit bacterial growth (bacteriostatic) and are effective only against multiplying microorganisms.[8] The widespread use of tetracyclines is thought to have contributed to an increase in the number of tetracycline-resistant organisms, in turn rendering certain infections more resilient to treatment.[8] *C. difficile*-associated diarrhea (CDAD) has been observed >2 months postantibiotic treatment. Tetracyclines are likely to cause photosensitivity, and patients taking this medication should use skin protection and avoid prolonged exposure to sunlight and ultraviolet light. Tetracyclines include *doxycycline* (Vibramycin), a common drug used to treat a wide range of infections, and *minocycline* (Minocin), a common drug used to treat respiratory and other infections.

Fluoroquinolones

The fluoroquinolones are a large group of broad-spectrum bactericidal antibiotics that are effective against both Gram-negative and Gram-positive bacteria. A common prototype fluoroquinolone is *ciprofloxacin* (Cipro), one of the most widely used antibiotics around the world.[31] Other examples of fluoroquinolones (the *-floxacins*) are *levofloxacin* (Levaquin) and *ofloxacin* (Floxin). *Ciprofloxacin* is commonly administered by team physicians for upper respiratory tract and sinus infections and gained notoriety in 2001 relating to concerns about widespread anthrax poisoning in the United States. An unusual potential adverse event associated with *ciprofloxacin* is its link to tendon pathology, including tendinitis and tendon rupture.[26] Concomitant administration of corticosteroids may potentiate the risk of tendinitis and tendon rupture associated with fluoroquinolone treatment.

RED FLAG

Tendon Rupture With Fluoroquinolones

To prevent a tendon-related adverse event secondary to fluoroquinolone use, these antibiotics should be used only to treat conditions that are proven or strongly suspected to be caused by bacteria and only if the benefits outweigh the risks. When working with patients taking fluroquinolones, at the onset of tendon pain, ATs should reduce the patient's exercise, consult with the prescriber,[29] and exclude eccentric exercises from rehabilitation programs during the course of medication.[20]

Patient Education for Use of Antibacterial Medications

In general, patient education for antibiotics is similar to that of most commonly prescribed antibacterial medications, with a few exceptions (table 10.2). When discussing antibiotic medications with a patient, in addition to providing the general reminders for antibiotic medications previously mentioned, the AT should do the following:

- Discuss specific use of the drug and side effects as they relate to treatment.

Evidence in Pharmacology

Risks Associated With Fluoroquinolones

Symptoms of fluoroquinolone-induced tendon injury may present within hours of starting antibiotic treatment and continue for up to 6 months after it has ceased. One theory for the cause of this type of injury is that medications in the fluoroquinolone category are linked with ischemia, degradation of the tendon matrix, and an adverse alteration of tenocyte activity that could reduce collagen development.[20] Although patients older than 60 years bear a greater risk, tendinopathy has been reported by people as young as 18 years old.[20,21] Comorbidities include concomitant use of oral or injectable corticosteroids and participation in sports.[21]

Although various fluoroquinolones have been associated with tendon injury, *ciprofloxacin* has specifically been implicated in many case reports. A review identified the Achilles tendon with an 88% incidence frequency.[20] Additionally, the FDA issued a black box warning in July 2008 for *ciprofloxacin* and other fluoroquinolones, in part due to 407 cases of tendon rupture and 341 cases of tendinitis that were associated with taking these medications.[29] Patients with pain, swelling, or inflammation of a tendon should be advised to stop taking the fluoroquinolone, avoid exercise and use of the affected area, and promptly contact their physician.

TABLE 10.2 Clinical Consideration for Antibiotics

Antibiotic	Clinical considerations
All types	Educate patient about signs of a significant reaction (e.g., wheezing; chest tightness; fever; itching; seizures; or swelling of face, lips, tongue, or throat). Have patient report immediately to prescriber any serious side or adverse effects.
Broad-spectrum *penicillin*	Administer medication around the clock to promote less variation in peak and trough serum levels. Extended release: Take within 1 hr of finishing a meal; do not chew or crush tablet.
Macrolides	Prescribers need to be aware of patients with history of cardiac arrythmia.
Tetracycline	Serious emergent signs of an allergic reaction to *doxycycline* include hives, difficulty breathing, swelling in face or throat, severe skin reaction, fever, sore throat, burning in eyes, skin pain, or red or purple skin rash that spreads and causes blistering and peeling. Patients should wear sunscreen when taking these medications because tetracyclines cause photosensitivity. These drugs should not be taken 1 hr before eating or 2 hr after consuming dairy products (e.g., milk, yogurt) or calcium-fortified juices, multivitamins, or antacids.
Fluoroquinolones	Can cause serious or disabling side effects that may not be reversible, such as tendon rupture or nerve problems, which may appear long after the therapy has been completed. These drugs should not be taken with dairy products (e.g., milk, yogurt) or calcium-fortified juices. Patients who regularly consume large quantities of caffeinated beverages may need to restrict caffeine intake if excessive cardiac or CNS stimulation occurs.

- Inform the patient that she may experience abdominal pain, diarrhea, headache, nausea, or vomiting while taking the antibiotic.
- Remind the patient that extended-release tablets should be swallowed whole and not crushed, chewed, or broken.
- Reinforce that the medication should be taken for the full prescribed length of time, even if symptoms quickly improve.
- Tell the patient to avoid skipping doses, which can increase the risk of infection that is resistant to medication.
- If taking certain antibiotics that can result in photosensitivity, the patient must wear sunscreen. The patient who spends significant amounts of time in the sun should discuss this with the prescriber.
- Remind the patient to immediately contact his prescriber about any serious adverse effects, including tachycardia, abnormal heartbeat, angina, difficulty breathing, hearing or vision changes, swollen glands, dizziness or passing out, signs of myasthenia gravis (i.e., muscle weakness, difficulty chewing, difficulty swallowing), signs of *C. difficile*-associated diarrhea, and signs of liver problems (e.g., dark urine, light-colored stools, jaundice).

Collateral Damage

Collateral damage refers to the development of resistance occurring in a patient's nontargeted antibacterial flora (microbiome) that may cause a secondary infection. For example, *clindamycin* may be used to treat Gram-positive cocci infections. However, this drug also readily selects for resistance in *C. difficile*, a nontargeted organism that may be present in the GI tract. Patients with diarrhea and indications of fever, abdominal pain, or frequent loose, watery, or bloody stools require prompt referral to the prescriber or urgent care. If several different antibacterials possess activity against a targeted pathogen, prescribers select the one that is least likely to be associated with collateral damage.[28] Antibiotics disturb the composition and function of the resident flora, which enables an overgrowth of the bacteria that can cause diarrhea.[11] Antibiotics most likely to cause antibiotic-induced diarrhea include the following:[1]

Antibiotic	% of Patients
Ampicillin	5% to 10%
Amoxicillin/clavulanate	10% to 25%
Cefixime	15% to 20%
Cephalosporins, fluoroquinolones	2% to 5%
Azithromycin, tetracycline	2% to 5%

RED FLAG

Antibiotic-Induced Diarrhea

Clostridium difficile (*C. difficile*) is a serious condition that mimics antibiotic-induced diarrhea and is a significant medical concern.[14] Patients with this condition present with the following signs and symptoms:[1,14]

- Fever >101°F (38.5°C)
- 10 watery stools per day, possibly with blood or pus
- Signs of significant dehydration
- Abdominal pain with evidence of colitis on CT scan or endoscopy

Antibiotic Resistance

The major problem threatening the continued success of antibacterial drugs is the development of resistant organisms. Antibiotic resistance mechanisms existed long before the clinical use of antibiotics, even resistance to synthetic drugs that were created in the 20th century. Because resistance mechanisms are already present in nature, an inevitable consequence of antibacterial use is the selection of resistant microorganisms. Since the start of the antibiotic era, antibiotic use in patients and animals has fueled a major increase in the prevalence of drug-resistant pathogens.[17]

Much attention has been focused on eliminating the misuse of antibiotics to slow the tide of resistance. Antibiotics are misused in a variety of ways, including prescription for patients who are unlikely to have bacterial infections, use over unnecessarily prolonged periods, and use of multiple agents or broad-spectrum agents when not needed. Large quantities of antibiotics have been used in agriculture to stimulate growth and prevent infection in livestock; this practice has added to the **selection pressure** that results in resistant organisms. The influence exerted by antibiotic use on natural selection promotes one group of organisms over another. In the case of **antibiotic resistance**, antibiotics cause a selective pressure by killing susceptible bacteria while allowing antibiotic-resistant bacteria to survive and multiply.[17]

Antibiotic resistance has many negative consequences. The prevalence of resistant organisms drives the use of broader-spectrum, less efficacious, or more toxic antibiotics. Not surprisingly, infections caused by antibiotic-resistant pathogens are associated with increased costs, morbidity, and mortality. The Centers for Disease Control and Prevention estimates that every year in the United States, at least 2 million people acquire and 23,000 people die from infections caused by resistant bacteria.[17] Prescribers are more discerning regarding treating infections with antibiotics because of the following:[22]

- Many infections are caused by viruses, so antibiotics are not effective.
- Antibiotics are often unlikely to speed up the healing process and can cause side effects.
- The more often antibiotics are used to treat trivial conditions, the more likely they are to become ineffective for treating more serious medical conditions.

Antibiotic Misuse and Clinician Stewardship

Athletic trainers can educate patients and parents on appropriate antibiotic use, which can improve their health literacy and augment efforts to improve antibiotic use. In collaboration with prescriber and

Evidence in Pharmacology

Antibacterial Drug Resistance

Up to half of antibiotic prescriptions may be unnecessary, poorly chosen, or dosed incorrectly. Indiscriminate use of broad-spectrum antibacterial agents is also believed to be a key contributor to emerging worldwide antibacterial drug resistance. The estimated additional hospital costs associated with drug-resistant hospital-acquired bacterial infections in the United States are estimated to be several billions of dollars annually. Prescribers should be familiar with the currently available antibiotics, their penetration into various tissues, their major adverse effects, and their spectrum of activity relative to local patterns of antibacterial resistance. When prescribing antibacterials, prescribers should also consider issues of cost and the potential for the emergence of resistance.[10]

pharmacist oversight, ATs and other health care providers (HCPs) can do the following in their education efforts:[25]

- **Use effective communications strategies to educate patients about when antibiotics are and are not needed.** For example, patients should be informed that antibiotic treatment for viral infections provides no benefit; thus, this practice should be avoided. Patients also should be informed that certain bacterial infections (e.g., mild ear and sinus infections) might improve without antibiotics. Explanations of when antibiotics are not needed can be combined with recommendations for symptom management.
- **Educate patients about the potential harms of antibiotic treatment.** Potential harms might include common and sometimes serious side effects of antibiotics, including nausea, abdominal pain, diarrhea, *C. difficile* infection, allergic reactions, and other serious reactions.
- **Provide patient education materials.** These materials might include information on appropriate antibiotic use, potential adverse drug events from antibiotics, and available resources regarding symptomatic relief for common infections. Educational materials for patients are found through high-quality online drug resources.

Summary

This chapter provides specific information that is necessary for discussing antibacterial medications with prescribers and other HCPs. Using the context of the patient's clinical presentation and manifestations of bacterial infections, ATs can appropriately make referrals and advocate on behalf of their patients. Best practices in antibiotic prescribing should be made on the basis of documented pathogen and susceptibility data whenever possible; this information also makes it possible to choose more targeted therapy, thereby reducing the risk of selection of resistant bacteria. Prescribers choose the antibacterial agent and duration of therapy according to the nature of the infection and the patient's response to treatment. Whenever possible, prescribers are informed by clinical studies with the understanding that shorter courses of medication are less likely than longer ones to promote the emergence of antibiotic resistance.[15]

Case Studies

Case Study 1

Coach Mike is the local high school's basketball coach and history teacher. The mid-winter flu season has been tougher than usual, and Coach Mike contracted something. He did not improve as quickly as he thought he would and complained of fatigue, low-grade fever (99.4°F; 37.4°C), and a sore throat. He felt this episode was more significant than when he had felt unwell in past seasons. Coach Mike saw his physician, Dr. Cal, who ordered a throat culture. The test came back positive, as Dr. Cal knew it would. Coach Mike, who is *penicillin* sensitive, was prescribed 250 mg of *azithromycin* for strep throat and a possible bacterial upper respiratory infection and received instructions to take the medication over the next 5 days. He asked his physician if there was anything stronger that could work faster, since he'd had good results in the past with the 500 mg dose. Dr. Cal opted to prescribe *azithromycin* 500 mg for use over 3 days with the warning that it may irritate his digestive tract. Coach Mike followed the 3-day protocol and felt improvement on the third day despite a mild case of stomach cramping.

Questions for Analysis

1. Do you think the physician was correct to change the prescription from 250 mg to 500 mg of the same medication? Why or why not?
2. What was the role of the rapid strep test in the diagnosis?

Case Study 2

Jimmy worked laying hardwood floor in renovated homes. As he was laying hardwood, he got a splinter in the index finger of his dominant hand but thought nothing of it. After a few days, the finger was warm, red, swollen, and stiff, with mild to moderate pain. Jimmy decided to see his company's workers' compensation medical clinic. He had a very brief visit with the nurse practitioner, was diagnosed with a mild infection, and given a prescription for *tetracycline*. After a few days of taking the medication, the infection was improving, so Jimmy decided to take some friends on a boat ride to enjoy the hot summer day. When they returned to the dock, Jimmy treated everyone to a barbecue and took his *tetracycline*. The next day, Jimmy woke up with a severe sunburn and diarrhea. He has a fair complexion and recalled that he had forgotten to use sunscreen the day before. He also realized he should have taken the medication either 1 hour before or 2 hours after eating rather than during the barbeque. When he finished his tetracycline prescription, both his finger infection and the diarrhea had improved, but he still had to manage the sunburn.

Questions for Analysis

1. Other than Jimmy's time in the sun without sunscreen, what could have contributed to his sunburn?
2. If it is accurate that the medication could have predisposed Jimmy to the sunburn, how could this have been prevented?

Drugs Described in This Chapter

Drug class	*generic* (pronunciation) Trade names	Therapeutic uses	Clinical concerns*
Broad-spectrum (β-lactam) *penicillin*	*amoxicillin* (a moks i SIL in) Amoxil, Moxatag Many brands and formulations of *amoxicillin* are available; not all brands are the same. The other β-lactams are the cephalosporins and carbapenems.	Many bacterial infections, such as tonsillitis, bronchitis, pneumonia, gonorrhea, and infections of the ear, nose, throat, skin, or urinary tract. *Amoxicillin* is also sometimes used with another antibiotic called *clarithromycin* (Biaxin) to treat stomach ulcers caused by *Helicobacter pylori* infection. Dosage: Immediate release—500 mg to 1 g taken orally every 8 to 12 hr Extended release—775 mg once daily	*Amoxicillin* can make birth control pills less effective. Female patients should be referred to the prescriber to discuss using a nonhormonal method of birth control (e.g., condom, diaphragm, spermicide) to prevent pregnancy while taking this medicine. Superinfection: Prolonged use may result in fungal or bacterial superinfection; for example, *C. difficile*-associated diarrhea (CDAD) has been observed >2 mo postantibiotic treatment.
Macrolide	*azithromycin* (a ZITH roe MYE sin) Zithromax, Z-pak *erythromycin* (er ITH roe MYE sin) Ery-Tab *clarithromycin* (kla RITH roe MYE sin) Biaxin	Oral or IV; used to treat acute otitis media, community-acquired pneumonia (CAP), uncomplicated skin and skin structure infections due to *Staphylococcus aureus* and other bacterial skin infections, and streptococcal pharyngitis/tonsillitis	Most commonly reported side effects include diarrhea/loose stools, abdominal pain, and nausea. Patients with side effects that are bothersome and do not go away need medical attention.
Tetracycline	*doxycycline*** (doks i SYE kleen) Adoxa, Doxy 100	Many different bacterial infections, such as acne, urinary tract infections, intestinal infections, respiratory infections, eye infections, gonorrhea, chlamydia, syphilis, and periodontitis (gum disease). Dosage depends on condition treated.	Common side effects: nausea, vomiting, headache, upset stomach, loss of appetite, mild diarrhea, skin rash or itching, darkened skin color, or vaginal itching or discharge. Different brands of *doxycycline* may have different instructions about taking the medication with or without food.

Drug class	*generic* (pronunciation) Trade names	Therapeutic uses	Clinical concerns*
Fluoroquinolone	*ciprofloxacin*** (sip roe FLOKS a sin) Cipro	Bacterial infections, including skin infections, bone and joint infections, respiratory or sinus infections, urinary tract infections, and certain types of diarrhea. It is also used to treat gonorrhea. Extended-release tablets and immediate-release formulations are not interchangeable. Unless otherwise specified, oral dosing reflects the use of immediate-release formulations. Dosage depends on condition treated.	May cause serious or disabling side effects that may not be reversible, such as swelling or tearing of a tendon, especially in the Achilles tendon. This can happen during treatment or up to several months after stopping this medicine. Tendon problems may be more likely in certain people (e.g., children, older adults, people who use steroid medicine or have had an organ transplant). Instruct the patient not to take the medication with dairy products, such as milk or yogurt, or calcium-fortified juice. Patients may eat or drink these products with meals but should not use them alone when taking *ciprofloxacin*, since this could make the medication less effective. Using caffeine while taking *ciprofloxacin* can increase the effects of the caffeine.

*Signs of an allergic or hypersensitivity reaction include rash; hives; itching; red, swollen, blistered, or peeling skin, with or without fever; wheezing; tightness in the chest or throat; trouble breathing, swallowing, or talking; unusual hoarseness; or swelling of the mouth, face, lips, tongue, or throat.

**These drugs could make the patient sunburn more easily. The patient should avoid sunlight and tanning beds and wear protective clothing and use sunscreen (SPF 30 or higher) when outdoors. Patient should report to prescriber if he has severe burning, redness, itching, rash, or swelling after being in the sun.

Note: This is not a comprehensive list of all side effects. The patient should be referred to the prescriber if there are questions.

PART III

Drugs for Treating Common Conditions

To this point, this text has introduced foundational concepts relating to the clinical use of medicines or drugs. Part II described large classes of medications commonly used in the sports medicine setting. Part III describes the use of pharmaceutical interventions for treating a variety of conditions in physically active people. Chapter 11 focuses on the drug treatment of asthma and other infectious and allergic respiratory conditions. Chapter 12 introduces drugs for cardiac conditions, both emergent and chronic. In chapter 13, drugs used to manage type 1 and type 2 diabetes mellitus are discussed. Drugs used to treat a variety of gastrointestinal conditions, including nausea, vomiting, and diarrhea, are discussed in chapter 14. Chapter 15 describes muscle relaxants and other drug treatments for muscular and neurological conditions, while chapter 16 details antifungal and antiviral medications used to treat dermatological conditions. Contraceptives and other medications used to treat reproductive concerns are described in chapter 17, while a variety of antidepressants and other medications used to treat mental health conditions are outlined in chapter 18. Finally, the final 4 chapters describe performance-enhancing drugs (chapter 19), cannabis and cannabinoids (chapter 20), drug testing in sport (chapter 21), and surgical medications (chapter 22). This last part of the text provides the athletic training student and practicing clinician with the necessary information on finding current recommendations and guidelines for these constantly evolving topics.

11

Drugs for Treating Asthma and Other Respiratory Conditions

OBJECTIVES

After reading this chapter, you will be able to do the following:

- Summarize the causes of common viral respiratory syndromes
- Differentiate between treatments for the common cold and influenza
- Describe supportive care for respiratory infections
- Explain the drugs for treating allergic rhinitis and other allergies
- Distinguish between acute asthma exacerbations and poor asthma control
- Describe pharmacologic strategies used for short- and long-term asthma control

Of all body systems, the respiratory system is extremely vulnerable in that it is constantly exposed to particles in the air, such as microorganisms and allergens. The respiratory system has effective defense mechanisms to cope with the numerous particulates and infectious agents inhaled on inspiration. The athletic trainer (AT) is most likely to encounter acute respiratory infections in otherwise healthy people >12 years old. This chapter and those that follow focus on this population, which is commonly encountered in the traditional athletic training setting, such as schools, clinics, factories, military settings, or performing arts centers.

Respiratory Infections

Although respiratory infections can be identified by the causative virus (e.g., influenza), these conditions are generally clinically classified according to syndrome (e.g., the common cold, bronchitis, pneumonia). The most common respiratory infections are caused by viruses. Although specific pathogens commonly cause characteristic clinical manifestations (e.g., rhinovirus causes the common cold, respiratory syncytial virus [RSV] causes bronchitis), each pathogen can cause various viral respiratory syndromes. Respiratory viruses are typically spread

Select Drugs Discussed in This Chapter

Drug class	Generic name	Trade name
Expectorants	*guaifenesin*	Mucinex, Robitussin
Antitussives	*dextromethorphan*	Delsym
Antivirals	*oseltamivir* *acyclovir*	Tamiflu Zovirax
Antihistamines		
Sedating (ethanolamine; first generation)	*diphenhydramine*	Benadryl
Nonsedating (second generation)	*loratadine*	Claritin
Nasal decongestants		
Alpha-adrenergic (or α-1 adrenergic) receptor agonists	*pseudoephedrine*	Sudafed
Alpha-adrenergic (or α-1 adrenergic) receptor agonists (nasal spray)	*phenylephrine oxymetazoline*	Neo-Synephrine Afrin Nasal Spray
Asthma rescue drugs		
Short-acting beta-agonists (or β-2 agonists)	*albuterol*	Proventil, ProAir, Ventolin
Anticholinergics	*ipratropium*	Atrovent
Combination drugs	*ipratropium* and *albuterol*	DuoNeb
Systemic corticosteroids	*prednisone*	Mainly generic
Long-term asthma control		
Inhaled corticosteroids	*fluticasone*	Flovent
Long-acting beta-adrenergic agonists (or β-2 adrenergic agonists)	*salmeterol*	Serevent Diskus

This list is not exhaustive, but rather contains drugs commonly encountered in the athletic training setting. Always consult up-to-date information, confirm with a pharmacist, or discuss the use of therapeutic medications with the prescriber of the medication.

from person to person by contact with infected respiratory droplets. Frequent and thorough handwashing or use of hand sanitizers is the best way to prevent the spread of infection.[30]

An **upper respiratory infection (URI)**, or **upper respiratory tract infection (URTI)**, is an illness caused by an acute infection involving the upper respiratory tract, which includes the nose, sinuses, pharynx, and larynx. This condition commonly includes viral infections such as the common cold, influenza, sore throat, and sinusitis. This section focuses on viral infections that commonly affect the upper respiratory tract. Lower respiratory tract infections, including bronchitis and pneumonia, are discussed in the section that follows.

The Common Cold

The common cold is an acute, usually afebrile, self-limited viral infection that causes upper respiratory symptoms, such as **rhinorrhea**, cough, and sore throat.[28] Many different respiratory viruses can cause the common cold, but rhinoviruses are the most common.[8] Rhinoviruses are most efficiently spread by direct person-to-person contact, although spread may also occur via large-particle aerosols, such as those emitted in a sneeze or cough. Several factors can increase risk for the common cold:[8]

- Exposure to someone with the common cold
- A weakened immune system (e.g., in someone who is recovering from surgery or taking drugs that weaken the immune system, such as *methylprednisolone* for a herniated disc)
- Season (i.e., colds are more common during the fall and winter)

Treatment for the Common Cold

Although antibiotics cannot treat infections caused by viruses, a variety of options exist to relieve some symptoms and help the patient feel better while a viral illness runs its course. For mild viral infections in otherwise healthy people, treating the symptoms and providing supportive care are important considerations. Rest, over-the-counter (OTC) medications, and other self-care methods provide symptomatic relief. A variety of OTC medications and products are available for upper respiratory tract infections, each with specific active ingredients to treat runny nose, cough, and nasal congestion. The AT should remind the patient to always use OTC products as directed.[8,28] Importantly, the AT must be mindful that many OTC products may interact with other medications that an athlete might be taking, and some may contain substances banned from sport (refer to chapter 21).

For cough related to the common cold or influenza, OTC cough syrups containing a combination of the expectorant *guaifenesin* and the antitussive *dextromethorphan* and the nasal decongestants *pseudoephedrine* or *phenylephrine* may be helpful for relieving symptoms (see table 11.1).

- **Expectorants** help loosen congestion in the chest and throat, facilitating cough out through the mouth.
- **Antitussive** drugs decrease the sensitivity of cough receptors and interrupt the cough impulse transmission by depressing the medullary cough center. Dilated blood vessels can cause nasal congestion (stuffy nose).
- **Nasal decongestants** are used to shrink blood vessels in the nasal passages to reduce nasal congestion.

Typical dosing in OTC cough syrups is *guaifenesin* 200 mg, *dextromethorphan* 20 mg, and *phenylephrine* 10 mg (10 mL) every 4 hours; maximum is 60 mL per 24 hours. *Guaifenesin* is an expectorant that is commonly available in granules (Theraflu), extended-release tablets, immediate-release tablets, or liquid preparations. Expectorants and antitussives, often combined with the analgesic *acetaminophen* or the nasal decongestant *phenylephrine*, are contained in a variety of OTC medications that are widely available at drug stores.

Influenza

Influenza is a viral respiratory infection causing fever, **coryza**, cough, headache, and **malaise**. Diagnosis is usually clinical and depends on local epidemiologic patterns[29] (the Centers for Disease Control and Prevention [CDC] posts updates on their website).[7] The incubation period for influenza ranges from 1 to 4 days, with an average of about 48 hours. After 2 or 3 days, acute symptoms rapidly subside, although fever may last for up to 5 days. Cough, weakness, sweating, and fatigue may persist for several days or occasionally for weeks.[7,29] Teammates who are in close contact, such as riding on a bus or sitting together in meeting rooms, are likely to pass the flu virus to one another. Frequent handwashing and cough etiquette are important in preventing the spread of viral illnesses.

Distinguishing Between Common Cold and Influenza

Since colds and flu share many symptoms, it can be difficult (or even impossible) for the AT in the prehospital setting to determine the difference between them based on symptoms alone. Diagnostic tests performed within the first few days of illness can indicate which virus is causing the illness. Distinguishing features of flu (see table 11.2) include abrupt onset, fever (or feeling feverish) and chills, body aches, headaches, and fatigue (tiredness). It is important to recognize that flu is contagious and can be a serious illness that makes the patient more vulnerable to complications. Cold symptoms are usually milder than the symptoms of flu. People with colds are more likely to have a runny nose or

TABLE 11.1 Common Over-the-Counter Cough and Cold Medicines

Generic drug	Drug class	Example products containing this drug
acetaminophen	Analgesic	Theraflu, Tylenol Cold + Head Congestion Severe
dextromethorphan	Antitussive	DayQuil, Delsym, Robitussin
diphenhydramine	Antihistamine and antitussive	Benadryl, Dimetapp, Theraflu
guaifenesin	Expectorant	Mucinex, Robitussin, Theraflu
phenylephrine	Nasal decongestant	Contac Cold, Neo-Synephrine, Triaminic
pseudoephedrine	Nasal decongestant	Sudafed

nasal congestion, with gradual increase in symptoms. Colds generally do not result in serious complications, such as pneumonia, bacterial infections, or hospitalization.[7]

Vaccination

According to the CDC, everyone older than 6 months should receive an annual influenza vaccination.[8] Flu vaccines cause antibodies to develop in the body about 2 weeks after the vaccination. These antibodies provide protection against infection with the viruses that are in the vaccine. The seasonal flu vaccine protects against the influenza viruses that research indicates will be most common during each upcoming flu season.

TABLE 11.2 Differentiating the Common Cold and Flu

Signs and symptoms	Cold	Flu
Symptom onset	Gradual	Abrupt
Fever	Rare	Usual
Aches	Mild to none	Moderate to severe
Chills	Uncommon	Fairly common
Fatigue, weakness	Sometimes	Usual
Sneezing	Common	Sometimes
Nasal congestion	Common	Sometimes
Sore throat	Common	Sometimes
Chest discomfort, cough	Mild to moderate	Common
Headache	Rare	Common

Based on Center for Disease Control and Prevention website (2019); Tesini (2019)

Clinical Application

H1N1 and COVID-19

The H1N1 virus (swine flu) that caused a **pandemic** in 2009 is now a regular human flu virus that continues to circulate seasonally worldwide.[7] Other viruses, specifically the common cold coronaviruses, cause severe acute respiratory syndrome (SARS) and Middle East respiratory syndrome (MERS). In late 2019, a novel coronavirus, now designated "severe acute respiratory syndrome coronavirus 2" (SARS-CoV-2), was identified as the cause of an outbreak of acute respiratory illness in Wuhan, a city in China. In February 2020, the WHO designated the disease "coronavirus disease 2019" (COVID-19).[35] People with COVID-19 experience a wide range of symptoms that range from mild symptoms to severe illness. Symptoms may appear 2 to 14 days after exposure to the virus.[9] The elderly, immunocompromised, and those with comorbid metabolic, pulmonary, and cardiac conditions are at a markedly greater risk of death from COVID-19.[13]

Our understanding of COVID-19 has evolved rapidly during the worldwide pandemic as therapies are tested and approved by the FDA.[1] Treatment of COVID-19 is mainly supportive. For each therapeutic agent, the benefits must be weighed against possible risks for the individual patient.[31] A COVID-19 vaccine is any of several different vaccines intended to provide acquired immunity against the disease. Previous work to develop a vaccine against the coronavirus diseases SARS and MERS established knowledge about the structure and function of coronaviruses, which accelerated the development during early 2020 of varied technology platforms for an FDA approved COVID-19 vaccine.[13] Future scientific discoveries on vaccines will continue from translational and clinical studies that could accelerate the diagnosis, management, and treatment of viral infections.[1]

Evidence in Pharmacology

Essential Information Regarding Tamiflu

One of the bedrock claims of *oseltamivir* is that it prevents hospitalizations or reduces complications from influenza in vulnerable patients, such as the elderly or those with chronic cardiac or respiratory comorbidities; however, results of a meta-analysis of published and unpublished clinical trials found no evidence of these outcomes.[14] The 2018 FDA guidelines are as follows:

> Tamiflu (*oseltamivir*) is an oral antiviral drug approved for the treatment of acute, uncomplicated influenza in patients 2 weeks of age and older whose flu symptoms have not lasted more than 2 days. This product is approved to treat Type A and B influenza; however, most patients included in the studies were infected with type A, the most common in the United States. Efficacy of Tamiflu in the treatment of influenza in vulnerable patients has not been established. Tamiflu is not a substitute for early influenza vaccination on an annual basis.[32]

This conclusion is based on data from 2,646 adult and adolescent subjects treated twice daily for influenza and 1,943 subjects treated once per day over a 6-week period of prophylaxis treatment. Also included is an FDA warning and precaution regarding the risk of neuropsychiatric events, particularly in adolescent patients.[32]

Treatment of most patients with influenza is symptomatic and supportive, including rest, hydration, and antipyretics as needed, but *aspirin* is avoided in patients ≤18 years old.[29] However, for people who have the influenza infection or suspected influenza infection and who are at high risk of serious flu complications, the CDC recommends prompt treatment with an antiviral medication.[7] Antiviral treatment reduces the duration of illness by about 1 day but is useful in preventing development of serious symptoms and can prevent serious flu complications, such as pneumonia. For people at high risk of serious flu complications, treatment with antiviral drugs can mean the difference between milder infection and a more serious illness that could possibly result in a costly hospital stay.[29]

It is important to remember that antiviral drugs are different from antibiotics, which fight against bacterial infections.[7] Antiviral drugs are neuraminidase inhibitor enzymes that cleave (cut) the glycosidic linkages of neuraminic acids found in a range of microorganisms. The best-known viral neuraminidase inhibitor is *oseltamivir* (Tamiflu), with a drug target for the prevention of the spread of influenza infection. This medication is obtained only by prescription and is available in various forms (pills, liquid, an inhaled powder, or intravenous solution). *Oseltamivir* is commonly administered by mouth as a pill or liquid suspension to be taken twice daily for 5 days. However, people hospitalized with influenza may need antiviral treatment for longer than 5 days. The most common side effects for *oseltamivir* are nausea and vomiting. Other less common side effects also have been reported.[7]

Sore Throat

Sore throat is pain in the posterior pharynx that occurs with or without swallowing. Most sore throats are caused by viral tonsillopharyngitis, a predominantly viral infection. The respiratory viruses (rhinovirus, adenovirus, influenza, coronavirus, respiratory syncytial virus) are the most common viral causes, but occasionally Epstein-Barr virus (the cause of mononucleosis) is involved.[15] It is difficult to clinically distinguish viral from bacterial causes of tonsillopharyngitis; laboratory diagnostic testing such as a throat culture is required. Cough, laryngitis, and stuffy nose are not characteristic of streptococcal pharyngitis infection; their presence suggests another cause (usually viral or allergic).[4]

Treatment of Sore Throat

For tonsillopharyngitis, supportive care is recommended, although symptomatic treatments such as warm saltwater gargles and topical anesthetics (e.g., *lidocaine*) may help temporarily relieve the pain of sore throat. Patients in severe pain may be prescribed short-term use of opioids or another analgesic. Corticosteroids (e.g., *dexamethasone* 10 mg IM) are occasionally prescribed to reduce inflammation if the tonsillopharyngitis appears to pose a risk of airway obstruction.[15] In the case of a bacterial infection confirmed by a throat culture, such as streptococcal pharyngitis, delaying treatment 1 or 2 days while waiting for laboratory confirmation of the specific infectious organism increases neither the duration of disease nor the incidence of complications. Pending culture results, patients with severe symptoms of tonsillopharyngitis may be prescribed a broad-spectrum antibiotic (e.g., *penicillin* or *amoxicillin*) or other antimicrobial medication.[4]

Sinusitis

Acute sinusitis often develops in people with immune systems weakened by stress, sleep deprivation, or poor nutrition, and is almost always viral (e.g., rhinovirus, influenza, parainfluenza). Chronic sinusitis involves many factors that combine to create chronic inflammation, including chronic allergies, nasal polyps, environmental irritants (e.g., airborne pollution, tobacco smoke), and other factors that interact with infectious organisms. Fever and chills suggest an extension of the infection beyond the sinuses.

Treatment of Sinusitis

Treatment of sinusitis is usually symptomatic to include local measures to enhance drainage (e.g., steam, topical vasoconstrictors). Steam inhalation; hot, wet towels over the affected sinuses; and hot beverages help alleviate nasal vasoconstriction and promote drainage. For temporary relief of nasal congestion, the alpha-adrenergic agonist *phenylephrine* (Neo-Synephrine Cold & Sinus) 0.25% nasal spray administered every 3 hours may be effective, but it should be used for a maximum of 5 days or for a repeating cycle of 3 days on and 3 days off until the sinusitis is resolved. Use of a humidifier or vaporizer at night is advised. Saline nasal irrigation devices, such as a neti pot, may help symptoms and be more appropriate for patients with recurrent sinusitis. Corticosteroid nasal sprays can help relieve symptoms, but typically take ≥10 days to be effective.[16]

Bronchitis and Pneumonia

Acute bronchitis is a common infection of the lower respiratory tract, commonly following a URI. The cause of acute bronchitis is viral in >95% of cases, but the pathogen is rarely identified. The most common symptom is cough, with or without fever, and possibly sputum production. Pneumonia is the most common and most frequent lower respiratory tract infection. Because pneumonia can be airborne, when inhaling this infection in the air, the particles enter the lungs and move into the air sacs. This infection quickly develops, spreads through the lower part of the lung, and fills the lung with fluid and excess mucus.

Treatment of Bronchitis and Pneumonia

Most cases of lower respiratory tract infections in healthy patients are treated with supportive care only to relieve symptoms without using antibiotics. Antiviral therapy may be indicated for select viral pneumonias;[26] for example, *acyclovir* (Zovirax) may be administered orally in the outpatient setting or the physician may admit the patient to the hospital for observation and more advanced care. In the hospital, the patient can receive supportive care in a more sterile environment, and may receive *acyclovir* 5 to 10 mg/kg IV every 8 hours. Although pure viral pneumonia does occur, **superimposed bacterial infections** are common and require antibiotics directed against *S. pneumoniae* or *H. influenzae*.

Allergic Rhinitis and Other Allergies

Allergic disorders are the most common upper respiratory disorders. **Allergy** is any exaggerated immune response to a foreign antigen, regardless of mechanism. **Atopy** is an exaggerated immunoglobulin E-mediated immune response; all atopic disorders are type I **hypersensitivity disorders**. Signs of allergic reactions may also include nasal turbinate edema, sinus pain during palpation, wheezing, conjunctival hyperemia and edema, **urticaria**, **angioedema**, dermatitis, and skin **lichenification**. Stridor, wheezing, and hypotension are signs of life-threatening anaphylaxis.[27]

Seasonal allergic rhinitis (hay fever) is most often caused by plant allergens, which vary by season. Causes also differ by region, and seasonal allergic rhinitis is occasionally caused by airborne fungal (mold) spores. **Perennial rhinitis** is caused by year-round exposure to indoor inhaled allergens (e.g., pollen, animal dander) or by strong reactivity to plant pollens in sequential seasons. Allergic rhinitis and asthma frequently coexist; it is unclear whether rhinitis and asthma result from the same allergic process or if rhinitis is a discrete asthma trigger.[12]

Treatment of Allergic Rhinitis and Other Allergies

Treatment of seasonal and perennial allergic rhinitis (hay fever) is generally the same, although attempts at removal or avoidance of allergens are recommended for perennial rhinitis. For allergic rhinitis, nasal drugs are often preferred to oral drugs because less of the drug is absorbed systemically. Intranasal saline, often forgotten, helps mobilize thick nasal secretions and hydrate nasal mucous membranes; various OTC saline solution kits and irrigation devices (e.g., neti pot, squeeze bottles, bulb syringes) are available or patients can make their own solutions.[12] The most effective first-line drug treatments for allergic rhinitis and allergy are as follows:

- Antihistamines
- Decongestants

Antihistamines

Antihistamines, or **histamine-1 receptor** antagonists (H1 blockers), are a mainstay of treatment for allergic disorders. Oral H1 blockers relieve symptoms of atopic and allergic disorders; however, they are less effective for allergic bronchoconstriction and systemic vasodilation. Antihistamine H1 blockers are classified as the following:[12,19]

- **Sedating (first-generation) antihistamines—** Widely available without prescription. The prevalence of allergic conditions and the relative safety of the drugs contribute to this heavy use. The prototypical drug is *diphenhydramine* (Benadryl). The sedative effect makes these OTC agents useful as sleep aids and unsuitable for daytime use. However, these drugs are a good choice for nighttime relief of allergic symptoms. The effects of sedation contribute to limitations of their use in sports or while driving; a better choice is second-generation antihistamines. Most have an effective duration of action of 4 to 8 hours following a 25 to 50 mg single dose.
- **Nonsedating (second-generation, nonanticholinergic) antihistamines—**These drugs are less sedating and are preferred except when sedative effects may be therapeutic. A common OTC drug is *loratadine* (Claritin), a long-acting H1 blocker. A 10 mg oral dose of this medication has an onset of action of 1 to 3 hours, with a peak effect of 8 to 12 hours. Since its $t_{1/2}$ is 8 hours, this long-acting medication is a good choice as a suppressant of allergy symptoms when used regularly.

Decongestants

Decongestants, such as the alpha- and beta-**adrenergic receptor** agonist *pseudoephedrine* (Sudafed), have been available OTC for years as a drug for reducing mucous membrane congestion. The use of *pseudoephedrine* as a precursor in the illicit manufacture of *methamphetamine* has led to restrictions on its sale. Additionally, this drug may be considered a banned substance for collegiate, professional, or international competition (see chapter 21). Nasal decongestants such as *phenylephrine* (Neo-Synephrine Cold & Sinus nasal spray) are alpha-adrenergic receptor agonists that reduce the discomfort of allergic rhinitis or the common cold. These medications work by decreasing the volume of the nasal mucosa by vasoconstriction, thus allowing less fluid to leave the blood vessels and enter the nose, throat, and sinus linings and decreasing inflammation of nasal membranes and mucus production. For a 60 mg immediate-release oral dose, the onset of action is 30 minutes and the peak effect occurs 1 to 2 hours later. Unfortunately, rebound hyperemia may follow topical use of these agents, and repeated use of high drug concentrations may result in ischemic changes in the nasal mucous membranes, probably as a result of vasoconstriction of nutrient arteries. Common OTC nasal decongestants containing the agent *phenylephrine* or the longer-acting *oxymetazoline* include the following:

- *phenylephrine* and *acetaminophen*: Sudafed PE Sinus Pressure + Pain, Tylenol Sinus + Headache, Robitussin Peak Cold Nasal Relief
- *oxymetazoline* (nasal spray): Afrin Nasal Spray, Mucinex Sinus-Max Full Force, Neo-Synephrine 12 Hour Spray, Vicks Sinex Severe

Additional medications that can be prescribed for allergic rhinitis are also important for the treatment of asthma. Inhaled nasal corticosteroids and mast cell stabilizers for the treatment of asthma are described in the following section.

Asthma

Asthma is a disease of diffuse airway inflammation caused by a variety of triggering stimuli, resulting in partially or completely reversible bronchoconstriction. Symptoms and signs include **dyspnea**, chest tightness, cough, and wheezing.[24] Most severe exacerbations of asthma that are treated in the emergency department resolve within 2 hours after presentation. The onset and duration of symptoms and the worsening of airflow obstruction before presentation are variable, but these problems usually occur over several hours. Even in fatal or near-fatal asthma attacks, there is potential for early recognition and aggressive treatment. Rarely, a patient has rapid, catastrophic onset of acute asthma, which can be fatal.[18]

RED FLAG

Fatal Asthma Attack

The following are signs and symptoms that may suggest a potentially fatal asthma attack:

Signs

- Use of accessory muscles of respiration
- Heart rate >120 beats/min or increasing
- Respiratory rate >25-30 breaths/min
- Difficulty speaking because of dyspnea or fatigue
- Altered level of consciousness
- Quiet chest in a patient who has dyspnea or reduced level of consciousness
- **Diaphoresis**
- Inability to lie in the supine position because of breathing distress
- Peak expiratory flow (PEF) <30% of predicted or forced expiratory volume (FEV_1) in 1 second or <25% of predicted volume 1-2 hours after initial therapy
- Oxygen saturation <90%
- Cyanosis

Symptoms

- Sense of progressive breathlessness or air hunger
- Sense of fear or impending doom
- Progressive agitation or anxiety

Treatment of Asthma

Medications for asthma are categorized into 2 general classes: quick-relief or rescue medications, which are used to treat acute symptoms and exacerbations, and long-term control medications, which are used to achieve and maintain control of

Clinical Application

Emergency Cases of Acute Asthma

Acute asthma is a common medical emergency that is often poorly managed. A survey of the management of asthma in children and adults in the emergency department revealed wide variations in care and substantial gaps in management in certain key areas.[20] These included poor adherence to a written asthma action plan, infrequent measurement of peak expiratory flow, infrequent use of systemic corticosteroids, and poor rates of referral to asthma educational services. The asthma action plan is developed in collaboration with the patient and her physician and guides efforts to control the patient's condition. The plan includes the following information:[34]

- How to know if the patient's symptoms are worsening
- Medicines to be administered when the patient is doing well and when there is an exacerbation
- What to do in an emergency
- Contact information for an emergency (e.g., physician, parents)
- How to control asthma triggers

The *NATA Position Statement on Management of Asthma in Athletes*[21] recommends use of a written asthma action plan that details the patient's daily regimen for asthma management (medications and environmental control strategies) and how to recognize and manage worsening asthma. A plan is particularly recommended for patients who have moderate or severe asthma, a history of severe exacerbations, or poorly controlled asthma. The written asthma action plan can be based on either symptoms or peak flow; evidence shows similar benefits for each. Referral to an asthma specialist for consultation or comanagement of the patient is recommended if there are difficulties achieving or maintaining control of asthma.[5,22]

persistent asthma. The next section describes the following:

- Short-acting rescue drugs for treatment of acute asthma exacerbations
- Long-acting drugs for long-term asthma control
- Process for assessing effectiveness of asthma medication
- Long-term strategies for controlling asthma

Drugs for Treatment of Acute Asthma Exacerbations

In the case of an acute asthma exacerbation, short-acting rescue drugs are effective in relieving symptoms and improving lung function.[5,22,24] **Short-acting rescue drugs** are inhaled bronchodilators that are the therapy of choice for relief of acute symptoms and prevention of symptoms. These drugs are the mainstay of asthma treatment in the prehospital setting and the emergency department. Short-acting rescue drugs include the following:

- Short-acting beta-agonists (SABA)
- Anticholinergics
- Systemic (oral) corticosteroids

Use of certain asthma medications may be restricted by drug testing agencies or sport governing bodies; therefore, it is important that anti-doping regulations are reviewed by the prescribing physician (see chapter 21).

Short-Acting Beta-Agonists Short-acting beta-agonists (SABAs; also short-acting β-2 agonists) relax bronchiole smooth muscle and are the first choice for quick relief of asthma symptoms. These bronchodilators are considered rescue inhalers because they relieve acute asthma symptoms or exacerbations by quickly opening the airways. The action of inhaled bronchodilators starts within minutes after inhalation and lasts for 2 to 4 hours. Short-acting bronchodilators are also used before exercise to prevent exercise-induced asthma (EIA).[5,34] *Albuterol* (Proventil) is a SABA that is administered by a metered-dose inhaler (MDI; see figure 11.1), often with a spacer.

Nebulized treatment is preferred for people who have difficulties coordinating MDIs and spacers. A nebulizer is a device that turns liquid medicine into a mist (figure 11.2). As the patient inhales, the mist of medicine is drawn into the lungs. When a nebulizer is used, it is called a breathing treatment or nebulizer treatment. Patients should be instructed on nebulizer use by their prescriber or pharmacist. ATs should be able to assist in the use of a nebulizer.

For acute asthma exacerbations, when possible, **peak expiratory flow (PEF)** should be measured (see section on Assessing Effectiveness of Asthma Medication) and symptoms assessed. Pharmacological intervention is necessary for patients who have PEF <80% of personal or predicted best (see section on Assessing Effectiveness of Asthma Medication),[23] lack of response to SABA treatment, and symptoms such as coughing, breathlessness, wheezing, chest

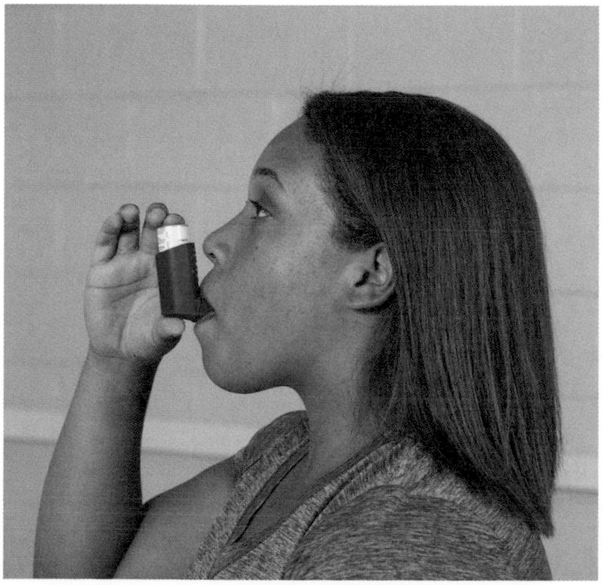

FIGURE 11.1 Metered-dose inhaler.

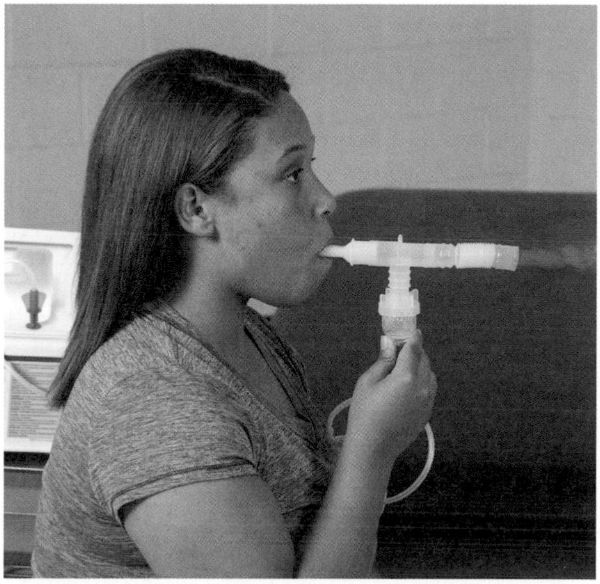

FIGURE 11.2 Nebulizer.

tightness, or use of accessory muscles for breathing. Recommendations from the *NATA Position Statement on Management of Asthma in Athletes* indicate that the AT should administer up to 3 puffs of SABA in 1 hour, reassessing the patient response to treatment every 5 to 10 minutes. If the episode is severe and response is poor (PEF <60% of personal or predicted best), the following are recommended:[21]

- Add prescribed oral corticosteroid drug.
- Repeat SABA treatment immediately.
- Add prescribed inhaled anticholinergic medication.
- Immediately transport the patient to a hospital emergency department.

When these short-acting rescue drugs are effective (symptoms are relieved and PEF returns to >80% of baseline), the acute exacerbation may be managed in the prehospital athletic training setting. Patients who do not respond or have severe symptoms or a PEF persistently <80% of baseline should be transported to the emergency department.[5]

Anticholinergics Anticholinergic medications reduce mucus and open airways by inhibiting muscarinic cholinergic receptors and reducing intrinsic vagal tone of the airway. Administration of anticholinergics provides additive benefit to SABAs in moderate to severe asthma exacerbations. These drugs take longer to be effective than SABAs but may be used as an alternative bronchodilator for patients who do not tolerate SABAs. Anticholinergics such as nebulized *ipratropium* (Atrovent) can be coadministered with nebulized *albuterol* for patients who do not respond optimally to *albuterol* alone. Additionally, anticholinergics can be administered with a soft mist inhaler (SMI), a new generation, propellant-free inhaler that generates a fine, slow-moving cloud (the soft mist) that can be easily inhaled. Based on recommendations, the prescription of *ipratropium* in combination with a SABA such as *albuterol* is an effective and recommended treatment in the management of patients with asthma exacerbation. Controlled trials and a meta-analysis have demonstrated that the addition of *ipratropium* to SABA therapy in the management of moderate to severe acute asthma exacerbations has been associated with a decreased risk of hospitalization and an improvement in lung function.[22]

Systemic (Oral) Corticosteroids Corticosteroid drugs work by reducing inflammation, swelling, and mucus production in the airways of a person with asthma. As a result, the airways are less inflamed and less likely to react to asthma triggers, allowing people with symptoms of asthma to have better control over their condition.[34] Systemic corticosteroids, although not short acting, are used for moderate and severe exacerbations and as an adjunct to SABAs to speed recovery and prevent recurrence of exacerbations. Oral systemic corticosteroids (such as *prednisone*) may be prescribed for all but the mildest acute exacerbation. These drugs are unnecessary for patients whose PEF normalizes after 1 or 2 bronchodilator doses. In general, higher doses of *prednisone* (50 to 60 mg once a day) are prescribed for the management of more severe exacerbations requiring in-patient care, while lower doses (40 mg once a day) are reserved for outpatient treatment of milder exacerbations. Although evidence about optimal dose and duration is weak, a treatment duration of 5 to 7 days is recommended as adequate by most guidelines and should be tailored to the severity and duration of an exacerbation (see the section Long-Term Strategies for Controlling Asthma).[22]

Drugs for Long-Term Asthma Control

Recommendations for long-term asthma control are that medications be taken daily on a long-term basis to achieve and maintain control of persistent asthma. Prescribers should select medication and delivery devices that meet the patient's needs and circumstances and then use a stepwise approach to identify appropriate treatment options. When choosing treatment, prescribers should consider patient risk, impairment, or both, as well as the patient's history of response to the medication and willingness and ability to use it. The most effective long-term-control medications are those that attenuate the underlying inflammation characteristic of asthma. Long-term control medications include asthma drugs that both help to control asthma and prevent asthma attacks, including the following:[22]

- Inhaled corticosteroids (ICS)
- Long-acting beta-agonists (LABAs)
- Inhaled mast cell stabilizers
- Leukotriene modifiers

Inhaled Corticosteroids Inhaled corticosteroids (ICS) are the most potent and consistently effective anti-inflammatory medications currently available for long-term control of asthma. These drugs block late-phase reaction to allergens, reduce airway hyperresponsiveness, and inhibit inflammatory cell migration and activation. The broad action of ICS on the inflammatory process may account for their efficacy as preventive therapy. Dosages of ICS in asthma inhalers vary, and the medication needs to be taken daily for best results. Some improvement in asthma symptoms can be seen 1 to 3 weeks after starting inhaled steroids, with the best results seen after 3 months of daily use. The clinical effects of ICS include the following:[22,34]

- Reduction in severity of symptoms
- Improvement in PEF, asthma control, and quality of life
- Diminished airway hyperresponsiveness
- Prevention of exacerbations
- Reduction in the need for systemic corticosteroid medications
- Reduced emergency department care, hospitalizations, and deaths due to asthma
- Possible attenuation of loss of lung function

Inhaled corticosteroid anti-inflammatory medications cause a reduction in inflammation in airway tissue or airway secretions and thus decrease the intensity of airway hyperresponsiveness. Because many factors contribute to the inflammatory response in asthma, many drugs may be considered anti-inflammatory. It is not yet established, however, which anti-inflammatory actions are responsible for their therapeutic effects. These medications are commonly prescribed as a hydrofluoroalkane (HFA) inhaler, also known as an MDI. The dosing guidelines depend on the severity or duration of an asthma exacerbation. Different dosing may be necessary in patients with mild to moderate asthma experiencing a mild flare in symptoms. Prescribers will modify dosage for patients with no prior history of life-threatening asthma exacerbations and for those with good self-management skills. *Fluticasone* (Flovent) is a common ICS medication used in the long-term treatment of asthma. Other common medications include a combination of corticosteroids and a long-acting bronchodilator drug (LABA), such as the following:

- *fluticasone* and *salmeterol* (Advair)
- *budesonide* and *formoterol* (Symbicort)

Long-Acting Beta-Agonists Long-acting beta-agonists (LABAs; also called long-acting beta-2 agonists or long-acting β-2 agonists) are bronchodilators that have a duration of bronchodilation of ≥12 hours after a single dose. LABAs are not to be used as monotherapy for long-term control of asthma but are used in combination with ICS for long-term control and prevention of symptoms in moderate or severe persistent asthma and with SABAs for management of acute symptoms. Frequent and chronic use of LABAs is discouraged because this may disguise poorly controlled persistent asthma. The use of LABA is not recommended as a rescue medication for the treatment of acute symptoms or exacerbations because their onset of action is >30 minutes.

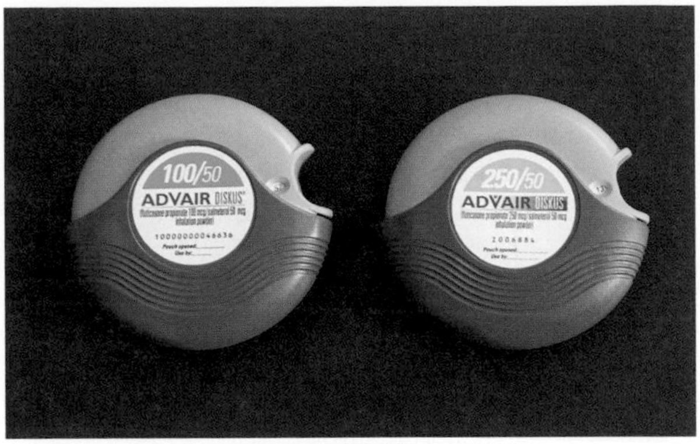

FIGURE 11.3 Dry powder inhaler.

Overuse of LABAs in treating acute asthma exacerbations has resulted in patient deaths. An example of a LABA is *salmeterol* (Serevent Diskus), an inhaled bronchodilator that has duration of bronchodilation of at least 12 hours after a single dose. LABA medications are available as a dry powder that is taken using a small, handheld device called a dry powder inhaler (DPI; see figure 11.3). Common examples are Advair, Flovent, or Serevent. DPIs deliver medication to the lungs as the patient inhales through the device. The DPI does not contain propellants or any other ingredients. It contains only the medication. The DPI Diskus contains up to 60 doses of medication and has a dose indicator that counts down the number of doses remaining.

Inhaled Mast Cell Stabilizers Mast cell stabilizers are an alternative, but not preferred, medication for the treatment of mild persistent asthma. These medicines are also used as preventive treatment prior to exercise or unavoidable exposure to known allergens. These agents stabilize **mast cells** and interfere with chloride channel function. The mast cell stabilizer *cromolyn sodium* (no brand name) may be used as a nebulized treatment prior to exercise or unavoidable exposure to known allergens.

Although experts do not currently recommend *cromolyn* for routine use for asthma due to its lower efficacy relative to other therapies, the drug may be considered for exercise-induced bronchospasm. However, regular controller therapy with ICS or a combination of SABAs and corticosteroids to be used as needed is preferred.[17]

Leukotriene Modifiers Leukotriene modifiers may be used for the treatment of certain conditions associated with allergic response or asthma. Leukotrienes are released from mast cells, basophils, and eosinophils. Leukotriene receptor occupation is the pathophysiology of asthma, including airway edema, smooth muscle contraction, and altered cellular activity associated with the inflammatory process, which contribute to the signs and symptoms of asthma. Leukotriene-receptor antagonists, such as *montelukast* (Singulair), prevent leukotrienes from binding to their receptors. Leukotriene modifiers are administered orally as tablets and have been shown to decrease the need for other asthma medications. These medications have also been shown to be effective in people with allergic rhinitis.[33]

However, *montelukast* (Singulair) has limited availability for use in the United States.[11] Because of its increased risk of adverse consequences, it must be monitored, which makes its use less desirable. The FDA issued a black box warning for *montelukast* in March 2020 to describe possible serious mental health side effects and recommended that *montelukast* be reserved only for treating allergic rhinitis in patients for whom other allergy medicines are ineffective or poorly tolerated.[33]

Assessment of the effectiveness of asthma medication is a key element of asthma care and should be employed on an ongoing basis, depending on the patient's clinical situation. Determining whether control of asthma is effective includes the use of objective measures, self-reported control, and regular visits to the patient's health care provider (HCP).[11]

Assessing Effectiveness of Asthma Medication

Asthma care involves long-term regular monitoring and an individualized written asthma control action plan. The patient's primary HCP should provide a written plan for monitoring the patient's asthma and treating changing symptoms or attacks. To assist the patient in adhering to his asthma action plan, the AT must determine the effectiveness of asthma medication by doing the following:[10,11]

- Assessing the severity of the asthma with lung function measures (e.g., spirometer)
- Recording vital signs (including pulse oximetry and peak flow meter readings)
- Performing a physical examination to identify signs and symptoms

Clinical skills for using a spirometer (**peak flow meter**) are provided in the text *Acute and Emergency Care in Athletic Training.*[10] For a patient in yellow or red zones (see the sidebar Determining Zones of Asthma Control) who has signs or symptoms of an asthma exacerbation, the AT should administer supplemental oxygen and inhaled SABA. Ideally, the AT will have a standing order that allows her to provide SABA to patients with an asthma exacerbation that is consistent with her legally authorized scope of practice and local medical directives. When administering bronchodilator treatment, the AT should not delay patient transport to hospital. Treatment can be repeated while transporting the patient but is limited to a maximum of 3 bronchodilator treatments during the first hour and then 1 per hour thereafter.[5]

The AT's role in the asthma patient's health care team cannot be overstated. In many cases, the AT is the HCP whom the patient encounters daily, allowing him to monitor the patient's response to long-term asthma control medications. Although the AT is not the primary HCP responsible for the asthma patient's care and should never change or stop treatment, his clinical judgment is important in evaluating the patient's response to therapy. The AT clinician must monitor the patient's response on several clinical parameters (e.g., symptoms, activity level, measures of lung function) and record data to report to the prescriber. Once asthma control is achieved and has been sustained ≥3 months, the prescriber can use the patient's data to reassess her medication and carefully titrate it down in a stepwise protocol to the minimum dose necessary for maintaining control.

Long-Term Strategies for Controlling Asthma

Guidelines for the diagnosis and management of asthma are updated regularly. However, asthma guidelines are rarely completely up to date because our knowledge about the pathophysiology and treat-

Determining Zones of Asthma Control

To assess the patient's need and response to asthma medication, find the patient's personal best peak flow meter assessment. The device should be used when asthma is under good control (e.g., the patient feels good and has no symptoms). To work with the patient in determining her individual personal best peak flow number, instruct her to take peak flow readings at the following times:

- At least twice a day for 2 to 3 weeks
- On waking in the morning and in late afternoon or early evening
- 15-20 minutes after taking her short-acting rescue inhaler
- Other times as directed by her prescriber

For each peak flow reading, the numbers should be used to determine the patient's personal best peak flow and to individualize 3 peak flow zones. These zones should be documented on the patient's asthma action plan. The zones are set up like a traffic light in green, yellow, and red to assist the patient in knowing what to do in each zone when her peak flow number changes (table 11.3).

TABLE 11.3 Zones of Asthma Control

Zone	% of personal best	Description
Green zone (go)	80% to 100%	Signals good control and no asthma symptoms. If the patient takes daily long-term control medicines (LABA), he should continue to follow the prescriber's instructions and keep taking them even when his peak flow number falls in the yellow or red zones.
Yellow zone (caution)	50% to 79%	Signals caution: The patient's asthma is getting worse. Follow the patient's written asthma plan and add quick-relief medicines (SABA). The prescriber may need to adjust asthma medicines.
Red zone (medical alert)	<50%	Signals medical alert! Add or increase quick-relief medicines (SABA) according to instructions in the written asthma action plan and call EMS immediately.

SABA = short-acting beta-agonists, LABA = long-acting beta-agonists

Based on Cloutier et al. (2020); National Heart, Lung, and Blood Institute (2020).

ment of asthma is continually evolving.[3] According to current asthma clinical practice guidelines, most people can effectively control their asthma with proper education and self-care.[6] Quality asthma care involves not only initial diagnosis and treatment to achieve asthma control, but also long-term regular follow-up care to maintain control. Asthma control focuses on the following:

- **Preventing exacerbation**—In particular, prevention focuses on EIA.
- **Reducing impairment**—Includes preventing asthma symptoms, reducing rescue medication use, maintaining lung function, and maintaining normal physical activity levels and attendance at work or school.
- **Reducing risk**—Minimizing the need for emergency department visits and hospitalizations and preventing repeated asthma attacks.

Achieving and maintaining asthma control requires providing appropriate medication, addressing environmental factors that cause worsening symptoms, helping patients learn self-management skills, and monitoring the asthma over the long term to assess control and adjust therapy accordingly. In general, patients with well-controlled asthma should fit the following profile:

- Few, if any, asthma symptoms
- Few, if any, awakenings during the night caused by asthma symptoms
- No need to take time off from school or work due to asthma
- Few or no limits on full participation in physical activities

Clinical Application

Preventing Exacerbation of Exercise-Induced Asthma

According to the *NATA Position Statement on Management of Asthma in Athletes*,[21] ATs should understand the various types of pharmacologic strategies used for short- and long-term asthma control and should be able to differentiate controller from rescue drugs or reliever medications. To prevent exacerbation of exercise-induced asthma (EIA) symptoms during practice and game participation, patients may be prescribed short- and long-acting beta-agonists. The recommendations include the following:[21,25]

- Encourage physical activity; for most patients, EIA should not limit participation in any activity they choose.
- Encourage an extended warm-up period; in cold weather, athletes should wear a mask or scarf over the mouth.
- Teach patients to take treatment before exercise. SABAs will prevent symptoms in most patients.
- For prophylaxis, use a rapid-acting SABA, such as *albuterol*, inhaled 10 to 15 minutes before exercise. The AT should be aware that excessive overuse of a SABA can lead to an increased tolerance to the medication, resulting in decreased effectiveness.
- The frequent need (≥3 times per day) for SABA therapy during practice or an athletic event should cause concern, and a physician should evaluate the patient before return to participation.
- ATs should understand the use, misuse, and abuse of SABAs. A history of cough, shortness of breath, chest pain or tightness, wheezing, or endurance problems during exercise suggests exercise-induced bronchospasm (EIB).
- Consider long-term control medication. EIB is often a marker of inadequate asthma control and responds well to regular anti-inflammatory therapy.
- Long-acting beta-2 agonists should, in general, be used only for asthma prophylaxis and control. They are usually combined with an inhaled corticosteroid.
- Frequent or chronic use of long-acting beta-agonists to prevent symptoms is discouraged, since it may disguise poorly controlled persistent asthma.

- No emergency department visits
- No hospital stays
- Few or no side effects from asthma medicines

Certified Asthma Educators

A certified asthma educator is typically a licensed HCP (e.g., nurse, respiratory therapist, pharmacist) with an additional certification in asthma education, but people who are not HCPs also can become certified if they have ≥1,000 hours of relevant experience and pass the National Asthma Educator Certification Board Exam. Multiple effective, economically sustainable programs implementing asthma control employ certified asthma educators. Additional information regarding certified asthma educators is available on the CDC's National Asthma Control Program website.[6]

Summary

The vulnerable respiratory system has multiple defense mechanisms that are found throughout the lining of the respiratory tract, the respiratory mucosa, and the respiratory epithelium.[2] ATs must have the knowledge and skills to recognize respiratory infections and a functional understanding of the various pathogens that invade the respiratory tract. This chapter discusses how particles in the air we breathe manifest into respiratory infections and allergic reactions, including asthma, and the pharmacological treatment for these common respiratory conditions. The discussion is focused on acute respiratory conditions in otherwise healthy people >12 years old. In this population, the AT is most likely to encounter the common cold and influenza and should be prepared to take steps to ensure that a sick person does not infect an entire team, performing troupe, or military platoon. Other common but less contagious respiratory infections include causes of sore throat, such as tonsillopharyngitis, pharyngitis, and strep throat. Sinusitis, bronchitis, and pneumonia can be caused by bacteria or viruses, and prescribers must use caution when prescribing antibiotics for an infection that could be viral in origin. For these conditions, the AT should recommend supportive care for treating the patient's symptoms and helping the patient feel more comfortable while the viral illness runs its course.

When treating patients with acute asthma exacerbations, prescribers use a stepwise approach to pharmacologic therapy to gain and maintain asthma control. In developing an asthma action plan, prescribers should consider the type, amount, and scheduling of medication, which is dictated by asthma severity and the level of asthma control. It is important to identify the minimum medication necessary for maintaining control, which requires patience and collaboration among members of the health care team. The AT has an essential role in assessing the effectiveness of medication, facilitating long-term strategies for controlling asthma, monitoring patient adherence to the asthma action plan, and referring the patient to the prescriber for follow-up.

Case Studies

Case Study 1

Arnie is sophomore football player who has been diagnosed with exercise-induced asthma (EIA). He routinely relies on 2 or 3 puffs of his Flovent inhaler in the morning and evening to minimize any effects of bronchospasm. However, when doing two-a-day conditioning sessions in the heat, Arnie has needed his prescribed Ventolin as a rescue inhaler when his wheezing exacerbated. One day, a teammate in respiratory distress approached Arnie and asked to borrow his Ventolin. Arnie gave it to him. Two days later, 4 other players said they were out of breath and needed something to help with it, so they wanted to use Arnie's Ventolin. The AT questioned these other 4 players and found they had never been diagnosed with asthma. The AT advised Arnie to not share his Ventolin with teammates.

Questions for Analysis

1. What is the purpose of Ventolin?
2. What is the problem with sharing the medication?

Case Study 2

Maurice and his younger brother Henri are high school teachers in the same district but at different schools. Flu season started early in their area, and each received their annual flu vaccine. In early January, Maurice started feeling the classic symptoms of the flu: body aches, congestion, low-grade fever, and fatigue. He thought he could manage it without seeking immediate medical attention, but after missing a day of school, he eventually did see his family physician. After a few days of rest and fluids, Maurice felt improved enough to return to school. About a week later, Henri felt what seemed to be the onset of the flu: unexplained body aches and more fatigue than usual. Henri saw his physician and was prescribed Tamiflu. He followed the course of medication established by his physician and was able to avoid any significant illness.

Questions for Analysis

1. Why was Tamiflu prescribed?
2. Tamiflu seemed to work for Henri. Would it have worked for Maurice if he had started it after experiencing flulike symptoms?

Drugs Discussed in This Chapter

Drug class	*generic* (pronunciation) Trade names	Therapeutic uses	Clinical concerns
Expectorants	*guaifenesin* (gwye FEN e sin) Mucinex	Oral cough expectorant (granules mixed in hot water): 200 to 400 mg every 4 hr as needed; maximum dosage: 2,400 mg/24 hr Extended-release tablet: 600 mg to 1,200 mg every 12 hr as needed; maximum dosage: 2,400 mg/24 hr Immediate-release tablet: 200 to 400 mg every 4 hr as needed; maximum dosage: 2,400 mg/24 hr Liquid: 200 to 400 mg every 4 hr as needed; maximum dosage: 2,400 mg/24 hr	Adverse reaction: Central nervous system issues include dizziness, drowsiness, nervousness, and re lessness.
Antitussives	*dextromethorphan* (deks troe meth OR fan) Robitussin	Oral: 10 to 20 mg every 4 hr or 20 to 30 mg every 6 to 8 hr Extended release: 60 mg twice daily; maximum dosage: 120 mg/24 hr	Adverse reaction: Central nervous system issues include dizziness, drowsiness, nervousness, and re lessness.
Antivirals	*oseltamivir* (oh sel TAM i vir) Tamiflu	Influenza type A and B treatment: 75 mg by mouth twice daily Influenza type A and B prophylaxis: 75 mg by mouth once daily for 7 days postexposure (or for a minimum of 2 wk for control of outbreaks in long-term care facilities and hospitals, and continue for up to 1 wk for last known case)	May cause occasional nausea and iting.
	acyclovir (ay SYE kloe veer) Zovirax	For viral pneumonia: 5 to 10 mg/kg IV every 8 hr	Although pure viral pneumonia do occur, superimposed bacterial inf tions are common and require an ics directed against *S. pneumonia influenzae*, and *S. aureus*.
Antihistamines: sedating (first generation)	*diphenhydramine* (dye fen HYE dra meen) Benadryl	Oral: 25 to 50 mg every 4 to 8 hr; maximum dosage: 300 mg daily	Central nervous system issues inc sedation, vertigo, ataxia, chills, co sion, dizziness, drowsiness, euph excitement, fatigue, headache, irr ity, and nervousness.
Antihistamines: nonsedating (second generation)	*loratadine* (lor AT a deen) Claritin	Oral: 10 mg once daily or 5 mg twice daily	Longer action; used at 5 mg dosag

g class	*generic* (pronunciation) Trade names	Therapeutic uses	Clinical concerns
sal decongestants: pha-adrenergic (α-1 drenergic) receptor gonists	*pseudoephedrine* (soo doe e FED rin) Sudafed	Oral: Immediate release: 60 mg every 4 to 6 hr Extended release: 120 mg every 12 hr or 240 mg every 24 hr; maximum dosage: 240 mg per 24 hr	Adverse reactions: Cardiovascular issues include cardiac arrhythmia, chest tightness, circulatory shock (with hypotension), hypertension, palpitations, and tachycardia.
	phenylephrine (fen il EF rin) Neo-Synephrine Cold & Sinus nasal spray	Intranasal 0.25% to 1% solution: Instill 2 or 3 sprays in each nostril no more than every 4 hr for ≤3 d.	Provides temporary relief of nasal congestion due to the common cold, hay fever, or other upper respiratory allergies (allergic rhinitis). For intranasal use only. Before using for the first time, prime the pump by firmly depressing the rim several times. Keep head upright and insert nozzle into nostril, depress rim firmly, and inhale deeply.
	oxymetazoline (oks i met AZ oh leen) Afrin Nasal Spray	Intranasal: Instill 2 or 3 sprays into each nostril twice daily for ≤3 d (maximum dose: 2 doses/24 hr)	Dry nose, nasal congestion (rebound; chronic use), nasal mucosa irritation (temporary), sneezing
thma rescue drugs: hort-acting beta-agnists (SABA)* or hort-acting β-2 agosts	*albuterol* (al BYOO ter ole) Proventil, ProAir, Ventolin	MDI: 90 mcg/puff	Inhalation powder: 1 or 2 inhalations (90 to 180 mcg) orally every 4 to 6 hr
		Nebulized solution: 5 mg/mL and 0.63, 1.25, and 2.5 mg/3 mL	2.5-5 mg every 20 min for 3 doses, then 2.5-10 mg every 1-4 hr as needed
thma rescue drugs: nticholinergics*	*ipratropium* (i pra TROE pee um) Atrovent	Nebulized solution: 500 mcg/2.5 mL (0.02%)	0.5 mg every 20 min for 3 doses, then every 2-4 hr as needed
thma rescue drugs: ombination drugs	*ipratropium* and *albuterol* (i pra TROE pee um) and (al BYOO ter ole) DuoNeb combination drug	SMI: 20 mcg *ipratropium* 100 mcg *albuterol*/puff	1 puff every 30 min for 3 doses, then every 2-4 hr as needed
		Nebulized solution: 0.5 mg *ipratropium* and 2.5 mg *albuterol* in a 3-mL vial	3 mL every 30 min for 3 doses, then every 2-4 hr as needed
thma rescue drugs: stemic corticosterds	*prednisone* (PRED ni sone) Mainly generic	Tablets: 1, 2.5, 5, 10, 20, and 50 mg Solution: 5 mg/mL	Tapering the dose is not needed if patients are also given inhaled corticosteroids.
ng-term asthma ontrol: inhaled cortiosteroids	*fluticasone* (floo TIK a zone) Flovent HFA	MDI: Initially based on previous asthma therapy and asthma severity. Take 88 mcg twice daily, approximately 12 hr apart. Higher dosages may provide additional asthma control. Maximum daily dosage: 1,760 mcg.	Each actuation delivers 44, 110, or 220 mcg of *fluticasone*. Not indicated for rapid relief of bronchospasm. Patients should contact their physicians immediately when episodes of asthma are not responsive to bronchodilators. During such episodes, patients may require therapy with oral corticosteroids.
ng-term asthma ontrol: long-acting eta-adrenergic (or β-2 drenergic) agonist	*salmeterol* (sal ME te role) Serevent Diskus	DPI: 1 inhalation (50 mcg) twice daily (~12 hr apart); maximum dosage: 2 inhalations per day.	For asthma control, long-acting beta-2 agonists (LABAs) should be used in combination with inhaled corticosteroids and not as monotherapy.

ount and timing of ongoing doses are dictated by clinical response.
referable to use a higher mcg/puff or mcg/inhalation formulation to achieve as low a number of puffs or inhalations as possible.
red-dose inhaler (MDI) dosages are expressed as the actuator dose, which is the amount leaving the actuator and delivered to the patient. Dry der inhaler (DPI) doses are expressed as the amount of drug in the inhaler following activation. Hydrofluoroalkane (HFA) inhalers, also called s, are administered using a nebulizer or soft mist inhaler (SMI).

12

Drugs for Treating Cardiovascular Conditions

OBJECTIVES

After reading this chapter, you will be able to do the following:

- Recognize red flag signs and symptoms that raise suspicion of a serious cardiac condition
- Summarize the drug classes used to treat cardiovascular conditions
- Identify example generic and trade drug names for each drug class

In the prehospital setting, unstable patients with abnormal vital signs, concerning ECG findings (if available), a history of prior coronary artery disease, multiple cardiovascular risk factors, or any abrupt, new, or severe chest pain or dyspnea should be treated quickly. The athletic trainer (AT) should identify and treat immediate life needs like supporting the airway, breathing, and circulation. Vital signs should be measured promptly and recorded at regular intervals. If pulse oximetry indicates O_2 saturation (O_2 sat) <95%, supplemental oxygen should be administered through a nasal cannula or non-rebreather face mask.[22] If any life-threatening signs or symptoms are present, the AT should activate the emergency action plan and arrange prompt transport of the patient to the emergency department for further evaluation and treatment.

RED FLAG

More Serious Etiology of Chest Pain

Certain findings raise suspicion of a more serious etiology of chest pain:[4,27]

- Abnormal vital signs: tachycardia, bradycardia, tachypnea, hypotension
- Signs of hypoperfusion: confusion, ashen color, diaphoresis
- Shortness of breath
- Hypoxemia on pulse oximetry, O_2 sat <95%
- Asymmetric breath sounds or pulses
- New heart murmurs
- **Pulsus paradoxus** >10 mmHg

Select Drugs Mentioned in This Chapter

Drug class	Generic name	Trade name
Antiatherogenic drugs		
Antiplatelet agents	*aspirin*	Bufferin, others
The statins	*atorvastatin*	Lipitor
Antihypertensive agents		
Loop diuretics	*furosemide*	Lasix
Thiazide diuretics	*hydrochlorothiazide*	HydroDIURIL
Beta-blockers (may also be used as antiarrhythmic or antianginal agents)	*labetalol* *metoprolol* *propranolol*	Normodyne Lopressor, Toprol-XL Inderal
ACE inhibitors	*lisinopril*	Prinivil, Zestril
Angiotensin II receptor blockers	*losartan*	Cozaar
Antianginal agents		
Nitrates	*nitroglycerin* (NTG)	Sublingual: Nitrostat SL Spray: Nitrolingual
Antiarrhythmic agents		
Cardiac glycosides	*digoxin*	Lanoxin, many others
Sodium channel blockers	*procainamide*	Generic only
Potassium channel blockers	*amiodarone*	Cordarone, Nexterone
Calcium channel blockers (maybe also used as antianginal and antihypotensive agents)	*verapamil*	Calan
Anticoagulants		
Blood thinners	*warfarin*	Coumadin

This list is not exhaustive, but rather contains examples of common drugs for treating cardiovascular conditions encountered in the athletic training setting.

In a stable patient, the AT should focus on the patient history and physical exam. A focused history should include symptoms, brief past medical history, and review of systems, seeking features of life-threatening causes of chest pain.[27] This chapter discusses pharmacological interventions for the most common cardiovascular conditions encountered in the athletic training setting.

Ischemic Chest Pain: Angina Pectoris

Angina pectoris is chest discomfort resulting from myocardial ischemia from an imbalance between myocardial oxygen supply and demand. If the demand for myocardial blood flow exceeds the capacity of obstructed coronary arteries to supply it, the discomfort lasts until the excessive demand for coronary flow is reduced.[8] Discomfort is more intense and lasts longer when coronary blood flow decreases markedly. Myocardial necrosis may occur, resulting in **myocardial infarction (MI)**; otherwise, the episode is one of acute coronary insufficiency, or preinfarction angina.[4]

Drugs for Managing Ischemic Chest Pain

Anti-ischemic drugs or short-acting nitrates, such as *nitroglycerin* (NTG), are the drugs of choice to reduce cardiac workload in patients with angina pectoris. *Nitroglycerin* dilates veins, arteries, and arterioles, resulting in reduced left-ventricular preload and afterload. As a result, myocardial oxygen demand is reduced, decreasing ischemia.[24] Current recommendations for patients who have previously been prescribed NTG are as follows:

- Take 1 dose of 0.4 mg NTG sublingually when pain starts.
- If pain does not improve after 5 minutes, the AT should call 911 before the patient takes any additional NTG.
- NTG can be repeated every 5 minutes up to 3 doses or until emergency medical services arrive.[4]

NTG may also be taken prophylactically several minutes before activities that regularly precipitate angina. Pain is usually relieved in 1 to 2 minutes. NTG tablets deteriorate in about 6 months once the original container has been opened. They must be dispensed in the original glass container, never in a plastic vial. Headache and sublingual tingling are common side effects of active, potent tablets.[4]

Atherosclerosis and Coronary Artery Disease

Atherosclerosis encompasses increased lipid deposition in blood vessels (early plaque), endothelial dysfunction, less vasodilation, increased risk of platelet adhesion, and narrowing of the blood vessel by increasing plaque formation. Taken together, important factors that determine the progress of **coronary artery disease** (CAD) are the concentration of lipids in the blood, endothelial function, blood pressure (BP), the activity of the inflammatory system, and the reactivity of pro- and antithrombotic systems.

Hyperlipidemia, or **dyslipidemia**, is elevation of plasma cholesterol, triglycerides, or both that contributes to the development of atherosclerosis and diabetes. Atherosclerosis is initially asymptomatic, often for decades. Symptoms and signs develop when lesions impede blood flow, leading to CAD and transient ischemic symptoms related to angina pectoris, as well as **transient ischemic attacks** (TIA). When unstable plaques rupture and acutely occlude a major artery, a thrombosis or embolism develops, resulting in MI, ischemic stroke or **cerebral vascular accident** (CVA), or sudden death without preceding stable or unstable angina pectoris.[26]

Drugs for Managing Atherosclerosis

The treatment of CAD resulting from atherosclerosis includes nonpharmacologic interventions such as risk factor reduction, lifestyle and dietary modifications, physical activity, and revascularization techniques (e.g., percutaneous coronary intervention, coronary artery bypass grafting). Drug therapy to treat CAD include the following:[5,8,18,25,26]

- **Antiplatelet agents**—Nonenteric-coated, chewable *aspirin* for acute chest pain; enteric-coated *aspirin* for long-term antiplatelet effects
- **Antiatherogenic agents**—The statins, such as *atorvastatin* (Lipitor)
- **Antiangina agents (nitrates)**—Such as *nitroglycerin* as needed for angina pectoris
- **Angiotensin-converting enzyme (ACE) inhibitors**—Such as *lisinopril* (Prinivil, Zestril)
- **Angiotensin II receptor blockers**—Such as *losartan* (Cozaar) and the *-sartans*
- **β-adrenergic blocking agents (beta-blockers)**—Such as *labetalol* (Normodyne), as described in the Hypertension and Hypertensive Crisis section; it is important for athletes who are subject to drug testing to discuss using beta-blockers with their prescriber
- **Anticoagulants**—Such as unfractionated *heparin* or *warfarin* (Coumadin)

These drugs are discussed further in the sections that follow.

Antiplatelet Agents: Aspirin

All patients who have CAD or are at high risk of developing CAD who present with chest pain are given *aspirin* 160 to 325 mg (not enteric coated), if not contraindicated (e.g., life-threatening active bleeding, allergy), at presentation and 81 mg (enteric coated) once daily indefinitely thereafter. Chewing the first dose before swallowing quickens absorption. *Aspirin* reduces short- and long-term mortality risk.[18]

Antiatherogenic Drugs: The Statins

The statins are hypolipidemic agents that inhibit an enzyme (HMG-CoA reductase) that blocks the metabolic pathway for synthesizing cholesterol in the liver. Low-density lipoproteins (LDL) are carriers of cholesterol and play a key role in the development of atherosclerosis and coronary heart disease. Statins are effective in lowering LDL cholesterol and are widely used for primary prevention in people at high risk of cardiovascular disease, as well as in secondary prevention for those who have already developed cardiovascular disease.[26]

Evidence in Pharmacology

Food–Drug Interactions

Grapefruit juice can interact with many medications, including statins. It is recommended that patients who are prescribed select statins avoid consuming grapefruit juice. Grapefruit juice contains a class of compounds, furanocoumarins, that prevents the complete breakdown of the statin by blocking the enzyme activity needed to break down the statin.[11,14] If the medication is not sufficiently metabolized, the resultant levels of medication in the body (greater than intended) could result in adverse side effects, such as statin-induced myopathy.[6] According to the Cleveland Clinic, the original research involved large quantities of grapefruit juice, >2 qt (1.9 L) per day.[6] A much smaller quantity is less likely to cause concern. Certain statins that are heavily metabolized by this enzyme, such as *atorvastatin*, *lovastatin*, and *simvastatin*, are more affected than other statins.[6]

Antiatherogenic drugs are prescribed to all patients with CAD without contraindications (e.g., statin-induced **myopathy**, liver dysfunction) to statin therapy. Examples of antiatherogenic drugs are the following:

- *atorvastatin* (Lipitor)
- *fluvastatin* (Lescol)
- *lovastatin* (Mevacor)
- *pravastatin* (Pravachol)
- *rosuvastatin* (Crestor)
- *simvastatin* (Zocor)

RED FLAG

Statin-Induced Myopathy

Atorvastatin (Lipitor) is prescribed for patients with CAD. Dosing should be titrated to achieve the patient's LDL goal as determined by the provider. Of concern to the AT is the major adverse effect associated with statin use, statin-induced myopathy. Myopathy refers to a broad spectrum of muscle complaints, ranging from mild muscle soreness, pain, or weakness (**myalgia**) to life-threatening **rhabdomyolysis**, as indicated by elevated creatine kinase (CK). The risk of muscle adverse effects increases in proportion to statin dose and plasma concentrations.[12]

Acute Coronary Syndrome

Acute coronary syndrome (ACS) refers to a spectrum of conditions that develop from coronary blood flow that is insufficient to meet the metabolic needs of the myocardium. ACS results from acute obstruction of a coronary artery, and its consequences depend on the degree and location of the obstruction. Individual patients may present differently, and great overlap in cardiac symptoms exists.

RED FLAG

Symptoms of Acute Coronary Syndrome

- Classic cardiac chest pain—Retrosternal left anterior chest crushing, squeezing, tightness, or pressure.
- Radiating chest pain—Moving to the arms, neck, or jaw; patient may experience diaphoresis, dyspnea, and nausea or vomiting.
- Exertional cardiac chest pain—Brought on or exacerbated by stress or exertion and relieved by rest.

Drugs for Treating Acute Coronary Syndrome

Prehospital interventions that can be performed by the AT or other health care provider (HCP) in the treatment of ACS include the following:[4,24]

- **Antiplatelet drugs**—The first and most important medication given to ACS patients presenting with acute chest pain is *aspirin*, administered as up to four 81 mg nonenteric-coated chewable tablets. Chewing the first dose before swallowing quickens absorption. *Aspirin* reduces short- and long-term mortality risk.

- **Supplemental oxygen**—If pulse oximetry indicates O_2 saturation is <95%, administer 2 L/min oxygen by nasal cannula.
- **Anti-ischemic drugs**—For patients with chest pain or hypertension who have been previously prescribed medications:
  - **Short-acting nitrates** such as *nitroglycerin* administered 0.4 mg sublingually or 1 spray delivered to the oral mucosa. Repeat if no effect occurs in 5 minutes, chest pain is not relieved, or SBP falls by 10%. Systolic blood pressure (SBP) should not drop below 90 mmHg.
  - **β-adrenergic blocking agents** such as *metoprolol* (Lopressor) administered 25 mg orally unless contraindicated (heart rate <60 beats/min, severe asthma, or chronic obstructive pulmonary disease). β-blocker use is recommended in first 24 hours of unstable angina.
- **Anticoagulants**—Prescriptions may include unfractionated *heparin* or *warfarin* (Coumadin), which are routinely administered to patients with ACS unless contraindicated by active bleeding or planned use of a **fibrinolytic** drug. These drugs are further described in the section Drugs for Treating Venous Thromboembolisms.

Hypertension and Hypertensive Crisis

Hypertension is the sustained elevation of resting systolic BP (≥130 mmHg), diastolic BP (≥80 mmHg), or both. Usually, no symptoms develop unless hypertension is severe or long standing. Very high BP without organ damage commonly occurs in highly anxious patients or those who have had very poor sleep quality over a period of weeks.[3] In the prehospital setting, a patient with suspected hypertensive urgency or hypertensive emergency requires immediate hospitalization.

Drugs for Managing Hypertension

Managing hypertension typically involves a combination of lifestyle changes and drugs. The AT may encounter these typical first-line drugs for managing hypertension:[3,4,9,24]

- **Diuretics**—Thiazides and thiazide-like diuretics such as *hydrochlorothiazide* (HydroDIURIL) and loop diuretics such as *furosemide* (Lasix)
- **β-adrenergic blocking agents (beta-blockers)**—Such as *propranolol* (Inderal)
- **Angiotensin-converting enzyme (ACE) inhibitors**—Such as *captopril* and many others with the suffix *-pril*
- **Angiotensin II receptor blockers**—The *-sartans*, such as *losartan* (Cozaar)
- **Calcium channel blockers**—Such as *verapamil* (Calan)

Diuretics

The AT should be familiar with common medications used to produce diuretic effects. A **diuretic** is any substance that promotes diuresis, the increased production of urine. All diuretics increase the excretion of water from the body (figure 12.1), although there are several categories of diuretics, each with a different mechanism of action. Conversely, an antidiuretic, such as *vasopressin* (an antidiuretic hormone, or ADH), is an agent that reduces the excretion of water in urine. A common strategy for the management of hypertension is to alter sodium balance by restriction of salt in the diet. Pharmacological alteration of sodium balance has an antihypertensive effect when using diuretic agents alone and can enhance the efficacy of virtually all other antihypertensive drugs. Thus, diuretics remain important in the treatment of hypertension. Many drugs are used as diuretics for the treatment of hypertension. The 2 major classes are as follows:[9]

- **Loop diuretics**—The prototype in this class used to treat edema is *furosemide* (Lasix). *Furosemide* works by decreasing the reabsorption of sodium in the thick ascending limb of the nephron loop (loop of Henle) of the kidneys. It has a secondary use to treat high blood pressure and can be administered by mouth or intravenously (IV). When taken by mouth, it typically begins working within an hour; when administered intravenously, it typically begins working within 5 minutes. Common side effects of *furosemide* include lightheadedness when standing, ringing in the ears, and sensitivity to light. Potentially serious side effects include decreases in magnesium, calcium, potassium, and sodium;

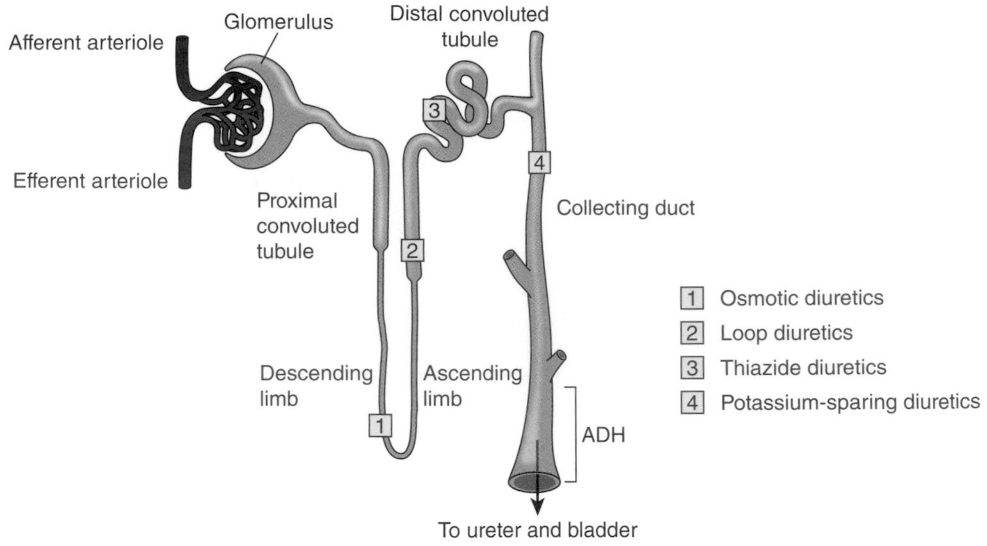

FIGURE 12.1 Sites of action for diuretics in the nephron loop of the kidneys.

low blood pressure; and hearing loss. Regular blood tests are recommended for those on this treatment. Loop diuretics are more potent than thiazides.

- **Thiazides and thiazide-like diuretics**—These drugs that act on the distal convoluted tubule of the nephron are the most frequently prescribed class of antihypertensive agents in the United States. *Hydrochlorothiazide* (HydroDIURIL) is one of the most widely used diuretics in the treatment of hypertension. Antihypertensive effects can be achieved with oral dosages of 25 to 100 mg taken once or twice daily. Common side effects include low blood potassium and magnesium, high blood glucose, dizziness, increased calcium and uric acid, and increased serum cholesterol.

β-*Adrenergic Blocking Agents (Beta-Blockers)*

Beta receptors are found on cells of the heart muscles, smooth muscles, airways, arteries, kidneys, and other tissues that are part of the sympathetic nervous system and lead to stress responses, especially when they are stimulated by epinephrine (adrenaline). β-adrenergic blocking agents (beta-blockers) are competitive antagonists that are predominantly used to manage abnormal arrhythmias and protect the heart from a second acute myocardial infarction (AMI) after a first one (secondary prevention).[3,9] These medications are widely used to treat hypertension, although they are no longer the first choice for initial treatment of most patients. The prototypical beta-blocker is *propranolol* (Inderal), which blocks sympathetic stimulation of the heart, reducing heart rate, cardiac contractility, conduction velocity, and relaxation rate, which in turn decreases myocardial oxygen demand and increases exercise tolerance. Heart rate and BP must be carefully monitored during treatment with beta-blockers. Dosage is reduced if bradycardia or hypotension develops.[24]

Clinical Application

Sudden Cardiac Death of an Athlete

Hank Gathers was an outstanding collegiate basketball player who was diagnosed with a cardiac condition after a syncopal episode during a game. Secondary to this, he was prescribed the beta-blocker Inderal (*propranolol*). Hank acknowledged difficulty adapting to the medication because he felt like it slowed him down, so the dose was reduced on 3 different occasions by his physicians.[28] During a game, Hank sustained a fatal sudden cardiac arrest. An autopsy indicated he had not taken his prescribed medication for at least 8 hours before his collapse.[1] Providers of critical cases must be certain that athletes understand the consequences of potential deviation from their drug protocol.

Angiotensin-Converting Enzyme (ACE) Inhibitors

An **angiotensin-converting enzyme** (ACE) inhibitor is a pharmaceutical drug used primarily for the treatment of hypertension, chronic kidney disease, and congestive heart failure. Angiotensin II is a hormone that causes blood vessels to constrict, resulting in increased BP and forcing the heart to work harder to pump blood. This group of drugs causes relaxation of blood vessels as well as a decrease in blood volume, which leads to lowered blood pressure and decreased oxygen demand from the heart. They inhibit the angiotensin-converting enzyme, an important component of the **renin–angiotensin system**. All ACE inhibitors block the conversion of angiotensin I to angiotensin II and have similar therapeutic indications, adverse-effect profiles, and contraindications.

Because hypertension usually requires lifelong treatment, quality-of-life issues are an important consideration in comparing antihypertensive drugs. ACE inhibitors reduce mortality risk in patients with myocardial infarction, especially in those with anterior infarction, heart failure, or tachycardia. The greatest benefit occurs in the highest-risk patients early during convalescence.[12,25]

A frequently prescribed ACE inhibitor is *lisinopril* (Prinivil, Zestril). Other examples of ACE inhibitors are drugs with the suffix *-pril*:[15]

- *benazepril* (Lotensin)
- *captopril* (Capoten)
- *enalapril* (Epaned, Vasotec)
- *perindopril* (Aceon)
- *ramipril* (Altace)
- *trandolapril* (Mavik)

Angiotensin II Receptor Blockers

All angiotensin II receptor blockers (ARBs) are approved for the treatment of hypertension. These drugs block this hormone, allowing relaxation of smooth muscle in arteries and veins and thus lowering BP. The efficacy of ARBs in lowering blood pressure is comparable with that of ACE inhibitors. ARBs have a favorable adverse-effect profile. Contraindications for ACE inhibitors and ARBs include hypotension, acute kidney failure, bilateral renal artery stenosis, pregnancy, and known allergy. The orally active, potent, and selective nonpeptide ARB *losartan* (Cozaar) was developed and approved for clinical use in the United States in 1995. Since then, several additional ARBs, the *-sartans*, have been approved:[15]

- *azilsartan* (Edarbi)
- *candesartan* (Atacand)
- *irbesartan* (Avapro)
- *olmesartan* (Benicar)
- *telmisartan* (Micardis)
- *valsartan* (Diovan)

Cardiac Arrhythmias

The heart normally beats in a regular, coordinated way because electrical impulses generated and spread by myocytes with unique electrical properties trigger a sequence of organized myocardial contractions. Arrhythmias (also known as dysrhythmia) and conduction disorders are caused by abnormalities in the generation or conduction of these electrical impulses. An arrhythmia is a rhythm disturbance resulting from cardiac abnormalities of impulse formation, impulse conduction, or both. The AT should carefully review each athlete's medical record for history of arrhythmia to ensure proper referral or monitoring. If left untreated, arrhythmia can lead to life-threatening complications, such as stroke, heart failure, or sudden cardiac arrest.[21]

Drugs for Treating Arrhythmias

Treatment of cardiac arrhythmia is directed at its causes and may include antiarrhythmic drugs.[21] Antiarrhythmic agents, also known as cardiac dysrhythmia medications, are a group of pharmaceuticals that are used to suppress abnormal rhythms of the heart. Many classes of antiarrhythmic medications exist, and each has different mechanisms of action and contains many different individual drugs. Although the goal of drug therapy is to prevent arrhythmia, nearly every antiarrhythmic drug has the potential to act as a proarrhythmic. Thus, these drugs must be carefully selected and used under medical supervision. Cardiologists and other HCPs treating patients with arrhythmias may use a variety of medications to manage the condition. Examples of medications used to treat cardiac arrhythmias include the following:[17,20,21]

- **Sodium channel blockers**—Such as *procainamide* (Pronestyl). These drugs block transmission of electrical signals, lengthen cell recovery periods, and make cardiac cells less excitable. However, they can increase risks of sudden cardiac arrest in people who have heart disease.

- **Calcium channel blockers**—Such as *verapamil* (Calan, among others). These drugs slow a rapid heart rate or the speed at which signals travel. Typically, they are used to control arrhythmias of the upper chambers. In some cases, calcium channel blockers can trigger ventricular fibrillation. They can also cause constipation, peripheral edema, and low blood pressure.
- **Potassium channel blockers**—Such as *amiodarone* (Cordarone, Nexterone). These drugs inhibit adrenergic stimulation (alpha- and beta-blocking properties); affect sodium, potassium, and calcium channels; prolong the action potential and refractory period in myocardial tissue; and decrease atrioventricular conduction and sinus node function. Contraindications include hypersensitivity to amiodarone, iodine, or any component of the formulation; sick sinus syndrome; second- or third-degree atrioventricular block; bradycardia leading to syncope without a functioning pacemaker; and cardiogenic shock.
- **Cardiac glycosides**—Such as *digoxin* (Lanoxin, among others). These medications are frequently used to treat a fast heart rate, atrial fibrillation, atrial flutter, and heart failure. *Digoxin* shortens atrial and ventricular refractory periods and is vagotonic, thereby prolonging cardiac conduction and refractory periods. It can trigger arrhythmias and cause nausea, loss of appetite, visual disturbances, and confusion. *Digoxin* toxicity includes nausea, vomiting, visual changes, and cardiac arrhythmias; toxicity is usually associated with digoxin levels >2 ng/mL, although symptoms may occur at lower levels.
- **β-adrenergic blocking agents (beta-blockers)**—Such as *propranolol* (Inderal). These drugs competitively block response to β1- and β2-adrenergic stimulation, which decreases heart rate, myocardial contractility, blood pressure, and myocardial oxygen demand. Beta-blockers are generally well tolerated. Adverse effects include **lassitude**, sleep disturbance, gastrointestinal upset, and sexual dysfunction. Beta-blockers can make some conduction disorders worse. These drugs are contraindicated in patients with asthma since they block β2 receptors. Some beta-blockers can cross the blood–brain barrier and produce an amnesic effect.
- **Anticoagulants**—This variety of blood-thinning medications reduces the risk of blood clots forming and helps prevent stroke. As with any blood-thinning drugs, there is a risk of bleeding. Patients with arrhythmia are often treated with blood thinners to reduce the risk of complications. These drugs are discussed in the section Drugs for Treating Venous Thromboembolisms.

Clinical Application

Treating Cardiac Arrhythmias

Treatment for cardiac arrhythmia may include a cardiac ablation and medication to regulate the cardiac rhythm. One such medication is *amiodarone* (Cordarone), which has been prescribed to professional and intercollegiate athletes diagnosed with an arrhythmia when planning to return to play following a cardiac event. A decision like this is made only after multiple consultations with cardiologists and extensive cardiac testing and with the consent of the patient. This drug has also been prescribed for those who have experienced supraventricular tachycardia.[10] This medication requires 1 to 3 weeks to establish a therapeutic blood level.[19] Athletic participation at an elite level while taking *amiodarone* is not contraindicated provided that the athlete receives medical clearance from the physicians involved in this decision.

If an athlete has been prescribed any arrhythmia medication, it is recommended that the AT have a back-up supply prescribed in the athlete's name. There may be occasions in which the athlete does not have her supply or inadvertently forgets to take it. Missing a dose is not ideal; thus the back-up supply is beneficial. If a dose is missed, it should not be doubled at the next opportunity; instead, the regular dosing schedule should be followed.[7]

Thromboembolisms

Blood must remain fluid within the vasculature and yet clot quickly when exposed to subendothelial surfaces at sites of vascular injury. Under normal circumstances, a delicate balance between coagulation and fibrinolysis prevents both thrombosis and hemorrhage. Alteration of this balance in favor of coagulation results in **thrombosis**. Thrombi (plural for **thrombus**), which are composed of platelet aggregates, fibrin, and trapped red blood cells, can form in arteries or veins.[16] **Thromboembolism** is the formation of a blood clot inside a blood vessel, obstructing the flow of blood through the circulatory system. Even when a blood vessel is not injured, blood clots may form in the body under certain conditions. A clot, or a piece of the clot, that breaks free and begins to travel around the body is known as an **embolus**.

Drugs for Treating Venous Thromboembolisms

Two classes of antithrombotic agents exist: **anticoagulants** and **antiplatelet** drugs. Anticoagulants slow down clotting, thereby reducing fibrin formation and preventing clots from forming and growing. Antiplatelet agents prevent platelets from clumping and clots from forming and growing (see Drugs for Managing Atherosclerosis). Fibrinolytics, or clot-busters, break up the clot once it is formed. All antithrombotic drugs increase the risk of bleeding (figure 12.2).[16] The AT may encounter patients on anticoagulation or antiplatelet therapy, or a patient may present with a hemorrhagic complication of anticoagulation or antiplatelet medications.[13] Therefore, it is important for the AT to be familiar with these medications and the risk of bleeding.

Antithrombotic drugs used to manage venous thromboembolism (VTE) include the following:

- **Anticoagulants (blood thinners)** such as the prototypical anticoagulant, *warfarin* (Coumadin).
- **Antiplatelet agents** such as *clopidogrel* (Plavix), which is used with *aspirin* to effectively prevent heart attack and stroke, prolong the lives of patients who have already had a heart attack,[2] or provide support after stent placement.
- **Fibrinolytics (clot-busters)** such as *alteplase* (Activase), which is a tissue plasminogen activator (tPA) administered in the emergency department, most commonly for the treatment of ischemic stroke. Many contraindications exist for fibrinolytic therapy because the major toxicity of all thrombolytic agents is hemorrhage.[16]

Whenever possible, the AT must be aware of athletes or others (e.g., coaches, referees, bystanders) involved in contact or collision sports who are taking medication specific to a risk for thromboembolism. All these medications can also increase risk of bleeding; therefore, in patients taking them, contusions or laceration sites will require more clotting time, which could exacerbate the condition.

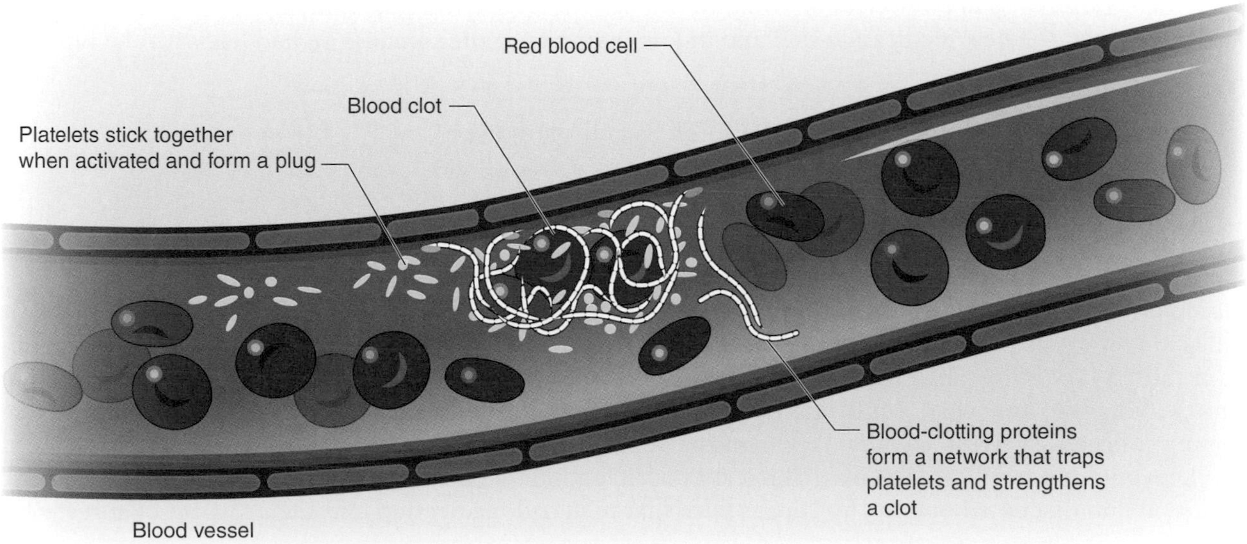

FIGURE 12.2 Antithrombotic drugs are anticoagulants (blood thinners), antiplatelets, and fibrinolytics (clot-busters).

Summary

The AT should be familiar with medications used to treat and manage common causes of cardiovascular dysfunction. Angina pectoris, a cause of ischemic chest pain, is readily treated in the prehospital setting with sublingual NTG in patients who have previously been prescribed this medication. Prehospital interventions by the AT in the treatment of ACS include having the patient chew nonenteric-coated *aspirin* and administering oxygen by nasal cannula. In a variety of settings, the AT may encounter patients with atherosclerosis or CAD and should be aware of the variety of drugs prescribed to treat this condition. He should also be aware of other cardiovascular conditions, including hypertension and thromboembolisms. Hypolipidemic agents, the statins, are commonly prescribed to manage CAD; however, these medications have occasional food–drug interactions and adverse effects. Hypertension is increasingly prevalent in the U.S. population and is managed with a plethora of medications, including those that interact with the renin–angiotensin system, beta-blockers, diuretics, and calcium channel blockers. The AT may provide care to an athlete with a cardiac arrhythmia and must work closely with the patient and her cardiologist, who will carefully select and prescribe medications used to treat these conditions. Finally, this chapter describes how the AT may be involved with patients on anticoagulant therapy that thin the blood, increase risk of bleeding, and could result in serious and potentially fatal sequelae.

Case Studies

Case Study 1

Albert is a 50-year-old former high school athlete who would like to get back into shape. Recently, he had a physical exam for the first time in several years. The results indicated BMI: 30, overall cholesterol: 230. His physician prescribed the statin Lipitor to treat Albert's high cholesterol and encouraged him to monitor his diet and exercise for the purposes of losing weight and lowering his cholesterol.

Albert knew he should start any exercise program slowly, but his goal was to run 1 mile (1.6 km) within 1 month, in time for his next medical exam. After 1 week of walking, Albert's legs and lower back were sore, which he had expected. However, he continued to experience moderate soreness that limited his exercise. He explained this to his physician at the 1-month exam. A cursory exam indicated no musculoskeletal dysfunction of his quadriceps group, hamstrings, or lower back, so his physician ordered more lab work. This test indicated that his creatine kinase was 549 (higher than the normal limit of 200); thus, Albert was diagnosed with rhabdomyolysis. Albert's physician changed his medication from Lipitor to *rosuvastatin* and scheduled a follow-up appointment in 1 month in order to ensure the rhabdomyolysis was under control. Albert tolerated the new medication well and did not experience the soreness he had felt with the Lipitor.

Questions for Analysis

1. Is there a relationship between muscle soreness and statin use?
2. Does rhabdomyolysis always occur with statin use?

Case Study 2

Nicco was an All-American high school basketball player looking forward to a career in college and on professional teams. He was very skilled and tall—6'10" (2.08 m) with a wingspan of 7'7" (2.3 m). During his collegiate preparticipation exam, the AT determined Nicco's wingspan-to-height ratio and identified significant thumb flexibility. She raised a concern that Nicco might have Marfan syndrome. Nicco was referred for a cardiology exam, which confirmed that his aorta was abnormally wide. Thus, he was disqualified from playing college basketball based on the diagnosis of Marfan syndrome. Nicco and his parents were shocked that he would not be allowed to play. The team physician reiterated that there was no cure for this genetic condition and discussed options for Nicco's care that included medication and the prospect of surgery for the aorta.

Questions for Analysis

1. Is there any medication that could reverse the symptoms of Marfan syndrome?
2. Although Nicco was disqualified to play intercollegiate basketball, could he play intramural basketball?

Drugs Described in This Chapter

Drug class	*generic* (pronunciation) Trade names	Therapeutic uses	Clinical concerns
Antiatherogenic drugs: antiplatelet agents	*aspirin* (AS pir in) Bufferin, many others	For stable angina: 75 or 81 mg PO (by mouth) once daily (enteric coated). Chewing the tablet before swallowing quickens absorption of the drug.	Recommended for all patients with CAD or at high risk of developing CAD unless *aspirin* is not tolerated or is contraindicated; used long term
		For ACS: 160-325 mg PO chewed (not enteric-coated), then 81 mg PO once daily long term after discharge	*Aspirin* reduces short- and long-term mortality risk. Higher doses do not provide greater protection and may increase risk of adverse effects.
Antiatherogenic drugs: the statins	*atorvastatin* (a TOR va sta tin) Lipitor (high-intensity therapy)	Initial treatment: 40 or 80 mg PO once daily. If 40 mg once daily is initiated and tolerated, increase to 80 mg once daily.	Major adverse effect: myopathy ranging from mild muscle soreness, pain, or weakness (myalgia) to life-threatening rhabdomyolysis
Antihypertensive agents: loop diuretics	*furosemide* (fyoor OH se mide) Lasix	20-40 mg twice daily; individualized according to patient response; use minimal dose necessary to maintain therapeutic response.	Alternative agent to thiazides. Serious side effects include electrolyte abnormalities, low blood pressure, and hearing loss. Regular blood tests are recommended for those receiving treatment.
Antihypertensive agents: thiazide diuretics	*hydrochlorothiazide* (hye dro klor o THY a zide) HydroDIURIL	25-100 mg PO once or twice daily.	Common side effects include low blood potassium, high blood sugar, dizziness, increased uric acid, and increased serum cholesterol.
Antihypertensive agents: beta-blockers	*labetalol* (la BET a lol) Normodyne	Initial dose: 100 mg PO twice daily (alone or added to a diuretic regimen) Maintenance dose: 200-400 mg PO twice daily	Serious side effects: low blood pressure, liver problems, heart failure, and bronchospasm. Also may be used as antiarrhythmic or antianginal agents.
Antihypertensive agents: ACE inhibitors	*lisinopril* (lise IN oh pril) Prinivil, Zestril	Initial dose: 5-10 mg PO once daily Maintenance dose: 20-40 mg PO once daily	ACE inhibitor cough (dry, hacking, nonproductive)

(continued)

Drugs Described in This Chapter *(continued)*

Drug class	*generic* (pronunciation) Trade names	Therapeutic uses	Clinical concerns
Antihypertensive agents: angiotensin II receptor blockers	*losartan* (loe SAR tan) Cozaar	25-50 mg once daily; evaluate response every 4-6 weeks and increase dose as needed up to 100 mg/day in 1 or 2 divided doses	May be used as an alternative in patients who cannot tolerate an ACE inhibitor (e.g., due to cough).
Antianginal agents: nitrates	*nitroglycerin* (nye troe GLI ser in) NTG	For immediate relief of chest pain; use as needed. Sublingual tablet or spray: 0.3-0.6 mg every 4 or 5 min; up to 3 doses	Recommended for patients who have unstable angina or persistent severe angina and continue to have anginal symptoms after the beta-blocker dose is maximized.
Antiarrhythmic agents: cardiac glycosides	*digoxin* (di JOKS in) Lanoxin, many others	IV: 0.25-0.5 mg over several min, with repeat doses of 0.25 mg every 6 hr. Maximum of 1.5 mg over 24 hr	Side effects: nausea, loss of appetite, trouble seeing, and confusion. *Digoxin* toxicity includes anorexia, nausea, vomiting, visual changes, and cardiac arrhythmias; toxicity is usually associated with digoxin levels >2 ng/mL, although symptoms may occur at lower levels.
Antiarrhythmic agents: sodium channel blockers	*procainamide* (pro KANE a mide) Pronestyl	IV: 10-15 mg/kg bolus at 25-50 mg/min, followed by a constant IV infusion of 1-4 mg/min	Follow ACLS guidelines: This drug increases risk of sudden cardiac arrest in people who have ACS or CAD. **Note:** Dose must be individualized and titrated to the patient's response.
		250-625 mg (rarely, up to 1 g) PO every 3 or 4 hr	Sustained-release preparations obviate the need for frequent dosing.
Antiarrhythmic agents: potassium channel blockers	*amiodarone* (a MEE oh da rone) Cordarone, Nexterone	Initial dose: 600-800 mg PO daily in divided doses for a total load of up to 10 g Maintenance dose: 200 mg PO once daily	This is the preferred antiarrhythmic for patients with structural heart disease.
Antiarrhythmic agents: calcium channel blockers	*verapamil* (ver AP a mil) Calan	For angina: Extended release 120-360 mg PO once daily. For arrhythmias: 40-120 mg PO 3 times/day For sustained-release form: 180 mg once daily to 240 mg twice daily	Recommended for patients with stable angina if symptoms persist despite nitrate use or if nitrates are not tolerated.
Anticoagulants	*warfarin* (WAR far in) Coumadin	Initial dosing must be individualized.	Recommended for primary prevention in patients at high risk of systemic emboli.

Prescribers may use different combinations of drugs depending on the type of cardiovascular disease that is present.
Note: This is not a comprehensive list of all side effects. The patient should be referred to the prescriber if there are questions.
ACE = angiotensin converting enzyme; ACS = acute coronary syndromes; ACLS = advanced cardiovascular life support; CAD = coronary artery disease

13

Drugs for Treating Diabetes and Disordered Glucose Metabolism

OBJECTIVES

After reading this chapter, you will be able to do the following:

- Describe the actions of *insulin* on glucose storage
- Explain glucose homeostasis and glycemic control
- Differentiate between the glucose metabolic disorders
- Identify common antidiabetic agents used in the management of type 1 and type 2 diabetes mellitus
- Summarize the recommendations for managing mild hypoglycemia
- Administer *glucagon* for patients with severe hypoglycemia

Select Drugs Mentioned in This Chapter

Drug class	Generic name	Trade name
Antihyperglycemic agents		
Biguanides	*metformin*	Glucophage
Sodium-glucose cotransporter-2 (SGLT-2) inhibitors	*empagliflozin*	Jardiance
Glucagon-like peptide-1 (GLP-1) receptor agonists	*dulaglutide*	Trulicity
Insulin secretagogue: sulfonylureas	*glipizide*	Glucotrol
Rapid-acting insulins	*insulin lispro*	Humalog
Short-acting (regular) insulins	*regular insulin*	Humulin R
Intermediate-acting insulins	*insulin isophane*	Humulin N
Long-acting insulins	*insulin glargine*	Toujeo, Lantus

This list is not exhaustive, but rather contains drugs commonly encountered in the athletic training setting. Always consult up-to-date information, confirm with a pharmacist, or discuss the use of therapeutic medications with the prescriber of the medication.

Disorders of carbohydrate (glucose) metabolism result from multiple etiologies, all of which are characterized by chronic hyperglycemia with disturbances of carbohydrate, fat, and protein metabolism that result from defects in insulin secretion, insulin action, or both.[28] **Diabetes** (also called diabetes mellitus) is a spectrum of metabolic disorders arising from myriad pathogenic mechanisms, all resulting in hyperglycemia. This chapter focuses on glucose homeostasis and related metabolic disorders.

Glucose Homeostasis

Blood glucose (sugar) levels reflect the difference between the amount of glucose released into the circulation by the liver and the amount of glucose removed from the blood by body tissues. Energy metabolism is controlled by several hormones, including insulin, glucagon, epinephrine, growth hormone, and the glucocorticoids. Of these hormones, only **insulin** has the effect of lowering the blood glucose level. Insulin facilitates the transport of glucose into body cells and decreases the liver's production and release of glucose into the bloodstream. Insulin also has the effect of decreasing lipolysis and the use of fats as a fuel source. The pancreas is primarily in hormonal control of blood glucose. The actions of insulin on glucose are as follows:[28]

1. Increases glucose transport into skeletal muscle and adipose tissue
2. Increases glycogen synthesis
3. Decreases gluconeogenesis

Serum insulin levels begin to rise within minutes after a meal, reach a peak in approximately 3 to 5 minutes, and then return to **basal state** within 3 hours.[28] The most important diagnostic test for all types of diabetes is **fasting blood glucose level**, or the blood glucose concentration after no caloric intake for ≥8 hours. Fasting glucose requirements are primarily provided by liver glycogen stores; conversion of other substrates into glucose accounts for the remainder. Insulin secretion is stimulated by food ingestion, nutrient absorption, and elevated blood glucose. The centrality of insulin in glucose metabolism is emphasized by the fact that all the forms of human diabetes have as a root cause some abnormality of insulin secretion or action.[29]

Broad categories of glucose homeostasis are defined as follows:[1,18,29]

- **Normal glucose homeostasis**—Fasting blood glucose 60 to 100 mg/dL
- **Euglycemia normal postprandial glucose**—Levels <140 mg/dL within 2 hours after a meal
- **Hypoglycemia**—Blood glucose levels <70 mg/dL
- **Hyperglycemia**—Excessive blood glucose >200 mg/dL
  - **Prediabetes**
    - **Impaired fasting glucose (IFG)**—Fasting plasma glucose (FPG) level between 100 and 125 mg/dL
    - **Impaired glucose tolerance (IGT)**—Glucose level between 140 and 199 mg/dL at 120 minutes after ingestion of 75 g liquid glucose solution (2-hour plasma glucose)
  - Diabetes
    - FPG >126 mg/dL
    - 2-hour plasma glucose ≥200 mg/dL

For the athletic trainer (AT) providing care to patients who have disorders of glucose homeostasis, the most important goal is to keep blood glucose levels at or as close to normal levels as possible without causing hypoglycemia. This goal requires the patient to maintain a delicate balance between hypoglycemia, euglycemia, and hyperglycemia. This is often more challenging for athletes due to the demands of physical activity and competition. However, effectively managing blood glucose, lipid, and blood pressure levels is necessary to ensuring the long-term health and well-being of the athlete with metabolic disorders. In conjunction with the NATA position statement *Management of the Athlete With Type I Diabetes Mellitus*,[18] recommendations in this chapter are intended to provide the AT with the specific knowledge and problem-solving skills necessary for treating athletes with these conditions. Athletic trainers have more contact with the athlete with diabetes than most other members of the diabetes management team and so must be prepared to assist the athlete as required.

Metabolic Disorders

Consistent, near-normal levels of blood glucose and blood pressure, as well as lipid control, are essential for preventing diabetes-related complications and improving the patient's quality of life. In the short term, hyperglycemia causes symptoms of increased thirst, urination, and hunger, as well as weight loss. However, in the long term, hyperglycemia causes diabetic complications, including **retinopathy** (damage to eyes leading to blindness), **nephropathy** (kidney damage leading to renal failure), and **neuropathy** (damage to nerves leading to impotence, pain, and foot disorders, possibly leading to amputation).[18,31] Uncontrolled hyperglycemia also increases the risk of heart disease, stroke, and insufficiency in blood flow to the legs. In general, good metabolic control prevents or delays these complications. Thus, the primary goal of treatment is to bring the elevated blood glucose down to a normal range, both to improve symptoms of diabetes and to prevent or delay diabetic complications. Achieving this goal requires a comprehensive, coordinated, patient-centered approach from the health care team.[31]

Both genetic and environmental factors contribute to the pathogenesis of metabolic disorders, which involve insufficient insulin secretion, reduced responsiveness to endogenous or exogenous insulin, increased glucose production, or abnormalities in fat and protein metabolism. The resulting hyperglycemia may lead to both acute symptoms and metabolic abnormalities. Although hyperglycemia is common to all forms of diabetes, the pathogenic mechanisms leading to diabetes are quite distinct.[28] The primary metabolic disorders discussed in this chapter are as follows:[1,5,28,31]

- **Type 1 diabetes mellitus (T1DM**—Usually develops in childhood and adolescence; patients require lifelong *insulin* injections for survival.
- **Type 2 diabetes mellitus (T2DM)**—Usually develops in adulthood and is related to obesity, lack of physical activity, and unhealthy diets. This is the more common type of diabetes (representing 90% of diabetic cases worldwide). Treatment may involve lifestyle changes and weight loss alone, oral medications, or even *insulin* injections.
- **Hypoglycemia**—A common problem in people who use *insulin* (i.e., those with T1DM or those with T2DM who must use *insulin* to control their blood glucose). Hypoglycemia (low blood sugar) is the most severe acute complication of intensive *insulin* therapy in diabetes.

The American Diabetes Association (ADA) and the World Health Organization (WHO) have adopted criteria for the diagnosis of diabetes based on fasting blood glucose, the glucose value following an oral glucose tolerance test, or the level of hemoglobin A1c (**HbA1c** or, more simply, A1c). The HbA1c level is related to exposure of proteins in the blood (including hemoglobin) to elevated glucose levels, resulting in **glycation** of proteins, including hemoglobin (Hb). Thus, the level of A1c represents a measure of the average glucose concentration to which the Hb has been exposed.[1,31] The desired outcome of **glycemic control** in both T1DM and T2DM (see table 13.1) is normalization of blood glucose as a means of preventing short- and long-term complications. Treatment plans involve dietary

TABLE 13.1 Characteristics of Types 1 and 2 Diabetes Mellitus

Characteristic	Type 1	Type 2
Age at onset	Most commonly <30 yr	Most commonly >30 yr
Associated obesity	Uncommon	Very common
Propensity to ketoacidosis requiring *insulin* treatment for control	Yes	No
Plasma levels of endogenous insulin	Extremely low to undetectable	Variable; may be low, normal, or elevated depending on degree of insulin resistance and insulin secretory defect
Pancreatic autoantibodies at diagnosis	Yes, but may be absent	No
Prone to develop diabetic complications (retinopathy, nephropathy, neuropathy, atherosclerotic cardiovascular disease)	Yes	Yes
Hyperglycemia responds to oral antihyperglycemic drugs	No	Yes, initially in many patients

Adapted from Porth and Gaspard (2015); Powers and D'Alessio (2017).

management (medical nutrition therapy), exercise, and antidiabetic agents. People with T1DM require *insulin* therapy from the time of diagnosis. In people with T2DM, weight loss and dietary management may be enough to control blood glucose levels. However, these patients require follow-up care because insulin secretion may decrease or **insulin resistance** may persist or worsen, in which case noninsulin agents are prescribed.[28]

Optimal control of both T1DM and T2DM is associated with prevention or delay of chronic diabetes complications.[28] Major sources of the morbidity of diabetes are the chronic complications that arise from prolonged hyperglycemia, including retinopathy, neuropathy, nephropathy, and cardiovascular disease. These chronic complications can be mitigated in many patients by sustained control of the blood glucose and treatment of comorbidities such as hypertension and dyslipidemia.[23,25] A wide variety of treatment options now exist for hyperglycemia that target different processes involved in glucose regulation or dysregulation.[24] Diabetes management typically involves the following:

- Patient education
- Blood glucose monitoring
- Dietary and nutrition management
- Exercise
- Drugs

Antidiabetic Agents for Managing Type 2 Diabetes Mellitus

Patients with T2DM are often initially treated with diet and exercise for glycemic control. For the management of T2DM when hyperglycemia cannot be managed with diet and exercise alone, patients may be prescribed oral antihyperglycemic drugs, injectable insulinlike drugs, *insulin*, or a combination of these drugs.[6,28] The antidiabetic (noninsulin) agents used in the treatment of T2DM are listed in table 13.2.

Antihyperglycemics: Biguanides

Biguanides are the first-line medication for the treatment of T2DM. *Metformin* (Glucophage) is a biguanide antihyperglycemic agent that works by doing the following:

- Decreasing hepatic glucose production
- Decreasing intestinal absorption of glucose
- Improving insulin sensitivity by increasing glucose uptake and use in target sites

Metformin is an oral medication that is generally well tolerated. Common side effects include diarrhea, nausea, and abdominal pain. *Metformin* has a very low risk of causing hypoglycemia. High level

TABLE 13.2 Antihyperglycemic and Antidiabetic Agents for Patients With Type 2 Diabetes

Class	Mechanism of action	Example
Antihyperglycemic agents		
Biguanides	Reduce insulin resistance by increasing the sensitivity of liver, muscle, and adipose tissue to insulin	*metformin* (Glucophage)
Sodium-glucose cotransporter-2 (SGLT-2) inhibitors	Reduce renal reabsorption of filtered glucose, thereby increasing urinary glucose excretion	*empagliflozin* (Jardiance)
Glucagon-like peptide-1 (GLP-1) receptor agonists	Enhance insulin secretion, slow gastric emptying, and reduce postprandial glucagon and food intake	*dulaglutide* (Trulicity)
Insulin secretagogues		
Sulfonylureas	Increase the amount of insulin secreted by the pancreas	*glipizide* (Glucotrol)

Based on Brutsaert (2019); Dungan and DeSantis (2019); Kennedy and Masharani (2017); Porth and Gaspard (2015).

of blood lactic acid is a concern if the medication is prescribed inappropriately or in overly large doses. It should not be used in patients with significant liver disease or kidney problems. Although no clear harm comes from its use during pregnancy, *insulin* is generally preferred for **gestational diabetes**.[2,6,28] The AT should be aware of relatively common drug interactions with certain medications, such as *insulin glargine* (Lantus) and the antibiotic *ciprofloxacin*.

RED FLAG

Potential Diabetic Drug–Drug Interactions

A major adverse drug–drug interaction has been identified between diabetic medications (particularly sulfonylureas) and quinolones.[30] For example, the antibiotic *ciprofloxacin* is listed as a drug that has a major drug interaction with the long-acting *insulin* Lantus *(insulin glargine)*; taking these 2 medications concomitantly can cause hypo- or hyperglycemia. The mechanism is unknown.[11] Patients with T2DM should be aware of this potential interaction if they are prescribed a quinolone antibiotic. Symptoms of hypoglycemia may include rapid heart rate, weakness, tingling in hands or feet, and hunger. Additionally, patients who experience increased thirst or urination while taking this drug combination should monitor their blood sugar and contact their prescribing physician promptly.[11,30]

Insulin Secretagogues: Sulfonylureas

Insulin and insulin secretagogues are known to cause hypoglycemia. Insulin **secretagogues** are antidiabetic medications used to treat T2DM. This medication class works to do the following:

- Stimulate insulin release from the pancreatic beta cells
- Reduce glucose output from the liver
- Improve insulin sensitivity at peripheral target sites

An insulin secretagogue and sulfonylurea, *glipizide* (Glucotrol) is an antidiabetic medication that is used together with a diabetic diet in the treatment of T2DM. Patients should not take *glipizide* if they are not going to eat a meal due to the risk of hypoglycemia; the effects of this oral medication generally begin within half an hour of administration and can last for up to 24 hours. Common side effects include nausea, diarrhea, low blood sugar, headache, sleepiness, skin rash, and shakiness. The dose may need to be adjusted for patients with liver or kidney disease. Use during pregnancy or when breastfeeding is not recommended.[19] The risk of hypoglycemia is increased when drugs such as *empagliflozin* (Jardiance) are used in combination with insulin secretagogues. Therefore, prescribers must consider prescribing a lower dose of insulin secretagogues and insulin to reduce the risk of hypoglycemia when they are used concomitantly with drugs such as *empagliflozin* (Jardiance; see Red Flag sidebar).

RED FLAG

Adverse Effects of Insulin Secretagogues

Empagliflozin (Jardiance) is an oral medication that lowers blood glucose. ATs must be able to recognize potential contraindications or side effects. *Empagliflozin* presents concerns for patients with kidney dysfunction and may cause hyperlipidemia. This medication is associated with dehydration symptoms such as dizziness, weakness, and a sense of being light-headed. This risk of dehydration is amplified if the patient is taking blood pressure medications or a diuretic. Although the risk of hypoglycemia is low when *empagliflozin* (Jardiance) is taken monotherapy (~0.4%), the risk for hypoglycemia significantly increases when it is taken concomitantly with *metformin* or *insulin* (anywhere from 1.2% to 28.4%).[12]

Antihyperglycemics: Sodium-Glucose Cotransporter-2 Inhibitors

Sodium-glucose cotransporter-2 (SGLT-2) is the predominant transporter responsible for reabsorption of glucose from the glomerular filtrate back into the circulation. The popular oral medication *empagliflozin* (Jardiance) is an inhibitor of SGLT-2.[12] By inhibiting SGLT-2, *empagliflozin* reduces renal reabsorption of filtered glucose and lowers the renal threshold for glucose, thereby increasing urinary glucose excretion. Like with all diabetes medications, *empagliflozin* is indicated as an adjunct to diet and exercise to improve glycemic control and reduce the risk of cardiovascular death in adults with T2DM. The use of *empagliflozin* is not recommended for patients with T1DM or for the treatment of diabetic **ketoacidosis**.

Antihyperglycemics: Glucagon-Like Peptide-1 Receptor Agonists

Glucagon-like peptide-1 (GLP-1) receptor agonists affect glucose control through several mechanisms, including enhancement of glucose-dependent insulin secretion, slowed gastric emptying, and reduction of postprandial glucagon and food intake.[14] These agents are administered subcutaneously and do not usually cause hypoglycemia in the absence of therapies that otherwise cause hypoglycemia. An example of a GLP-1 agonist is *dulaglutide* (Trulicity); it is indicated as an adjunct to diet and exercise regimens to improve glycemic control in adults with T2DM. *Dulaglutide* (Trulicity) is recommended as adjunct therapy to the first-line agent *metformin* therapy for patients who have inadequate glycemic control with diet and exercise regimens alone. Prescribers should provide *dulaglutide* only to patients for whom the potential benefits outweigh the risk.[13]

Insulin for Managing Type 1 and Type 2 Diabetes Mellitus

People living with T1DM always require treatment with *insulin*, and many people with T2DM eventually require *insulin* therapy. *Insulin* is destroyed in the GI tract and must be administered by injection or other parenteral routes.[6,28] *Insulin* replacement in people with T1DM should ideally mimic pancreatic beta-cell function by providing basal and **prandial** requirements (physiologic replacement); this approach requires close attention to diet and exercise as well as to *insulin* timing and dose. When insulin is needed for patients with T2DM, glycemic control can often be achieved with a combination of basal *insulin* and noninsulin antihyperglycemic drugs, although prandial *insulin* may be needed in some patients. Most *insulin* preparations are **recombinant human analogs**, which has practically eliminated the allergic reactions to *insulin* that were common when it was extracted from animal sources.[6] Its manufacture uses recombinant deoxyribonucleic acid (DNA) technology. More recently, several analogs to human insulin have become available that offer even better and more reproducible release characteristics.[28] These drugs were created by modifying the human insulin molecule that alters absorption rates and duration and time to action.[6]

Types of *Insulin*

Human *insulin* preparations are commonly categorized by their time to onset and duration of action; however, these parameters vary within and among patients, depending on many factors (e.g., site and technique of injection, amount of subcutaneous fat, blood flow at the injection site). All forms of *insulin* have the potential to produce hypoglycemia or insulin reaction as a side effect.[28] Four *insulin* types are classified by length and peaking of action: short acting, rapid acting, intermediate acting, and long acting (figure 13.1).[6,19,28]

- **Rapid-acting *insulins***—These *insulins*, such as *insulin lispro* (Humalog), are rapidly absorbed and often begin to reduce plasma glucose within 15 minutes, but have short duration of action (<4 hours). They are best used at mealtime to control postprandial spikes in plasma glucose. Inhaled regular *insulin* is a newer, rapid-acting *insulin* that is taken with meals.
- **Short-acting (regular) *insulin***—*human insulin r* (Humulin R) has a slightly slower onset (30 to 60 minutes) than *insulin lispro* but lasts longer (6 to 8 hours). This is the only *insulin* form for IV use; after subcutaneous injection, it leads to more rapid absorption into the circulation.[19]
- **Intermediate-acting *insulins***—*Insulin isophane* (Humulin N, Novolin N), also known as NPH, has an onset of action about 2 hours

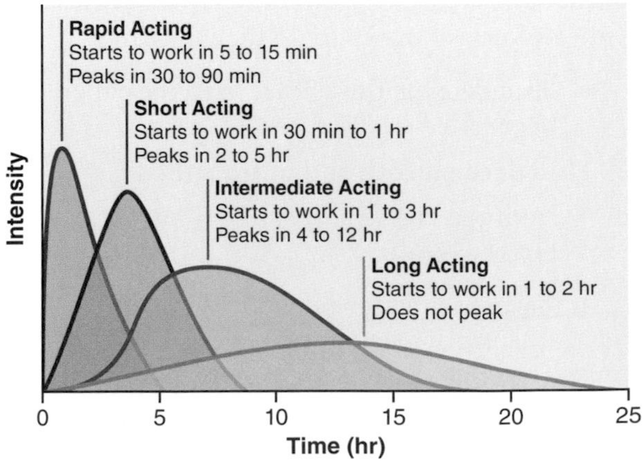

FIGURE 13.1 Types of *insulin* and duration of action.

after injection, peak effect of 4 to 12 hours after injection, and duration of action of 18 to 26 hours. Concentrated regular *insulin* U-500 has a similar peak and duration of action (peak 4 to 8 hours; duration 13 to 24 hours) and can be dosed 2 or 3 times per day.

- **Long-acting *insulins*—**Such as *insulin glargine* (Toujeo and others), these *insulins* have no discernible peak of action and provide a steady basal effect over 24 hours.
- **Premixed combinations—**Combinations such as *regular insulin* + *insulin isophane* are commercially available in premixed preparations.

Insulin Dosing Regimens and Delivery Devices

Insulin dosing regimens closely simulate the normal pattern of insulin secretion by the body. With each method, a basal insulin level is maintained, and bolus doses of short- or rapid-acting *insulin* are delivered before meals.[28] The choice of management is determined by the person with diabetes in collaboration with the health care team.[28] With multiple daily injections, the basal *insulin* requirements are met by an intermediate- or long-acting *insulin* administered once or twice daily.

Insulin Pen

Many prefilled *insulin* pen injection devices (figure 13.2) are available as an alternative to the conventional vial-and-syringe method. *Insulin* pen injectors may be used away from home and may be preferable for patients with limited vision or manual dexterity. Spring-loaded self-injection devices (for use with a syringe) may be useful for the occasional patient who is fearful of injection, and syringe magnifiers are available for patients with limited vision.[6]

Insulin Pump

The continuous subcutaneous *insulin* infusion (CSII) method uses an *insulin* pump. A small device, often the size of a pager, is worn on a belt or in the clothing, with thin plastic tubing coming from the pump to a needle that penetrates the skin, usually in the abdomen (figure 13.3). It is in place 24 hours a day, and this device is as close as one can get to the constant gradual administration of insulin that is taking place in the body. With this method, the basal insulin requirements are met by continuous infusion of subcutaneous *insulin*, the rate of which can be varied to accommodate diurnal variations. The computer-operated pump then delivers 1 or more set basal amounts of *insulin*. In addition to the basal amount delivered by the pump, a bolus amount of *insulin* may be delivered when needed (e.g., before a meal) by pushing a button. Self-monitoring of blood glucose levels is a necessity when using the CSII method of management.[28]

Insulin pumps are increasingly common in the physically active population. Continuous subcutaneous *insulin* infusion pumps can eliminate the need for multiple daily injections, provide maximal

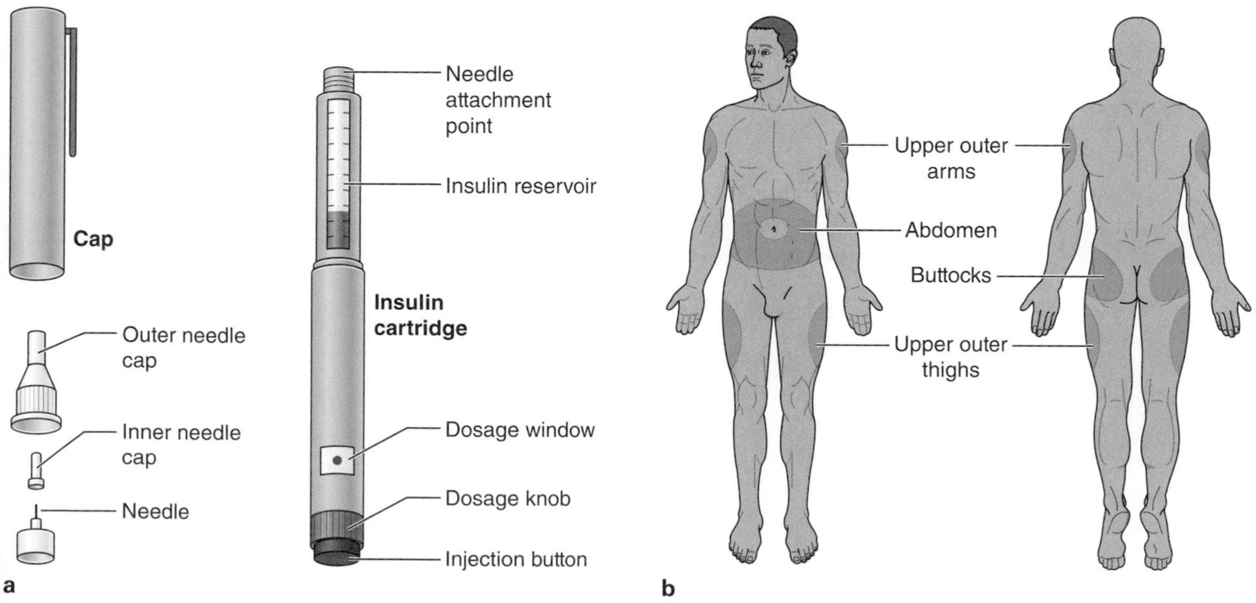

FIGURE 13.2 Using an *insulin* pen injector: *(a)* parts of an *insulin* pen and *(b) insulin* injection sites.

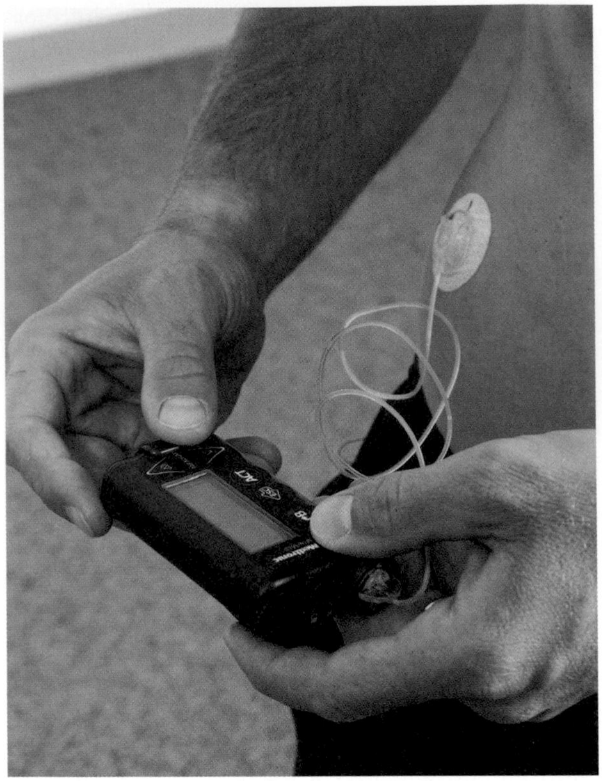

FIGURE 13.3 Basic *insulin* pump with glucose sensor and infusion set

flexibility in the timing of meals, and substantially reduce variability in glucose levels. Disadvantages include cost, mechanical failures leading to interruptions in insulin supply, and the inconvenience of wearing an external device.[6,27] Pump failure can lead to hyperglycemia and ketotic episodes, and needle-site complications such as catheter clogging and infections at the needle site also are possible. Candidate selection is crucial to the successful use of the *insulin* pump.[17,28] Frequent and meticulous self-monitoring and close attention to pump function are necessary for safe and effective use of the *insulin* pump.[6,17,27]

Diabetes Care Plan

Proper management of blood glucose levels during practices and games allows the athlete with diabetes to compete in a safe and effective manner. Maintaining a near-normal blood glucose level (100 to 180 mg/dL) reduces the risk of dehydration, lethargy, hypoglycemia, and autonomic counterregulatory failure. This goal is best achieved through a team approach to providing support for patients with diabetes. In the secondary school setting, the team should include the AT, school nurse, coach, and school administrators. In adult athletes, diabetes is best managed by a team that includes several health care professionals. Creating this team requires a deliberate, well-designed plan that defines the role of each person involved in the supervision and care of the athlete with diabetes. All members of the team should be trained and willing to assist an athlete who is experiencing a diabetes-related emergency.

Critical roles for the AT include prevention, recognition, and immediate care of hypoglycemia and hyperglycemia (with and without ketoacidosis); exercise; nutrition; hydration; and counseling. The AT should also help the athlete recognize the intensity of the exercise session and adjust glucose and insulin levels accordingly. The AT also facilitates communication among the other members of the diabetes management team.[9,18] The plan should identify blood glucose targets for practices and games, including exclusion thresholds; strategies to prevent exercise-associated hypoglycemia, hyperglycemia, and **ketosis**; a list of medications used for glycemic control or other diabetes-related conditions; signs, symptoms, and treatment protocols for hypoglyce-

Evidence in Pharmacology

Exercise and Type 1 Diabetes

Each type 1 diabetic patient must follow *insulin* and dietary management suggestions in conjunction with exercise. Adjustments to *insulin* administration are necessary with exercise to prevent hypo- or hyperglycemia.[20] A hyperinsulinemia state with inadequate calorie intake can lead to hypoglycemia during or after exercise. Thus, prior to exercise, athletes with type 1 diabetes should reduce their exogenous *insulin* by 20% to 50%, depending on intensity and duration of exercise. Consistent exogenous *insulin* administration can be achieved through an *insulin* pump. The pump administers continuous *insulin* via a subcutaneous catheter.[20] Removing the pump for exercise requires adjustments in *insulin* timing and administration.

mia, hyperglycemia, and ketosis; and emergency contact information. The athlete must have access to supplies for managing glycemic emergencies at all times. When the athlete requires assistance, the AT or other members of the diabetes management team (e.g., coach) must have immediate access to these supplies. The athlete or parent or guardian should provide the necessary supplies and equipment.[9,18] Specifically, the plan should include the following:[8,9,18,20]

- **Blood glucose monitoring guidelines**—Address frequency of monitoring and pre-exercise exclusion values.
- **Insulin therapy guidelines**—Include the type of *insulin* used, dosages and adjustment strategies for planned activity types, as well as *insulin* correction dosages for high blood glucose levels.
- **List of other medications**—Include those used to assist with glycemic control or to treat other diabetes-related conditions.
- **Guidelines for hypoglycemia recognition and treatment**—Include prevention, signs, symptoms, and treatment of hypoglycemia, including instructions on the use of *glucagon*.
- **Guidelines for hyperglycemia recognition and treatment**—Include prevention, signs, symptoms, and treatment of hyperglycemia and ketosis.
- **Emergency contact information**—Includes telephone numbers for the patient's parents or other family members, physician's telephone number, and consent for medical treatment (for minors).
- **Identification**—Athletes with diabetes should have a medic alert tag with them at all times.

Managing Hypoglycemia

Hypoglycemia is the most severe acute complication of intensive *insulin* therapy in diabetes, and exercise is its most frequent cause. Mild hypoglycemia is blood glucose levels <100 mg/dL, whereas severe hypoglycemia is blood glucose <70 mg/dL; both require action according to the diabetes care plan to bring it back into the target range. Under most circumstances, hypoglycemia is the result of the patient skipping a meal or snack, eating less than usual, or being more physically active than usual.[3] Athletes with T1DM who have achieved superior levels of performance have established patterns of carbohydrate feedings and *insulin* therapy that work for them. Individual experiences and trial and error with manipulations of diet and *insulin* administration must occur if such an athlete is to establish reliable glucose control.[15] For people with T1DM or those with T2DM who must use *insulin* to control their blood glucose, hypoglycemia is a common problem. The most important thing for managing diabetes is monitoring blood glucose levels regularly, especially before exercise. The AT should be competent at using a blood glucose meter and assisting the athlete with managing glycemic conditions. Clinical skills for using a glucometer (blood glucose meter) are provided in the text *Acute and Emergency Care in Athletic Training.*[7]

Managing blood glucose levels during practices and games and preventing hypoglycemia are challenges. The athlete and the health care team should work together to prevent hypoglycemia and be prepared to manage mild episodes of hypoglycemia during and after practices and games (see table 13.3).[18] Athletes with diabetes must drink plenty of fluids while being physically active to prevent dehydration. T1DM or T2DM athletes who are prescribed *insulin* may find it particularly helpful to check blood glucose levels before they are physically active. It is important that blood glucose is not too low while being physically active. Hypoglycemia during or after physical activity is more likely when the athlete does the following:[3,4,18]

- Takes *insulin* or an insulin secretagogue
- Skips meals
- Exercises for a long time
- Exercises strenuously

Patients with severe hypoglycemia may present with symptoms of brain neuronal glucose deprivation and may have blurred vision, fatigue, difficulty thinking, loss of motor control, aggressive behavior, seizures, convulsions, and loss of consciousness; if hypoglycemia is prolonged and severe, brain damage and even death can result. Symptoms of hypoglycemia can be unique from person to person.[18] A patient with severe hypoglycemia may need *glucagon* if he presents with blood glucose <70 mg/dL, is unable to eat or drink safely because of confusion or disorientation, is unconscious, or is having seizures.[3,18,22] In cases of severe hypoglycemia, an intramuscular injection of *glucagon* remains the preferred method of treatment.[2]

TABLE 13.3 Treatment Guidelines for Hypoglycemia

Mild hypoglycemia: blood glucose <100 mg/dL	Severe hypoglycemia: blood glucose <70 mg/dL
Signs and symptoms: headache, hunger, sweating, irritability, dizziness, nausea, fast heart rate, feeling anxious or shaky	Signs: blurred vision, fatigue, difficulty thinking, loss of motor control, aggressive behavior, seizures, convulsions, and loss of consciousness
Patient is conscious and able to follow directions and swallow.	Patient is unconscious or unable to follow directions or swallow.
Remove patient from activity and follow the 15/15 rule: 1. Administer 15 g of fast-acting carbohydrate: e.g., 4 to 8 glucose tablets, 2 Tbsp of raisins, or 1/2 c of fruit juice or regular soda (not diet). 2. Measure blood glucose level again. 3. Wait approximately 15 min and remeasure blood glucose. 4. If blood glucose level remains low, administer another 15 g of fast-acting carbohydrate. 5. Recheck blood glucose level in approximately 15 min. 6. If blood glucose level does not return to the normal range after second dosage of carbohydrate, activate the emergency medical system. 7. Once blood glucose level is in the normal range, the athlete may wish to consume a snack (e.g., sandwich, bagel).	1. Activate the emergency medical system. 2. Prepare *glucagon* for injection following the steps listed in the Clinical Application sidebar. 3. *Glucagon* administration may cause nausea or vomiting when the athlete wakes up. 4. Place the athlete on his side to prevent aspiration. 5. The athlete should become conscious within 15 min of administration. 6. Once the athlete is conscious and able to swallow, follow the 15/15 rule.

Based on American Diabetes Association (2018); American Diabetes Association (2019); Jimenez et al. (2007).

Clinical Application

The 15/15 Rule

The 15/15 rule for treating low blood sugar is to eat 15 g of carbohydrate and wait 15 minutes.[21] The following foods will provide about 15 g of carbohydrate:

- 4 glucose tablets
- 1/2 c (4 fl oz or 120 mL) of fruit juice or regular soda
- 6 or 7 hard candies
- 1 Tbsp (15 g) of sugar

After consuming the carbohydrate, the patient should wait about 15 minutes for the sugar to get into her blood. If the patient does not feel better within 15 minutes, she can consume more carbohydrate. The patient's blood sugar should be checked to determine if it is within a safe range.

The athletic training staff should be familiar with athlete-specific symptoms of hypoglycemia and be prepared to act appropriately.[18] Unfortunately, many people believe that ATs aren't permitted to administer any sort of injectable medication or perform any invasive procedure.[16] In many states, regulatory policies prevent ATs or other prehospital health care providers (HCPs) from administering or carrying *glucagon*, which makes treating patients experiencing severe hypoglycemia with loss of consciousness far more complicated and slower than necessary.[16] In addition to difficulties with *glucagon* availability, ATs must perform blood glucose testing (i.e., finger sticks), which makes the identification and treatment of hypoglycemia even more challenging. Although many patients who use *insulin* receive training on the use of *glucagon*, in many settings, ATs and patients do not have access to *glucagon*. The AT should work with the directing physician or the patient's physician to obtain an emergency *glucagon*

Clinical Application

Administering a *Glucagon* Injection

Before administering a *glucagon* injection, check the patient's blood glucose level.
The patient may need *glucagon* if she presents with blood glucose <70 mg/dL and any of the following:

- Unable to eat or drink safely because of confusion or disorientation
- Unconscious
- Having seizures

Once the patient has been determined to require *glucagon*, retrieve the *glucagon* emergency kit (figure 13.4) and activate Emergency Medical Services by calling 911. A *glucagon* emergency kit contains the following:

- Vial of sterile glucagon powder
- Syringe of sterile diluting agent with needle attached
- Instructions for use

Other necessary supplies include the following:

- Latex-free gloves
- Alcohol swabs
- Blood glucose meter and test strips
- Sharps container

An unconscious patient will usually wake up during the first 15 minutes after the injection. Once the patient is awake and able to drink, give him sips of fruit juice or regular soda. This will help restore the glucose in his liver and prevent his blood sugar from dropping again.

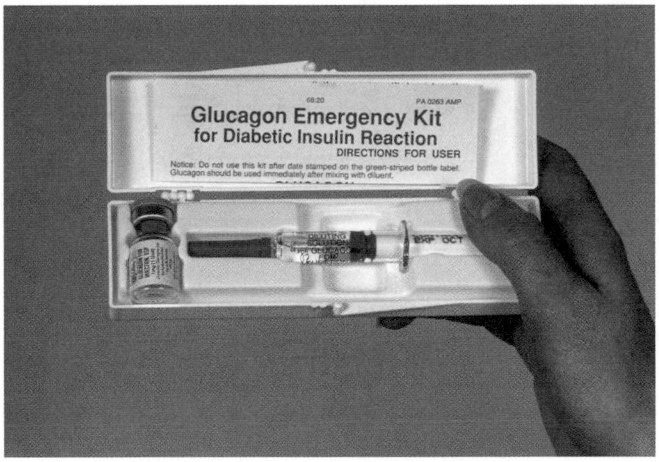

Southern Illinois University/Science Source

FIGURE 13.4 Glucagon emergency kit.

Based on American Diabetes Association, *ADA Position Statement: Pharmacologic Approaches to Glycemic Treatment* (2018); American Diabetes Association, *Low Blood Glucose (Hypoglycemia)* (2018); Farrell (2019); Jimenez et al. (2007); Memorial Sloan Kettering Cancer Center (2016).

kit and supplies for prehospital treatment of severe hypoglycemia. *Glucagon* emergency kits are routinely provided to families and patients and used without any complications in these settings. Furthermore, ATs are already permitted (in many areas) to use intramuscular *epinephrine* (EpiPen) as well as *naloxone*. *Glucagon* should be considered similarly simple to use. All prehospital HCPs should have access to and use this lifesaving drug.[16]

Managing Hyperglycemia

In patients with T1DM who are insulin deficient and ketotic (due to missed or insufficient insulin), hyperglycemia can be worsened by exercise; however, very few people with T2DM develop such a profound degree of insulin deficiency. High-intensity anaerobic exercise is frequently the cause of dramatic exercise-induced hyperglycemia and places a theoretical risk of exercise-induced ketoacidosis in the patient with inappropriately low basal insulin concentrations. In the patient without diabetes, these processes often lead to hyperglycemia, but normal secretion of insulin provides a rapid reduction in blood glucose. For the athlete with diabetes, high-intensity exercise performed until exhaustion (at 80% of maximal oxygen-carrying capacity) often leads to elevated blood glucose levels after exercise that remain high for a significantly longer period of time than in control subjects without diabetes.[26] Therefore, people with T2DM generally do not need to postpone exercise because of high blood glucose, provided that they are feeling well. People with T2DM may engage in physical activity, using caution when exercising with blood glucose levels >300 mg/dL without symptoms of ketosis, provided that they are feeling well and are adequately hydrated.[9,10]

Summary

Athletic trainers have more contact with the athlete with diabetes than most members of her diabetes management team and so must be prepared to assist the athlete as required. This chapter addresses the steps necessary for ensuring the long-term health and well-being of athletes with metabolic disorders. Throughout, it describes recommendations for pharmacological interventions consistent with those provided by the American Diabetic Association, the American College of Sports Medicine, and the NATA position statement *Management of the Athlete With Type I Diabetes Mellitus*.[18] The recommendations described in this chapter are intended to provide the AT with the specific knowledge and problem-solving skills for appropriately managing athletes with hypo- or hyperglycemia. The AT must have the supplies and be prepared to assist a patient with an injection of *glucagon* or *insulin* or with the use of an *insulin* pump. As part of a long-term plan for managing diabetes, patients must exercise regularly to have continued benefits. Most people with T1DM and T2DM can perform exercise safely as long as they follow certain precautions,[9,10] including monitoring blood glucose concentration and following their diabetic care plan. The inclusion of an exercise program or other means of increasing overall physical activity is critical for optimal health in people with diabetes.

Case Studies

Case Study 1

Tom is 58 years old and mildly overweight. In his routine physical exam, his fasting blood glucose level was 120 mg/dL. His physician diagnosed him as prediabetic and started him on 500 mg *metformin* (Glucophage) twice daily. Also, the physician recommended that Tom lose weight and add exercise to his daily routine. At a 6-month follow-up, his blood glucose level was 140 mg/dL. Tom was prescribed *insulin glargine* (Toujeo) daily and advised to continue the *metformin*.

Questions for Analysis

1. Why was the *metformin* prescribed during Tom's prediabetic phase?
2. Why was *insulin glargine* added?

Case Study 2

Jamie is an elite baseball player and a type 2 diabetic who takes Levemir, a recombinant human *insulin* analog, to manage his diabetes. His routine is to administer a 10-unit injection nightly from a preloaded syringe, followed by taking 1,000 mg *metformin* each morning. When Jamie reported to batting practice at 11:00 a.m., he told his AT, George, that he felt very fatigued, thirsty, and slightly light-headed but did not know why. George knew Jamie's history and was concerned about him being hyperglycemic. Jamie said he had overslept and skipped both eating breakfast and taking his *metformin* this morning prior to practice. Also, he admitted that he had forgotten to administer the Levemir the past 2 nights. George helped Jamie find his Levemir in his backpack and assisted him in giving himself a subcutaneous injection and taking his *metformin* according to his diabetes care plan. George held Jamie out of practice and monitored his vital signs and blood glucose level until he stabilized.

Questions for Analysis

1. What is a potential complication of missing insulin?
2. What is the significance of Jamie presenting as thirsty and fatigued?

Drugs Described in This Chapter

Drug class	*generic* (pronunciation) Trade name	Therapeutic uses	Clinical concerns
Antihyperglycemics: biguanides	*metformin* (met FOR min) Glucophage	Initial: 500 mg orally once or twice daily or 850 mg once daily Usual maintenance dosage: 1 g twice daily or 850 mg twice daily Maximum: 2.55 g/d	For patients who are not meeting glycemic targets despite following diet and exercise regimens and taking *metformin*, combination therapy is necessary to achieve optimal results.
Antihyperglycemics: sodium-glucose cotransporter-2 (SGLT-2) inhibitors	*empagliflozin* (EM pa gli FLOE zin) Jardiance	10 mg orally once daily in the morning, taken with or without food. In patients tolerating Jardiance, the dose may be increased to 25 mg. In patients with dehydration, correcting this condition prior to initiation of Jardiance is recommended.	This drug can cause dehydration, which may cause feelings of weakness or dizziness, especially when standing up. Dehydration should also be a cause for concern in people exercising in the heat.
Antihyperglycemics: GLP-1 receptor agonists	*dulaglutide* (DOO la GLOO tide) Trulicity	Initial: 0.75 mg subcutaneous injection once weekly. May be increased to 1.5 mg once weekly for additional glycemic control. Maximum recommended dose: 1.5 mg once weekly.	In animal studies, Trulicity caused thyroid tumors or thyroid cancer. It is not known whether these effects would occur in people using regular doses.
Insulin secretagogue: sulfonylureas	*glipizide* (GLIP i zide) Glucotrol	Initial: 2.5 mg orally once daily administered 30 min before a meal (preferably before breakfast)	Stimulates the pancreas to release insulin and increases tissue sensitivity to insulin

14

Drugs for Treating Digestive Disorders

OBJECTIVES

After reading this chapter, you will be able to do the following:

- Summarize common symptoms related to common gastrointestinal (GI) tract conditions and disorders
- Recognize warning symptoms of severe GI conditions
- Identify examples, therapeutic uses, and clinical concerns for drug classes commonly used to treat GI conditions
- Provide patient instructions for taking medications for GI conditions that are administered orally or rectally as an enema or suppository
- Describe the mechanisms of action for common gastric acid–reducing medication

The gastrointestinal (GI) tract is an organ system responsible for nutrient absorption, waste excretion, and immunity. The primary organs of the digestive system include the following:[27]

- **Upper GI tract**—Oral cavity, esophagus, stomach, and duodenum
- **Lower GI tract**—Small intestine, cecum, colon, rectum, and anus
- **Associated glandular organs**—Gallbladder, pancreas, and liver

Abdominal pain is a common and frequent GI complaint that is often inconsequential. In patients with minor complaints, a medical history and physical examination are all that is required.[24] Acute and severe abdominal pain, however, is almost always a symptom of an intra-abdominal condition that may be emergent; the patient must be referred for medical exam swiftly (see Red Flag). This chapter describes how to recognize common GI tract–related conditions and the therapeutic medications used treat physically active patients with these conditions. It also describes the pharmaceutical management of several common gastrointestinal disorders.

RED FLAG

Signs of Severe GI Disorders

During the primary survey, the athletic trainer (AT) should rapidly screen for certain findings that in an otherwise healthy person raise suspicion of a more serious etiology:[2,8,9,15,17,28]

- **Signs of shock**—Tachycardia, hypotension, diaphoresis, and confusion are indications of an emergent medical condition.

(continued)

Select Drugs Mentioned in This Chapter

Drug class	Generic name	Trade name
Antiemetics		
Antihistamines	*dimenhydrinate*	OTC: Dramamine
Phenothiazine derivatives	*promethazine* *prochlorperazine*	Rx: Phenadoz Rx: Compazine, Compro
Serotonin antagonists	*ondansetron* *metoclopramide*	Rx: Zofran Rx: Metozolv ODT, Reglan
Antidiarrheals	*bismuth subsalicylate* *loperamide*	OTC: Pepto-Bismol OTC: Imodium
Laxatives		
Bulking agents	*psyllium* *methylcellulose*	OTC: Metamucil OTC: Citrucel
Stool softeners	*docusate sodium*	OTC: Docusil, Colace
Stimulants	*senna* *sennosides* *magnesium citrate* *bisacodyl*	OTC: Senokot OTC: Ex-Lax OTC: Citroma OTC: Dulcolax
Acid reducers		
Absorbable antacids	*calcium carbonate*	OTC: Tums, Rolaids
Nonabsorbable antacids	*aluminum hydroxide* and *magnesium hydroxide* suspension	OTC: Maalox
Proton pump inhibitors	*omeprazole* *esomeprazole* *lansoprazole*	OTC: Prilosec OTC: Nexium OTC: Prevacid
Histamine (H2) blockers	*famotidine* *cimetidine*	OTC: Pepcid OTC: Tagamet
Prostaglandin E1 analog	*misoprostol*	Rx: Cytotec
Corticosteroid: inhaled	*budesonide*	Rx: Pulmicort

This list is not exhaustive, but rather contains drugs commonly encountered in the athletic training setting. Always consult up-to-date information, confirm with a pharmacist, or discuss the use of therapeutic medications with the prescriber of the medication.

(continued)

- Fever—Low-grade fever (rectal temperature 37.7°C to 38.3°C [100°F to 101°F]) is common in **appendicitis**.
- Severe pain—Particularly in a patient with a silent abdomen who is lying as still as possible, suggesting **peritonitis**.
- Tenderness in the abdomen—Suggests etiology, depending on location (e.g., right upper quadrant suggesting **cholecystitis**, right lower quadrant suggests appendicitis), but may not be diagnostic.
- Acute bloody diarrhea with or without hemodynamic instability—Suggests an enteroinvasive infection. Inflammatory bowel disease, diverticular bleeding, and ischemic colitis also manifest with acute bloody diarrhea.

Presence of any of these signs and symptoms indicates a serious medical condition and dictates urgent referral to the emergency department.

Evidence in Pharmacology

Antibiotics for Treating Appendicitis

Appendectomy has been the gold standard of care for acute appendicitis for over a century.[22] This surgical procedure, along with antibiotics and fluid administration, is still usual and customary treatment.[5] However, modern considerations for treating acute and uncomplicated appendicitis involve treatment with antibiotics only, rather than surgery. Research in Finland over a 3-year period demonstrated successful results when opting for a conservative approach using antibiotics only. In a randomized control trial, patients with appendicitis were divided equally into surgical and antibiotic cohorts.[22] Over the course of 90 days, some patients within the antibiotic group did need surgery, but those without appendicolith (calcified deposit within the appendix present in a large number of children with acute appendicitis) were more successfully treated with antibiotics only. It was concluded that for appendicitis, antibiotic treatment alone was noninferior to surgery based on a standard health-status measure.[22] This information is valuable for ATs who want to discuss possible nonsurgical options for managing appendicitis with their patient's directing physician.

Nausea and Vomiting

Nausea, the unpleasant feeling of needing to vomit, represents awareness of afferent stimuli to the vomiting center in the brain stem. Vomiting is the forceful expulsion of gastric contents caused by involuntary contraction of the abdominal musculature when the gastric fundus and lower esophageal sphincter are relaxed.[18] **Emesis** and the sensation of nausea that frequently accompanies it are generally viewed as components of a protective reflex that serves to rid the stomach and intestine of toxic substances and prevent further ingestion.[30] Nausea is a frequent side effect of medications as well as a common feature in a number of systemic conditions, disorders of the central nervous system (CNS), and GI conditions.[19,30] A comprehensive history and physical examination, as well as the use of various diagnostic tests, may be needed to determine the cause of the nausea and its complications.[19] The most common causes of nausea and vomiting are as follows:[18]

- Gastroenteritis
- Drugs or toxins
- Motion sickness and other labyrinthine disturbances
- Pregnancy

Drugs for Treating Nausea and Vomiting

If vomiting is severe and a surgical condition has been excluded, an antiemetic may be beneficial in adult patients.[18,19,30] In actively vomiting patients, parenteral agents should be used. Antihistamines are effective for the prevention of **motion sickness** as well as nausea and vomiting associated with migraines and **vertigo** (labyrinthine disturbances that are vestibular in origin). A common side effect (or intended effect in some cases) of antihistamines is drowsiness.[13,18,19] Many antihistamines are commonly available for the prevention or treatment of mild nausea, vomiting, and vertigo associated with motion sickness, migraine, and other labyrinthine disturbances. The prototypical drug in this class is *dimenhydrinate* (Dramamine), which is available in oral (PO), intravenous (IV), or intramuscular (IM) forms. To prevent motion sickness, this drug should be administered 30 to 60 minutes prior to boarding the vehicle.

If vomiting is the main cause of fluid loss, **metabolic alkalosis** with **hypochloremia** can occur. If diarrhea is more prominent, **metabolic acidosis** is more likely. Both vomiting and diarrhea can cause **hypokalemia**. **Hyponatremia** may develop, particularly if hypotonic fluids are used in fluid replacement therapy.[4] Specific conditions, including dehydration, should be treated. Even without significant dehydration, IV fluid therapy often leads to reduction of symptoms. Various antiemetics are effective, depending on the cause and severity of symptoms.[13,18] A potent antiemetic, *promethazine* (Phenadoz), is a phenothiazine derivative histamine (H1) antagonist. *Promethazine* is used for active and prophylactic treatment of motion sickness as well as for prevention and control of nausea and vomiting associated with certain types of anesthesia and surgery. It is commonly administered IM and IV and has an onset of action of 20 minutes and 5 minutes, respectively. This drug has limited oral bioavailability because it largely undergoes first-pass metabolism. The effects of this drug usually last 4 to 6 hours (≤12 hours).

For **psychogenic vomiting**, the AT should give the patient reassurance, showing an awareness of the patient's discomfort and a desire to work toward relief of symptoms, regardless of cause. Brief symptomatic treatment with antiemetics may be prescribed. If long-term management is necessary, regular visits to a specialist may be needed to resolve an underlying problem.[18] A common antiemetic, *prochlorperazine* (Compazine, Compro) is a phenothiazine derivative available as a generic, oral tablet, IM injection, IV, or rectal suppository. In severe cases of vomiting, a suppository may be an option to introduce the medication into the body. The onset of action for the oral medication is 30 to 40 minutes and for rectal is about 60 minutes. The medication lasts 3 to 4 hours for oral and 3 to 12 hours for rectal administration. The $t_{1/2}$ is 6 to 10 hours for a single oral dose and 14 to 22 hours for repeated dosing.

Ondansetron (Zofran) is prototypical serotonin antagonist drug in this class that has therapeutic effects against **hyperemesis** of pregnancy and, to a lesser degree, postoperative nausea, but not against motion sickness.[30] *Ondansetron* is absorbed well from the GI tract and has a rapid onset of action. This drug is extensively metabolized in the liver and has a $t_{1/2}$ of 3 to 6 hours. The antiemetic effects of the drug persist long after it disappears from the circulation, and the drug can be administered effectively just once a day. This medication is available as tablets, oral solution, and IV preparations for injection.[30] In general, this drug is very well tolerated; the most common adverse effects are constipation or diarrhea, headache, and light-headedness.[30] Another common drug with this mechanism of action is *metoclopramide* (Metozolv ODT, Reglan), which is rapid and well absorbed when administered orally.

Diarrhea

Diarrhea, from the Greek *dia* ("through") and *rhein* ("to flow or run"), does not require any definition to people who suffer from "the too rapid evacuation of too fluid stools."[30] Diarrhea is defined as stool weight >200 g per day.[17] Several basic mechanisms are responsible for most clinically significant diarrheas: increased osmotic load, increased secretions, and decreased contact time or surface area. In many disorders, >1 mechanism is active. For example, diarrhea in inflammatory bowel disease results from mucosal inflammation, exudation into the intestinal lumen, and secretions and bacterial toxins that affect enterocyte function.[17] Severe GI conditions should be suspected in the following cases:[4,17]

- **Acute, watery diarrhea in an otherwise healthy person**—Likely to be of infectious etiology, particularly when travel, possibly tainted food, or an outbreak with a point source is involved. Antibiotic-associated diarrhea, such as diarrhea induced by *Clostridium difficile* (*C. difficile*), is a common adverse effect of recent antibiotic use.
- **Acute bloody diarrhea with or without hemodynamic instability in an otherwise healthy person**—Suggests an enteroinvasive infection. Diverticular bleeding and ischemic colitis also manifest with acute bloody diarrhea. Recurrent bouts of bloody diarrhea in a younger person suggest inflammatory bowel disease.
- **Diarrhea that consistently follows ingestion of certain foods (e.g., fats)**—Suggests food intolerance.

Many patients with sudden onset of diarrhea have a benign, self-limited illness that does not require treatment or evaluation. Acute diarrhea is frequently due to infection with bacteria, viruses, or protozoa. Therefore, oral rehydration therapy is a cornerstone treatment for patients with acute illnesses that result in significant diarrhea. Oral electrolyte replacement contains water and electrolytes that link sodium absorption to glucose uptake by the enterocyte; this is followed by movement of water in the same direction. A balanced mixture of glucose and electrolytes in volumes matched to losses can therefore prevent dehydration. This can be provided by many commercial premixed formulas using glucose-electrolyte (Pedialyte) or rice-based physiological solutions.[30] Pedialyte is lower in sugars than most sports drinks, containing 100 calories per L compared to approximately 240 calories per L in Gatorade. It contains more sodium (1,035 mg/L vs. 465 mg/L in Gatorade) and potassium (780 mg/L vs. 127 mg/L in Gatorade). Pedialyte does not contain sucrose, which has the potential to make diarrhea worse by drawing water into the intestine, increasing the risk of dehydration. In its flavored formulations, Pedialyte uses the synthetic sweeteners sucralose and acesulfame potassium.[1]

Drugs for Treating Diarrhea

Complications may result from diarrhea of any etiology. These include fluid loss with consequent dehydration and electrolyte loss (sodium, potassium, magnesium, chloride). Diarrhea is a symptom of another disorder. When possible, the underlying disorder should be treated, but symptomatic treatment is often necessary. Pharmacotherapy of diarrhea in adults should be reserved for patients with significant or persistent symptoms. Nonspecific antidiarrheal agents typically do not address the underlying pathophysiology responsible for the diarrhea. Many of these agents act by decreasing intestinal motility and should be avoided in acute diarrheal illnesses caused by invasive organisms. In such cases, these agents may mask the clinical picture, delay clearance of organisms, and increase the risk of systemic invasion by the infectious organisms.[4]

Antidiarrheal agents are safe for adult patients with watery diarrhea (as shown by a heme-negative stool). However, antidiarrheals may cause deterioration of patients with *C. difficile* or *E. coli O157:H7* infection (see Evidence in Pharmacology sidebar) and thus should not be given to any patient with recent antibiotic use or heme-positive stool, pending specific diagnosis.[4]

Compounds containing *bismuth subsalicylate* (Pepto-Bismol) are used to treat a variety of GI disorders, although their mechanism of action remains poorly understood. *Bismuth subsalicylate* is a popular over-the-counter (OTC) preparation that consists of trivalent bismuth and salicylate suspended in a mixture of magnesium aluminum silicate clay. In the low pH of the stomach, the *bismuth subsalicylate* reacts with hydrochloric acid to form bismuth oxychloride and salicylic acid.[30] Bismuth is thought to have antisecretory, anti-inflammatory, and antimicrobial effects. It also relieves nausea and abdominal cramps. The clay in *bismuth subsalicylate* and generic formulations may have some additional benefits in diarrhea, but this is not clear. *Bismuth subsalicylate* is used for the prevention and treatment of **traveler's diarrhea**, but it also is effective in other forms of episodic diarrhea and acute gastroenteritis.[30]

The recommended dose of *bismuth subsalicylate* (30 mL of regular-strength liquid or 2 tablets) contains approximately equal amounts of bismuth and salicylate (262 mg each). For control of indigestion, nausea, or diarrhea, the dose is repeated every 30 to 60 minutes, as needed, up to 8 times a day. Dark stools (sometimes mistaken for **melena**) and black staining of the tongue in association with bismuth compounds are caused by bismuth sulfide, which is formed in a reaction between the drug and bacterial sulfides in the GI tract. Although 99% of the bismuth passes unaltered and unabsorbed into the feces, the salicylate is absorbed in the stomach and small intestine. Thus, the product carries the same warning regarding Reye's syndrome as other salicylates and may also cause CNS side effects, hearing loss, and tinnitus.[30] Additionally, *bismuth subsalicylate* products are contraindicated for patients with a salicylate allergy or a stomach ulcer.[30]

Antimotility and antisecretory agents such as the opioid *loperamide*, the prototype antidiarrheal, are widely used in the treatment of diarrhea. These

Evidence in Pharmacology

Probiotics

The human microbiome of the GI tract contains a vast and complex commensal microflora necessary for health. Alterations in the balance or composition of the microflora are responsible for antibiotic-associated diarrhea and possibly other disease conditions. Probiotic preparations containing a variety of bacterial strains have shown some degree of benefit in acute diarrheal conditions, antibiotic-associated diarrhea, and infectious diarrhea. In clinical trials, preparations containing *Lactobacillus GG* and *Saccharomyces boulardii* are effective for these conditions.[12,30]

Clinical Application

Treating Traveler's Diarrhea

Antimicrobial treatment of traveler's diarrhea, bacterial diarrhea, and diarrhea with more severe conditions is appropriate under some conditions, based on the severity of diarrhea and the duration of the symptoms. The first-line therapy for acute (most commonly, traveler's) diarrhea in adults is oral *ciprofloxacin* (500 mg twice daily for up to 3 days).[30]

medications are used to decrease the frequency of diarrhea, particularly in GI conditions such as gastroenteritis, inflammatory bowel disease, and short bowel syndrome. However, treatment of diarrhea from an underlying GI disorder with blood in the stool is contraindicated. Antimotility and antisecretory agents can affect the following:[4,30]

- Intestinal motility
- Intestinal secretion
- Absorption

Loperamide (Imodium), the prototypical antidiarrheal, increases small intestinal and mouth-to-cecum transit times and anal sphincter tone.[30] *Loperamide* is available OTC in capsule, solution, and chewable tablet forms and is often preferred over opioids that penetrate the CNS.[30] It acts quickly after an oral dose, with peak plasma levels achieved within 5 hours. It has a $t_{1/2}$ of about 11 hours and undergoes extensive hepatic metabolism.[30]

The therapeutic adult dose of *loperamide* is 4 mg, initially followed by 2 mg after each subsequent loose stool, up to 16 mg per day. If clinical improvement in acute diarrhea does not occur within 48 hours, *loperamide* should be discontinued and the patient should be referred to the next level care provider. *Loperamide* is effective against traveler's diarrhea, used alone or in combination with antibiotics. It is used as adjunct treatment in many forms of chronic diarrheal disease (initially as for acute diarrhea, but with typical divided daily doses of 4 to 8 mg per day), with few adverse effects. *Loperamide* has abuse potential, and overdose can result in constipation, CNS depression, and **paralytic ileus**. In patients with active inflammatory bowel disease involving the colon, *loperamide* should be used with great caution, if at all, to avoid development of **toxic megacolon**.[3,4,30]

Constipation

Patients use the term *constipation* not only for decreased frequency but also for difficulty in initiation or passage of firm or small-volume feces or a feeling of incomplete evacuation.[16,21,30,41] Constipation is often one of several symptoms (abdominal pain, nausea, fatigue, anorexia) of an underlying problem (e.g., irritable bowel syndrome, depression). Constipation has many reversible or secondary causes, including lack of dietary fiber, drugs, hormonal disturbances, neurogenic disorders, and systemic illnesses.[16,30]

In most patients with constipation, the chief complaint is sluggish movement of stool through the colon.[16] Water normally accounts for 70% to 85% of total stool weight. The daily challenge for the gut is to extract water, minerals, and nutrients from the luminal contents, leaving behind a manageable pool of fluid for proper expulsion of waste material via the process of defecation.[30] With decreased motility and excess fluid removal, feces can become thickened and impacted, leading to constipation.

Initially, constipation should be corrected by adherence to a fiber-rich (20-35 g daily) diet, adequate fluid intake, appropriate bowel habits and training, regular exercise, and avoidance of constipation-causing drugs.[21] Patients with constipation that is suspected to be related to medications should be examined by the prescriber, who may prescribe alternative drugs where possible or adjust the dosage.

Drugs for Treating Constipation

If nonpharmacological measures alone are inadequate, various drugs are available for treating constipation. Medications that are the least disruptive (bulking agents, stool softeners) should be used first. More potent medications, such as stimulant laxatives, may be used, although they should be administered at the lowest effective dosage and for the shortest possible period of time to avoid dependency.[16] Drugs for treating constipation include bulking agents, stool softeners, and stimulant laxatives.

Bulking agents, also considered dietary fiber supplementation, are particularly effective in treating normal-transit constipation. Bulk-forming laxatives absorb liquid in the intestines and create a bulky, more liquid-like stool that is softer and easier to pass. Common bulk-forming laxatives include *psyllium* (Metamucil) and *methylcellulose* (Citrucel). These soluble fibers are helpful when started with an initial dose of 2.5 to 4 g (1-3 tsp in 250 mL of fruit juice). The dose is then titrated upward until the desired goal is reached. The onset of action of these bulk-forming laxatives is generally between 12 and 72 hours. Bloating is the most common side effect of soluble fiber products (due to colonic fermentation), but it usually decreases with time.[20,30]

Stool softeners (also called emollient laxatives) are laxatives that work gently to lubricate the stool and draw water into the stool, making it softer and more comfortable to pass. The primary active ingredient in OTC stool softener products is *docusate sodium* (Docusil, Colace). Most stool softener products should soften the stool and trigger the urge for a bowel movement within 72 hours.

Stimulant laxatives should be used judiciously, since some bind drugs and interfere with absorption. Rapid fecal transit may rush some drugs and nutrients beyond their optimal absorptive state. Contraindications to laxatives are as follows:[16]

- Acute abdominal pain of unknown origin
- Inflammatory bowel disorders
- Intestinal obstruction
- GI bleeding
- Fecal impaction

Stimulant laxatives typically induce defecation by stimulating peristaltic activity on the intestine through direct action on intestinal mucosa or nerve plexus, therefore increasing motility. These drugs can be dangerous under certain circumstances. Prolonged use of stimulant laxatives can create drug dependence by damaging the colon's haustral folds, making the user less able to move feces through the colon on his own.[30] Common stimulant laxatives are anthraquinones, which are laxative derivatives of plants such *senna* (Senokot) and *sennosides* (Ex-Lax). A potent laxative, *magnesium citrate* (Citroma) promotes bowel evacuation by causing osmotic retention of fluid, which distends the colon with increased peristaltic activity. When administered as an oral solution, this drug produces a laxative effect in 0.5 to 6 hours. Another common stimulant laxative is *bisacodyl* (Dulcolax). *Bisacodyl* can be taken by oral tablet or as an **enema** or **suppository** forms, which are administered in the rectum (see Evidence in Pharmacology sidebar). Common laxatives administered rectally include sodium phosphate enemas and glycerin suppositories.

Gastroesophageal Reflux Disease

Gastroesophageal reflux (GER) involves **incompetence** of the lower esophageal sphincter that allows reflux of gastric contents into the esophagus, causing burning pain. Prolonged reflux may lead to esophagitis, stricture, and, rarely, **intestinal metaplasia** or cancer.[23,25] Gastroesophageal reflux disease (GERD), also known as acid reflux, is a more serious and long-lasting form of GER. GERD is a long-term condition in which stomach contents rise up into the esophagus, resulting in either symptoms or complications. Other conditions known as GERD include the following:

- Acid indigestion
- Acid reflux
- Acid regurgitation
- Heartburn
- Reflux

The most prominent symptom of GERD is heartburn, with or without regurgitation of gastric contents into the mouth. Other symptoms include the

Evidence in Pharmacology

Opioid-Induced Constipation

Opioids bind to the mu-opioid receptor in the GI tract, resulting in opioid-induced constipation (OIC), along with possible nausea, vomiting, or **pruritus**. Opioids are critical to pain management;[31] however, after commencing opioid therapy, 40% to 90% of patients experience a reduction of spontaneous bowel movement from baseline to typically <3 bowel movements per week.[31,32] This condition is associated with multiple medications used for both cancer and noncancer care, including *acetaminophen* with *hydrocodone*, *morphine*, *oxycodone*, *acetaminophen* with *oxycodone*, and *tramadol*.[31]

OIC generally does not respond well to traditional laxatives, which often results in increased physician visits and reduced productivity and prompts some patients to curtail their opioid use in order to stimulate bowel activity. Peripherally acting mu-opioid receptor agonists (PAMORAs) are prescription medications developed to reverse OIC.[32] Examples of these medications are *methylnaltrexone* (Relistor), *lubiprostone* (Amitiza), and *naloxegol* (Movantik). They should be administered 1 hour before or 2 hours after meals. Although these agents are FDA approved for the treatment of OIC, they are not used first line and are usually reserved for patients who have first failed other bowel regimen therapies. PAMORAs are contraindicated for anyone with a GI tract obstruction or hepatic impairment and should be ceased if opioid use ends.[31]

taste of acid in the back of the mouth, bad breath, chest pain, vomiting, breathing problems, and wearing away of the teeth from exposure to gastric acid.[23] Gastric acid is secreted by parietal cells in the proximal two-thirds (body) of the stomach. Gastric acid aids digestion by creating the optimal pH for pepsin and gastric lipase and stimulating pancreatic bicarbonate secretion.[29,37]

Drugs for Decreasing Gastric Acidity

Drugs for decreasing gastric acidity are important for treating GERD, peptic ulcers, many forms of gastritis, and, in some in regimens, *Helicobacter pylori* infection. Drugs that decrease gastric acidity include the following:[23,29,33]

- Antacids
- Proton pump inhibitors
- Histamine-2 (H2) receptor blockers

Antacids

Antacids are OTC medications used to relieve heartburn, indigestion, or an upset stomach by neutralizing gastric acid and reducing pepsin activity (which diminishes as gastric pH rises). In addition, some antacids adsorb pepsin. Antacids contain alkaline ions that chemically neutralize stomach gastric acid, reducing damage and relieving pain. Absorbable antacids such as *calcium carbonate* (Tums, Rolaids) provide rapid, complete neutralization, but may cause alkalosis and thus should be used only briefly (1 or 2 days). Nonabsorbable antacids, such as *aluminum hydroxide* and *magnesium hydroxide* suspension (Maalox), have fewer systemic adverse effects and are preferred. Antacids may interfere with the absorption of other drugs (e.g., *tetracycline*, *doxycycline*, *fluroquinolones*, *digoxin*, iron products). Antacids are relatively inexpensive but must be taken 5 to 7 times per day. The total daily dosage of antacids should provide 200 to 400 mEq neutralizing capacity. Antacids can have side effects, including diarrhea and constipation.[23,33]

Proton Pump Inhibitors

Proton pump inhibitors (PPIs) are a group of drugs with the mechanism of action of blocking the final step in gastric acid production. These medications provide a pronounced and long-lasting reduction of stomach acid production (up to 48 hours) and are the most potent inhibitors of acid secretion available. They have a short plasma $t_{1/2}$ of about 0.5 to 3 hours.[29] Many PPIs are available OTC, such as *esomeprazole* (Nexium) or *lansoprazole* (Prevacid), and all have equivalent efficacy at comparable doses. Although there may be some concern for this practice, PPIs are commonly recommended for long-term use, but the dose should be adjusted to the minimum required to prevent symptoms, including intermittent or as-needed dosing.[23,29,33]

> **RED FLAG**
>
> **Interaction of Antacids and Antibiotics**
>
> Certain medications have efficacy concerns when administered with antacids. Simultaneous administration of *aluminum hydroxide* with *tetracycline* or *ciprofloxacin* can reduce the effectiveness of the antibiotic.[26] To avoid substantially affecting the other drug therapy's efficacy, a general rule of thumb is to take the antacid 1 hour before or 2 hours after the interacting drug so as to allow the stomach to sufficiently empty. Consideration should be taken when administering an antacid simultaneously with a nonsteroidal anti-inflammatory drug (NSAID) due to its associated gastric irritation. There is a distinct interaction between *indomethacin* and antacids. Simultaneous administration of antacids with a base of *aluminum hydroxide* and *magnesium hydroxide* and *indomethacin* reduces the effectiveness of *indomethacin* by up to 35%.[26]

Histamine (H2) Blockers

Histamine (H2) blockers are competitive selective histamine H2 receptor antagonists that suppress gastrin-stimulated acid secretion, reduce the volume of gastric juice, and decrease histamine-mediated pepsin secretion. Many H2 blockers, such as *famotidine* (Pepcid) and *cimetidine* (Tagamet), are available without a prescription in the United States. These drugs are less potent than PPIs but still suppress 24-hour gastric acid secretion by about 70%.[29] H2 blockers are well absorbed from the GI tract, with onset of action occurring 30 to 60 minutes after ingestion and peak effects at 1 to 2 hours. Duration of action is proportional to dose and ranges from 6 to 20 hours.[29,33] All the H2 blockers are well tolerated; however, *cimetidine* has some significant drug–drug interactions.

Gastritis and Peptic Ulcer Disease

Gastritis is inflammation of the gastric mucosa caused by any of several conditions, including infection (*Helicobacter pylori*), drugs (NSAIDs, alcohol), stress, and autoimmune phenomena (**atrophic gastritis**). Many cases are asymptomatic, but **dyspepsia** and GI bleeding sometimes occur.[34] A peptic ulcer is an erosion in a segment of the GI mucosa that penetrates through the muscularis mucosae in the stomach (gastric ulcer) or the first few centimeters of the duodenum (duodenal ulcer).[35] Peptic ulcer disease (PUD) is considered an imbalance between mucosal defense factors (bicarbonate, mucin, prostaglandins, and other peptides and growth factors) and injurious factors (acid and pepsin). Although patients with PUD have normal or even diminished acid production, ulcers rarely, if ever, occur in the complete absence of acid. Factors that interfere with these mucosal defenses (particularly NSAIDs and *H. pylori* infection) predispose a patient to gastritis and PUD.[37] Up to 60% of peptic ulcers are associated with *H. pylori* infection of the stomach.[11,29]

In addition, NSAIDs promote mucosal inflammation and ulcer formation (sometimes with GI bleeding) when administered both topically and systemically. By inhibiting prostaglandin production via blockage of the enzyme cyclooxygenase (COX), NSAIDs reduce gastric blood flow, mucus, and bicarbonate secretion and decrease cell repair and replication. Also, because NSAIDs are weak acids and are nonionized at gastric pH, they diffuse freely across the mucus barrier into gastric epithelial cells, where H^+ ions are liberated, leading to cellular damage.[37] *Misoprostol* (Cytotec) is a synthetic prostaglandin E1 analog that reduces stomach acid and helps protect the stomach from damage that can be caused by taking NSAIDs. This medication has minor side effects, including nausea, stomach cramps, or diarrhea; however, in pregnant women, this medication can cause serious adverse effects, including birth defects, premature birth, miscarriage, and dangerous uterine bleeding.

Drugs for Treating *Helicobacter Pylori* Infection

H. pylori is a spiral-shaped, Gram-negative organism that has adapted to thrive in acid. It commonly causes chronic infections and is usually acquired during childhood. In the United States, infection is less common among children, but incidence increases with age: About 50% of people aged 60 and over are infected. Infection is most common among Black, Hispanic, and Asian people. The organism has been cultured from stool, saliva, and dental plaque, which suggests oral–oral or fecal–oral transmission.[36] The American College of Gastroenterology's guidelines for the management of *H. pylori* infection[7] recommend multiple therapies to eradicate the bacteria. Triple therapy is the most frequently prescribed regimen for *H. pylori* infection and involves drugs given for 10 to 14 days:[7,10,14,36]

- A proton pump inhibitor (*omeprazole* 20 mg PO BID, *esomeprazole* 40 mg PO once/day, or *lansoprazole* (30 mg PO BID)
- *Amoxicillin* (1 g PO BID) or *metronidazole* (250 mg QID)
- *Clarithromycin* (500 mg PO BID)

Gastroenteritis

Gastroenteritis is inflammation of the lining of the stomach and small and large intestines. Most cases are foodborne, waterborne, or spread via person-to-person infection, although gastroenteritis may occur after ingestion of drugs and chemical toxins (e.g., metals, plant substances). In the United States, an estimated 1 in 6 people contracts foodborne illness each year. Gastroenteritis is usually uncomfortable but self-limited. Electrolyte and fluid loss are usually little more than an inconvenience to an otherwise healthy adult, but can be grave for people who are very young, elderly, or immunocompromised or have serious concomitant illnesses.[4] Symptoms include anorexia, nausea, vomiting, diarrhea, and abdominal discomfort. Treatment is symptomatic, although some parasitic and some bacterial infections require specific anti-infective therapy.[4]

Viruses are the most common cause of gastroenteritis in the United States. They infect enterocytes in the villous epithelium of the small bowel. The result is transudation of fluid and electrolytes into the intestinal lumen; sometimes, malabsorption of carbohydrates worsens symptoms by causing osmotic diarrhea. Diarrhea is watery. Inflammatory diarrhea (dysentery), with fecal white blood cells (WBCs) and red blood cells (RBCs), or gross blood, is uncommon. Four categories of viruses cause most gastroenteritis, and norovirus and rotavirus cause most cases of viral gastroenteritis (see Clinical Application sidebar).[4]

Clinical Application

Management of Norovirus Infection

The norovirus is generally found among groups who maintain close contact and eat from a common dining hall. A college basketball team is the perfect breeding ground for norovirus—for example, the case of a team that was infected with norovirus during their postseason tournament. In this case, all members of the team's travel party ate the same food in the same dining area, players were housed 2 per hotel room, and everyone took the same bus to and from games and practices. The initial patient, a player, presented with nausea and vomiting from an unknown cause. Initially, these symptoms did not raise concern from the team's medical staff, and the patient was considered an isolated incident. He was treated with an OTC medication to relieve diarrhea symptoms. Soon thereafter, patient 2, another player, and patient 3, a coach, also presented with the same symptoms. Within a matter of hours, other players and staff members complained of gastric distress, fatigue or weakness, and loss of appetite. Some patients also presented with a low-grade fever, but none spiked a fever >102°F (39°C), as would be associated with food poisoning.[6] For each case, symptoms came on fast and generally resolved within 72 hours. Conversely, other members of the travel party followed the same meal and travel routines as those who became ill but were not affected.

Norovirus is a challenge to ATs and other health care providers for many reasons. One reason is that the pathogen is a virus and thus cannot be treated with antibiotics. Also, antivirals are generally unsuccessful in treating this infection. The reflexive thought is to rely on OTC antidiarrhea medication, but in the case of norovirus, the medication could delay excretion of the virus. The best course of action is to isolate affected people away from the group and emphasize frequent handwashing by everyone. Affected people should do their best to maintain hydration, rest, and monitor themselves for more significant medical conditions such as bloody stools.

Treatments for Gastroenteritis

Supportive treatment is all that is needed for most patients (see section on Supportive Care and General Management of Digestive Disorders).[4] If *C. difficile* or *E. coli O157:H7* infection is not suspected, antidiarrheal agents should be considered. Antibiotics are generally administered only in select cases. Empiric antibiotics are generally not recommended except for certain cases of traveler's diarrhea or when suspicion of *Shigella* or *Campylobacter* infection is high (e.g., contact with a known case). In proven bacterial gastroenteritis, antibiotics are not always required. Antibiotics are also often ineffective against toxic gastroenteritis (e.g., *S. aureus*, *B. cereus*, *C. perfringens*). As discussed in chapter 10, indiscriminate use of antibiotics fosters the emergence of drug-resistant organisms. However, certain infections do require antibiotics.[4]

Functional Bowel Disorders: Inflammatory Bowel Disease

Functional bowel disorders (FBD) are a spectrum of chronic GI disorders characterized by predominant symptoms or signs of abdominal pain, bloating, distention, or bowel habit abnormalities (e.g., constipation, diarrhea, or mixed constipation and diarrhea).[21] A common FBD, inflammatory bowel disease (IBD)—which includes Crohn's disease, ulcerative colitis, and irritable bowel syndrome (IBS)—is characterized by a relapsing and remitting condition with chronic inflammation at various sites in the GI tract, resulting in diarrhea and abdominal pain. Inflammation results from a cell-mediated immune response in the GI mucosa. NSAIDs may exacerbate IBD.[38]

Drugs for Treating Inflammatory Bowel Disease

In many patients, IBD can be managed with dietary restrictions, notably by avoiding **fermentable oligo-di-monosaccharides and polyols (FODMAPs)**, lactose, or gluten. Treatment of bowel symptoms (either diarrhea or constipation) is predominantly symptomatic and nonspecific, using the agents discussed previously.[30] Several classes of drugs are helpful for IBD:[39,40]

- **5-Aminosalicylic acid (5-ASA)**—Blocks production of prostaglandins and leukotrienes and has other beneficial effects on the inflammatory cascade.

- **Corticosteroids**—Such as the inhaled corticosteroid *budesonide* (Pulmicort), these can be useful for acute flare-ups of most forms of IBD and Crohn's disease when 5-ASA compounds are inadequate.
- **Immunomodulating drugs**—Certain antimetabolites such as *methotrexate* are also used in combination therapy with biologic agents.
- **Biologic agents (anticytokine drugs)**—Antibodies to tumor necrosis factor (TNF), such as *infliximab*, *certolizumab*, and *adalimumab*, are useful in Crohn's disease and are beneficial in ulcerative colitis.
- **Antibiotics and probiotics**—These may be helpful in Crohn's disease but are of limited use in ulcerative colitis. *Metronidazole* and *ciprofloxacin* are recommended in combination. Various nonpathogenic microorganisms (e.g., commensal *Escherichia coli*, *Lactobacillus* species, *Saccharomyces*) given daily serve as probiotics and may be effective in IBD, but other therapeutic roles have yet to be clearly defined.

Supportive Care and General Management of Digestive Disorders

Supportive treatment is all that is needed for most patients with GI symptoms. Bed rest with convenient access to a toilet or bedpan is desirable. Taking oral glucose-electrolyte solutions as well as broth or bouillon may prevent dehydration or treat mild dehydration. Even if vomiting, the patient should take frequent small sips of such fluids; vomiting may abate with volume replacement.[4] To manage chronic GI conditions, most patients and their families are interested in diet and stress management. Although there are anecdotal reports of clinical improvement on certain diets, controlled trials have shown no consistent benefit. Stress management may be helpful.[39] Avoiding raw fruits and vegetables limits trauma to the inflamed colonic mucosa and may reduce symptoms. A dairy-free diet may help, but it need not be continued if no benefit is noted. *Loperamide* 2 mg orally 2 to 4 times a day is indicated for relatively mild diarrhea; higher oral doses (4 mg in the morning and 2 mg after each bowel movement) may be required for more intense diarrhea. All patients with IBD should be advised to take appropriate amounts of calcium and vitamin D.[38]

Summary

Practically everyone has experienced a GI condition at some point, and most people are familiar with many of the symptoms and treatments. Nausea and vomiting are very common and are caused by a variety of etiologies, including motion sickness, migraines, and vertigo. Diarrhea and constipation are several GI symptoms (abdominal pain, nausea, fatigue, anorexia) that may be an indication of an underlying problem (e.g., gastroenteritis, irritable bowel syndrome, depression). Fortunately, many conditions that cause nausea, vomiting, diarrhea, and constipation are reversible, self-limiting, or benign. Treatment can include OTC antiemetics, antidiarrheals, bulking agents, stool softeners, or other commonly available OTC medications. In less common cases, GI symptoms have secondary causes, including lack of dietary fiber, drugs, hormonal disturbances, neurogenic disorders, and systemic illnesses. Potentially serious chronic GI conditions, such as GERD, PUD, and IBD, may require a variety of treatments to prevent or heal damaged tissues. The challenge for the AT is to provide supportive care to the patient, accurate drug information, and advice to help the patient and her family with diet and stress management.

Case Studies

Case Study 1

Raul is a 45-year-old executive and a recreational athlete. He recently sustained a torn ACL while skiing and had reconstructive surgery at an appropriate time. As part of his postoperative pain management, Raul was prescribed *acetaminophen* with *hydrocodone* as needed and up to 4 times daily. Raul was still experiencing pain secondary to the surgery, but noticed a sense of constipation that was becoming annoying and uncomfortable. After 1 week of bowel irregularity, he contacted his pharmacist to see if this made sense. The pharmacist referred him back to his physician, who considered the condition opioid-induced constipation. The physician recommended that Raul take a course of OTC laxatives, increase fiber in his diet, and switch his pain management routine to OTC *acetaminophen*, NSAIDs, and ice therapy.

Questions for Analysis

1. Was Raul's concern a figment of his imagination or a legitimate concern?
2. Was the prescribed course of action from the physician prudent?

Case Study 2

Many Olympic, professional, and intercollegiate athletic teams regularly travel overseas for competitions. Typically, a team physician accompanies the team to care for all members of the travel party, which includes the team, administration, and guests. Precautions are taken to minimize the risk of traveler's diarrhea, which can affect people who travel internationally, particularly if the trip is to a developing nation.

Questions for Analysis

1. What is the role of prophylactic medication in this case?
2. Other than medication, what else can be done to prevent traveler's diarrhea?

Drugs Described in This Chapter

Drug class	*generic* (pronunciation) Trade name	Therapeutic uses	Clinical concerns
Antiemetic agents: antihistamines	*dimenhydrinate* (dye men HYE dri nate) Dramamine	50 mg PO q 4-6 hr; *dimenhydrinate* is available PO, IV, and IM.	Used to treat vomiting of labyrinthine etiology (e.g., motion sickness, labyrinthitis). A common side effect is drowsiness.
	promethazine (proe METH a zeen) Phenadoz	Oral, IM, IV, rectal: 12.5-25 mg every 4-6 hr, as needed.	A potent antiemetic, used for active and prophylactic treatment of motion sickness as well as for prevention and control of nausea and vomiting associated with certain types of anesthesia and surgery.
	prochlorperazine (proe klor PER a zeen) Compazine, Compro	Oral (tablet): 5-10 mg 3 or 4 times/d; usual maximum: 40 mg/d Rectal: 25 mg twice daily	Larger doses may rarely be required for resistant nausea or vomiting.
Antiemetic agents: serotonin antagonists	*ondansetron* (on DAN se tron) Zofran	Prophylaxis: 0.25 mg IV as a single dose 30 min before needed; acutely: 4-8 mg PO or IV q 8 hr.	Well tolerated; common side effects include constipation and dizziness. Uncommon side effects include headache. Rare cases of anaphylaxis have been reported.

Drug class	*generic* (pronunciation) Trade name	Therapeutic uses	Clinical concerns
Antidiarrheals	*bismuth subsalicylate* (BIZ muth sub sa LISS i late) Pepto-Bismol	Acute diarrhea, nausea and abdominal cramping, heartburn, indigestion, and upset stomach. Shake the liquid medicine well and measure a dose. Do not take >8 doses in 1 d (24 hr). Chewable tablet must be chewed before swallowing.	Contains salicylate; do not administer with blood thinners or other salicylate-containing products, such as *aspirin*. This medication should not be given to a child or teenager who has a fever, especially if the child also has flu symptoms or chicken pox. Salicylates can cause Reye's syndrome in children. Do not use with stomach ulcer, a recent history of stomach or intestinal bleeding, or allergy to salicylates. Can cause constipation, dark-colored stools, or black or darkened tongue.
	loperamide (loe PER a mide) Imodium	For acute nonspecific diarrhea and control and symptomatic relief of chronic diarrhea associated with inflammatory bowel disease. Acute diarrhea: Oral form Initial dose: 4 mg, followed by 2 mg after each loose stool (maximum: 16 mg/d)	Limit use to 10 d. Use adjunctive therapy with antibiotics for traveler's diarrhea to decrease duration of diarrhea.
Laxatives: bulk forming	*psyllium* (SIL i yum) Metamucil, many others	Constipation: Take 10-15 g/d in divided doses of 2.5-7.5 g.	Softens feces in 1-3 days. Side effects include bloating and flatulence.
	methylcellulose (METH il SEL yoo los) Citrucel, many others	Constipation: Take 6-9 g/d in divided doses of 0.45-3.0 g.	Less bloating than with other fiber agents.
Laxatives: stool softeners	*docusate sodium* (DOK ue sate) Docusil, Colace	For mild constipation: Oral: 50-360 mg once daily or in divided doses. Rectal: 283 mg per 5 mL: 283 mg (1 enema) 1-3 times daily.	Ineffective for severe constipation. Oral softens stool in 12 to 72 hr; rectal softens stool in 2 to 15 min.
Laxatives: stimulants, anthraquinones	*senna* (SEN ah) Senokot *sennosides* (SEN oh sides) Ex-Lax	Occasional constipation (irregularity). Oral: *senna leaf extract*: 10-15 mL (352-528 mg) once daily (preferably at bedtime); may increase to 10-15 mL (352-528 mg) twice daily if needed; maximum daily dose: 30 mL/d.	For sennosides, chew tablet well before swallowing. Causes bowel movement in 6-12 hr.
	magnesium citrate (mag NEE zhum SIT rate) Citroma	Oral: Solution: 195-300 mL given once or in divided doses.	OTC labeling: When used for self-medication, do not use if on a low-salt diet.

(continued)

Drugs Described in This Chapter *(continued)*

Drug class	*generic* (pronunciation) Trade name	Therapeutic uses	Clinical concerns
	Bisacodyl (bis AK oh dil) Dulcolax	For constipation; available as oral tablet, rectal suppository, or enema.	Taken by mouth should produce a bowel movement within 12 hr. Rectal suppository produces a bowel movement within 60 min; rectal enema produces a bowel movement within 20 min.
Gastric acid reducers: absorbable antacids	*calcium carbonate* (KAL see um KAR boe nate) Tums, Rolaids	For acid reflux and indigestion. Provide rapid, complete neutralization, but may cause alkalosis and thus should be used only briefly (for 1 or 2 d).	OTC; generally well tolerated
Gastric acid reducers: nonabsorbable antacid	*aluminum hydroxide, magnesium hydroxide,* and *simethicone* suspension (a LOO mi num hye DROX ide; mag NEE see um hye DROX ide; sye METH i kone) Maalox	For heartburn and indigestion. Measure liquid as directed.	Fewer systemic adverse effects than absorbable antacids and are preferred. May interfere with the absorption of other drugs. Take after meals and at bedtime. Shake well before use.
Gastric acid reducers: proton pump inhibitors (PPIs)	*omeprazole* (oh MEP ra zol) Prilosec	For gastroesophageal reflux disease (GERD) or heartburn that occurs ≥2 d per wk.	Must be taken as a course on a regular basis for 14 d in a row. Patients may be more likely to fracture bone while taking the medication long term or more than once per d.
	esomeprazole (ee so MEP ra zol) Nexium	For GERD; prevent gastric ulcer caused by *H. pylori* infection or by the use of NSAIDs.	OTC forms for acid reflux. Not for immediate relief of heartburn symptoms.
	lansoprazole (lan SOE pra zol) Prevacid	NSAID-associated gastric ulcer. Short-term (up to 8 wk) treatment of symptomatic GERD. Part of a multidrug regimen for *H. pylori* eradication.	Administer 30-60 min before a meal. Gastric acid suppression in 1-3 hr. Generally well tolerated. Patients may be more likely to fracture bone while taking long term or more than once per d.
Gastric acid reducers: histamine (H2) blockers	*famotidine* (fam OH ti deen) Pepcid	Heartburn (OTC only): Relief of heartburn, acid indigestion, and sour stomach. Also for GERD, peptic ulcer disease (PUD; active duodenal or gastric ulcers).	Oral: Within 3 hr (dose dependent). If symptoms persist after 2 wk of taking 20 mg twice daily, refer the patient to the prescriber and consider PPI therapy.
	cimetidine (sye ME ti deen) Tagamet	Heartburn (OTC only): Relief and prevention of heartburn associated with acid indigestion and sour stomach. Relief of symptoms: 200 mg PO daily; maximum: 400 mg per 24 hr.	Also treats GERD and PUD (active gastric and duodenal ulcers). Risk of drug–drug interactions (cytochrome P450 inhibition) and gynecomastia.

15

Drugs for Treating Common Musculoskeletal and Neurological Conditions

OBJECTIVES

After reading this chapter, you will be able to do the following:

- Distinguish between different causes of articular (joint) pain
- Provide examples of medications used to treat joint pain
- Differentiate between the different classes of drugs for treating arthritis
- Discuss advantages and disadvantages of drugs used to treat musculotendinous pain
- List drugs for treating neck and back pain
- Provide examples of drugs for treating fibromyalgia and complex regional pain syndrome
- Identify drugs for treating headache disorder

The athletic trainer (AT) encounters many conditions of the nervous and musculoskeletal systems; indeed, the International Classification of Diseases (ICD) lists hundreds of diagnoses that affect nerves, muscles, bones, joints, and associated tissues, such as tendons, ligaments, and bursae. These conditions range from those that are acute, such as fractures, sprains, and strains, to lifelong conditions associated with chronic pain and disability, such as migraine, rheumatoid arthritis, and fibromyalgia.[51]

This chapter presents examples of drugs used to treat arthralgia and pain as a result of injury, acute infectious arthritis and **osteomyelitis**, **gout**, osteoarthritis (OA) or degenerative joint disease, rheumatoid arthritis (RA), and systemic lupus erythematosus (SLE). It covers pain relating to musculotendinous structures, as well as neck and back pain. This chapter also discusses systemic, nontraumatic causes of musculoskeletal pain, including fibromyalgia and complex regional pain syndrome (CRPS). It closes with a section on pharmacological treatment of neurological sources of pain, such as headache disorder.

Articular (Joint) Pain

Articular sources of pain originate within the joint and periarticular pain originates in structures surrounding the joint (e.g., tendons, ligaments, bursae, muscles). **Arthralgia** is pain that originates within a joint and may be caused by **arthritis** (joint inflammation) or other triggers like a trauma. Pain in or

Select Drugs Mentioned in This Chapter

Drug class	Generic name	Trade name
Antiarthritic agents		
Antigout drugs	*colchicine*	Colcrys, others
Hyaluronate injection	*sodium hyaluronate*	Euflexxa, others
Antirheumatic agents		
Antimalarials	*hydroxychloroquine*	Plaquenil
Immunosuppressants	*methotrexate*	Trexall, others
Neuropathic pain		
Muscle relaxants	*cyclobenzaprine*	Flexeril
Anticonvulsants	*gabapentin*	Neurontin, others
Antimigraine agents		
Ergotamines	*dihydroergotamine*	Migranal
Triptans	*sumatriptan*	Imitrex

This list is not exhaustive, but rather contains drugs commonly encountered in the athletic training setting. Always consult up-to-date information, confirm with a pharmacist, or discuss the use of therapeutic medications with the prescriber of the medication.

around a single joint is referred to as *monoarticular pain*,[46] which can result from **synovitis**, injury, or OA. Polyarticular pain may be caused by systemic conditions such as inflammation, which can result from bone infection, gout (crystal-induced arthritis), or systemic inflammatory disorders such as rheumatoid arthritis.[46]

Rheumatic diseases are systemic autoimmune conditions causing musculoskeletal disease that occur when the immune system attacks the joints, muscles, and bones, which in turn causes pain, inflammation, stiffness, and deformity. A myriad of diseases and disorders exist that affect the musculoskeletal system; however, this chapter focuses on the pharmacological management of the systemic or inflammatory causes of joint and musculotendinous pain that ATs most commonly encounter.

Acute Infectious (Septic) Arthritis and Osteomyelitis

Acute infectious (or **septic**) **arthritis** is a joint infection that evolves over hours or days. Septic arthritis is an emergency that may lead to disability or death. *Methicillin*-resistant *Staphylococcus aureus* (MRSA) has become a major cause of septic arthritis.[33,34] Symptoms include rapid onset of pain, effusion, and restriction of both active and passive range of motion—usually within a single joint—and require prompt referral to a physician.[36] Osteomyelitis is inflammation and destruction of bone caused by bacteria, mycobacteria, or fungi (figure 15.1). Trauma, ischemia, and foreign bodies can predispose a patient to osteomyelitis. Contiguous spread from adjacent infected tissue or open wounds (from contaminated open fractures or bone surgery) causes about 80% of osteomyelitis; it is often polymicrobial. *Staphylococcus aureus* (including both *methicillin*-sensitive and *methicillin*-resistant strains) is present in ≥50% of patients. Although osteomyelitis is an uncommon cause of joint pain, ATs should suspect the condition in patients with localized peripheral bone pain, fever, and malaise or tenderness, particularly for those who have recently had **bacteremia**.[35] Similarly, prosthetic joints (e.g., joint replacements) are also at risk of acute and chronic infection, which can cause sepsis, morbidity, or mortality.

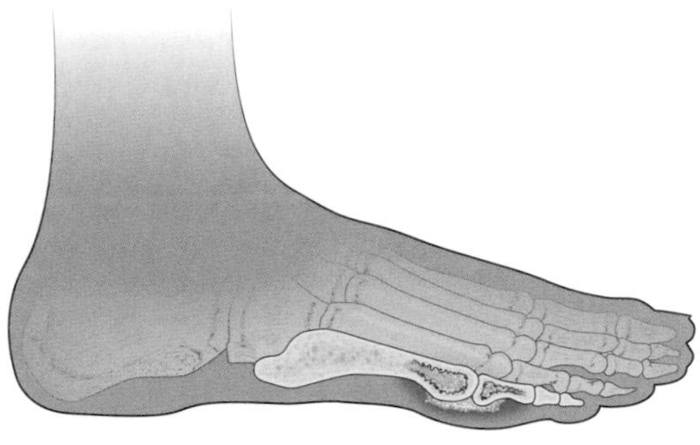

FIGURE 15.1 Osteomyelitis.

Drugs for Treating Acute Infectious Arthritis and Osteomyelitis

Prompt management by the appropriate health care provider (HCP) includes drainage and intravenous

(IV) antibiotics; sometimes operative joint **lavage** may be required to minimize permanent joint damage and prevent sepsis and death. Septic arthritis treated with antibiotic courses of 3 to 4 weeks are usually adequate for uncomplicated bacterial arthritis.[34] Severe septic arthritis is usually treated with IV antibiotics that target Gram-positive organisms (e.g., *vancomycin, cefazolin, nafcillin, oxacillin*). In some patients, a Gram-negative organism grows from the synovial fluid; this condition would be treated with a cephalosporin antibiotic (e.g., *ceftriaxone, ceftazidime, cefotaxime, cefepime*). For osteomyelitis arising from a contiguous soft tissue, treatment involves **debridement** and IV antibiotics that are effective against anaerobic organisms in addition to Gram-positive and Gram-negative aerobes. In these cases, IV *ampicillin* and *sulbactam* (Unasyn) may be used to control infection, and *vancomycin* twice daily may be added when infection is severe or MRSA is prevalent. Antibiotics must be administered parenterally for 4 to 8 weeks and tailored to results of appropriate cultures.[1,35]

Crystal-Induced Arthritis (Gout)

Gout is a crystal-induced arthritic disorder caused by **hyperuricemia** (serum urate >6.8 mg/dL) that results in the precipitation of monosodium urate crystals in and around joints, most often causing recurrent acute or chronic arthritis. The initial attack (flare) of gout is usually monoarticular and often involves the first metatarsophalangeal joint (figure 15.2). Symptoms of gout include acute or severe pain, tenderness, warmth, redness, and swelling. Diagnosis requires identification of crystals in synovial fluid.[12]

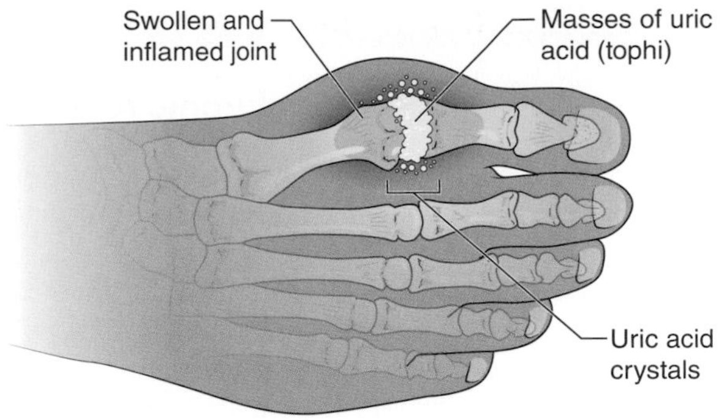

FIGURE 15.2 Inflamed first metatarsophalangeal joint in gout.

Drugs for Treating Gout

Treatment of acute gout attacks with nonsteroidal anti-inflammatory drug (NSAIDs) or *colchicine* (Colcrys) is effective and generally well tolerated. However, both NSAIDs and *colchicine* can cause GI upset and bleeding. Virtually any NSAID used in anti-inflammatory (high) doses is effective and likely to exert an analgesic effect in a few hours. To prevent relapse, treatment should be continued for several days after the pain and signs of inflammation have resolved. Supplementary analgesics, rest, ice application, and splinting of the inflamed joint may be helpful.[9,11]

Osteoarthritis

Osteoarthritis (also called *degenerative joint disease, osteoarthrosis*, or *hypertrophic osteoarthritis*) is a chronic arthropathy characterized by disruption and potential loss of joint cartilage along with other joint changes (figure 15.3), including bone hypertrophy (osteophyte formation). As OA progresses,

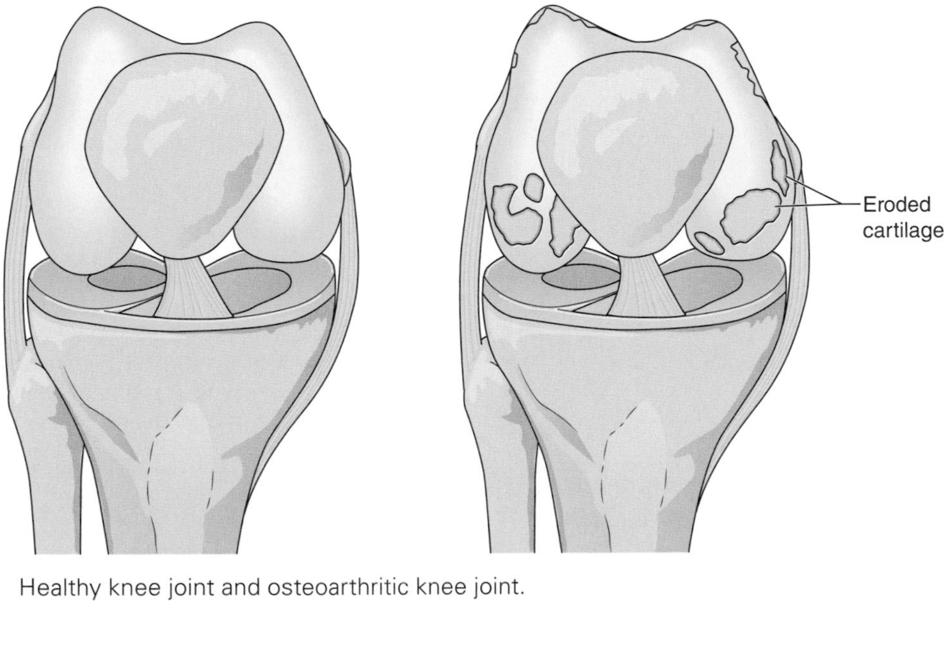

FIGURE 15.3 Healthy knee joint and osteoarthritic knee joint.

Evidence in Pharmacology

Hyaluronic Acid Injections for Knee Arthritis

Hyaluronic acid (HA) is an endogenous component of synovial fluid that decreases in osteoarthritis conditions. Theoretically, HA enhances lubrication of the inflamed joint in patients with OA. Despite equivocal results in clinical studies, general protocols involve weekly injections of this supplement directly into the joint over 3 consecutive weeks. A review of patient-rated outcome scales of patients who were administered an injection of *sodium hyaluronate* and derivatives (Supartz FX) indicated moderate improvement of knee function, pain, and stiffness after 2 injections rather than 3 injections.[14] This evidence was not deemed clinically significant, and the efficacy of HA use is considered inconclusive. The evolution of HA products has resulted in higher doses (and prices) with little or no increase in efficacy. Other single-dose regimens are available, and the average course of therapy costs >$1,000 USD.

joint motion becomes restricted and tenderness and crepitus or grating sensations develop. Tenderness on palpation and pain on passive motion are relatively late signs, and muscle spasm and contracture may add to the joint pain.[19]

Drugs for Treating Osteoarthritis

OA treatment goals are relieving pain, maintaining joint flexibility, and optimizing joint and overall function. As an adjunct to the rehabilitation program, pharmacological intervention may be considered.[19] In general, pharmacologic therapy depends on the joints affected, but the recommended first-line agents are topical analgesics or *acetaminophen*. If unsuccessful, additional pharmacologic interventions can be recommended for the initial management of patients with OA. Chapter 9 details drug interventions and common supplements for OA, such as NSAIDs and analgesics. Additional pharmacologic options are described in table 15.1.

Rheumatoid Arthritis

Rheumatoid arthritis (RA) is a chronic systemic autoimmune disease that primarily involves inflammation of the synovial membrane, which becomes inflamed and thickened. Next, fluid builds up and joints erode and degrade, causing pain, swelling, and deformity (figure 15.4). Although RA involves auto-

TABLE 15.1 Pharmacologic Interventions Recommended for Management of Patients With OA

Agent	Example	Clinical application
Muscle relaxants	*cyclobenzaprine* (Flexeril)	Usually prescribed in low doses. May relieve pain that arises from muscles strained by attempting to support OA joints; however, it may cause more adverse effects than relief.
Cartilage supplement injection	*sodium hyaluronate* and derivatives injection (Supartz, Euflexxa, others)	*Hyaluronic acid* formulations can be injected into the joint and may provide some pain relief in some patients for prolonged periods of time. The treatment is a series of 1-5 weekly injections but should not be used more often than every 6 mo. Efficacy in patients with X-ray evidence of severe OA is absent or limited; in some patients, local injection can cause an acute severe inflammatory synovitis. Studies have shown that these agents have a strong placebo effect.
Supplements*	*glucosamine* (Genicin, OptiFlex-G) *chondroitin* (OptiFlex-C)	Oral 1,500 mg once daily has been suggested to relieve pain and slow joint deterioration; chondroitin sulfate 1,200 mg once daily has also been suggested for pain relief. Studies to date have shown mixed efficacy in terms of pain relief and no strong effect on preservation of cartilage.

*No regulated manufacturing standards are in place for many herbal compounds, and some marketed supplements have been found to be contaminated with toxic metals or other drugs. Herbal or health supplements should be purchased from a reliable source to minimize the risk of contamination.

Based on Bobacz (2013); Harvard Health Publications (2019); Hochberg et al. (2012); McAlindon et al. (2014); National Collaborating Centre for Chronic Conditions (2008).

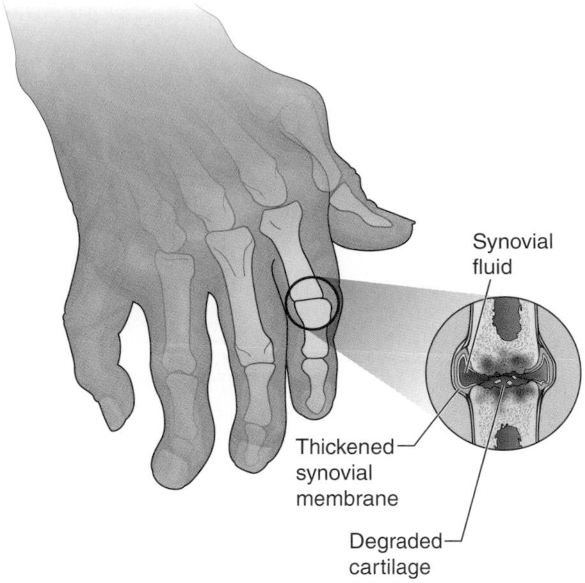

FIGURE 15.4 Rheumatoid arthritis.

immune reactions, the precise cause is unknown; many factors may contribute to it. Characteristically, peripheral joints (e.g., wrists, metacarpophalangeal joints) are symmetrically inflamed, leading to progressive destruction of articular structures, usually accompanied by systemic symptoms.[20]

Drugs for Treating Rheumatoid Arthritis

Treatment of RA involves a balance of rest and exercise, adequate nutrition, physical measures, drugs, and sometimes surgery. The goal is to reduce inflammation as a means of preventing erosions, progressive deformity, and loss of joint function. Almost all patients are treated early and primarily with drugs that modify disease activity. **Disease-modifying antirheumatic drugs (DMARDs)** are used to treat RA. The traditional DMARD is the immunosuppressive drug *methotrexate* (Trexall, Rheumatrex) administered 7.5 mg orally (PO) once a week (with folic acid 1 mg PO once daily).[40] NSAIDs are of some help for the pain of RA, but they do not prevent erosions or disease progression and may increase cardiovascular risk; thus, they should be used only as adjunctive therapy. Low-dose systemic corticosteroids (*prednisone* <10 mg once daily) may be added to control severe polyarticular symptoms, usually with the objective of replacement with a DMARD. Intra-articular depot corticosteroids can control severe symptoms, but with chronic use, they may have adverse metabolic effects, even in low doses. Combination therapy with a DMARD and a biologic may be used in patients if initial DMARD therapy fails.

Musculotendinous Pain

The most common cause of periarticular pain is injury, including overuse pain relating to the musculotendinous structures. Common musculotendinous disorders include bursitis, tendinitis, epicondylitis (e.g., lateral epicondylitis), fasciitis, and tenosynovitis. Periarticular infection is less common. Pain primarily occurs with active joint movement; minimal pain occurs during passive movement and joint compression. Point tenderness and sometimes swelling or erythema are found over the bursa, tendon insertion site, or other periarticular structure (e.g., fascia). In cases of tendinitis, there is inflammation of a tendon, often developing after degeneration (tendinopathy). Tenosynovitis involves tendinitis with inflammation of the tendon sheath lining. Symptoms usually include pain with motion and tenderness with palpation. Chronic deterioration or inflammation of the tendon or tendon sheath can cause scars that restrict motion. Diagnosis is clinical and is sometimes supplemented with imaging.[3,5,46]

Drugs for Treating Musculotendinous Pain

Pain is relieved by rest or immobilization (splint or sling) of the tendon, application of heat (usually for chronic inflammation) or cold (usually for acute inflammation), followed by exercise. Analgesics, such as *acetaminophen*, or high-dose NSAIDs are typically administered for 5 to 7 days. However, for pain that persists after a seemingly minor injury, the AT should refer the patient to a sports medicine specialist for evaluation to see if additional or more severe injuries are present. These injuries are treated as appropriate with NSAIDs and sometimes with oral or injectable corticosteroids.[3,5]

RED FLAG

Corticosteroids and Tendon Rupture

Corticosteroids should be injected by a skilled practitioner and only given when necessary. Corticosteroids should not be injected into a tendon because they can delay soft-tissue healing and weaken injured tendons and muscles. Additionally, the frequency of corticosteroid injections should be monitored because too-frequent injections may increase the risk of tissue degeneration and ligament or tendon rupture.

Injecting a sustained-release corticosteroid (e.g., *betamethasone* 6 mg/mL or *methylprednisolone* 20 to 80 mg/mL) in the tendon sheath may help with pain and inflammation. Injection is usually indicated if pain is severe or the problem has been chronic. Specialized clinicians should be careful to not inject the tendon (which can be recognized by marked resistance to injection); doing so may weaken it, increasing risk of rupture. Patients are advised to rest the adjacent joint to reduce the risk of tendon rupture. Infrequently, symptoms can worsen for up to 24 hours after the injection. Additional injections and symptomatic treatment may be required.[3,5]

Neck and Back Pain

Neck pain and back pain are among the most common reasons for acute and chronic musculoskeletal pain (with or without radicular pain). Depending on the underlying cause, neck or back pain may be accompanied by neurologic symptoms. If a nerve root is affected, pain may radiate distally along the distribution of that root (**radiculopathy**), resulting in radicular pain, weakness, numbness, or difficulty controlling specific muscles. Strength, sensation, and reflexes of the area innervated by that root may also be impaired. If the spinal cord is affected, strength, sensation, and reflexes may be impaired at the affected spinal cord level and all levels below (segmental neurologic deficits). Any painful disorder of the spine may also cause reflex tightening (spasm) of paraspinal muscles, which can be excruciating.[26]

Drugs for Treating Neck and Back Pain

In addition to treating and correcting underlying causes of neck and back pain, initial management with nonmedication-based treatments is recommended, and normal activity should be continued as much as the pain allows. Whether the neck and back pain is acute, subacute, or chronic, management is similar and should start with nonpharmacologic measures. These range from massage and mindfulness-based stress reductions to physical rehabilitation. Symptoms will improve in most patients with acute or subacute back pain with time, either with or without treatment. Medication use should be limited to patients who have had an inadequate response to nonpharmacologic therapy, particularly those with chronic lower back pain.[41] However, if these interventions are not sufficiently effective, medications are recommended for the duration that they are helpful.[29,32]

A wide range of medications are used to treat acute and chronic neck and back pain. Some are available over the counter (OTC); others require a physician's prescription. According to guidelines,[41] no evidence supports the use of *acetaminophen* for chronic lower back pain. NSAIDs and skeletal muscle relaxants are now prescribed as pharmacologic agents for acute lower back pain. For chronic lower back pain, NSAIDs are considered to be first-line therapy; however, other options are available based on the patient's history and presentation. In general, the following are the main types of medications used for nonspecific lower back pain:[18,26,29,32,41]

- **Topical creams or sprays**—Counterirritants applied to the skin stimulate cutaneous nerves in the skin to provide feelings of warmth or cold in order to dull the sensation of pain. Topical analgesics reduce inflammation and stimulate blood flow.
- **NSAIDs**—NSAIDs such as OTC *ibuprofen* (Advil, Motrin) or *naproxen* (Aleve, Naprosyn) can relieve pain and inflammation related to lower back pain. Because NSAIDs alter the way the body processes or eliminates other medications, many other drugs should be taken at the same time.
- **Muscle relaxants**—For example, *cyclobenzaprine* (Flexeril) is effective in the management of nonspecific lower back pain, but the adverse effects of such muscle relaxants require that they be used with caution. Muscle relaxants should be restricted to patients with visible and palpable muscle spasm and used for ≤72 hours. Trials are needed that evaluate whether muscle relaxants are more effective than analgesics or NSAIDs.[44]
- **Corticosteroids**—In patients with severe radicular symptoms and lower back pain, some clinicians recommend a course of oral corticosteroids or early referral to a specialist for epidural injection therapy.
- **Antidepressants**—Serotonin and norepinephrine reuptake inhibitors, such as *duloxetine* (Cymbalta), are commonly prescribed for chronic lower back pain. However, their benefit for nonspecific lower back pain is unproven, according to a review of studies assessing their benefit. Limited evidence exists that antidepressants are more effective

than placebo in the management of patients with chronic lower back pain.[43]

- **Opioids**—Because of their potential for addiction, opioids should be used only for a short period of time and under a physician's supervision. Some evidence (very low to moderate quality) exists for short-term efficacy (for both pain and function) of opioids to treat chronic lower back pain compared to placebo.[7] Physicians should exercise extreme caution in prescribing a trial of opioids for long-term pain management due to the potential risks of opioid abuse.[8]

Fibromyalgia

Fibromyalgia (myofascial pain syndrome) is a common nonarticular disorder of unknown cause characterized by generalized aching (sometimes severe), widespread tenderness of muscles or muscle stiffness, fatigue, mental cloudiness, poor sleep, and a variety of other somatic symptoms.[4] Symptoms and signs of fibromyalgia are generalized (figure 15.5); this contrasts with localized soft-tissue pain and tenderness (myofascial pain syndrome), which is often related to overuse or microtrauma. Stiffness and pain frequently begin gradually and diffusely and the pain has an achy quality.[49]

Clinical Application

Challenge of Treating Fibromyalgia

Fibromyalgia, classified as a chronic widespread pain syndrome, is generally treated following the clinical guidelines of the American Pain Society.[8] Patients suffering from fibromyalgia may have concomitant conditions that enhance the brain's response to pain. Pharmacologic intervention complements nonpharmacologic therapies and assists the patient's ability to cope with his symptoms. Antidepressants may be beneficial for the patient with chronic pain or sleep disturbance, whereas traditional analgesics may be less effective. NSAIDs and opioids are essentially ineffective. Pharmacologic treatment of fibromyalgia pain is challenging and requires continued monitoring by the patient's prescriber.

Drugs for Treating Fibromyalgia

Nonpharmacological interventions, such as stretching exercises, aerobic exercises, sufficient sound sleep, local applications of heat, and gentle massage may provide relief. Overall stress management (e.g., deep breathing exercises, meditation, psychologic support, counseling if necessary) is important.

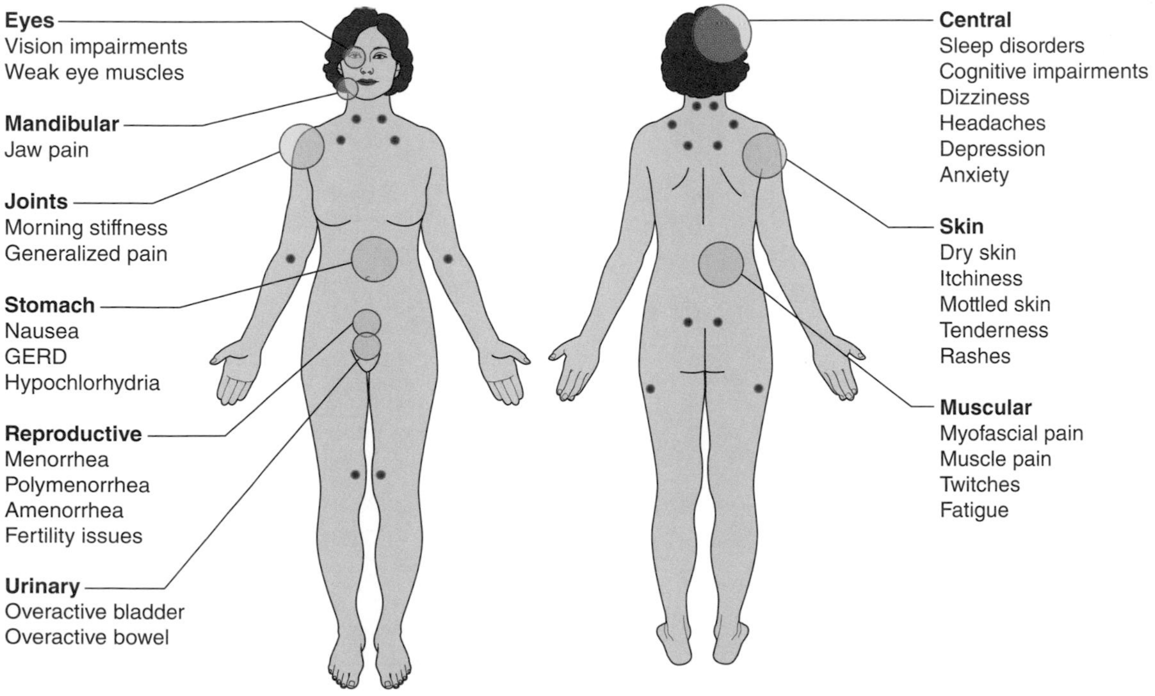

FIGURE 15.5 Signs and symptoms of fibromyalgia.

Improving sleep is critical. Sedating drugs can be taken at night, but only to improve sleep. Low-dose oral tricyclic antidepressants at bedtime such as *amitriptyline* (Elavil)[27] or a muscle relaxant such as *cyclobenzaprine* (Flexeril) may be prescribed to promote deeper sleep and decrease muscle pain. The lowest effective dose should be used to minimize side effects, including drowsiness, dry mouth, and other adverse effects.[27,47] *Acetaminophen* or NSAIDs may help some patients. No evidence exists that opioids such as *oxycodone* have any efficacy in pain in fibromyalgia, so they should be avoided.[13] Occasional injections of 0.5% *bupivacaine* or 1% *lidocaine* 1 to 5 mL are used to treat incapacitating areas of focal tenderness, but such injections should not be relied on as primary treatment because evidence does not support their regular use.[4]

Complex Regional Pain Syndrome

Complex regional pain syndrome (CRPS), formerly called *reflex sympathetic dystrophy* or *causalgia*, is chronic neuropathic pain that follows soft-tissue or bone injury or nerve injury and lasts longer and is more severe than what is expected for the original tissue damage.[30,48] The key symptom of CRPS is prolonged severe pain that may be constant. The pain can be described as a burning or pins and needles sensation or the feeling that someone is squeezing the affected limb. There is often increased sensitivity in the affected area (allodynia), in which normal contact with the skin is experienced as very painful. People with CRPS also experience changes in skin temperature or swelling of the affected limb. The skin on the affected limb may change color, becoming blotchy and blue, purple, pale, or red.[30]

Drugs for Treating Complex Regional Pain Syndrome

In addition to a variety of nonpharmacologic and alternative therapies, some evidence exists that early treatment (i.e., within the first few months of symptoms) might help improve CRPS symptoms. Often, a combination of different treatments, individualized to the specific patient case, are necessary. Medication options include the following:[22]

- **NSAIDs**—If OTC medications are not helpful, opioids might be an option if they are taken in appropriate doses for controlling pain.
- **Antidepressants and anticonvulsants**—Sometimes antidepressants, such as the tricyclic antidepressant *amitriptyline*, and anticonvulsants, such as *gabapentin* (Neurontin), are used to treat pain that originates from a damaged nerve (neuropathic pain).
- **Corticosteroids**—Steroid medications, such as *prednisone*, may reduce inflammation and improve mobility in the affected limb.
- **Sympathetic nerve-blocking medication**—Injection of an anesthetic to block pain fibers in the affected nerves may relieve pain in some people.
- **Anesthetics**—Low doses of IV or intranasal *ketamine* (Ketalar), a strong anesthetic in a medical setting, may substantially alleviate pain. However, despite pain relief, there is generally no improvement in function.

Headache Disorders

Headache is pain in any part of the head. Headache disorders, which are characterized by recurrent headache, are among the most common disorders of the nervous system.[50] Headache is a result of the activation of pain-sensitive structures in or around the brain, skull, face, sinuses, or teeth.[37] Some causes of headache are common; others are important to recognize because they are dangerous, require specific treatment, or both.

RED FLAG

Indications of a Neurological Emergency

Any of the following signs or symptoms may indicate a more serious medical problem and should prompt immediate referral to the emergency department:[24,38]

- An abrupt, severe headache that strikes suddenly like a thunderclap
- Headache with fever, stiff neck, mental confusion, seizures, double vision, weakness, numbness, or trouble speaking
- Headache after a head injury, especially if the headache worsens
- A chronic headache that is worse after coughing, exertion, straining, or a sudden movement
- New headache pain after age 50

Clinical Application

Concussion-Related Headache

Headache is a common symptom following a sport-related concussion. Mild traumatic brain injury can result from a direct hit to the skull or a contrecoup action. Aspirin and NSAIDs have anticoagulant, or blood-thinning, properties. Therefore, these medications should be avoided when managing post-concussion headache out of concern that an intracranial bleed could be exacerbated by the medication. Opioids for post-concussion headache should be avoided because these medications may mask other symptoms or alter the patient's mental state.[2] The safest option for treating a post-concussion headache is *acetaminophen*.[23] This medication, which offers relief from headache pain, has no anticoagulant properties and does not alter the patient's mental status.

A special consideration for athletes is concussion-related headache. Appropriate treatment of concussion-related or other headache disorders requires ATs to recognize the general cause of the headache and refer the patient to an appropriate prescriber. The post-concussion patient should receive treatment with cost-effective medications, simple lifestyle modifications, and patient education. The main classes of drugs for treating non-concussion-related headache disorders include analgesics, antiemetics, specific antimigraine medications, and prophylactic medications.[50]

Migraine Headache

Migraine is an episodic primary headache disorder with symptoms that typically last 4 to 72 hours and may be severe. Pain is often unilateral, throbbing, worse with exertion, and accompanied by symptoms such as nausea and sensitivity to light, sound, or odors. **Auras** occur in about 25% of patients, usually just before but sometimes after the headache. Preventive regimens include lifestyle modifications (e.g., sleeping habits or diet) and drugs.[38]

Drugs for Treating Migraine Headache

Migraine is a common, disabling condition, and many sufferers choose not to or are unable to seek professional help, relying instead on OTC analgesics. Cotherapy with an antiemetic should help to reduce the nausea and vomiting commonly associated with migraine headaches.[17] Medications used to relieve migraine pain work best when taken at the first sign of an oncoming migraine—as soon as the signs and symptoms of a migraine begin.[24] When deciding which medication to prescribe for acute therapy of a migraine attack, prescribers should consider the evidence base for medication, along with potential medication side effects, potential adverse events, patient-specific contraindications to use of a particular medication, and drug–drug interactions.[21] According to a systematic review of the literature,[21] specific combination medications within several classes are considered effective for the acute therapy of migraine. Patients who do not experience adequate relief should try an alternative therapy.[17] Drugs that are effective for treating migraine headache include the following:[17,21,24,31,38]

- **Combination medications**—Medication containing a combination of *caffeine*, *aspirin*, and *acetaminophen* (Excedrin Migraine) may be helpful, but it is usually only useful for mild migraine pain.
- **Oral NSAIDs**—For example, OTC or prescription pain relievers, such as *aspirin* or *ibuprofen* (Advil, Motrin), may help with migraine.
- **Emergency use *ketorolac* (Toradol) injection**—This NSAID is often administered in the emergency department. When taken for too long, the injection might cause medication-overuse headaches and possibly ulcers and bleeding in the gastrointestinal tract. Toradol must be used in a medically supervised setting because it has numerous black box warnings, precautions, and contraindications.[10]
- **Triptans**—Vasoconstrictors, such as *sumatriptan* (Imitrex), are effective for treating migraine because they block pain pathways in the brain. However, they might not be safe for patients at risk of a stroke or heart attack. Triptans are given once and then repeated once if needed according to the maximum daily limit.

- **Dihydroergotamines**—Vasoconstrictors, such as *dihydroergotamine* (Migranal), are most effective when taken shortly after the start of migraine symptoms that tend to last longer than 24 hours. Side effects can include worsening of migraine-related vomiting and nausea. People with coronary artery disease, high blood pressure, or kidney or liver disease or those who are pregnant should avoid *dihydroergotamine*. *Dihydroergotamine* cannot be used concurrently with triptans and has a black box warning that it must not be taken with macrolide antibiotics.
- **Antinausea drugs**—For example, *metoclopramide* (Reglan) can help a migraine with aura that is accompanied by nausea and vomiting.

Tension Headache

Tension headaches may be episodic or chronic. Episodic tension headaches occur <15 days per month; indeed, episodic tension headache is very common. Episodic headaches may last for as little as 30 minutes or as long as several days. They typically start several hours after waking and worsen as the day progresses. They rarely awaken patients from sleep. Chronic tension headaches occur ≥15 days per month. Although they may vary in intensity throughout the day, they are almost always present. Tension headache pain is usually mild to moderate and is often described as viselike. These headaches originate in the occipital or frontal region bilaterally and spread over the entire head. Unlike migraine headaches, tension headaches are not accompanied by nausea and vomiting and are not made worse by physical activity, light, sounds, or smells. Potential triggers for chronic tension headache include sleep disturbances, stress, temporomandibular joint dysfunction, neck pain, and eye strain.[39]

Drugs for Treating Tension Headache

Most patients with episodic tension headache obtain relief with OTC analgesics and do not seek medical attention. For most mild to moderate tension headaches, OTC analgesics can provide relief. Massaging the affected area may help. Although *ibuprofen* 400 mg is one choice for treatment of tension headache, available evidence indicates that this dose is probably not much different from any other treatment.[45] *Acetaminophen* 1,000 mg may relieve headache pain, but the chance of the pain being relieved entirely in 2 hours is low.[42] For chronic tension headache, behavioral and psychologic interventions (e.g., relaxation and stress management techniques) are common and effective, especially when combined with drug treatment.[39]

Summary

Chronic musculoskeletal and neurological conditions can cause long-term pain and disability. A working knowledge of the pathophysiology and medications used to treat these conditions will allow the practicing AT to manage these conditions and improve patient outcomes. This chapter describes conditions commonly encountered in the AT setting and includes a basic overview of the medications used in the treatment of arthralgia and musculotendinous pain as a result of injury. It provides an overview of the drugs used to treat joint pain as a result of bone infection, including acute infectious arthritis and osteomyelitis. It also discusses treatment of gout, osteoarthritis, rheumatoid arthritis, and fibromyalgia. Common causes of chronic musculotendinous pain are treated with a variety of therapeutic interventions, including corticosteroids, while neck and back pain are often treated with muscle relaxants. Finally, this chapter discusses the serious headache disorders of migraine and tension headache, paying special attention to red flag symptoms and concussion-related headache.

Case Studies

Case Study 1

Gordie is a bouncer at a local night spot that is popular with young people. He is well known for his strength and patience. One evening, a group of underage youths tried to enter the club. Gordie stopped them for an identification check. One of them took a swing at Gordie, who responded by punching the youth in the face. Once the situation calmed down, Gordie noticed that his hand was bleeding significantly and went to the local hospital. He was diagnosed with a third metacarpal fracture, and a piece of a tooth was irrigated out of his hand. One week later, Gordie complained of pain at the fracture site and warmth emanating from the area of his wound. He was diagnosed with a bone infection.

Questions for Analysis

1. What is the protocol for a bone infection?
2. What is the correct diagnosis of a bone infection?

Case Study 2

Carl is in his first year as the head athletic trainer at a local community college and was working providing medical services during an early-season soccer game. Kyle, a rookie defensive player, sustained a kick to the head and asked Carl to evaluate him for a possible concussion. During this evaluation, Kyle's mother came to the bench area and strongly recommended that Kyle take the Tylenol with Codeine that she had been prescribed for her own dental pain. The assistant coach also came over and recommended *ibuprofen* because that's what he had always taken when he'd had concussions. Carl expressed his sincere thanks to both the mother and the assistant coach and said his decision was to start Kyle on *acetaminophen*, per the institution's approved concussion protocol.

Questions for Analysis

1. What prompted Carl's decision to administer *acetaminophen*?
2. Regardless of the efficacy of an opioid for this condition, is it appropriate to use someone else's medication?

Drugs Described in This Chapter

Drug class	*generic* (Pronunciation) Trade name	Therapeutic uses	Clinical concerns
Antigout agent	*colchicine* (KOL chi seen) Colcrys, others	FDA-approved drug for treating or preventing gout in adults	Affects the way the body responds to uric acid crystals, thus reducing swelling and pain. Suitable for prophylaxis and treatment of acute gout flares when taken at the first sign of a flare.
Antiarthritic agents	*sodium hyaluronate* solution (hye al yoor ON ate) Euflexxa, others	2.5 mL by intra-articular injection into the knee once weekly for 5 wk	Most side effects are related to local reactions such as injection site pain, swelling, effusion, or redness of the joint. Other side effects include fever and headache.
Antirheumatic agents: immunosuppressant	*methotrexate* (meth oh TREX ate) Trexall, others	Indicated for patients with active RA that is unresponsive to or intolerant of first-line therapy, including full-dose NSAIDs.	This medication is a disease-modifying antirheumatic drug (DMARD) and immunosuppressant agent. *Methotrexate* is the preferred initial DMARD for most early or established RA patients and for moderate to severe systemic lupus erythematosus.
Antirheumatic agents: antimalarials	*hydroxychloroquine* (hye drox ee KLOR oh kwin) Plaquenil	Indicated for all patients with systemic disease. Dividing doses, taking with food, and, if appropriate, gradually escalating the dose may improve tolerability.	Interferes with function within sensitive malarial parasites. For treatment of rheumatic disease, the patient may require several weeks to respond. GI upset (nausea, vomiting, diarrhea) is a common adverse effect.

(continued)

Drugs Described in This Chapter *(continued)*

Drug class	*generic* (Pronunciation) Trade name	Therapeutic uses	Clinical concerns
Muscle relaxants	*cyclobenzaprine* (sye kloe BEN za preen) Flexeril	For fibromyalgia and muscle spasm: As an adjunct to rest and physical therapy for short-term (2 to 3 wk) relief of muscle spasm associated with acute, painful musculoskeletal conditions. Usual: 15 mg/d; some patients may require up to 30 mg/d.	Pharmacologically related to tricyclic antidepressants; reduces tonic somatic motor activity, influencing both alpha and gamma motor neurons. Do not use longer than 3 wk. Common side effects are blurred vision, dizziness, drowsiness or lightheadedness, and dry mouth.
Neuropathic pain, anticonvulsants	*gabapentin* (GA ba PEN tin) Neurontin	Safe and effective for treatment of neuropathic pain, including complex regional pain syndrome. For patients who do not respond to or tolerate preferred agents, this is an alternate agent for the pain and sleep disturbances associated with fibromyalgia.	Common side effects are ataxia, dizziness, drowsiness, fatigue, fever, nystagmus disorder, sedated state, and viral infection.
Antimigraine agents	*dihydroergotamine* (dye HYE droe er GOT a meen) Migranal	Injection IM, SQ: 1 mg at first sign of headache; repeat hourly to a maximum dose of 3 mg/d Intranasal: 1 spray (0.5 mg) into each nostril; repeat after 15 min for a total of 4 sprays (2 mg). When migraine attack is complicated by vomiting or severe nausea, use of a nonoral preparation is recommended, since oral agents may be ineffective.	Causes vasoconstriction or inhibition of proinflammatory neuropeptide release. Most effective when taken shortly after the start of migraine symptoms that tend to last longer than 24 hr. Common side effects are nausea and vomiting or application site reaction for oral medication and nausea, vomiting, and altered sense of smell for nasal spray. See the black box warning on the nasal solution.
	sumatriptan (SOO ma TRIP tan) Imitrex	Oral: Take 50-100 mg once; may repeat once after ≥2 hr. Nasal spray: 10 mg once in 1 nostril Subcutaneous injection: 6 mg once. If initial dose was partially effective or headache recurs, may repeat the dose once after ≥1 hr. Triptans are given once, then repeated if needed, but all have maximum daily limits.	Causes vasoconstriction and reduces the neurogenic inflammation associated with migraine. However, this medication might not be safe for patients at risk of a stroke or heart attack. It should not be used for common tension headache or a headache that causes loss of movement on 1 side of the body. Common side effects are dizziness, injection site reaction, vertigo, nausea and vomiting, flushing sensation, tingling sensation, and unpleasant taste.

Black box warning: Risk exists for the following: medication errors; addiction, abuse, and misuse; risk evaluation and mitigation strategy (REMS); life-threatening respiratory depression; accidental ingestion; neonatal opioid withdrawal syndrome; cytochrome P450 3a4 interaction; problems from concomitant use with benzodiazepines or other CNS depressants; and monoamine oxidase inhibitors (MAOIs) interactions.

16

Drugs for Treating Dermatological Conditions

OBJECTIVES

After reading this chapter, you will be able to do the following:

- Describe basic principles of topical dermatological pharmacology
- Identify medications for treating common skin diseases in athletes
- Apply current recommendations about therapeutic medications used in the management of common skin diseases in athletes
- Distinguish between medications used to treat bacterial, viral, and fungal skin infections
- Summarize antipruritic agents used to treat atopy and allergic skin reactions
- Recognize signs and symptoms of a severe skin reaction or infection and know when to promptly refer a patient to a higher-level care provider

Select Drugs Mentioned in This Chapter

Drug class	Generic name	Trade name
Antibiotics: topical	*neomycin*, *bacitracin*, and *polymyxin B*	Triple Antibiotic, Neosporin
Antibiotics: systemic	*clindamycin*	Cleocin
Antipruritics: topical corticosteroids	*hydrocortisone topical*	Cortaid, Cortizone-5, others
Antipruritics: local anesthetic	*pramoxine topical*	Gold Bond, Blistex
Antipruritics: nonsedating antihistamines	*loratadine*	Claritin
Antipruritics: sedating antihistamines	*diphenhydramine*	Benadryl

This list is not exhaustive, but rather contains drugs commonly encountered in the athletic training setting. Always consult up-to-date information, confirm with a pharmacist, or discuss the use of therapeutic medications with the prescriber of the medication.

People involved in athletic activities that involve being with others in close quarters and promote skin-to-skin and bodily secretion contact (e.g., football, wrestling, rugby) can be particularly vulnerable to contracting skin diseases. The athletic trainer (AT) should have an understanding of basic etiology, clinical features, and swift management of common skin diseases, which is essential in preventing the spread of common and serious skin infections.[32] Inflammatory conditions of the skin are often characterized by itching, which can be intense, and lesions, which can be recurrent. Although most skin conditions are benign and self-limiting, some skin infections (e.g., *Methicillin*-resistant *Staphylococcus aureus*, or MRSA) can lead to septic shock, which can be life threatening. This chapter outlines the current recommendations and clinical guidelines from the National Athletic Trainers' Association (NATA)[32,40] and the American Academy of Dermatology[19] to provide comprehensive recommendations for the AT in identifying and treating microbial, autoimmune, and other skin diseases in athletes at all levels.[32] Further, the AT must be able to educate athletic program staff and athletes about minimizing disease transmission, preventing the spread of infectious agents, and improving the recognition and management of common skin conditions. The AT is in the unique position of monitoring the healing process, often on a daily basis, and must be able to recognize the signs and symptoms of a severe skin reaction or infection and promptly refer the patient to a higher-level care provider.

Protective Barriers of the Skin

Epidermal barriers protect the body against various physical, chemical, and microbial assaults from the outside and keep water and solutes from the inside from leaking out. Cells are continuously turned over to renew the epidermis and its barriers. The skin is an efficient physicochemical, microbial, and immunological barrier that exerts several protective functions, many of which are in the epidermis. Skin barrier biology and immune mechanisms closely interact. The 2 major pathophysiological processes involve the following:[4,37]

- Injury or infection that disrupts the antimicrobial properties of the skin
- Autoimmune responses to antigens and the anti-inflammatory properties of the skin

Antimicrobial Properties of the Skin

Controlling the microbiota that the skin encounters is important for preventing bacterial and fungal infections. The skin is equipped with immunologic barriers to the innate and acquired immune systems. Antimicrobial proteins are a diverse group of proteins that form a chemical barrier against microorganisms on the surface of the epidermis.[27] Continuous turnover of epidermal cells by **desquamation** (daily detachment of dead skin cells) prohibits colonization of microorganisms on the skin. The physical properties of the skin's surface itself—that is, low carbohydrate and water content and weakly acidic pH (a pH of 5.6 to 6.4)—prevent bacterial growth. Antimicrobial proteins of the epidermis show broad antibacterial activity against both Gram-positive and Gram-negative bacteria; some even show antifungal or antiviral activity.[27]

Anti-Inflammatory Properties of the Skin

Epidermal barrier disruptions and skin inflammation are mutually reinforcing processes. Cutaneous inflammation and immune dysregulation affect epidermal structure and function. Poor epidermal barrier function is related to defects of structural proteins, inherited factors, and environmental exposures, such as to soaps, detergents, and exogenous proteases (e.g., from mite allergens); repetitive scratching might also impair various aspects of barrier function.[37]

Principles of Topical Dermatological Pharmacology

Dermatological therapy can include oral or systemic medications, such as antimicrobials, but topical agents are often helpful in treatment of skin disorders. The dosage form of the medication is the therapeutical vehicle; it influences the effectiveness of a treatment and may itself cause adverse effects (e.g., contact or irritant dermatitis). Generally, aqueous and alcohol-based preparations are drying because the liquid evaporates; they are used in acute inflammatory conditions. Oil-based (**petrolatum**) preparations are moisturizing and are preferred for chronic inflammation. Many dosage forms exist as over-the-counter (OTC) options for the AT to administer and as prescription medication for the provider to use as indicated. Elements to factor into the decision of which dosage form to select include location of application, cosmetic effects, and convenience (table 16.1).[5,26,37]

Dressings Used in Dermatological Pharmacology

Dressings protect open lesions, facilitate healing, increase drug absorption, and protect the patient's clothing. Examples of dressings used with dermatological therapy are provided in table 16.2.[5,26,37]

TABLE 16.1 Common Topical Pharmaceutical Vehicles and Dosage Forms

Dosage form	Description
Baths and soaks	Useful when therapy must be applied to large areas, such as with extensive contact dermatitis or atopic dermatitis.
Combination vehicles	These usually contain oil and water, but may also contain propylene or polyethylene glycol.
Creams	These are semisolid emulsions of oil and water. They are used for moisturizing and cooling and when exudation is present. They vanish when rubbed into skin.
Emollients	These water-based emulsions are easily applied to hairy skin. Lotions cool and dry acute inflammatory and exudative lesions, such as contact dermatitis, tinea pedis, and tinea cruris.
Foams	These alcohol- or emollient-based aerosolized preparations tend to be rapidly absorbed and may be favored in hair-bearing areas of the body.
Gels	Ingredients are suspended in a solvent that is thickened with polymers. Gels are often more effective for controlled release of topical agents. They are often used in treating acne, rosacea, and psoriasis of the scalp.
Ointments	These petrolatum- or oil-based products contain little, if any, water. Ointments are optimal lubricants and increase drug penetration because of their occlusive nature; a given concentration of drug is typically more potent in an ointment. Ointments are less irritating than creams for erosions or ulcers. They are usually best applied after bathing or dampening the skin with water.
Powders	May be mixed with active agents (e.g., antifungals) to deliver therapy. Prescribed for lesions in moist or intertriginous areas.
Solutions	Ingredients are dissolved in a solvent, usually ethyl alcohol, propylene glycol, polyethylene glycol, or water. Solutions are convenient to apply (especially to the scalp for disorders such as psoriasis or seborrhea), but tend to be drying.

Clinical Application

Removing Keloids

A **keloid** is a hypertrophic scar or a raised overgrowth of a scar site that differs from mature scars in areas such as surgical incisions.[24] Keloids are more common in African Americans and occur more frequently in patients between the ages of 10 and 30 years old.[24] Treatment includes invasive and noninvasive options. Invasive treatment options, such as intralesional injections of *triamcinolone* or *verapamil*, have been successful in reducing keloids. Noninvasive topical silicone gel is a safe, effective treatment that reduces itching and discomfort. An ultra-thin layer of silicone gel is self-drying and works over a 24-hour daily span; this product may be applied by an AT. The gel increases hydration of the stratum corneum, protects the scar tissue from bacterial infection, and helps restore balance between scar tissue formation and breakdown.[34]

TABLE 16.2 Common Dressings and Indications for Use

Dressing	Description	Indication
Gauze dressings and nonadherent pads	The most common nonocclusive dressings, these maximally allow air to reach the wound, which is at times preferred in healing, and the lesion to dry. Examples include sterile woven and nonwoven gauze and Curad or Telfa nonadherent dressings.	Use for abrasions, avulsions, blisters, incisions, lacerations, or punctures.
Nonocclusive dressings: • Wet to dry • Wet to moist	Dressings wetted with solution, usually saline, are used to help cleanse and debride thickened or crusted lesions. Examples include gauze, natural or synthetic bandages, cotton, rayon, polyester, and wool dressings used to prevent wounds from becoming contaminated.	Wet-to-dry dressings are applied wet and removed after the solution has evaporated (i.e., wet to dry), with materials from the skin adhering to the dried dressing. Wet-to-moist **debridement** can be achieved with woven gauze with superficial to full-thickness abrasions, avulsions, blisters, incisions, and lacerations.
Occlusive film dressings	Transparent films such as polyethylene (plastic household wrap) or flexible, transparent, semipermeable dressings that seal off a wound or increase the absorption and effectiveness of topical therapy. Examples include Nexcare Tegaderm waterproof transparent dressing, Bioclusive, and Polyskin.	Can be applied over topical corticosteroids to increase absorption; sometimes used to treat psoriasis, atopic dermatitis, and other skin lesions. Also used to protect and help heal open wounds, such as burns; special silicone dressings are sometimes used for keloids.[26]
Foams	Use a propellant or air-spray foam pump to generate a liquid that forms a continuous film as a consequence of the solvent's evaporation on the skin. Examples include Allevyn, PolyMem, and Tegaderm foams.	Can be used for superficial- to partial-thickness abrasions, avulsions, blisters, incisions, lacerations, and punctures.
Hydrocolloid and hydrogel dressings	Draw out fluid from the skin to form a gel; can be applied with a gauze cover. Examples include AquaHeal, Tegaderm, and Duoderm.	Used in patients with cutaneous ulceration or other lesions. Can also be used for full-thickness traumatic and postoperative incisions.
Dermal adhesives	Adhesives include sticky strips of tape used to pull together the edges of minor skin wounds and skin glue for topical application to hold closed easily approximated skin edges of wounds from surgical incisions. Example products include Steri-Strips, Leukostrips, and Dermabond skin glue.	Used for partial- to full-thickness lacerations and traumatic and postoperative incisions in areas of low skin tension.

Topical Agents: Cleansing, Moisturizing, and Drying

ATs commonly use dermatological cleansing agents, including soaps, detergents, and solvents. Soap is the most popular cleanser, but synthetic detergents are also used. However, acutely irritated, weeping, or oozing lesions are most comfortably cleansed with water or **isotonic saline**.[5,26] Normal saline and potable tap water should be used as cleansing agents with superficial- to full-thickness abrasions, incisions, and lacerations. Topical organic solvents (e.g., acetone, petroleum products, propylene glycol) can be drying and irritating and may cause allergic contact dermatitis.[5,26]

Moisturizers (**emollients**) restore water and oils to the skin and help maintain skin hydration. These topical agents typically contain glycerin, mineral oil, or petrolatum and are available as lotions, creams, ointments, and bath oils. Stronger moisturizers contain 2% to 47% urea, 5% to 12% lactic acid, and 10% glycolic acid (higher concentrations of glycolic acid are used as **keratinolytics**). Moisturizers are most effective when applied to already moistened skin (i.e., after a bath or shower). Cold creams are moisturizing OTC emulsions of fats (e.g., beeswax) and water.[26] Moisturizing agents are used to treat a variety of dry skin conditions and can serve as a vehicle for applying medications over areas of skin.

Drying agents decrease excessive moisture in **intertriginous areas** (e.g., between the toes; between folds of skin) that can cause irritation and **maceration**. Powders dry macerated skin and reduce friction by absorbing moisture. Cornstarch and talc are most often used. Although talc is more effective, it may cause granulomas if inhaled and is no longer used in baby powders. Cornstarch may promote fungal growth. Aluminum chloride solutions are another type of drying agent (often useful in **hyperhidrosis**). Superabsorbent powders (i.e., extremely absorbent powders) are occasionally required to dry very moist areas (e.g., to treat **intertrigo**).[26] Medicated powders containing drugs such as *miconazole*, *clotrimazole*, *tolnaftate*, *undecylenic acid*, and *nystatin* are helpful for treating or preventing fungal infections.

Bacterial Skin and Soft Tissue Infections

Skin and soft tissue infections (SSTIs) are among the most common bacterial infections, posing considerable diagnostic and therapeutic challenges. Humans are natural hosts for many bacterial species that colonize the skin as normal flora. Predisposing factors to infection include minor trauma, preexisting skin disease, poor hygiene, and depressed immune system of the host.[14,40] The primary pathogens in SSTI are *Streptococcus* and *Staphylococcus* species, including *methicillin*-resistant *Staphylococcus aureus* (MRSA).[14] The more common bacterial SSTIs found in the athletic training setting are as follows:

- *Methicillin*-resistant *Staphylococcus aureus* infection
- Nonpurulent skin and soft tissue infections: impetigo and ecthyma (further discussed in the section Nonpurulent Skin Infections: Impetigo and Ecthyma)
- Purulent skin and soft tissue infections: folliculitis, furuncles, carbuncles
- Cutaneous abscesses

The diagnosis of bacterial infections is primarily based on the history and characteristic appearance of the lesions. Specimens for culture and antimicrobial susceptibility should be obtained from any questionable lesions. Guidelines[35] for the diagnosis and management of bacterial skin and soft tissue infections are that a skin condition is considered severe if patients have signs of systemic toxicity and **bacteremia** or **systemic inflammatory response syndrome (SIRS)**. Development of hypotension or GI symptoms (abdominal pain, nausea, vomiting, diarrhea) suggests sepsis or septic shock. **Septic shock** develops in 25% to 40% of patients with significant bacteremia. Sustained bacteremia may cause metastatic focal infection or sepsis.[8] ATs should be able to recognize bacterial infections and refer the athlete to a knowledgeable sports medicine practitioner who can skillfully perform incision and drainage when necessary and prescribe oral antibiotics.[40]

RED FLAG

Signs of Systemic Toxicity

Should a patient present with these signs and symptoms, an immediate referral for bacteremia or SIRS is indicated, requiring parenteral (IV) antibiotic therapy:[8,13,14,30,35]

- Body temperature >38°C or <36°C
- Tachypnea (>24 breaths per minute)
- Tachycardia (>90 beats per minute)
- Delirium
- Extensive soft tissue involvement
- Rapid progression of clinical manifestations or symptoms after 48 to 72 hours of oral therapy
- Proximity of soft tissue infection to an indwelling device (i.e., surgical hardware) if it originates on the skin directly overlying the site

All bacterial infections must be carefully monitored; suspicious lesions should be cultured and tested for antimicrobial sensitivity before the athlete returns to competition.

TABLE 16.3 Topical Antibiotic Agents Used to Prevent or Treat Skin Infections

Drug or agent	Usual regimen	Prescription or OTC
Combination of *neomycin*, *bacitracin*, and *polymyxin B* (Triple Antibiotic, Neosporin)	3 dose/d for 1 wk	OTC
clindamycin 1% to 2% (Cleocin)	1-2 dose/d	Prescribed as needed
mupirocin 2% ointment (Bactroban)	3 dose/d for 10 d	Prescription only
retapamulin 1% ointment (Altabax)	2 dose/d for 5 d	Prescription only

Systemic antibiotic use is determined on a case-by-case basis, based on culture and sensitivity of lesion, until information is available on antibiotic susceptibilities in the local community.

Data from Keri (2019); Zinder et al. (2010).

Topical Antibiotic Agents

Topical antimicrobial agents may effectively reduce rates of infection with acute skin trauma (table 16.3).[5] Topical antibiotics such as *clindamycin* (Cleocin) are used as primary or adjunctive treatment for **acne vulgaris** in patients who do not warrant or tolerate oral antibiotics. *Mupirocin* (Bactroban) has excellent Gram-positive (mainly *Staphylococcus aureus* and *streptococci*) coverage and can be used to treat **impetigo** when deep tissues are not affected (further discussed in the section Nonpurulent Skin Infections: Impetigo and Ecthyma). OTC topical antibiotics such as *bacitracin* and *polymyxin B* have been replaced by topical petrolatum for postoperative care of a skin biopsy site and to prevent infection in scrapes, minor burns, and **excoriations**.[26] According to the NATA position statement *Management of Acute Skin Trauma*,[5] topical antibiotic agents such as the combination of *neomycin*, *bacitracin*, and *polymyxin B* (Neosporin) and *mupirocin* 2% ointment (Bactroban) may effectively reduce rates of infection with acute skin trauma. Topical antimicrobials decrease infection rates among superficial- and partial-thickness abrasions, lacerations, punctures, and sutured lacerations compared to topical preparations without an antibiotic. There were no differences in rates of infection among triple antibiotic, *mupirocin*, *bacitracin zinc* ointment, and *povidone-iodine* cream.[36] However, the period of use should be limited to help prevent emergence of resistant bacterial strains, hypersensitivity reactions, and adverse effects on wound healing.[5]

Methicillin-Resistant *Staphylococcus Aureus* Infection

Methicillin-resistant *Staphylococcus aureus*, also called staph infection, is caused by a bacterial strain that has acquired a specific gene that makes it resistant to antibiotic treatment with common penicillin and other drugs in the extended-spectrum penicillin family. MRSA infection initially presents as standard bacterial infection and is commonly confused with spider bites. Reports of spider bites (figure 16.1) should be considered a possible sign for community-associated MRSA.[40] Particularly because MRSA can be resistant to multiple antibiotics, recommended antibiotics for bacterial skin and soft tissue infections depend largely on the local prevalence and resistance patterns of MRSA.[14,40]

ATs must understand the proper recognition, disposition, and management of MRSA infections. The physician, who should maintain close contact with the AT in such cases, should abide by the evolving guidelines for the management of these infections. Individual treatment should be guided by local susceptibility data because prevalence of resistance to antimicrobial agents varies geographically and is likely to change over time.[40] The Centers for Disease Control and Prevention (CDC) website provides current, up-to-date information on the MRSA strains presenting in emergency departments.

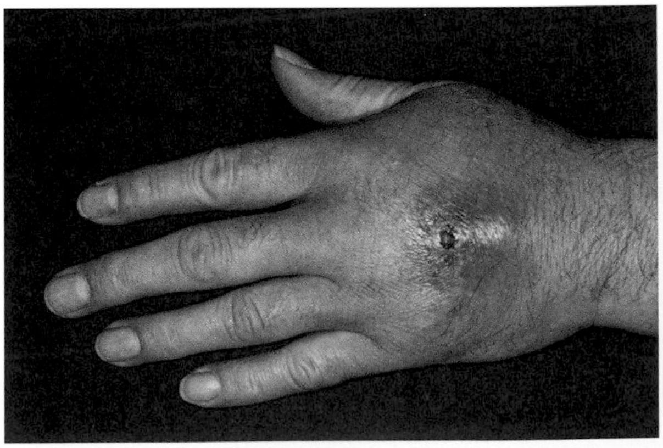

Scott Camazine/Science Source

FIGURE 16.1 MRSA infection.

Drugs for Treating MRSA Infection

Given the potential for rapid development of resistance, some antimicrobial agents are discouraged for the treatment of MRSA. Specifically, these agents include the fluoroquinolones (i.e., *ciprofloxacin*) and the macrolides and azalides (*erythromycin*, *clarithromycin*, and *azithromycin*).[40] Treatment of MRSA bacteremia consists of prompt source control (such as removal of an implicated prosthetic and drainage of **purulent** collections, if present) and prompt initiation of appropriate antimicrobial therapy.[31]

For treatment of MRSA in outpatients with SSTI, oral antibiotic options should include the following prescription antibiotics:[30]

- *Clindamycin* (Cleocin)
- *Trimethoprim* + *sulfamethoxazole* (Bactrim, Septra)
- A tetracycline such as *doxycycline* (Vibramycin) or *minocycline* (Minocin)
- *Linezolid* (Zyvox)

Due to the communicable nature of bacterial infections, the AT must not allow patients with active lesions to participate in sports, even when the lesions are covered. The AT is often required to monitor affected athletes, who must complete a course of directed antibiotic therapy for ≥72 hours.[32,40]

Nonpurulent Skin Infections: Impetigo and Ecthyma

Impetigo is a common and contagious superficial bacterial infection characterized by thin-walled sacs of fluid that rupture into a honey-colored crust, often occurring on the face.[35] Impetigo is caused by *streptococci*, *staphylococci*, or both.[15,35] It usually occurs in warm, humid conditions and is easily spread among people who are in close contact.[40] Ecthyma is an ulcerative form of impetigo.[15,35] The painful fluid- or pus-filled sores cause redness of the skin, usually on the arms and legs, and may become ulcers that penetrate deeper into the dermis. Ecthyma may be accompanied by swollen lymph nodes in the affected area.[15,35,40] Impetigo and ecthyma cause mild pain or discomfort, and pruritus is common; scratching may spread infection, inoculating both adjacent and nonadjacent skin.[15,35,40] The AT must be able to identify serious nonpurulent skin infections and refer the patient to his primary health care provider (HCP) or dermatologist.

Drugs for Treating Nonpurulent Skin Infections

Although impetigo has no standard therapy, Gram staining and culture of the pus or exudates from the skin lesions of impetigo and ecthyma are recommended to help identify whether *Staphylococcus aureus* or a *streptococcus* bacterium is the cause. The management guidelines[35] include culture of suspicious lesions and treatment with appropriate topical or oral (or both) antibiotics. When *streptococci* alone are the cause, *penicillin* is the drug of choice.[35] Evidence suggests that topical *mupirocin* (Bactroban) or *retapamulin* (Altabax) ointments are as effective or more effective and have fewer side effects than oral antibiotics. If the athlete is allergic to penicillins, *erythromycin* or *clindamycin* may be used effectively.[40] Clinical experience suggests that systemic therapy is preferred for patients with numerous lesions or in outbreaks affecting several people to decrease transmission of infection.[35]

Purulent Skin Infections: Folliculitis, Furuncles, and Carbuncles

Folliculitis is a purulent superficial infection of the hair follicles characterized by redness and the presence of fluid- or pus-filled sacs at the base of hair follicles. Furuncles (or boils) are deeper infections of the hair follicle characterized by inflamed nodules that drain fluid; these can join together to form larger nodules called carbuncles.[40] Furuncles are different from folliculitis, in which the inflammation is more superficial and pus is limited to the epidermis. Infection involving several adjacent follicles produces a carbuncle, a coalescent inflammatory mass with pus draining from multiple follicular orifices. Carbuncles develop most commonly on the back of the neck and are typically larger and deeper than furuncles. Purulent bacterial skin infections are usually caused by *S. aureus*, in which **suppuration** (pus) extends through the dermis into the subcutaneous tissue, where a small abscess forms.[35]

Drugs for Treating Purulent Skin Infections

Athletes with purulent skin infections should be referred to a higher-level care provider for culture of purulent perifollicular lesions and prescription for appropriate antibiotics. Simple furuncles may be treated with warm compresses to promote drainage, but more **fluctuant** furuncles and carbuncles require incision and drainage. For most cases, topical antiseptic treatment is adequate for most cases and may include the following OTC topical antibiotics:[40]

- *mupirocin* (Bactroban)
- *neomycin + polymyxin B + bacitracin* (Neosporin)

Systemic antimicrobials are usually unnecessary for purulent skin infections; however, the AT must monitor the patient for fever or other evidence of systemic infection.[35] The decision to prescribe antibiotics directed against *S. aureus* as an adjunct to incision and drainage should be made based on the presence or absence of SIRS. An antibiotic active against MRSA is recommended for patients with carbuncles or abscesses who have failed initial antibiotic treatment or have signs of SIRS.[35]

Cutaneous Abscesses

Cutaneous abscesses are collections of pus within the dermis and deeper skin tissues. They are usually painful, tender, and fluctuant red nodules, often surmounted by a pustule and encircled by a rim of erythematous swelling. Cutaneous abscesses can be polymicrobial, containing regional skin flora or organisms from the adjacent mucous membranes, but *S. aureus* alone causes a large percentage of skin abscesses, with a substantial number due to MRSA strains.[35] The AT must be able to identify serious skin infections such as cutaneous abscesses and refer the patient to her primary HCP or dermatologist.

Drugs for Treating Cutaneous Abscesses

A higher-level HCP such as a dermatologist may perform surgical incision, evacuation of pus and debris, and probing of the cavity to break up **loculations** as effective treatment of cutaneous abscesses. The AT is involved in covering the surgical site with a dry dressing while inspecting for signs of infection, which is the most effective treatment of the wound. The AT may be required to follow up on surgeries to close the wound with sutures or pack it with gauze or other absorbent material. However, packing may cause more pain and may not improve healing compared to just covering the incision site with sterile gauze.[35] The addition of systemic antibiotics to incision and drainage of cutaneous abscesses does not improve cure rates, even in cases due to MRSA. However, systemic antibiotics should be prescribed to patients with severely impaired host defenses or signs or symptoms of SIRS. The AT should monitor the patient for multiple abscesses, extremes of age, and lack of response to incision and drainage alone, which are additional criteria where systemic antimicrobial therapy should be considered.[35] The AT must promptly notify the patient's provider of signs and symptoms of MRSA or SIRS to implement antimicrobial therapy.

Fungal Skin Infections

Dermatophytes—fungal organisms living in soil or on animals or humans—include a group of fungi that infect and survive mostly on dead keratin cells in the stratum corneum of the epidermis.[2,32,40] Approximately 40 different species of fungi can cause dermatophytosis, or ringworm, which is a misnomer, since the condition is not caused by parasitic worms. The most common dermatophytoses in the athletic training setting are as follows:[2,10,40]

- **Tinea capitis**—Common fungal infection of the scalp manifested by gray scaly patches and accompanied by mild hair loss in many cases (figure 16.2*a*).
- **Tinea corporis**—Fungal infection on the body, commonly referred to as ringworm (name gleaned from its characteristic ringlike appearance) (figure 16.2*b*).
- **Tinea cruris**—Fungal infection in the groin area, commonly referred to as jock itch (figure 16.2*c*).
- **Tinea pedis**—The most common fungal infection that affects the feet, commonly referred to as athlete's foot (figure 16.2*d*).

Antifungal Agents

Antifungals are used to treat candidiasis, a wide variety of dermatophytoses, and other fungal infections (discussed in the section on Drugs for Treating Fungal Skin Infections). Common topical and systemic antifungal agents are presented in table 16.4.

Drugs for Treating Fungal Skin Infections

Treatment of dermatophytosis varies by site but always involves topical or oral antifungals (refer to table 16.4). Identification of specific organisms by culture is unnecessary; however, culture may also be useful when overlying inflammation and bacterial infection are severe or accompanied by **alopecia**.[2] Athletes who participate in noncontact

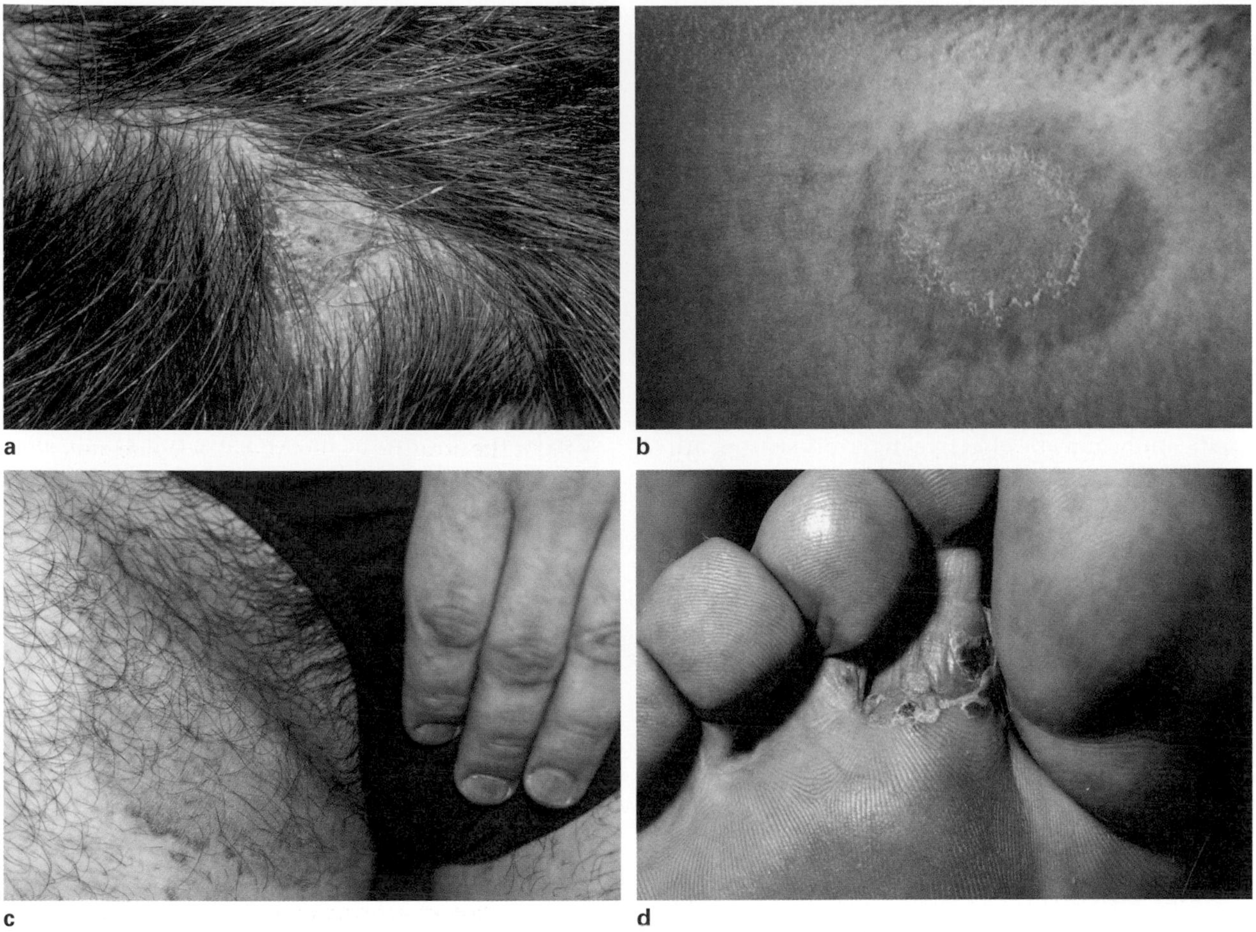

FIGURE 16.2 Common fungal skin infections: *(a)* tinea capitis, *(b)* tinea corporis (ringworm), *(c)* tinea cruris (jock itch), and *(d)* tinea pedis (athlete's foot).

a Dr P. Marazzi/Science Source; *b* DermPics/Science Source; *c* Dr Harout Tanielian/Science Source; *d* Dr H.C. Robinson/Science Source

TABLE 16.4 Topical and Systemic Agents for Treating Fungal Infections

Drug or agent	Usual regimen*	Prescription or OTC
Topical antifungals		
terbinafine 1% cream (Lamisil)	2 doses/d for 2-4 wk	Available OTC
clotrimazole 1% cream (Lotrimin AF)	1 dose/d for 2-4 wk	Available OTC
ketoconazole 2% cream (Nizoral)	1 dose/d for 2-4 wk	Available OTC
naftifine 1% cream (Naftin)	2 doses/d for 2-4 wk	Prescription only
oxiconazole 1% cream (Oxistat)**	2 doses/d for 2-4 wk	Prescription only
ciclopirox 0.77% cream (Loprox)**	2 doses/d for 2-4 wk	Prescription only
Systemic antifungals		
terbinafine oral (Lamisil)	250 mg/d for 2-4 wk	Prescription only
ketoconazole oral (Nizoral)	200 mg/d for 2-4 wk	Prescription only
fluconazole oral (Diflucan)	100-200 mg/d for 2-4 wk	Prescription only
itraconazole oral (Sporanox)	100-200 mg/d for 2-4 wk	Prescription only

*Depends on specific condition treated.
**Often used in combination twice a day.
OTC = over the counter

Data from Aaron (2018); Centers for Disease Control and Prevention (2018); Centers for Disease Control and Prevention (2019); Zinder et al. (2010).

sports or have localized cases of fungal infections may initially be treated with topical preparations for 2 to 4 weeks. More widespread, inflammatory, or otherwise difficult-to-treat cases may require the use of systemic antifungal drugs, which can have substantial side effects.[32]

Oral antifungals are used for most nail and scalp infections and resistant skin infections and are useful for patients unwilling or unable to adhere to prolonged topical regimens; doses and duration differ by site of infection. Recommended are topical creams containing the antifungals *terbinafine, naftifine, oxiconazole, or ciclopirox*. Although these topical medications may be effective in the off-season, athletes in the middle of a competitive season should be treated immediately with oral antifungals (the *-azoles*), such as *fluconazole* (Diflucan), *ketoconazole* (Nizoral), or *itraconazole* (Sporanox). Topical treatment is typically required through the entire course of the athletic season for 2 to 4 weeks in the off-season.[40] Corticosteroids may be prescribed in addition to antifungal creams to help relieve itching and inflammation. However, combining topical corticosteroids and antifungal creams should be avoided when possible because topical corticosteroids promote fungus growth.[2]

Tinea Capitis

Treatment of tinea capitis with systemic antifungal medication is required, since topical antifungal products are ineffective for treatment. Scalp lesions can be particularly difficult to eradicate, so systemic therapy with oral medications such as *terbinafine* (Lamisil) or 1 of the oral antifungals such as *fluconazole* (Diflucan) may be prescribed for up to 6 weeks. Additionally, daily use of an antifungal shampoo containing *ketoconazole* (Nizoral) may be required in particularly virulent scalp infections in athletes.[10,40] Athletes with tinea capitis must take systemic antifungal therapy for ≥2 weeks to be considered infection-free.[33,40]

Tinea Corporis and Tinea Cruris

Tinea corporis and tinea cruris are usually treated with OTC antifungal products. For tinea corporis, antifungal treatments include topical agents such as *terbinafine* (Lamisil), *clotrimazole* (Lotrimin), or the OTC 1% shampoo *ketoconazole* (Nizoral) used daily until symptoms resolve. Patients with more diffuse inflammatory conditions should be referred to a next-level provider for treatment with prescription oral systemic antifungal medication or a combination of topical and systemic antifungal medications.[10,40] Topical treatments should be continued for a further 7 days after resolution of visible symptoms to prevent recurrence. The AT must be aware that for sport participation, athletes with tinea corporis must have used the topical fungicide for ≥72 hours and must adequately cover any lesions with a nonocclusive dressing followed by underwrap and stretch tape.[33,40]

Tinea Pedis

Athlete's foot can usually be treated with OTC topical antifungal products; topical *terbinafine* (Lamisil) appears to be most effective, but other agents can also be used. Chronic or extensive tinea pedis may require treatment with prescription oral antifungal agents such as *fluconazole* (Diflucan) or *itraconazole* (Sporanox). In addition, chronic tinea pedis may require adjunctive therapy such as foot powder or talcum powder to prevent skin maceration.[10] Topical antifungal products or talcum powder may also be used to prevent tinea pedis. Refer to table 16.4 for a summary of common topical and systemic agents for treating fungal infections.

Candidiasis

Candida is a ubiquitous yeast that resides harmlessly on skin and mucous membranes until dampness, heat, and impaired local and systemic defenses provide a fertile environment for it to grow. Infections can occur anywhere and are most common in skinfolds, digital web spaces, nails, genitals, cuticles, and oral mucosa (also called thrush). The AT should consider candidiasis in patients who have erythematous, scaling, pruritic patches in intertriginous areas (between folds of skin or between fingers or toes), and lesions in the mucous membranes, around the nails, or at the corners of the mouth.[1]

Drugs for Treating Candidiasis

Candida auris is an emerging fungus and a multidrug-resistant organism that presents a serious global health threat. According to the CDC,[12] *C. auris* is resistant to multiple antifungal drugs that are commonly used to treat candida infections. Most cases of candidiasis are treated by the prescriber with *clotrimazole* (Lotrimin) **troches** (medicated lozenges), *nystatin* (Mycostatin) oral suspension, or a systemic antifungal agent. Candidal **paronychia** (inflammation of the nail fold) is treated by protecting the area from wetness and giving topical or oral antifungals. These infections are often resistant to treatment. For extended care or difficult conditions, the patient should be referred to the next-level care provider for treatment with prescription medications. *Thymol* 4% in alcohol applied to the affected area twice daily is often helpful. Oral candidiasis can be treated by dissolving a *clotrimazole* 10 mg troche (lozenge) in the mouth 4 or 5 times per day for 14 days. Chronic mucocutaneous candidiasis requires long-term oral antifungal treatment with oral *fluconazole* (Diflucan).[1]

Viral Skin Infections: Herpes Simplex and Molluscum Contagiosum

Two primary viral infections prevalent in athletic populations are herpes simplex and molluscum contagiosum. Herpes simplex virus (HSV) infection is common among athletes, especially those engaged in activities with full skin-on-skin contact, such as wrestling and rugby (i.e., herpes gladiatorum).[40] **Mucocutaneous infection** is the most common HSV infection, causing recurrent infection that affects the skin, mouth, lips, eyes, and genitals. HSV causes painful clusters of small fluid-filled sacs on a base of red skin. Viruses may remain dormant in the body for years, manifesting themselves during situations of depressed immunity and stress.[25,40] When HSV infection is suspected, the AT must refer the patient to his primary care provider for diagnosis, requiring either a culture of lesion scrapings or a Tzanck smear, which may give more rapid and accurate results.

Molluscum contagiosum is a highly infectious and contagious viral condition that commonly causes localized chronic infection. Transmission is by direct contact, and spread occurs via **fomites** (e.g., towels, bath sponges) and bath water. Athletes acquire the infection via close skin-to-skin contact with an infected person (e.g., wrestling, rugby).[16,40]

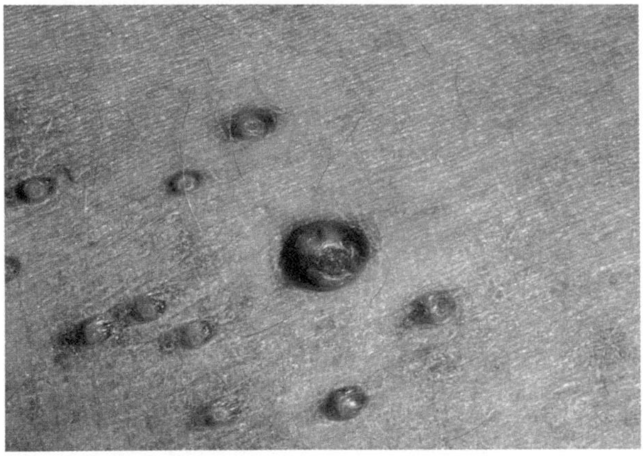

DR P. MARAZZI/Science Source

FIGURE 16.3 Molluscum contagiosum.

Molluscum contagiosum infection (figure 16.3) is usually a benign, mild skin disease that is characterized by lesions appearing anywhere on the body. The lesions, known as **mollusca**, are small and raised with a dimple or pit in the center; they are usually white, pink, or flesh colored and may have a pearly appearance. The mollusca may become itchy, sore, red, or swollen.[9] With treatment, molluscum contagiosum typically resolves without scarring after 6 to 12 months, but recovery may take as long as 4 years.[9]

Drugs for Treating Herpes Simplex

Isolated HSV infections often go untreated without consequence. For recurrent or primary symptomatic infections, the AT should refer the patient to her primary care provider for treatment with prescribed antiviral therapy such as *acyclovir* or *valacyclovir*, which are most effective if begun early.[25] Secondary bacterial infections are treated with OTC topical antibiotics (e.g., *neomycin + bacitracin*) or, if severe, with prescription oral systemic antibiotics (e.g., penicillinase-resistant beta-lactams). The AT may

Clinical Application

Herpes Gladiatorum

Herpes gladiatorum (HG), a herpes simplex virus, was responsible for 40.5% of all lost-time conditions sustained by NCAA wrestlers between 1993 and 2004.[39] This cutaneous infection presents as painful vesicles that lead to moist ulcerations and crusted plaques; it is transmitted skin to skin. Oral antivirals should commence within 24 hours of HG being detected. *Valacyclovir* 500 mg BID for 7 days is effective in decreasing the HG lesion. *Acyclovir* and *famciclovir* are also viable options for treatment of this contagious skin condition. Prophylactic treatment with *valacyclovir* is 500 mg per day for athletes with >2 years of HG history and 1,000 mg per day for athletes with <2 years of history.[39]

recommend systemic analgesics such as *acetaminophen* to help with pain and discomfort. Once the lesions are fully formed, ruptured, and crusted over, antiviral medications are no longer effective.[40] New, active lesions may be treated with an oral antiviral medication, such as prescription *valacyclovir*, to shorten the duration of the infection and reduce the chance of transmission.[25,40]

Drugs for Treating Molluscum Contagiosum

Patients with molluscum contagiosum infection should be referred to a dermatologist for treatment, which often involves surgical destruction of the lesions with a sharp curette or antiviral medications.[16,32,40] When extensive, mollusca lesions can be a reason for an athlete's disqualification from participation; however, solitary lesions can be appropriately covered or curetted before competition. Although an evidence-based medicine review failed to determine any standard effective therapies, the most efficient way to clear this infection rapidly and return the athlete to participation is simple **curettage** of lesions.[40] The AT providing care for the competitive athlete with molluscum contagiosum must monitor treatment and, since it is a contagious skin condition, prevent the spread to others.

Autoimmune Inflammatory Skin Conditions

Common inflammatory skin diseases, such as urticaria, contact and atopic dermatitis, and psoriasis, present with skin lesions and signs and symptoms in multiple body regions and are related to stimulation of the immune response. Most inflammatory skin diseases, such as mild urticaria or irritant contact dermatitis, can be managed clinically and are generally self-limiting. However, other skin conditions, such as atopic dermatitis, eczema, and psoriasis, are inflammatory dermatoses that often have an atypical presentation or do not respond to OTC treatments; these require referral to a dermatologist for treatment. According to the American Academy of Dermatology,[3] autoimmune diseases that manifest in the skin should not be treated with oral antibiotics unless there is clinical evidence of infection. The presence of high numbers of the *Staphylococcus aureus* (staph) bacteria on the skin of people with atopic dermatitis is quite common. The routine use of oral antibiotics can also cause side effects, including hypersensitivity reactions (exaggerated immune responses, such as allergic reactions), or contribute to the development of antibiotic resistance.

Anti-Inflammatory Agents

Corticosteroids are the mainstay of treatment for most noninfectious inflammatory skin disorders (table 16.5). Topical corticosteroids are available as aerosols, creams, gels, lotions, solutions, and tapes that contain corticosteroids and are applied externally to the scalp or the skin, depending on the condition being treated. Similar to systemic corticosteroids, topical corticosteroids counter inflammation by mimicking the naturally occurring corticosteroid hormones produced by our adrenal glands. In addition to reducing inflammation in the

TABLE 16.5 Topical Anti-Inflammatory Agents for Treatment of Inflammatory Skin Conditions

Drug	Description	Indications
hydrocortisone topical (Cortaid, Cortizone-5, many others)	Topical corticosteroid in dosage forms of creams, lotions, gel, or ointment combined for management of inflammatory dermatoses.[18]	Useful on the face and in intertriginous (between skinfolds) areas. Gels are useful on the scalp and in management of contact dermatitis. Ointments are useful for dry scaly areas and when increased potency is required.
betamethasone (Diprosone, Valisone)	Corticosteroid ointment, cream, lotion, gel, and aerosol (spray) in various strengths for use on the skin and as a foam to apply to the scalp.	Used to treat itching, redness, dryness, crusting, scaling, inflammation, and discomfort of various skin conditions.

area where they are applied, topical corticosteroids also suppress the immune response, reduce cell turnover, and constrict blood vessels.[21] Optimal response depends on choosing a vehicle that is appropriate for the body location and lesion characteristics, as well as the patient's preference.

Topical corticosteroids are generally applied 2 or 3 times a day, but high-potency formulations may require application only once a day or even less frequently. Most dermatoses are treated with mid-potency to high-potency formulations; mild formulations are better for mild inflammation and for use on the face or intertriginous areas where systemic absorption and local adverse effects are more likely. High-potency formulations may cause adrenal suppression when applied over extensive skin surfaces or for long periods. Relative contraindications include conditions in which infection plays an underlying role.[26]

RED FLAG

Adverse Effects of Topical Corticosteroids

Systemic absorption of topical corticosteroids may occur and cause adrenal suppression when high-potency formulations are applied over extensive skin surfaces or for long periods of time. Local adverse effects of topical corticosteroids such as *hydrocortisone* cream (when used for >1 month) include the following:[18,26]

- Skin irritation
- Development of **miliaria**
- Skin atrophy
- **Striae**
- Bacterial infections
- Fungal growth

Antipruritic Agents

Itching (pruritus) is usually a symptom of an underlying skin disorder or systemic allergic reaction, but it can result from a widespread systemic disorder (see sidebar) such as a food or drug allergy. Itching leads to scratching, which can cause inflammation, skin degradation, and possible secondary infection.[7,26] Itching can be relieved with topical or systemic drugs.[7] Corticosteroids are effective in relieving the itch caused by inflammation, but should be avoided for conditions that have no evidence of inflammation. Mid- to high-potency topical corticosteroids (e.g., *triamcinolone* 0.1% ointment) are indicated for inflammatory itching. Oral corticosteroids (e.g., *prednisone* 60 mg once a day for 7 to 14 days) can be prescribed for severe blistering or extensive disease. Systemic antihistamines (e.g., *hydroxyzine*, *diphenhydramine*) also help relieve pruritus.[28]

Topical options include lotions or creams that contain *camphor* or *menthol*, *capsaicin*, *diphenhydramine*, or corticosteroids.[7] *Calamine* (combination of zinc oxide and 0.5% ferric oxide) lotion is a medication used to treat mild itch. *Calamine* works by causing a cooling sensation as it evaporates on the skin, usually leaving a thin film on the surface. *Calamine* also dries oozing or weeping from minor skin irritation. *Calamine* lotion is used to treat itching and skin irritation caused by chicken pox and insect bites or stings, among other common skin conditions.[17]

Itching is caused less often by systemic disorders than by skin disorders; however, if skin lesions are not evident, systemic causes should be investigated. In systemic disorders, itching may occur with or without skin lesions. However, when itching is prominent without any identifiable skin lesions, systemic disorders and drugs should be suspected. Drug reactions can cause itching as an allergic reaction or by directly triggering histamine. Regular skin care, including limiting bathing, avoiding irritants, moisturizing regularly, and humidifying the environment, is usually helpful for preventing or treating itching.[7]

Common Skin and Systemic Disorders That Cause Pruritis (Itching)

Skin-Related

- Dry skin
- Contact or irritant contact dermatitis
- Atopic dermatitis (eczema)
- Fungal skin infections

Systemic Skin Disorders

- Allergic reaction (e.g., to foods, drugs, and insect bites and stings)
- Drug reactions (most commonly morphine, some IV contrast agents)

Urticaria

Urticaria can be caused by allergic or nonallergic mechanisms. Most acute cases are caused by an allergic reaction to a specific substance. Most chronic cases are idiopathic or result from autoimmune disease. Treatment is based on severity; nonsedating antihistamines and avoidance of triggers are first-line options. Topical corticosteroids and topical antihistamines are not beneficial. Concomitant systemic symptoms require a thorough evaluation for the etiology.[6]

Drugs for Treating Urticaria

Antihistamines remain the mainstay of treatment and must be taken on a regular basis, rather than as needed. Newer (second-generation) oral antihistamines often are preferred because of once-daily dosing and because some are less sedating. Appropriate systemic oral antihistamines for treating allergic urticaria include the following:[6]

- Nonsedating (second-generation) antihistamines
  - *loratadine* (Claritin), available OTC
  - *cetirizine* (Zyrtec), available OTC
  - *fexofenadine* (Allegra), available OTC
  - *levocetirizine* (Xyzal), available OTC or by prescription
- Sedating (first-generation) antihistamines
  - *hydroxyzine* (Vistaril), available by prescription only
  - *diphenhydramine* (Benadryl), available OTC or by prescription

Systemic corticosteroids (e.g., *prednisone* 30 to 40 mg PO once/day) are prescribed for severe symptoms, but they should not be used long term. Patients with angioedema involving the oropharynx or any involvement of the airway should be administered an autoinjectable *epinephrine* pen (EpiPen) or subcutaneous *epinephrine* 0.3 mL of 1:1000 solution injection and be admitted to the hospital. On discharge, patients should be supplied with and trained in the use of an EpiPen.[6]

Contact Dermatitis

Contact dermatitis is acute inflammation of the skin caused by irritants or allergens. The primary symptom is pruritus. Irritant contact dermatitis (ICD) accounts for 80% of all cases of contact dermatitis. In ICD, the immune system is not activated; it is a nonspecific inflammatory reaction to substances contacting the skin. Prior exposure to the offending agent is not necessary, and the reaction develops in minutes to a few hours. Chronic low-grade irritant dermatitis is the most common type of ICD, and the most common area of involvement is the hands. The most common irritants encountered are chronic wet skin, chemicals, or soaps that come in contact with the skin.[22]

Nonspecific dermatitis, or irritant contact dermatitis, causes a localized itchy or burning rash or irritation of the skin where it has come in contact with a foreign substance. Only the superficial regions of the skin are affected in contact dermatitis. Inflammation of the affected tissue is present in the epidermis and the outer dermis. The rash may take anywhere from several days to weeks to heal. Chronic ICD can develop when the removal of the offending agent no longer provides expected relief.[22] The clinical lesions of ICD may be acute (wet and edematous) or chronic (dry, thickened, and scaly), depending on the persistence of the contact with the irritating substance.[29] Irritant contact dermatitis is usually confined to the area where the trigger actually touched the skin and presents with the following signs and symptoms:[7,22,29]

- **Red rash**—Usual reaction that appears immediately after contact with the irritant.
- **Blisters, wheals (welts), and urticaria (hives)**—Often form a pattern where skin was directly exposed to the irritant.
- **Itchy, burning skin**—More painful than itchy.

Drugs for Treating Contact Dermatitis

The first intervention for ICD involves identification, withdrawal, and avoidance of the offending agent. The second treatment is symptomatic relief while decreasing skin lesions. Cold compresses help soothe and cleanse the skin; they are applied to wet or oozing lesions, removed, remoistened, and reapplied every few minutes for 20 to 30 minutes. If the affected areas are already dry or hardened, wet dressings applied as soaks (without removal for 20 to 30 minutes) will soften and hydrate the skin; soaks should not be used on acute exudating lesions. *Calamine* lotion or 5% aluminum acetate (Burow's or Domeboro) solution, available OTC, relieves the itching and stinging of irritated, inflamed skin and helps stop the growth of bacteria and fungus.[22] Oatmeal baths or moisturizers may be used to prevent dryness and skin fissuring.[22,28] Wet-to-dry dressings can soothe oozing blisters, dry the skin, and promote healing.[22] Topical corticosteroids provide relief for excessive itching and are the mainstay of treatment.[29] Systemic drugs are indicated for ICD with generalized itching or local ICD that is resistant to topical agents. Systemic antihistamines, such as *hydroxyzine*, are effective; however, newer nonsedating antihistamines such as *loratadine*, *cetirizine*, *fexofenadine*, and *levocetirizine* can be useful for treating contact dermatitis.[7]

According to clinical guidelines from the American Academy of Dermatology,[3] systemic (oral or injected) corticosteroids should not be prescribed as a long-term treatment for atopic dermatitis. The potential complications of long-term treatment with oral or injected corticosteroids outweigh the potential benefits. Although the short-term use of systemic corticosteroids is sometimes appropriate for providing relief of severe symptoms, long-term treatment could cause serious short- and long-term adverse effects.

Atopic Dermatitis and Eczema

Atopic dermatitis (also known as atopic eczema) is a chronic, pruritic inflammatory skin disease that is characterized by intense itching and recurrent eczematous lesions.[19,23,37,38] Common triggers include airborne allergens (e.g., pollen, dust), sweat, harsh soaps, rough fabrics, and fragrances. Atopic dermatitis often improves by adulthood.[23]

Drugs for Treating Atopic Dermatitis and Eczema

Atopic dermatitis cannot be cured at present; thus, the aim of management is to improve symptoms and achieve long-term disease control with a multistep approach, as outlined in national and international guidelines from the American Academy of Dermatology.[3,19] The goals of treatment are to reduce symptoms (pruritus and dermatitis), prevent exacerbations, and minimize therapeutic risks. Standard treatment modalities for the management of these patients are centered around the use of topical anti-inflammatory preparations and moisturization of the skin.[19,37,38] Treatment of atopic dermatitis focuses on restoration of epidermal barrier function, which is best achieved through the use of emollients. Topical corticosteroids are still the first-line therapy for acute flares, but they are also used proactively along with topical calcineurin inhibitors to maintain remission. The main principles of long-term treatment are continuous epidermal barrier repair with emollients, avoidance of individual trigger factors, and anti-inflammatory therapy with topical corticosteroids or calcineurin inhibitors.[37]

Psoriasis

Psoriasis manifests most commonly as well-circumscribed, erythematous papules and plaques covered with silvery scales. Patches are typically found on the elbows, knees, scalp, lower back, face, palms, and soles of the feet, but can affect other places (fingernails, toenails, and mouth). Symptoms are usually minimal, but mild to severe itching may occur.

Drugs for Treating Psoriasis

Patients with limited psoriasis are initially treated with topical corticosteroids, emollients, vitamin D_3 analogs, topical retinoids (*tazarotene*), coal tar, anthralin, and phototherapy.[11,20] In severe cases of psoriasis, systemic drugs (e.g., *methotrexate*, retinoids, immunomodulatory agents) may be necessary.[20] The AT should monitor the patient with psoriasis for worsening of the symptoms or adverse effects of medication and refer her to the appropriate provider.

Summary

Dermatological conditions result when the skin is injured or infected with microorganisms that can cause pain, discomfort, itching, and other symptoms. The barrier of healthy skin provides protection from physicochemical, microbial, and immunological intrusions into the body. The most common pathophysiological processes involved in dermatological conditions result from injury or infection that disrupts the antimicrobial properties of the skin. Additionally, in people prone to allergy or atopy, the skin has autoimmune responses to antigens, causing inflammatory reactions in the skin.[4,37] ATs and other athletic team HCPs must be able to identify and prevent transmission of common skin diseases in athletes. Many sports have requirements for managing patients with skin lesions that promote healing and prevent the spread of infection in the patient's own body as well as to others coming into contact with infected skin. To assist the AT, this chapter provides the current recommendations about therapeutic medications that are important in minimizing disease transmission, preventing the spread of infectious agents, and improving the management of common skin diseases in athletes.

Case Studies

Case Study 1

Charlie is a first-year intercollegiate cross country runner. Part of his team's recovery routine is to soak in a cold tub after practice. The first time Charlie sat in the tub, he tolerated it for only 2 minutes. He noticed that his skin itched and that he had a mild tingling in his mouth, but these sensations seemed to dissipate soon after rewarming. The next time he sat in the tub, he tolerated it a bit longer, but noticed welts on his skin and felt swelling around his lips and tongue. He reported this to his athletic trainer, who felt he was presenting with an anaphylactic reaction to the cold contact on the skin. She contacted the team physician, who recommended immediate treatment and physician referral for cold urticaria.

Questions for Analysis

1. What is cold urticaria?
2. What is the treatment?

Case Study 2

While trying out his new moped, Tony failed to navigate a sharp corner well and crashed. The result was several abrasions, also known as road rash, on his left arm and leg. He tried to care for the abrasions himself over the next few days, but they were not improving, so he went for evaluation and treatment at a local urgent care clinic. The provider started Tony on an oral antibiotic out of concern for MRSA and covered the largest abrasion with a hydrogel dressing.

Questions for Analysis

1. Which oral antibiotic is likely to have been prescribed?
2. What is a hydrogel dressing and how does it work?

Drugs Discussed in This Chapter

Drug class	*generic* (pronunciation) Trade name	Therapeutic uses	Clinical concerns
Topical antibiotics	*neomycin + bacitracin + polymyxin B* (NEE oh MYE sin; BAS i TRAY sin; POL ee MIX in B) Triple Antibiotic, Neosporin	Topical ointment applied 3 times daily for 1 wk	Common side effects are itching, skin rash, redness, swelling, or other signs of irritation that did not present before use of this medicine.
Antipruritics: topical corticosteroids	*hydrocortisone topical* (hye droe KOR ti sone) Cortaid, Cortizone-5, many others	In general, start with the lowest-potency agent appropriate for the severity of the condition and application site. Potency depends on vehicle, concentration, site of application, and use of occlusive dressings.	For relief of inflammatory and pruritic manifestations of corticosteroid-responsive dermatoses. Common side effects are burning, itching, irritation, dryness, and folliculitis.
Antipruritics: local anesthetic	*pramoxine topical* (pra MOX een TOP i kal) Gold Bond, Blistex	Apply as needed, 4-6 times daily as a lip balm, gel, lotion, ointment, or solution.	Can cause dryness or irritation at application site.

Drug class	*generic* (pronunciation) Trade name	Therapeutic uses	Clinical concerns
Systemic antihistamines nonsedating (second generation)	*loratadine** (lor AT a deen) Claritin	Initial: 10 mg PO once daily. For urticaria (acute and chronic spontaneous): If symptom control is inadequate, may increase to 10 mg twice daily. Limited evidence exists for larger doses. Prescriber should reevaluate necessity for continued treatment periodically.	For treating skin hives and itching in people with chronic skin reactions. The most commonly reported side effects include headache, somnolence, nervousness, and fatigue.
Sedating (first generation)	*diphenhydramine** (DYE fen HYE dra meen) Benadryl	25-50 mg PO every 4-6 hr as needed. Maximum dose: 300 mg/d	The most commonly reported side effects include sedation, somnolence, or sleepiness; drowsiness; unsteadiness; dizziness; and headache. Symptomatic relief of allergic dermatosis; adjunct to epinephrine in the treatment of anaphylaxis.
Systemic antibiotics	*clindamycin* (klin da MYE sin) Cleocin	Tablet or suspension: 300 mg PO 3 or 4 times daily.	For treatment of septicemia caused by *S. aureus*, streptococci (except *E. faecalis*), and susceptible anaerobes. For treatment of skin and skin structure infections caused by *Streptococcus pyogenes*, *S. aureus*, and susceptible anaerobes. May cause *Clostridium difficile*-induced diarrhea.
	trimethoprim + sulfamethoxazole (trye METH oh prim; SUL fa meth OX a zole) Bactrim, Septra	Double-strength tablets: 1 or 2 tablets twice daily. Contains *sulfamethoxazole* 80 mg and *trimethoprim* 16 mg per mL.	May cause nausea, vomiting, rash, or photosensitivity.
	doxycycline (doks i SYE kleen) Vibramycin	100-200 mg/d, in 1 dose or divided into 2 doses.	May cause nausea, photosensitivity, and deposition in teeth and bones.

*Also described in chapter 11.
MRSA = *Methicillin*-resistant *Staphylococcus aureus*; VRE = *Vancomycin*-resistant *enterococcus*

17

Drugs for Treating Reproductive and Genitourinary Concerns

OBJECTIVES

After reading this chapter, you will be able to do the following:

- Describe sexual health and the medications used to prevent pregnancy
- Summarize the black box warnings for the use of hormonal contraceptives
- Discuss the advantages and disadvantages of long-acting reversible contraception
- Summarize the medications used to treat bacterial and viral sexually transmitted infections
- Discuss treatments for common reproductive and urogenital concerns

Select Drugs Mentioned in This Chapter

Drug class	Generic name	Trade name
Short-acting hormonal contraception		
Oral combination hormone pill	*ethinyl estradiol* + *norgestrel* pill	Cryselle, many others
Oral progestin-only pill (mini pill)	*norethindrone* pill	Camila, many others
Contraceptive patch	*ethinyl estradiol* + *norelgestromin* transdermal patch	Xulane
Contraceptive: vaginal ring	*ethinyl estradiol* + *etonogestrel* vaginal ring	NuvaRing
Long-acting reversible contraception		
Contraceptive implant	*etonogestrel* subdermal implant	Nexplanon
Intrauterine devices (IUDs)	copper intrauterine contraceptive	Paragard
Contraceptive implant		
Hormonal IUD	*levonorgestrel*-releasing intrauterine device	Skyla, Mirena
Hormonal contraceptive injection	*medroxyprogesterone* injection	Depo-Provera

This list is not exhaustive, but rather contains drugs commonly encountered in the athletic training setting. Always consult up-to-date information, confirm with a pharmacist, or discuss the use of therapeutic medications with the prescriber of the medication.

Reproductive health refers to the diseases, disorders, and conditions that affect the functioning of the male and female reproductive systems during all stages of life.[52] **Sexual health** addresses contraception, sexually transmitted infections (STIs), and erectile dysfunction. The athletic trainer (AT) must be able to educate athletes and other physically active people about the most common reproductive and sexual health considerations and conditions encountered in a traditional AT setting. This chapter focuses primarily on the conditions and challenges encountered by healthy adolescents and young adults 10 to 24 years old, although most of the information also translates to physically active nonathletes across the life span. The chapter is organized by concern or condition and then describes the medications used for each, including the mechanism of action, accessibility to patients, and safety. It discusses medications used for common reproductive health concerns and disorders of the genitourinary (GU) system. The information provided in this chapter should allow the AT to provide patient education, recognize adverse effects of medication, and identify conditions that require urgent or immediate referral to the patient's primary health care provider or pharmacist.

Family Planning and Contraception

ATs and other health care providers (HCPs) should always appropriately refer people considering family planning options to their student health center, primary care provider, or **gynecologist**.[12] The content in this chapter is not intended to be a substitute for professional medical advice for individual patients. ATs serve as sources of information for patients regarding overall reproductive health. The AT may also work with people who encounter complications from participating in athletics while using contraception. In these cases, the AT provides education, information, support, and referral for reproductive and GU concerns.

Contraceptive Method Effectiveness

The effectiveness of a contraceptive method is critical for minimizing the risk for an unintended pregnancy. It depends both on the inherent effectiveness of the method itself and on how consistently and correctly the contraception is used. The AT should be able to inform athletes considering using contraception about the range and effectiveness (figure 17.1) of contraceptive options available for which they are medically eligible so that they can identify the optimal method for their specific situation.[12,13]

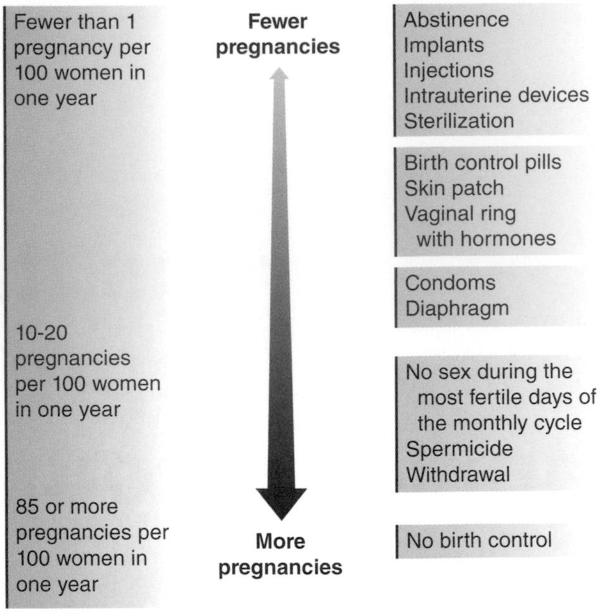

FIGURE 17.1 Effectiveness of various contraceptives, in decreasing order.

Classification of Contraceptive Methods

Contraception, also called birth control, is the deliberate use of a medicine, device, or a technique to prevent pregnancy.[18] Many types of contraceptives are available. For example, the use of the birth control pill is common among people who work with ATs.[62] The AT should be able to describe classifications and characteristics for the use of the following specific contraceptive methods:[12,13,18]

- Short-acting hormonal contraceptives
  - Combination oral contraceptives
  - Progestin-only oral contraceptives
  - Contraceptive patch
  - Contraceptive vaginal ring
- Long-acting reversible contraception
  - Contraceptive hormone injection
  - Intrauterine devices (copper only or with hormones)
  - Subdermal contraceptive implants
- Barrier methods
  - Contraceptive sponge
  - Cervical cap or diaphragm

  - Female condom
  - Male condom
  - Spermicide alone
- Emergency contraception

Short-Acting Hormonal Contraceptives

Several differences exist between contraceptives. Hormone-containing contraceptives have more side effects than nonhormonal contraceptives. Combination hormonal contraceptives are contraceptive products that contain an estrogen combined with a progestin. Hormonal contraceptives can be safely used by most women. ATs must reiterate to patients that no hormonal contraceptives protect against STIs, including HIV.

Combination Oral Contraceptives

Combination oral contraceptives are medications that require a prescription and contain an estrogen and a progestin. Oral contraceptives (OCs) mimic ovarian hormones. Once ingested, they inhibit the release of gonadotropin-releasing hormone (GnRH) by the hypothalamus, thus inhibiting the release of the pituitary hormones that stimulate ovulation.[9] Pregnancy is prevented by suppressing ovulation (the release of an egg from an ovary), thinning the lining of the uterus (endometrium) and thus preventing a fertilized egg from implanting, and thickening the cervical mucus, making it impenetrable to sperm.[2,45]

OCs may contain either a combination of the hormone estrogen and a progestin or a progestin alone. Oral contraceptives are available in different mixtures of active and inactive pills, depending on how frequently a menstrual cycle is desired.[18,21] Most combination OCs contain 10 to 35 mcg of *ethinyl estradiol*. Low-dose OCs are usually preferred to high-dose OCs (50 mcg of estrogen) because they appear equally effective and have fewer adverse effects, except for a higher incidence of irregular vaginal bleeding during the first few months of use.[9,61] The pill must be swallowed at the same time every day, regardless if the person has had sex. If 1 or more pills is missed or a pill pack is started late, the patient should use another method of birth control, like a condom and spermicide.[45] All combination OCs have similar efficacy; the pregnancy rate after 1 year is 0.3% with perfect use and about 9% with typical (i.e., inconsistent) use.[9,45] Refer to the Adverse Effects section and to the table at the end of this chapter (Drugs and Medical Devices Described in This Chapter) for clinical concerns with the use of contraception. The AT should be able to provide information about side effects and adverse effects while assisting the patient in learning more about the prescribed medication.

Beneficial Effects

OCs have some very important health benefits. High- and low-dose combination OCs decrease the risk of endometrial cancer and ovarian cancer by about 50% for ≥20 years after OCs are stopped. They also decrease the risk of benign ovarian tumors, abnormal vaginal bleeding, dysmenorrhea, osteoporosis, premenstrual dysphoric disorder, iron deficiency anemia, benign breast disorders, and functional ovarian cysts. Ectopic pregnancy and **salpingitis** (infection and inflammation in the fallopian tubes), which can impair fertility, occur less frequently in OC users.[9] Some questions exist about the use of OCs as performance-enhancing drugs; see Clinical Application sidebar for more information.

Clinical Application

Oral Contraceptives as Performance-Enhancing Drugs

It has been suggested that estrogen may have an anabolic effect, that progesterone may have a catabolic effect, and that oral contraceptives negatively affect athletic performance. A study comparing isokinetic knee strength, hand-grip strength, and hop testing indicated no significant difference between times of OC use and non-OC use, comparing the two conditions in the same patients.[26] Little evidence exists correlating hormone fluctuations of an OC cycle with aerobic performance, but ventilation and oxygen consumption may be influenced by OC progestogen content. No evidence exists that OCs influence anaerobic power, and modern OC formulas do not offer a sufficient androgenic effect on muscle strength.[56]

Adverse Effects

All combination OCs are equally effective; formulations with a low estrogen dose are preferred because they have fewer adverse effects. Hormonal contraceptives may be contraindicated for women >35 years who smoke because these patients are at higher risk of serious side effects, such as heart attack, blood clots, or stroke. Although these effects are very rare, they can be serious enough to cause death.[45] It is not common, but some women who take the pill develop high blood pressure or experience blood clots, heart attacks, or strokes.[58]

Serious side effects of hormonal contraceptives include the following:[2,4]

- Blurred vision
- Severe stomach pain
- Severe headache
- Swelling or pain in the legs (from blood clots)
- Cardiovascular complications such as chest pain, heart attack, blood clots, stroke

Common side effects include the following:[9,45]

- Abdominal cramping or bloating
- Spotting between periods
- Breast pain, tenderness, or swelling
- Possible weight gain
- Dizziness
- Nausea and vomiting
- Swelling of ankles and feet
- Unusual tiredness or weakness

Hormonal contraceptives are not recommended in women who have certain types of cancer or are at higher risk of clotting disorders or strokes, liver disease, severe headaches, undiagnosed vaginal bleeding, uncontrolled high blood pressure, or heart disease. Thus, the provider needs a thorough history when discussing therapeutic options with the patient. The association between OC use and the subsequent risk of breast cancer has been well studied. A scientific specialist review panel agreed that there was sufficient evidence for an association between OC use and breast cancer risk in humans. However, this assessment found inconsistent results for women who had previously used OCs versus those who had never used OCs. The increased risk was noted only for women who were current or recent OC users, particularly those who were <35 years of age at diagnosis.[34,57]

Progestin-Only Oral Contraceptives

Women who are sensitive to hormones may benefit from taking a lower-dose pill rather than a combination oral contraceptive, which contains estrogen and progestin. Progestin-only pills (POPs), or the mini pill *norethindrone* (Camila, many others), contain only the hormone progestin and can be safely used by most women. These contraceptives work by thickening cervical mucus, which helps block sperm from entering the uterus, and thinning the endometrium, which prevents a fertilized egg from implanting. In some cycles, POPs also suppress ovulation, but this effect is not their primary mechanism of action.[9] Mini pills must be taken within the same 3-hour time frame every day and are available only in a single mixture or formulation—all the pills in each pack are active.[61] Lower-dose pills may cause more **breakthrough bleeding** (i.e., bleeding or spotting between periods) than do higher-dose pills. Pregnancy rates with perfect and typical use of progestin-only oral contraceptives are similar to those with use of combination OCs.[9]

Contraceptive Patch

The contraceptive patch, or the *norelgestromin* and *ethinyl estradiol* transdermal system (Xulane), has 2 hormones (estrogen and progestin) that stop the ovaries from releasing eggs and thicken the cervical mucus, which keeps sperm from getting to the egg. Due to the risk of venous thromboembolism (VTE), *norelgestromin* has an FDA black box warning; thus, the patient and provider should have an appropriate discussion if this medication is prescribed.[24]

Contraceptive Vaginal Ring

In the United States, only 1 vaginal ring, that contains *ethinyl estradiol* and *etonogestrel* (NuvaRing), is currently available. This vaginal ring is flexible, soft, and transparent; it comes in 1 size, which is 58 mm in diameter and 4 mm thick. Each ring releases 15 mcg of *ethinyl estradiol* (estrogen) and 120 mcg of *etonogestrel* (progestin) daily. These hormones are absorbed through the vaginal epithelium. When a vaginal ring is used, hormone blood levels are relatively constant.[10] The ring is typically left in place for 3 weeks, then removed for 1 week to allow for **withdrawal bleeding**. Contraceptive efficacy and adverse effects with vaginal rings are similar to those in use of OCs, but adherence may be better than with pills taken daily because the user inserts the ring just once a month. The NuvaRing has an

FDA black box warning indicating that women who are >35 years old and smoke cigarettes are at risk of developing significant heart- and blood-related side effects.[23]

Long-Acting Reversible Contraception

Long-acting reversible contraceptives are methods that last for several years; they may be removed anytime to resume fertility.[58] A prescription is required for these types of contraception; however, once started, this type of birth control is highly effective and easy to use. The AT should be able to provide information on options for the following forms of long-acting reversible contraception:

- Contraceptive hormone injections
- Subdermal contraceptive implants
- Intrauterine devices (copper only or with hormones)

Contraceptive Hormone Injection

Depot *medroxyprogesterone acetate* (Depo-Provera contraceptive injection) is a long-acting injectable formulation of 150 mg that is administered every 3 months (13 weeks) by deep intramuscular injection in the gluteal or deltoid muscle, using strict aseptic technique and rotating the sites with every injection. Effective contraceptive hormonal serum levels are usually attained as early as 24 hours after the injection and are maintained for ≥14 weeks (levels may remain effective for up to 16 weeks).

The most common adverse effect of Depo-Provera is irregular vaginal bleeding. In the 3 months after the first injection, about 30% of women have **amenorrhea**. Because Depo-Provera has a long duration of action, ovulation may be delayed for up to 18 months after the last injection. After ovulation occurs, fertility is usually rapidly restored. Depo-Provera contraceptive injection has a black box warning that users may lose significant bone mineral density.[64]

Subdermal Contraceptive Implants

Progestin-only subdermal implants are a type of long-acting contraception.[61] The *etonogestrel* implant (Nexplanon) is the only progestin implant available in the United States; it is a long-acting (up to 3 years), reversible hormonal contraceptive method. This 4-cm, match-sized single-rod implant can be subdermally inserted with a **trocar** at a point 8 to 10 cm above the medial epicondyle, avoiding the groove between the bicep and tricep.[16] This location is intended to avoid the large blood vessels and nerves lying within and surrounding the sulcus, and no skin incision is required. The implant contains 68 mg of *etonogestrel* (ETG, a progestin), which is released at an average rate of 50 mcg per day at 12 months. The implant provides effective contraception for up to 3 years. (In some studies, however, efficacy persisted up to 5 years.)

The most common adverse effects are similar to those experienced with use of other progestins, including irregular vaginal bleeding, amenorrhea, and headache. Some women experience changes in menstrual bleeding patterns, weight gain, and acne. Less common risks involve complications of insertion and removal of the implant, including pain, bleeding, scarring, infection, movement of the implant to another part of the body, ectopic pregnancy, and ovarian cysts. Rarely, some women will have blood clots, heart attacks, or strokes.[58]

Intrauterine Devices

An intrauterine device (IUD) is a small T-shaped device that is inserted through the vagina into the uterus (figure 17.2) by a trained HCP to prevent implantation of a fertilized egg. IUDs provide contraception for 3 to 10 years, depending on the type. IUDs do not protect against STIs, including HIV.[11,25,27] The AT should be familiar with the 2 types of IUDs and be able to explain how they intervene in the pregnancy process:

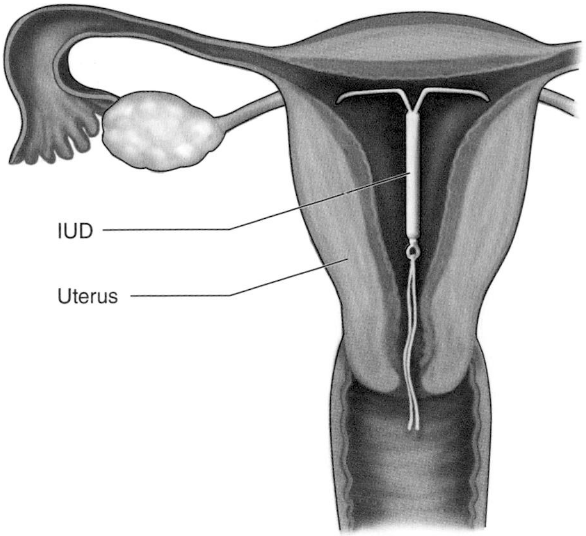

FIGURE 17.2 Placement of intrauterine device.

- **Copper-bearing IUD (Paragard)**—Effective for 10 years and has a cumulative 12-year pregnancy rate of <2%.[11]
- ***Levonorgestrel*-releasing IUDs (Skyla, Mirena)**—Can be used for 3 (Skyla) to 5 years (Mirena).[25,27] Vaginal bleeding stops completely within 1 year of insertion in 6% of women using the 3-year IUD (Skyla) and in 20% of women using the 5-year IUD (Mirena).[11]

Barrier Methods

Barrier methods with spermicide are interventions used by men and women to prevent sperm from entering the uterus. Most spermicides contain *nonoxynol-9*, which immobilizes or kills sperm before they can enter the uterus by damaging sperm cell membranes, thus preventing fertilization.[42] The following barrier methods are available over the counter (OTC):[42]

- **Spermicide**—Most spermicides contain *nonoxynol-9*, which provides a chemical barrier to sperm by damaging sperm cell membranes and prevents fertilization.
- **Contraceptive sponge**—This soft, disk-shaped polyurethane foam contains spermicide, which blocks or kills sperm. It acts as both a barrier device and a spermicidal agent. Complications or side effects of the contraceptive sponge and the spermicide it releases include the following:
  - Vaginal irritation or dryness
  - Urinary tract or vaginal infection
  - Increased risk of contracting STIs
  - Toxic shock syndrome (see Red Flag sidebar)

RED FLAG

Signs and Symptoms of Toxic Shock Syndrome

Toxic shock syndrome is a condition that can escalate quickly to a life-threatening emergency with little or no warning. The AT should be aware of the signs and symptoms that would prompt an urgent referral or emergency care, which include the following:

- A sudden high fever (39°C to 40.5°C) that remains elevated
- Low blood pressure (hypotension), which can be refractory
- Diffuse macular erythroderma (i.e., a rash resembling a sunburn, particularly on the palms and soles) occurs between 3 and 7 days after onset
- Vomiting or diarrhea
- Confusion
- Muscle aches
- Redness of the eyes, mouth, and throat
- Seizures
- Headaches

Emergency Contraception

Emergency contraception (EC), or postcoital contraception, may involve either use of the emergency contraceptive pill (ECP), sometimes called the morning-after pill (available OTC), or insertion of a copper-bearing IUD after unprotected sex.[18] Emergency contraception can prevent up to 95% of pregnancies when taken within the 5 days after intercourse.[63] Emergency contraception methods cannot interrupt an established pregnancy or harm a developing embryo.[18,63]

Recommendations for Exercise During Pregnancy

The role of the AT is important because the AT is often the first HCP to recognize that an athlete may be pregnant or the first person the athlete approaches in confidence. As such, the AT should be well versed in the institution's pregnancy policies and able to access resources easily. Before such an event, it is important to discuss medical issues around pregnancy and parenting with the directing or team physician and institutional administrators. If the institution lacks a pregnancy and parenting policy, the AT should collaborate with the physician and institutional administrators to develop one and participate in periodic reviews. It may be helpful to use the *Model Pregnancy and Parenting Policy* from the National Collegiate Athletic Association's (NCAA) sports medicine resources website.[51]

The AT should help the patient feel supported by avoiding asking judgmental questions and giving her time to work through emotions and decisions. The AT should reassure each patient seeking counsel that he will maintain confidentiality within the medical team as long as it is medically safe to do so and that there are few risks to athletic participation in uncomplicated pregnancies, particularly in the first trimester. However, the patient should be referred to an appropriate maternal health care provider, such as the student health clinic staff, primary care provider, or gynecologist. A few warning signs should be reported immediately if encountered during exercise (see Red Flag sidebar).[1,51]

RED FLAG

Warning Signs to Stop Exercise While Pregnant

- Vaginal bleeding
- Shortness of breath before exercise
- Dizziness
- Headache
- Chest pain
- Calf pain or swelling
- Preterm labor
- Decreased fetal movement
- Amniotic fluid leakage
- Muscle weakness

Sexually Transmitted Infections

In 2006, in the United States, approximately 1 million adolescents and young adults aged 10 to 24 years were reported to have chlamydia, gonorrhea, or syphilis.[29] Also in the United States, 25% of females aged 15 to 19 years and 45% of those aged 20 to 24 years had evidence of infection with human papillomavirus during 2003 and 2004.[29] STIs are a variety of clinical syndromes and infections caused by pathogens that can be acquired and transmitted through sexual activity. Physicians and other HCPs play a critical role in preventing and treating STDs.[14,60] Table 17.1 provides general guidelines for the pharmacological interventions for STIs to assist ATs in advising and educating patients for the prevention and treatment of these reproductive conditions.

Reproductive and Urogenital Concerns

Women have pathologies relating to their menstrual, obstetric, or gynecologic histories, such as endometriosis, urinary tract infections, and osteoporosis. This section discusses erectile dysfunction, which affects men specifically, as well as kidney stones, which can occur in women but are more common in men. The AT generally serves as a health educator for the patient. Although the AT does not prescribe medication, she should have a general knowledge of common medications used to treat reproductive and urogenital concerns in advising patients about their conditions. Most importantly, the AT must be able to identify adverse effects of medications, recognize signs and symptom of adverse effects, and refer patients to their primary care provider or pharmacist.

Urinary Tract Infections

The urinary tract, which spans the kidneys to the urethral meatus, is normally sterile and resistant to bacterial colonization, despite frequent contamination of the distal urethra with bacteria from the colon and anus (*Escherichia coli*). The major defense against cystitis or urinary tract infection (UTI) is complete emptying of the bladder during urination. About 95% of UTIs occur when bacteria ascend the urethra to the bladder and ascend the ureter to the kidney (**acute pyelonephritis**).

Women are at greater risk of developing a UTI than men because of the short distance between the urethra and both the anus and the urethral opening to the bladder. Infection limited to the bladder can be painful and annoying; however, serious consequences can occur if a UTI spreads to the kidneys (kidney infection or acute pyelonephritis).[35,40] Sexual intercourse may lead to cystitis, but a person does not have to be sexually active to develop a UTI.

Prescribers typically treat UTIs with antibiotics.[35,40] Often, symptoms resolve within a few days of antibiotic treatment, most commonly with *trimethoprim* with *sulfamethoxazole* (Bactrim, Septra, others) or *nitrofurantoin* (Macrodantin, Macrobid). In some cases, the fluoroquinolones such as *ciprofloxacin* (Cipro) are necessary, but these are not commonly recommended. The patient may also be prescribed a pain medication (analgesic) that numbs the bladder and urethra to relieve burning experienced while urinating, but pain usually is relieved

TABLE 17.1 Sexually Transmitted Infections: Signs and Symptoms and Medications for Treatment

Pathogen: disease	Signs and symptoms	Medication options
Bacterial infections		
Chlamydia	Abdominal pain, dysuria, testicular pain, discharge from vagina or penis, dyspareunia for women	*azithromycin*, *erythromycin*, or *doxycycline*
Pelvic inflammatory disease (PID)	Spectrum of inflammatory disorders of the upper female genital tract,[31] including sexually transmitted bacteria, especially *N. gonorrhoeae* and *C. trachomatis*	IM *ceftriaxone* and oral *doxycycline* 100 mg BID for 2 weeks
Gonorrhea	Men: urethral infection that requires treatment as soon as it is experienced Women: asymptomatic infections or symptoms that do not present until there is a concurrent PID	*ceftriaxone* plus *doxycycline* or *azithromycin*
Syphilis	Common manifestations include genital ulcers, skin lesions, meningitis, aortic disease, and neurologic syndromes.	*penicillin*; *doxycycline* or *tetracycline* if allergic to *penicillin*
Trichomoniasis	Men: asymptomatic urinary tract infection Women: possibly asymptomatic or possible urethritis or cystitis; possible yellow-green vaginal discharge, soreness of vulva and perineum, dysuria, and **dyspareunia**	*metronidazole* or *tinidazole* 2 g
Viral infections		
Human papillomavirus (HPV)	Persistent infection with some HPV types can cause cancer and genital warts.	Vaccines are available to protect against many of the HPV strains that can cause genital warts and cancer.
Herpes simplex virus (HSV)	Small red bumps, blisters (vesicles), or open sores (ulcers) in the genital, anal, and nearby areas; pain or itching begins within a few weeks after exposure to an infected sexual partner.	Antivirals: *acyclovir*, *valacyclovir*, or *famciclovir*
Human immunodeficiency virus (HIV)	Acute retroviral syndrome develops in 50% to 90% of people within the first few weeks after they become infected with HIV; the syndrome is characterized by nonspecific symptoms, including fever, malaise, lymphadenopathy, and skin rash.	Antiviral treatment aims to suppress HIV replication by using combinations of ≥3 drugs; treatment can restore immune function in most patients if suppression of replication is sustained.

Based on Cachay (2019); Goje (2019); Morris (2019); Workowski (2015).

soon after starting an antibiotic.[40] For patients with troublesome **dysuria**, the AT should serve as a patient educator on prevention and treatment of UTI and refer the patient to the appropriate provider for examination and treatment, including possible prescription medication. *Phenazopyridine* (available OTC as 95 mg tablets or by prescription in 100 mg or 200 mg tablets) may help control symptoms until the antibiotics do (usually within 48 hours).

Osteoporosis and Osteopenia

Osteoporosis is a disease identified by low bone mass and structural deterioration of bone tissue (figure 17.3); **osteopenia** is a term that defines bone density that is abnormal but not as low as that seen in osteoporosis. Although osteoporosis is often associated with women, among men >50 years old, 4% to 6% are diagnosed with osteoporosis and 33% to 47% have osteopenia.[36] As of 2018, >53 million people in

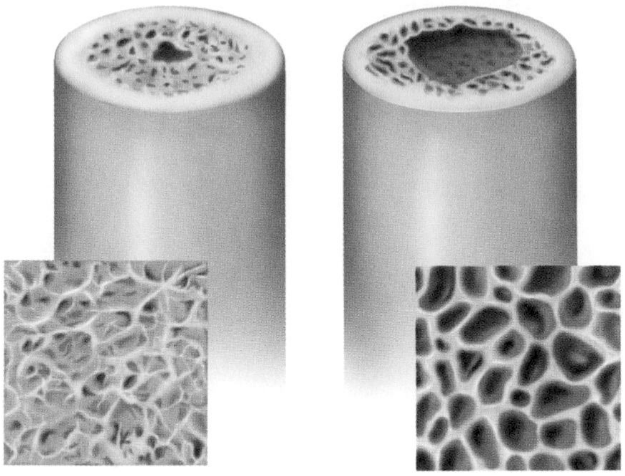

FIGURE 17.3 Normal and osteoporotic bone.

the United States have osteoporosis or are at risk of developing it due to low bone mass. Osteoporosis is considered a silent disease because patients are generally asymptomatic until sustaining a fracture, such as after a sudden fall.[53] Severe back pain, lost height, or spinal deformities such as kyphosis also are indicators of this disease.[41] Both exogenous and endogenous risk factors exist relative to the development of osteoporosis. Endogenous factors cannot be changed, whereas exogenous factors can be modified through various means.

The primary treatment options for osteoporosis include supplementation with vitamin D (described in chapter 19) and calcium, as well as specific prescription medications. The 2 categories of prescription medications for treating osteoporosis are as follows, based on the patient's history, images, presentation, and physician preference:

- **Bisphosphonates or RANK ligand inhibitors**—Medications such as *alendronate* (Fosamax) and *denosumab* (Prolia) are the common antiresorptive medication options that slow down osteoclast breakdown of bone to prevent bone loss and, subsequently, strengthen bones.[20]
- **Osteoanabolics**—Medications such as *teriparatide* (Forteo) produce rapid increases in bone formation and remodeling, which increases bone mass and improves bone microarchitecture.[37] *Teriparatide* is the only osteoanabolic approved by the FDA to treat osteoporotic men, and the results have paralleled postmenopausal women relative to reduction in vertebral fractures.[50] Patients taking *teriparatide* must supplement with vitamin D since this drug causes decreased vitamin D synthesis.

Off-label application of medications intended to treat osteoporosis have been suggested to treat bone marrow edema and stimulate fracture healing. Bone marrow edema is a symptom of an intra-articular or extra-articular bone contusion. Mobility of 64% of patients with bone marrow edema improved within 2 weeks of application of a bisphosphonate, and patients with an early diagnosis and rapid treatment had shortened time for return to activity. Also, case reports of athletes with metatarsal fracture nonunion have cited that *teriparatide* increased bone formation through stimulation of osteoblasts to optimize the healing process.[47] However, the benefits of treating bone edema and fracture healing with medications must be discussed with the patient and provider and balanced with the potential adverse effects of these medications.

Endometriosis and Endometritis

Endometriosis occurs when bits of the tissue that lines the uterus (endometrium) grow on other pelvic organs, such as the ovaries or fallopian tubes (figure 17.4). Outside the uterus, endometrial tissue thickens and bleeds, just as the normal endometrium does during the menstrual cycle.[43] **Endometritis** occurs when the uterine lining becomes inflamed from infection. Endometritis is likely to be a shorter-term condition that is easier to treat than endometriosis. Symptoms depend on the location of the tissue and may include dysmenorrhea, dyspareunia, infertility, dysuria, and pain during defecation. ATs need to be familiar with the signs, symptoms, and history of gynecological dysfunction and able to provide information and refer patients appropriately. Contemporary approaches to gynecological dysfunction include conservative surgical resection or ablation of endometriotic tissue, with or without drugs.[38] Pharmacological treatments for endometriosis suppress ovarian function to inhibit the growth and activity of endometriotic implants. The following are commonly used:[19,38]

- **Hormonal contraceptives**—These include cyclic or continuous methods, usually oral, such as birth control pills like *norethindrone*; injections like *medroxyprogesterone*; and patches and vaginal rings, which may slow disease progression.

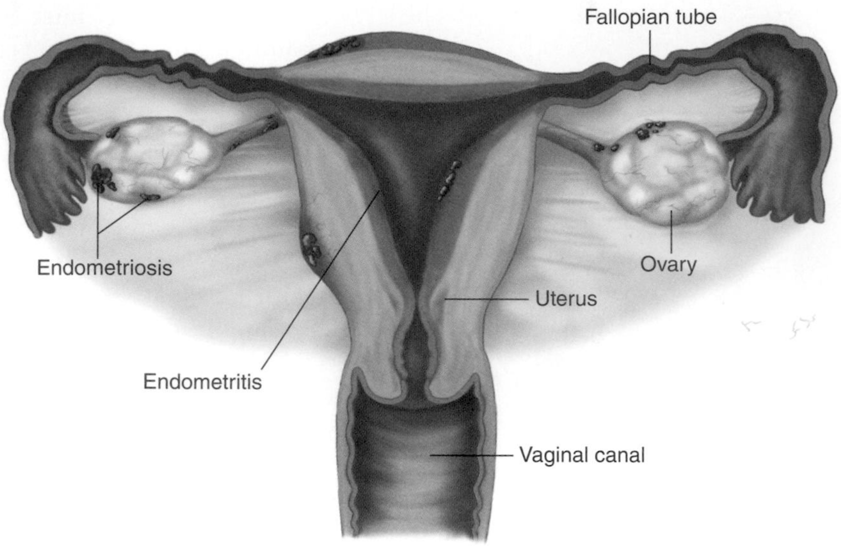

FIGURE 17.4 Endometriosis and endometritis.

- **NSAIDs**—Options include *ibuprofen* or *naproxen* for pain, which can be used with contraceptives for more moderate pain.
- **Gonadotropin-releasing hormone (GnRH) analogs**—These temporarily suppress estrogen production by the ovaries.
- **Cannabis**—Use may be helpful for some women.

Kidney Stones

Kidney stones (renal lithiasis, nephrolithiasis) are hard deposits (*calculi* is plural and *calculus* singular) made of minerals and salts that form inside the kidneys.[44] Calculi vary in size from microscopic crystalline foci to several centimeters in diameter. During passage, calculi may irritate the ureter and become lodged, obstructing urine flow and affecting renal function. Typically, a calculus must have a diameter >5 mm to become lodged; calculi ≤5 mm are likely to pass spontaneously. Severe pain, often accompanied by nausea and vomiting, usually occurs when calculi pass into the ureter and cause acute obstruction. Stones can cause fever, chills, and blood in the urine (**hematuria**).[44,55] Initial treatment is likely to be OTC pain relievers and NSAIDs; however, advance treatment of urinary calculi primarily involves analgesia for pain, including opioids such as *morphine* and, for a rapid onset, *fentanyl*. For persistent or infection-causing calculi, complete removal using primarily endoscopic techniques may be performed.[55]

Erectile Dysfunction

Erectile dysfunction (ED)—formerly called impotence—affects up to 20 million men in the United States. The prevalence of partial or complete ED is >50% in men aged 40 to 70 years and increases with age. The most common vascular cause of ED is atherosclerosis of cavernous arteries of the penis, often caused by smoking and diabetes. Atherosclerosis and aging decrease the capacity for dilation of arterial blood vessels and smooth muscle relaxation, limiting the amount of blood that can enter the penis. Diabetic neuropathy and surgical injury are particularly common causes of ED.[33]

Effective treatments are available for ED, many of which involve resolving underlying causes; however, the AT should have a general understanding of first-line treatment of ED, usually with an oral phosphodiesterase (PDE5) inhibitor. These include *sildenafil* (Viagra), *vardenafil* (Levitra), *tadalafil* (Cialis), and *avanafil* (Stendra). These treatments are less effective in men with neurological causes of impotence.[32,33] For men who have abnormally low levels of the hormone, testosterone replacement may enhance sexual desire, but will not improve ED.[32] The AT must inform the patient of the adverse effects of ED medications, including the potential for the following:[30]

- Decreased blood pressure
- **Priapism**
- Headaches

Evidence in Pharmacology

Viagra as a Performance-Enhancing Drug

Athletes have been reported to use ED medication as a performance-enhancing drug.[54] Unscientific reports in pop culture sources promote Viagra as an adjunct to a strength training regimen, spreading the idea that increased muscular blood flow will enhance the weightlifting pump. Also, there is the presumption that the nitrous oxide (NO) element of ED medications will be beneficial for muscle development.[30] A drug information database of self-reported information collected between 2006 and 2008 in the United Kingdom indicated that PDE 5i use was acknowledged on the same level as antibiotics, pain relievers, and alcohol.[54] Some benefit of PDE 5i may have been experienced by athletes in endurance sports.[15]

- Cardiac arrythmia
- Potential myocardial infarction secondary to lower blood pressure

Summary

This chapter discusses diseases, disorders, and conditions that affect the functioning of the male and female reproductive systems during all stages of life. It describes pharmacological treatment of some of the more common reproductive and sexual health considerations and conditions the AT encounters in a traditional AT setting. ATs do not need to be experts on all these topics, but as a primary care provider often treating healthy adolescents and young adults, they should be prepared to address questions related to contraception, including hormonal, oral, nonoral, and long-acting reversible methods as well as common barrier methods. Occasionally, depending on the patient and the setting, the AT may be asked about emergency contraception or provide information about exercising while pregnant. The AT should reassure these patients that their health information is confidential and refer them to the student health clinic, primary care provider, or gynecologist. Medications used in treating reproductive and genitourinary health conditions in this population are discussed, including STIs, UTIs, endometriosis, kidney stones, and erectile dysfunction.

Case Studies

Case Study 1

Al, an athlete at a local university, visited Mack, the director of a local gym where many clients are confirmed anabolic steroid users. Al wanted Mack's advice on getting bigger, but he wished to avoid steroids out of concern for positive drug test. Mack suggested a popular erectile dysfunction medication. He said it would increase Al's testosterone to stimulate muscle growth. Mack also said that the medication is available on various Internet sites and that Al would not need a physical exam to get the drug.

Questions for Analysis

1. Is an ED medication a viable anabolic agent that sidesteps a drug test? Why or why not?
2. Would it have been wise for Al to procure this medication without a prescription? Why or why not?

Case Study 2

Maria is a university first-year student who is living in the dorm and away from home for the first time. Midway through her first semester, Maria recognized an irregular schedule of her menstrual period to the point that she consulted with a student health physician. Maria was started on a low-estrogen birth control pill for treatment of her current situation as well as to prevent potential future menstrual concerns. Maria explained this to her mother, who was confused as to why this medication was prescribed and worried that it could promote promiscuous behavior.

Questions for Analysis

1. Is it common to use oral contraceptives for noncontraception purposes? Why or why not?
2. What future concerns could be minimized by using OCs?

Drugs and Medical Devices Described in This Chapter

Drug class	*generic* (pronunciation) Trade name	Therapeutic uses	Clinical concerns
Short-acting (oral) hormonal contraceptive options	[a]*ethinyl estradiol + norgestrel* (ETH in il ess tra DYE ol; nor JESS trel) Cryselle, many others	For the prevention of pregnancy in women who elect to use this product as a method of contraception 1 tablet PO once daily	Combination progestin and estrogen pill Correct and consistent use can result in low failure rates. Withdrawal bleeding usually occurs within 3 d after discontinuing active tablets.
	norethindrone (nor eth IN drone) Camila, many others	For the prevention of pregnancy in women who elect to use this product as a method of contraception 1 tablet PO once daily	Progestin-only birth control pills (mini pills); for use in patients who are breastfeeding or at high risk for blood clots
Short-acting (nonoral) hormonal contraceptive options	[a,b]*ethinyl estradiol + norelgestromin* (EH thi nil ESS tra DYE ol; nor ell JESS tro min) transdermal patch, Xulane	Apply 1 patch once a week (on the same day every week) for the first 3 wk, then use no patch in week 4 to allow menstruation (withdrawal bleeding). Repeat this each month.	Failure rate is 1% if used correctly; may be less effective in women who weigh >198 lbs (90 kg). May result in lighter periods and less cramping. Cost is roughly $100 to $150 USD per month, but insurance may cover. Can cause skin irritation. Stop use if pregnancy should occur.
	[b]*ethinyl estradiol + etonogestrel* (ETH in il es tra DYE ole; et oh noe JES trel) NuvaRing	Vaginal ring is inserted by patient and worn continuously for 3 weeks, then removed for 1 week to allow menses (withdrawal bleeding).	Failure rate is 1% if always used correctly. Prescription is required but no fitting is needed; do not use if pregnant. Use barrier method of contraception if ring is out for >3 continuous hr until a new ring has been used continuously for ≥7 d. Common side effects include vaginal infections, irritation, or secretion.

Drug class	*generic* (pronunciation) Trade name	Therapeutic uses	Clinical concerns
Long-acting reversible contraception	[c]*medroxyprogesterone* injection (me DROX ee proe JES ter one) Depo-Provera	Intramuscular injection of progestin-only hormone given every 13 wk	May lighten or eliminate menstrual periods. Failure rate <1% if used as directed. May initially cause irregular bleeding. Should not be used as a long-term birth control method (i.e., >2 yr) unless other birth control methods are considered inadequate.
	etonogestrel subdermal implant (e toe noe JES trel) Nexplanon Implant	Progestin-only implant. Health care provider inserts a match-sized rod under the skin of the upper arm. Implant should be replaced after 3 yr but may be removed at any time; do not use if pregnant.	Effective for 3 yr; <1% failure rate; not known if equally effective in very overweight women. May cause irregular periods initially; may lighten or eliminate periods.
	levonorgestrel-releasing intrauterine device (LEE voe nor jes trel) Skyla	Prevention of pregnancy for up to 3 yr Initially releases *levonorgestrel* ~14 mcg/d after 24 d, then rate subsequently decreases; mean release rate over 3 yr is *levonorgestrel* ~6 mcg/d.	Users may experience irregular bleeding; 6% will have amenorrhea after 1 yr. Insertion should be performed by a trained health care provider thoroughly familiar with the product and procedure.
	levonorgestrel-releasing intrauterine device (LEE voe nor jes trel) Mirena	Initially releases *levonorgestrel* 20 mcg/d, then rate subsequently decreases to half of that after 5 yr. Do not leave device in place for >5 yr.	Prevention of pregnancy for up to 5 yr.
	Copper intrauterine device Paragard	A single intrauterine copper contraceptive should be placed at the fundus of the uterine cavity.	Should be removed on or before 10 yr from the date of insertion.

[a]Smoking cigarettes while using ethinyl estradiol raises the chance of serious heart- and blood-related side effects. This chance is increased in women >35 years of age. It is also increased with the number of cigarettes smoked. It is strongly advised that patients taking these medications not smoke; these drugs should not be prescribed in women who smoke and are >35 years of age.

[b]Risk of venous thromboembolism (VTE) among women aged 15 to 44 who used the norelgestromin + ethinyl estradiol transdermal system compared to women who used several different oral contraceptives was assessed in 5 U.S. epidemiologic studies using electronic health care claims data. The relative risk estimates ranged from 1.2 to 2.2; 1 of the studies found a statistically significant increased relative risk of VTE for current users of the norelgestromin + ethinyl estradiol transdermal system.[49]

[c]Women who use Depo-Provera contraceptive injection may lose significant bone mineral density. Bone loss is greater with increasing duration of use and may not be completely reversible. It is unknown if use of Depo-Provera contraceptive injection during adolescence or early adulthood, a critical period of bone accretion, will reduce peak bone mass and increase the risk for osteoporotic fracture in later life.

Based on Anderson (2019); Casey (2018); Drugs.com. *Vasectomy* (2019); Drugs.com. *Essure* (2019); Food and Drug Administration (2019); WebMD.com. (2019).

18

Drugs for Treating Mental Health Conditions

OBJECTIVES

After reading this chapter, you will be able to do the following:

- Describe treatment for common mental health disorders
- Define commonly prescribed medications for mental health conditions
- Recognize conditions in which mental health disorders can be a secondary symptom

Select Drugs Mentioned in This Chapter

Drug class	Generic name	Trade name
Antidepressants		
Selective serotonin reuptake inhibitors (SSRIs)	*fluoxetine* *sertraline*	Prozac Zoloft
Norepinephrine and dopamine reuptake inhibitors (NDRIs)	*bupropion*	Wellbutrin
Anxiolytics (sedatives)		
Benzodiazepines	*diazepam*	Valium
Hypnotics		
Benzodiazepine-like medications	*zolpidem*	Ambien
Stimulants		
Dopamine reuptake inhibitors	*methylphenidate*	Ritalin
Mixed amphetamines	*amphetamine* and *dextroamphetamine*	Adderall
Drugs for treating substance use disorders		
Alcohol metabolism blocker	*disulfiram*	Antabuse

This list is not exhaustive, but rather contains drugs commonly encountered in the athletic training setting. Always consult up-to-date information, confirm with a pharmacist, or discuss the use of therapeutic medications with the prescriber of the medication.

Patients with mental health complaints or concerns or disordered behavior present in a variety of clinical settings, such as primary care and emergency department settings. Although these concerns are not recognized frequently in the sports medicine practice, athletic trainers (ATs) may encounter athletes with complaints or concerns that may be new or a continuation of a history of **mental health conditions.**[11] Athlete complaints may be related to direct or secondary effects of physical conditions, such as injury or concussion. When evaluating an athlete for a potential mental illness, the AT may have to focus on more immediate history, symptoms, and behavior to make a management decision.

Increasingly, sports medicine practitioners are treating patients with a diagnosed mental health challenge. Although the AT is not the primary mental health caregiver, he should recognize the signs and symptoms of common mental health conditions and be familiar with the range and purpose of medications for treating patients with these conditions. This text does not aim to provide specific medical advice, but rather to present information to help clinicians better understand mental health disorders and the therapeutic medications used to treat mental health conditions. The AT should always consult with a qualified health care provider for diagnosis, treatment, and management of a patient with a mental health condition. This chapter briefly describes the mental health disorders most commonly found in the physically active population and the medications often prescribed for these conditions.

Mental Health Conditions

The American Psychiatric Association Diagnostic and Statistical Manual of Mental Disorders, 5th edition (DSM-5),[1] defines a **mental disorder** as a syndrome characterized by a clinically significant disturbance in a patient's cognition, emotional regulation, or behavior that reflects a dysfunction in the psychological, biological, or developmental process underlying mental functioning. The definition further states that mental disorders are usually associated with significant distress or disability in social, occupational, or other important activities.[1]

Mental illnesses are common in the United States, with nearly 1 in 5 adults living with a mental illness (46.6 million in 2017). Mental illnesses include many different conditions that vary in degree of severity, ranging from mild to severe. Two broad categories can be used to describe these conditions: any mental illness (AMI) and serious mental illness (SMI). AMI encompasses all recognized mental illnesses and is defined as a mental, behavioral, or emotional disorder. See table 18.1 for a summary of AMIs and other common mental health conditions that ATs may encounter. SMI is a smaller and more severe subset of all mental illnesses, such as dissociative disorder, obsessive compulsive disorder, and personality disorders. SMIs are mental, behavioral, or emotional disorders that result in serious functional impairment that substantially interferes with or limits 1 or more major life activities.[11,26]

A variety of mental health professionals are qualified to assess, diagnose, and provide treatment for patients with mental health concerns. Their job titles, specialties, and scope of practice vary by state;[23] some have the authority to prescribe medications for the treatment of mental disorders. Mental health professionals often work in inpatient facilities, such as general hospitals and psychiatric facilities, as well as in outpatient facilities, such as community mental health clinics, schools, and private practices. Other professionals connected with this field include certified peer specialists, who are often (but not always) trained or certified to assist with recovery by providing support, mentoring, and guidance. ATs should refer patients to appropriately credentialed and licensed mental health professionals who have specialized expertise and training.

Several National Collegiate Athletic Association (NCAA) institutions have either incorporated a

Mental Health Professionals

With Prescribing Authority

- Psychiatrists (MD or DO)
- Psychiatric or mental health nurse practitioner (NP) or physician assistant (PA)
- Psychiatric pharmacists (PharmD)

Without Prescribing Authority

- Psychologists (PhD or PsyD)
- Counselors, clinicians, therapists (MS or MA)
- Clinical social workers (MSW)
- Pastoral counselors
- Sport psychologists

TABLE 18.1 Common Mental Health Conditions

Common mental disorders	Examples	Description	Treatment and common drugs
Mood disorders[9]	Major depressive disorder (MDD) Bipolar disorder	Emotional disturbances consisting of prolonged periods of excessive sadness, excessive joyousness, or both	Antidepressants Mood stabilizers Cognitive behavior therapy
Anxiety disorders[4]	Generalized anxiety disorder (GAD) Panic attack Panic disorder	Distressing, unpleasant emotional state of nervousness and uneasiness; can be anticipatory before a threat, persist after a threat has passed, or occur without an identifiable threat. Often accompanied by physical changes and behaviors like those caused by fear.	Initial support, cognitive behavior therapy Anxiolytics or sedatives (benzodiazepines) Antidepressants
Stressor-related disorders[5]	Post-traumatic stress disorder (PTSD) Acute stress disorder (ASD)	PTSD consists of intrusive recollections occurring within 4 wk of witnessing or experiencing an overwhelming traumatic event; to have PTSD, symptoms must last >1 mo.	Cognitive behavior therapy SSRIs or other antidepressants
Sleep or wakefulness disorders[28]	Insomnia	Neurological condition, not a mental illness. Difficulty falling or staying asleep, early awakening, or a sensation of unrefreshing sleep.	Hypnotics
Neurodevelopmental disorders[31]	Attention-deficit/hyperactivity disorder (ADD, ADHD)	Not considered a mental illness. Disorder marked by an ongoing pattern of inattention or hyperactivity and impulsivity that interferes with functioning or development.	Psychotherapy Stimulants Antidepressants
Eating disorders[3]	Anorexia nervosa Avoidant/restrictive food intake disorder (ARFID) Binge eating disorder Bulimia nervosa	Persistent disturbance of eating or behavior related to eating that alters consumption or absorption of food and significantly impairs physical health or psychosocial functioning	Intense psychiatric management Certain antidepressants
Substance-related disorders[18]	Substance use disorders (includes 10 classes of drugs and substances)	Pathologic pattern of behaviors in which patients continue to use a substance despite experiencing significant problems related to its use	Varies depending on substance and circumstances
Suicidal behavior and self-injury[8]	Suicidal ideation Nonsuicidal self-injury (NSSI)	Thinking about, considering, or planning suicide	Call police, EMS, or the National Suicide Prevention Lifeline Psychotherapy

full-time licensed counseling or clinical psychologist within the athletic medicine or academic services department or established a mechanism for student-athlete psychological referrals as needed.[7] Social workers (BA or BS) provide case management, inpatient discharge planning services, placement services, and other services to support healthy living. Pastoral counselors are clergy members with training in clinical pastoral education in diagnosing and providing counseling. Sports psychologists specialize in the study of how psychology influences sports, athletic performance, exercise, and physical activity. Sports psychologists may work with professional or elite athletes and coaches to improve performance, increase motivation, and help patients recover from injuries.

Behavioral Health Emergencies

Patients who are experiencing severe changes in mood, thoughts, or behavior or severe, potentially life-threatening adverse drug effects need urgent assessment and treatment. An AT must be able to identify when a patient's mood, thoughts, or behavior is highly unusual or disorganized and is required to report if she has determined that the patient is a threat to himself or others. A threat to self can include, but is not limited to, the following:

- Suicidal ideation or attempts
- **Self-neglect** or failure to attend to basic needs, including nutrition, shelter, and needed medication

As health care providers, ATs are also required to report patients who pose a threat to others—those who are actively violent (i.e., actively assaulting staff members, throwing and breaking things), those who appear belligerent and hostile (i.e., potentially violent), and those who do not appear threatening to the AT or staff members, but express **intent to harm** another person (e.g., spouse, neighbor, public figure). Danger to others includes the following:

- Expressing homicidal intent
- Placing others in peril
- Failing to provide for the needs or safety of dependents

When dealing with a patient who has expressed or indicated an intent or plan to harm herself or others or has attempted suicide, the AT should not attempt to determine the seriousness of the thought, gesture, or attempt. Nonspecialists, such as ATs, coaches, or teammates, are often the first people contacted in the prehospital or outpatient setting and are mandated to immediately report such cases to the emergency department, team physician, or other emergency response service (see Clinical Application sidebar).[12] Most college campuses have a counseling center staff member who can offer guidance or referral, and many counseling centers offer walk-in or emergency services.[19]

Clinical Application

Mandatory Reporting

In most jurisdictions, knowledge of intent to commit suicide requires the AT to act immediately to prevent the suicide by calling either 911 to notify the police or the National Suicide Prevention Lifeline (in the United States, 1-800-273-8255). ATs are also mandatory reporters for patients posing a threat to others or indicating intent to harm. The AT is required to notify security or the police.

The AT must ensure that a suicidal patient is not left alone. A coach or other staff member may stay with the patient during transport to an on-campus counseling center or until a mental health evaluation has been completed.

For patients who may have overdosed on recreational, OTC, or prescription drugs or other substances, ATs should activate EMS by calling either 911 or the American Association of Poison Control Centers at 1-800-222-1222.

Treatment Options for Mental Health Disorders

Treatment of mental health disorders is multifaceted. In some cases, long-term conditions require years of treatment. Unfortunately, the delay between the onset of symptoms and treatment of mental health conditions can exceed 10 years.[26] Complicating the issue is that 2 different patients with the same diagnosis may present with differing symptoms or respond differently to the same medication. Pharmacological intervention is a key component of mental health disorders care but is not the only treatment regimen available to prescribers.

Initial Support

For mental disorders, in addition to referral to an appropriate mental health professional, the AT may need to provide initial support while gathering assistance from the health care team. Until a full evaluation, diagnosis, treatment, and improvement are initiated, the AT may need to check in on patients daily or weekly to provide support and education and monitor progress. While monitoring the patient's progress and noting any difficulties with treatment, with permission, the AT can be an important liaison between the patient and the prescriber.

Psychotherapy

Psychotherapy involves working with a therapist to reduce symptoms of a variety of mental health concerns. The aim of psychotherapy is to help a person cope with painful memories and manage emotional and physical reactions to stress. A variety of techniques can be helpful.[25] Regardless of the technique used, education about human responses to trauma is valuable. Psychotherapy and education can help family members understand the patient's mental disorder and cope with its effects.

Mood Disorders

A **mood disorder** is characterized by prominent and prolonged disturbances of mood that are generally inappropriate to the person's life situation; depression and mania are considered the primary syndromes. Symptoms could include insomnia, suicidal thoughts, anorexia, and feelings of being a burden to others in people with depression and euphoria, irritability, decreased need for sleep, and hyperactivity in people with mania.[4] Cases of intense sadness are termed **depression**, and intense elation is termed mania. **Depressive disorders** are characterized by depression; bipolar disorders are characterized by varying combinations of depression and mania. Depression and bipolar disorder are the most common mood disorders encountered by the AT in the sports medicine setting.

Drugs for Treating Mood Disorders: Antidepressants

Mood disorders are treated by several drugs in different categories, including antidepressants and mood stabilizers. An antidepressant is a medication that can help relieve the symptoms of depression and other mood disorders. Antidepressants help to relieve the symptoms of depression such as low mood, irritability, feelings of worthlessness, restlessness, anxiety, and difficulty in sleeping. Distinct differences exist between the various classes of antidepressants available because they have different mechanisms of action. In addition to depression, certain antidepressants may also be used to treat a range of other conditions.[3,21]

Antidepressants are classified into different types depending on their chemical structure and mechanism of action. At least 7 categories of antidepressant exist,[21,29] including the following:

- **Selective serotonin reuptake inhibitors (SSRIs)**—These medications increase levels of serotonin in the brain by preventing its reuptake by the nerves. Common examples of SSRIs are *fluoxetine* (Prozac) and *sertraline* (Zoloft).
- **Norepinephrine and dopamine reuptake inhibitors (NDRIs)**—These medications block the reuptake of norepinephrine and dopamine, increasing the concentration of these 2 neurotransmitters in the nerve synapse. An example of an NDRI is *bupropion* (Wellbutrin).

SSRIs, the most commonly prescribed antidepressant, are widely accepted as a first-line medication

Evidence in Pharmacology

Concussion and Depression

Retired American football players who sustain concussions while playing are more likely to present with depression symptoms than players who have not been concussed. Symptoms may be summarized as common medical disorders, such as anxiety, depression, and sleep disturbances.[15] Antidepressants are a viable treatment option, although psychotherapy may be preferred. An SSRI is likely to be a first-line medication; if a change is necessary, a serotonin–norepinephrine reuptake inhibitor (SNRI) would be next, although tricyclic antidepressants (TCAs) could also be considered.[29] When treating patients 48 hours after they had sustained a concussion, sports medicine physicians prescribed tricyclic antidepressants 46% of the time and SSRIs 24% of the time.[30]

for depression and are generally not addictive.[21] When taken at the recommended dosage, antidepressants are considered safe. However, some SSRIs have been associated with severe side effects, some of which are potentially fatal. Women reported more psychiatric adverse reactions than men did (71% to 24%, respectively), and they are more prone to an allergic reaction to an SSRI than are men.[10] Patients may experience an increase in suicidal thoughts and behaviors when taking SSRIs, particularly people under the age of 25 years. This effect is most likely to occur when starting the drug therapy. There is also an increased risk of seizures in people with a history of seizures.[13]

When patients abruptly discontinue or interrupt antidepressant therapy, they may experience **discontinuation syndrome**. Symptoms arising may vary with each antidepressant medication, but commonly include nausea, sweating, chills, tremors, paresthesia, **somnolence**, and sleep disturbances (e.g., vivid dreams, insomnia).[13] Patients should be closely monitored for clinical worsening and emergence of suicidal thoughts and behaviors. Mental health professionals should advise families and caregivers such as ATs to closely observe the patient and communicate with the prescriber.

One complication with antidepressant use is **serotonin syndrome**, a potentially life-threatening condition that can occur when 2 antidepressants are taken simultaneously.[21] Serotonin syndrome is caused by excessive levels of serotonin in the body and is more likely to occur with higher dosages of SSRIs or when SSRIs are administered with other medications that also release serotonin or block its reuptake. Symptoms include agitation, hyperthermia, clonus, confusion, sweating, tremor, hypertonia, hyperreflexia, and a rapid heart rate.[13] Additionally, excess serotonin can occur when antidepressants are administered in conjunction with the nutritional supplement St. John's wort (see Red Flag sidebar).[21]

RED FLAG

Unintended Drug–Drug Interaction

St. John's wort is a plant that grows in the wild and has been used to treat depression for centuries.[24] The herb is a nutritional supplement sold in various retail and digital marketplaces. Unintended consequences could occur if a patient takes St. John's wort concurrently with some sedatives or hypnotics (e.g., benzodiazepines) because the herb can induce the metabolism of these drugs to the point that it can compromise the medication's effectiveness if taken simultaneously.[20] Also, St. John's wort can increase the serotonin level, which places the patient at risk of developing serotonin syndrome, especially when the herb is taken concomitantly with other medications that cause serotonin syndrome, such as SSRIs.

Anxiety Disorders

Anxiety disorders are among the most prevalent psychiatric conditions worldwide.[1] Generalized anxiety disorder (GAD), panic attack, and panic disorders are anxiety disorders that cause nightmares, obsessive thoughts, and a fear of leaving one's house (see the sidebar). **Anxiety** refers to the presence of fear or apprehension that is out of proportion to the situation.

Drugs for Treating Anxiety Disorders: Anxiolytics or Sedatives

Anxiolytics or **sedatives** are central nervous system agents that relieve anxiety, aid sleep, or have a calming effect. The main class of anxiolytic and sedative drugs are the **benzodiazepines** (or "benzos"), although >20 benzodiazepine derivatives exist and some can be all 3: anxiolytics, sedatives, and hypnotics.[14] Other anxiolytic drugs include the SSRIs, SNRIs, tricyclic antidepressants, and other medications that may be prescribed off-label. These drugs are often preferred over benzodiazepines for anxiety because they are unlikely to cause dependence; however, they may not work as quickly as benzodiazepines and may initially worsen anxiety.[14] Discontinuation of benzodiazepines has caused symptoms to worsen and is sometimes fatal; thus, extreme caution should be exercised when these medications are used. Overdose of benzodiazepines can be lethal.[25] The following list highlights benzodiazepines (the *-ams*) that have been approved to treat mental health conditions:[14,25]

- Anxiety disorders: *diazepam* (Valium), *lorazepam* (Ativan)
- Panic disorder: *alprazolam* (Xanax)

These medications carry a risk of addiction that may limit their long-term use; the most common side effects of benzodiazepines are related to their

Common Anxiety Disorders

- **Agoraphobia**—A type of anxiety disorder in which the patient fears and often avoids wide open spaces or uncontrolled social conditions that might cause panic and make him feel trapped, helpless, or embarrassed.
- **Anxiety disorder**—A chronic condition characterized by an excessive and persistent sense of apprehension and stress and physical symptoms, such as sweating and palpitations.
- **Generalized anxiety disorder (GAD)**—A disorder characterized by excessive or unrealistic anxiety about ≥2 aspects of life (e.g., work, social relationships, financial matters), often accompanied by symptoms such as palpitations, shortness of breath, or dizziness. It often occurs along with other anxiety disorders or depression.
- **Panic disorder**—Repeated episodes of sudden feelings of intense anxiety and fear or terror that reach a peak within minutes (panic attacks).
- **Social anxiety disorder (social phobia)**—Involves high levels of anxiety, fear, and avoidance of social situations due to feelings of embarrassment, self-consciousness, and concern about being judged or viewed negatively by others.

sedating and muscle-relaxing action and include drowsiness, dizziness, and decreased alertness and concentration. With benzodiazepines, care must be taken not to overdose because they can cause dangerous deep unconsciousness. When combined with other central nervous system depressants, such as alcohol and opioids, the potential for toxicity and fatal overdose increases.[14]

Stressor-Related Disorders

Post-traumatic stress disorder (PTSD), a serious stressor-related disorder, involves distressing symptoms that occur after 1 or more frightening incidents or traumatic events that affects a person's ability to function normally at home, at work, or in social situations. The DSM-5 describes a person with PTSD as one who has personally experienced or witnessed a traumatic event. The person may also have learned about violence to a close loved one. The event must have involved serious physical injury or the threat of serious injury or death. **Acute stress disorder (ASD)** is an anxiety response with some form of reexperiencing of or reactivity to the traumatic event; symptoms develop within the first month after a traumatic event.[1]

Treatment of Stressor-Related Disorders

In addition to various psychotherapeutic interventions that are recommended for the treatment of stressor-related disorders in at-risk people, several psychopharmacology recommendations exist. For acute stress disorder, SSRIs and other antidepressants are reasonable clinical interventions for the following reasons:[21]

- Effective treatments for psychiatric disorders that are frequently comorbid with PTSD (e.g., depression, panic disorder, social phobia, and obsessive-compulsive disorder)
- May reduce clinical symptoms (such as suicidal, impulsive, and aggressive behaviors) that often complicate the management of PTSD
- Have relatively few side effects

RED FLAG

Treating PTSD With SSRIs

Military veterans returning from combat may have comorbidities of physical and emotional dysfunction. Conservative management of these physical conditions could include opioid therapy, and some patients may need surgery while using a SSRI to manage depression. Concurrent administration of surgical anesthesia and pain management medications could lead to serotonin syndrome, an adverse reaction that causes excessive serotonergic receptor activity in the central and peripheral nervous systems. This reaction enhances the depression symptoms secondary to PTSD.[27] ATs must understand the comorbidities and polypharmacy involved in this type of case and advocate for other pain management options when a patient must undergo anesthesia.

Sleep or Wakefulness Disorders

Almost half of all people in the United States report sleep-related problems. Although they are technically a neurological condition, sleep disorders are treated with drugs used for mental health conditions. Disordered sleep can cause emotional disturbance, memory difficulty, poor motor skills, decreased work efficiency, and increased risk of traffic accidents. It can even contribute to cardiovascular disorders and mortality. The most commonly reported sleep disorders are the following:[28]

- **Insomnia**—Difficulty falling or staying asleep, early awakening, or a sensation of unrefreshing sleep.
- **Excessive daytime sleepiness (EDS)**—The tendency to fall asleep during normal waking hours.
- **Sleep apnea**—Episodes of partial or complete closure of the upper airway that occur during sleep and lead to breathing cessation (defined as a period of apnea or hypopnea >10 sec).
- **Parasomnias**—Abnormal sleep-related events (e.g., night terrors, sleepwalking).

Drugs for Treating Sleep or Wakefulness Disorders: Hypnotics

Hypnotics are prescribed for patients who need rapid relief and who have insomnia with daytime effects, such as EDS and fatigue. In most cases, these drugs must not be used indefinitely. Hypnotics differ primarily in elimination half-life and onset of action. Drugs with a short half-life are used for sleep-onset insomnia; an example is low-dose *zolpidem* (Ambien), which has a very short duration of action and can be taken in the middle of the night during a nocturnal awakening as long as patients stay in bed for ≥4 hours after use. Drugs with a longer half-life are useful for both sleep-onset and sleep maintenance insomnia. Examples of hypnotic medications include the following:[28]

- *zolpidem* (Ambien)
- *zaleplon* (Sonata)
- *eszopiclone* (Lunesta)

Patients who experience daytime sedation, incoordination, or other daytime effects should avoid activities that require alertness (e.g., driving, contact sports), and the prescriber should adjust the dose or stop the use of the drug. Other adverse effects include amnesia, hallucinations, incoordination, and falls, which are a significant risk when taking hypnotics.[28]

Neurodevelopmental Disorders: Attention-Deficit/Hyperactivity Disorder

Attention-deficit/hyperactivity disorder (ADHD) is a persistent pattern of inattention or hyperactivity and impulsivity that interferes with functioning or development.[1] ADHD is not as clearly defined or diagnosed in adults as it is in children, but it presents as a combination of problems relative to attention span or impulsive behavior, among other traits. Adult ADHD can lead to low self-esteem and poor work performance and may interfere with daily functioning and maintaining stable relationships.[22] Adults who have been diagnosed with ADHD also present with comorbidities; 30% to 50% also have depression and 40% to 60% have anxiety.[17]

Drugs for Treating Attention-Deficit/Hyperactivity Disorder

Treatment of ADHD can involve medication and psychotherapy. For adults with ADHD, the pharmacological approach involves stimulants and nonstimulants that are available in a variety of different formulations, including patches and extended-release products. The stimulant approach for adults has a 70% to 80% response rate, and the medication alleviates difficulties with attention span, impulse behavior, hyperactivity, and restlessness. Side effects of oral formulations include insomnia, weight loss, and nervousness. In addition to some nonstimulant options, the primary pharmacological interventions for ADHD include the following stimulants:[17]

- **NDRIs**—*Methylphenidate* (Ritalin) is historically the first line of treatment; it is absorbed rapidly and has a first-pass hepatic metabolism.
- **Mixed amphetamine salts**—*Amphetamine* and *dextroamphetamine* (Adderall), *dextroamphetamine* (Dexedrine, ProCentra, Zenzedi), and *lisdexamfetamine* (Vyvanse) are CNS stimulants that affect the chemicals in the brain and nerves that contribute to hyperactivity and impulse control.

Eating Disorders

Eating disorders involve a persistent disturbance of eating or behavior related to eating that alters the consumption or absorption of food and significantly impairs physical health or psychosocial functioning.[3] Disordered eating is best conceptualized along a continuum of pathogenic eating and weight control behaviors that encompass a full spectrum of clinical and subclinical classifications. For the purposes of this discussion, *disordered eating* is the preferred term when reference is made to the entire spectrum of abnormal behaviors, whereas the term *eating disorders* is preferred when there is a definite clinical classification of abnormal behaviors.[6]

Treatment of Eating Disorders

The National Athletic Trainers' Association (NATA) provides guidelines for creating the necessary team infrastructure, collaborative relationships, and strategies for preventing, detecting, and managing patients with disordered eating.[2,3,6]

ATs should have knowledge of the psychotropic medications that are commonly prescribed to treat the symptoms that accompany eating disorders, including their potential side effects. They should also be able to recognize symptoms of missed doses or overdose.[6] In general, treatment of anorexia nervosa may require life-saving short-term intervention to restore body weight. Outpatient treatments may include varying degrees of support and supervision and commonly involve a team of practitioners. Once nutritional, fluid, and electrolyte status have been stabilized, long-term treatment begins. Outpatient psychologic therapy is the cornerstone of treatment. Intervention and treatment should continue for a full year after weight is restored. Medications for **anorexia nervosa** include antidepressants to treat persistent depression or anxiety following weight restoration.[2] Results are best in adolescents who have had the disorder <6 months.[2,3]

For **bulimia nervosa**,[2,3] in addition to the psychotherapy treatment options previously mentioned, medications are helpful for depression, anxiety, obsessions, and certain impulse disorder symptoms, as well as for patients with a suboptimal response to appropriate psychosocial therapy. Prescribers may consider SSRIs, which have the most evidence for efficacy and the fewest difficulties with adverse effects. Dosages may need to be higher than those used to treat depression (e.g., 60-80 mg/day of *fluoxetine*). Typical side effects include insomnia, nausea, **asthenia**, and sexual side effects.[2]

Substance-Related Disorders

Substance use disorders involve a pathologic pattern of behaviors in which patients continue to use a substance despite experiencing significant problems related to its use. There may also be phys-

Classes of Addictive Substances

Classification of substances involved in substance use disorder is not based on whether a drug is legal (e.g., alcohol, caffeine), illegal (e.g., hallucinogens), or available by prescription (e.g., *morphine*, *lorazepam*). Addictions to substances in these different classes are presented as separate disorders, but they are not fully distinct because all drugs taken in excess activate the brain's reward circuitry and their co-occurring use is common. The classes of addictive substances are as follows:[1,18]

- Alcohol
- Caffeine
- Cannabis
- Hallucinogens (e.g., LSD, phencyclidine [PCP], psilocybin)
- Inhalants of volatile hydrocarbons (e.g., paint thinner, certain glues)
- Opioids (e.g., *fentanyl*, *morphine*, *oxycodone*)
- Sedatives, hypnotics, and anxiolytics (e.g., *diazepam*, *lorazepam*)
- Stimulants (e.g., *amphetamine*, *methamphetamine*, *methylphenidate*, *cocaine*)
- Tobacco
- Other (e.g., anabolic steroids)

iologic manifestations, including changes in brain circuitry. The common terms *addiction*, *abuse*, and *dependence* are too loosely and variably defined to be very useful in systematic diagnosis; *substance use disorder* is more comprehensive and has fewer negative connotations.[16,18] Substance-related disorders involve drugs that directly activate the brain's reward system, which typically causes feelings of pleasure; the specific pleasurable feelings evoked vary widely depending on the drug. These drugs are divided into 10 different classes (see sidebar) that have different, although not completely distinct, pharmacologic mechanisms. Drugs in these classes vary in how likely they are to cause a substance use disorder. The likelihood is termed *addiction liability* and depends on a combination of factors:[18]

- Route of administration
- Rate at which the drug crosses the blood-brain barrier and stimulates the reward pathway
- Time to onset of effect
- Ability to induce tolerance or withdrawal symptoms

Treatment of Substance Use Disorders

Treatment of substance use disorders varies depending on the substance and the circumstances. Different treatment phases may be managed with drugs, counseling and support, or a combination of the two.[18] Formulation and implementation of a treatment plan involves using specific pharmacological and psychosocial treatments in the context of an organized treatment program that combines different treatment modalities. In addition to psychosocial treatments (e.g., behavioral therapy, 12-step facilitation, group therapy), pharmacological treatments may be helpful for select patients. Therapeutic medications may be used to decrease or eliminate withdrawal symptoms in an effort to reduce craving and risk of relapse. Prescribers may consider use of medications such as the following:[16]

- ***disulfiram*** **(Antabuse)**—Discourages alcohol use by the patient's knowledge of its unpleasant drug–drug interaction.
- ***naltrexone*** **(Vivitrol, ReVia)**—Decreases alcohol craving, presumably through the antagonistic effects of kappa-opioid receptors in mediating the reinforcing effects of alcohol.
- ***acamprosate*** **(Campral)**—Promotes abstinence from alcohol use by decreasing neuronal hyperexcitability.
- ***bupropion*** **(Wellbutrin)**—Decreases nicotine craving and the urge to smoke.
- ***methadone***—Reduces withdrawal symptoms from opioid use disorder (discussed in chapter 8).

Summary

Mental health disorders affect a significant percentage of the population; in addition to treatment options such as initial support and psychotherapy, pharmacological interventions are an effective approach for many patients. Sports medicine practitioners may have patients who have been prescribed these medications following a concussion or secondary to an athletic injury that led to depression or anxiety. These patients or others exhibiting signs or symptoms of mental health disorders or a behavioral emergency should be appropriately referred to a mental health professional. A plethora of medications treat mental health conditions such as mood disorders. In some cases, patients may need multiple medications; in other cases, patients with similar diagnoses will respond differently to the same medication. Risks are associated with these medications for mental health disorders, and providers must monitor patients. ATs should be aware of the black box warnings relating to suicidality and antidepressant drugs as well as the risk of misuse and abuse of amphetamines.

Case Studies

Case Study 1

Frank is a very successful and highly driven stockbroker. The emotional volatility associated with this line of work caused him to seek out medical assistance for anxiety. Frank was prescribed the antianxiety medication Xanax by his family practice physician. While rushing to get to work, Frank stepped on a crack in the sidewalk, fell, and sustained a compound fracture of his ulna and radius. In his frustration and pain, Frank did not give a full accounting of his medical health at the emergency department and forgot to inform HCPs that he was taking Xanax. Frank underwent an open reduction internal fixation of his fractures and was prescribed a combination of *hydrocodone* and *acetaminophen* for his postsurgical pain.

Questions for Analysis

1. Could the combination of the antianxiety medication and pain reliever be problematic?
2. What pharmacological options are available for Frank's postsurgical care?

Case Study 2

Irma is a 5th year senior and All-American gymnast who has missed an entire season due to depression. Over the past year, she had academic problems, grieved the death of a close friend, and developed an eating disorder, all of which led her into depression and forced her to miss the competitive season. She has been under the care of the institution's psychiatrist, who prescribed Zoloft approximately 4 months previously. Irma felt that her depression was improving. She recently resumed practice with the team and sustained a knee injury, which resulted in a torn anterior cruciate ligament and lateral meniscus. She needs surgery approximately 3 weeks after the injury that will involve reconstruction of the anterior cruciate ligament and repair of the lateral meniscus; this will cause her to miss her final season.

Questions for Analysis

1. What should the orthopedic surgeon know about the medication Irma takes for her mental health?
2. What accommodations should the orthopedic surgeon make for Irma's antidepressant?

Drugs Discussed in This Chapter

Drug class	*generic* (pronunciation) Trade name	Therapeutic uses	Clinical concerns
Antidepressants: selective serotonin reuptake inhibitors (SSRIs)	*fluoxetine* (floo OX e teen) Prozac	For depression: Doses > 20 mg/d may be given in divided doses (i.e., in the morning and at noon). The full effect may be delayed until after ≥4 wk of treatment.	Used to treat major depressive disorder (MDD), bulimia nervosa, obsessive-compulsive disorder, panic disorder, and premenstrual dysphoric disorder (PMDD).
Norepinephrine and dopamine reuptake inhibitors (NDRIs)	*bupropion* (byoo PRO pee on) Wellbutrin	Doses of IR oral tablets should be given ≥6 hr apart, SR oral tablets should be given ≥8 hr apart, and ER oral tablets should be given ≥24 hr apart.	May be also used to treat seasonal affective disorder and aid in smoking cessation.
Anxiolytics (sedatives): benzodiazepines	*diazepam* (dye AZ e pam) Valium	Oral: 2 to 10 mg orally 2 to 4 times daily	Used for anxiety, sedation, alcohol withdrawal, muscle spasm, and seizure disorders.

(continued)

Drugs Described in This Chapter *(continued)*

Drug class	*generic* (pronunciation) Trade name	Therapeutic uses	Clinical concerns
Hypnotics: nonbenzodiazepines	*zolpidem* (zole PI dem) Ambien CR, Intermezzo (sublingual)	Oral at bedtime: 6.25-12.5 mg CR delivers half the dose immediately and half the dose 4 hr later. 1.75-3.5 mg lasts 4 hr for middle of the night awakening.	Effective for sleep-onset insomnia only. May cause a severe allergic reaction.
Stimulants	*methylphenidate* (METH il FEN i date) Ritalin	For treatment of attention-deficit/hyperactivity disorder (ADHD)	**Warning:** Has high potential for abuse and dependence. This is a mild CNS stimulant that blocks the reuptake of norepinephrine and dopamine and stimulates the brain in a manner similar to amphetamines. Common side effects are insomnia, nausea, headache, vomiting, decreased appetite, and dry mouth.
Drugs for treating substance use disorders	*disulfiram* (dye SUL fi ram) Antabuse	Used together with behavior modification, psychotherapy, and counseling support to help the patient stop drinking alcohol.	Produces very unpleasant side effects (severe nausea and vomiting) when combined with alcohol in the body.

CR = controlled release; IR = immediate release; SR = sustained release; ER = extended release

19

Drugs and Supplements to Enhance Performance

OBJECTIVES

After reading this chapter, you will be able to do the following:

- Explain the FDA approval process for supplements intended to treat or cure health conditions
- Describe supplements and performance-enhancing drugs that athletes may be tempted to use
- Advise athletes about banned and potentially illegal substances
- Use appropriate resources (pharmacist, prescriber, Natural Medicines Database) to provide information to athletes about supplements used for treating musculoskeletal or neurological conditions
- Describe how athletes might manipulate approved medications to enhance performance

Select Supplements Mentioned in This Chapter

Drug class	Examples
Performance-enhancing drugs	Anabolic-androgenic steroids (*testosterone*) Human growth hormone (hGH) Creatine monohydrate (Cr)
Supplements for treating skeletal conditions	Glucosamine and chondroitin sulfate Omega-3 fatty acids Vitamin D Cannabinoids (*marijuana*)
Manipulation of approved medications to enhance performance	Erythropoietin (EPO) Beta-blockers
Stimulants	*ma huang*, *ephedra*, *ephedrine*, and *pseudoephedrine*

This list is not exhaustive, but includes supplements and performance-enhancing drugs commonly encountered in the athletic training setting. Always consult up-to-date information, confirm with a pharmacist, or discuss the use of therapeutic medications with the prescriber of the medication.

Products that claim to prevent, treat, or cure health conditions such as Alzheimer's disease, diabetes, and cancer are being illegally marketed as new drugs. The claims of these products, many of which are marketed as dietary supplements, have not been proven, nor have the products been approved by the U.S. Food and Drug Administration (FDA). To help ensure that supplements are safe and effective for their intended medical use, products intended to treat any health condition must gain FDA approval before being sold to consumers. A new dietary ingredient (NDI) notification allows the FDA to evaluate the safety of a new ingredient before it becomes available to consumers.

Athletes use nutritional and dietary supplements to enhance both general nutrition and performance. Since the era of Roman gladiators, athletes have ingested herbs with the hope of gaining a competitive edge.[3] A 2009 study illustrated this commitment to win: 52% of a cohort of competitive athletes indicated that they would take a drug guaranteeing success even if it resulted in their death within the next 5 years.[4] Conversely, some rationale may exist for use of nutritional supplements for injury care. Some supplements used primarily for ergogenic purposes cross over to treat medical conditions that may not be associated with athletic ability. This chapter focuses on the supplements and **performance-enhancing drugs (PEDs)** that athletes may be tempted to use. The AT should have a working knowledge of banned and potentially illegal substances.

Clinical Application

An Emergency Medical Situation Caused by a Supplement

Tom Gugliotta, a skilled professional basketball player, was looking for a product to help him sleep after games. He found *gamma-butyrolactone* (GBL), which was marketed on the Internet as a sleep aid that enhances muscle recovery. Following a game, Tom added 5 mL of GBL to a drink. Soon after, he had a seizure and nearly stopped breathing on the team bus before it left the arena. Tom received immediate care from emergency personnel and was subsequently hospitalized.[15] What Tom didn't know was that GBL converts to *gamma-hydroxybutyrate* (GHB), the date rape drug, which can be lethal. *Gamma-butyrolactone* was eventually removed by the FDA, partly because of this situation.

Substances Banned for Competition

Although many nutritional supplements are used for general health, some athletes use them to become bigger, faster, or stronger. Much of the ergogenic-related substance abuse of supplements pertains to those that enhance performance through strength development. An athlete, by accident or design, might indulge in a substance that is banned by the various agencies that oversee performance-enhancing drugs. The World Anti-Doping Agency (WADA) is the primary agency that has developed a list of banned substances that may give athletes a competitive edge or enhance their performance. This list, which is reviewed annually, outlines the substances that disrupt the level field of competition and serves as an international standard.[7]

The United States Anti-Doping Agency (USADA) is the domestic governing body that oversees American competitions that subscribe to drug testing to prevent or detect doping. Most major competitive sports leagues in the United States subscribe to all or part of the WADA philosophy and use their model of banned substances for their respective competitors.

WADA Prohibited Substance List

The banned substance list is divided into the following categories (additional details in chapter 21):[7]

Substances Prohibited at All Times

- Nonapproved substances
- Anabolic agents
- Peptide hormones, growth factors, and related substances
- Beta-2-agonists
- Hormone and metabolic modulators
- Diuretics and other masking agents

Substances Prohibited During Competition

- Stimulants
- Narcotics
- Cannabinoids
- Corticosteroids

Substances Prohibited in Particular Sports

- Alcohol
- Beta-blockers

Supplements for Enhancing Musculoskeletal Performance

This section describes supplements and PEDs that are commonly used by athletes and other physically active people to facilitate muscle hypertrophy and strength, including **anabolic-androgenic steroids** (AAS), human growth hormone (hGH), and creatine monohydrate (Cr).

Anabolic-Androgenic Steroids

Anabolic steroids gained popularity following the 1954 world weightlifting championships and expanded to other international competitions during the 1960s.[20] In 1972, male and female athletes from the German Democratic Republic (the former country East Germany), who did particularly well in strength-dependent events, were purported to have used anabolic steroids. In 2004, the United States Drug Enforcement Administration (DEA) enacted the Anabolic Steroid Control Act, which defines *anabolic steroid* as any drug or hormonal substance that is chemically and pharmacologically related to testosterone (other than estrogens, progestins, corticosteroids, and dehydroepiandrosterone). The legislation revised the definition of anabolic steroids for inclusion in the class of Schedule III controlled substances by eliminating the requirement that an AAS improve muscle growth. It lists 59 specific substances as anabolic steroids, including the following:[6]

- *testosterone*
- *androstenediol*
- *norandrostenedione*

Despite contemporary protocols for drug testing and education, anabolic steroid use has been prevalent in elite international, professional, and intercollegiate sports. A review of WADA-approved laboratories indicated that 45% of all 2006 drug tests were positive for anabolic steroids.[24] In 2012, the National Athletic Trainers' Association (NATA) considered it vital that sports medicine practitioners understand the nature of AAS and recommended that these practitioners serve as resources of accurate and reliable information regarding the effect of anabolic steroids on health.[23] The risks and benefits of AAS use are well documented. However, despite the potential for adverse events, anabolic steroid use to enhance performance or for cosmetic purposes remains a common, if clandestine, activity. Use is influenced by athletes' sense of invulnerability and advice received from other athletes, popular literature, and steroid gurus.[24]

The FDA classifies AAS as Schedule III drugs, acknowledging that these steroids carry a moderate to low risk of physical and psychological dependence.[9,23] Anabolic steroids are manufactured derivatives of testosterone, the endogenous hormone responsible for the development and maturation of secondary male sexual characteristics.[20] Research has established that fat-free mass, muscle size, strength, and power correlate with serum testosterone concentration, which is the philosophic basis of the role of AAS as performance-enhancing agents.[24] Because of the potential strength gains associated with AAS, clinical applications exist for select medical conditions. AAS use can compromise various metabolic systems, which could be deleterious to the athlete's health.

The clinical application of AAS use is limited, but it focuses on the benefits of increased weight, lean body mass, and strength. Although these substances may have promising clinical results, most research lacks scrutiny and strong evidence. Initially, some medical professionals felt that AAS would be beneficial for women with osteoporosis, but this treatment option was supplanted by bisphosphonates.[20] It was also thought that incorporating AAS into clinical treatment would be beneficial for patients with human immunodeficiency virus (HIV), renal failure, or severe burns, conditions where standard nutritional therapy had not been successful.[24] Unfortunately, clinical evidence is lacking and more well-designed research is needed. Other conditions related to bone health were presumed to benefit from AAS treatment, but results were moderate at best.[23]

The **ergogenic** benefits of AAS have been well documented. In general, the primary benefit is strength gains that could result in enhanced performance. More specifically, benefits of AAS include increased lean mass, protein synthesis stimulation that promotes recovery between workouts, and increased pain tolerance.[20] However, the most apparent result is an increase in strength as determined by improved weightlifting metrics. Despite the actual or anticipated ergogenic benefits of AAS, the list of adverse effects is lengthy and significant, with dose- and duration-related effects. Athletes seeking ergogenic gains generally use doses that are many times beyond what is considered therapeutic and are thus more likely to experience severe adverse effects from overuse. Body systems adversely affected by AAS use include the following:[23]

- **Cardiovascular:** general cardiac dysfunction
- **Hematologic:** increased cholesterol
- **Hepatic:** jaundice, liver dysfunction

- **Neuroendocrine:**
  - Men: testicular atrophy, sexual dysfunction, **gynecomastia**, libido changes, prostate hypertrophy
  - Women: general virilization, clitoral hypertrophy, menstrual dysfunction
- **Renal:** kidney stones, renal cell cancer, focal segmental glomerulosclerosis

Another significant health risk is the effect of AAS on the central nervous system, specifically on mental and behavioral health. Studies have identified that ≤60% of AAS users report some form of aggression or irritability.[20] This increase in aggression, termed *roid rage*, may be considered a benefit in contact sports.[24] Other psychological effects of AAS use could include mood swings, psychosis, addiction, and depression.

RED FLAG

Addiction Concerns of Androgenic Anabolic Steroids

The diagnosis of AAS dependence has met the standard of the Diagnostic and Statistical Manual for Mental Disorders (DSM) for substance use disorders. Although the DSM criteria was not intended for AAS dependence, research has identified that approximately 30% of steroid users met the DSM criteria. People dependent on AAS had a lifetime prevalence of childhood conduct disorder, lower levels of educational attainment, and a higher frequency of abusing other substances, particularly opioids. An initial driving force behind the onset of AAS dependence is a body image disorder. People with muscle dysmorphia see a normally healthy muscular body as being weak and small; this mental health condition has been described as reverse anorexia nervosa.[14]

Human Growth Hormone

Human growth hormone is a naturally occurring peptide hormone secreted by the pituitary gland that fluctuates in concentration throughout the day.[35] It is affected by factors such as sleep, stress, and exercise and is at its highest levels during puberty. Under normal circumstances, hGH plays a crucial role in human physiology. This hormone stimulates skeletal and organ growth, regulates lean body mass, and assists in regulating the immune system.[36] Some people interested in performance enhancement or bodybuilding are attracted to the potential for increase in muscle mass or decrease in lean mass that could result from hGH use. Numerous professional baseball players have abused hGH to enhance performance.[13] In addition, hGH is popular among female athletes who use AAS to avoid the symptoms associated with steroid use.[35] hGH is sold by vendors, such as anti-aging clinics, and has been used by athletes at various levels.[13,36]

hGH is not recognized by the FDA as a viable treatment for athletic injury care and has been banned by all major drug testing agencies and sport governing bodies. The penalties for a positive hGH test are significant and severe; however, conducting hGH testing is challenging. The hGH half-life is approximately 4 hours for a subcutaneous injection and 22 minutes for IV administration.[36] The pulsatile nature of its physiological delivery through the body allows for various concentrations of endogenous growth hormone throughout the day. hGH is 100 to 1,000 times less concentrated in urine than in blood, and blood testing must be conducted within 24 hours of hGH administration in order to have the best chance of detecting the substance.[35,36]

Clinical Application

Risks of hGH

Human growth hormone (hGH) is unique in that off-label use is expressly prohibited by the FDA. Only 5 accepted clinical diagnoses indicate therapeutic use of hGH, and all but 1 have to do with shortness of stature or tissue wasting due to HIV or AIDS. Neither aging nor unsatisfactory athletic performance is an acceptable diagnosis for hGH use, and some physicians have had their licenses revoked for prescribing it. The significant risk of hGH use is developing **acromegaly**. Symptoms of this condition include coarsened facial appearance, cardiomyopathy, and impotence, as well as joint pain, fluid retention, and excessive sweating.[35]

Creatine Monohydrate

Creatine monohydrate (creatine or Cr) became popular in the 1990s as a supplement that increases muscle mass without the side effects of anabolic steroids. Cr is an endogenous substance that is synthesized naturally in the liver, kidney, and pancreas. The substance is found naturally in meat or fish products and can also be ingested as a nutritional supplement.[21,34] Cr may have a role in the resynthesis of adenosine triphosphate (ATP) during exercise.[21]

Although performance enhancement was the initial purpose for using Cr, both science and contemporary culture associate the supplement with enhanced recovery for the following conditions:

- **Parkinson's disease**—Patients with mild to moderate Parkinson's disease who supplemented with creatine monohydrate had improved lean mass, local muscle endurance, and chair rise performance compared to the control group.[18]
- **Spinal cord injury**—In general, Cr supplementation contributed to increased upper-extremity work capacity and oxygen uptake based on ergometry training and testing.[21]
- **Sport-related concussion**—Based on a systematic review, animals supplemented with Cr exhibited a resilience to traumatic brain injury that may be similar to traumatic brain injury in humans.[28] However, as of 2017, no conclusive evidence has been found that nutritional supplements have a neuroprotection role in humans.[28]

Supplements for Treating Skeletal Conditions

Osteoarthritis (OA) is the most common form of arthritis and presents as pain and swelling as a result of gradual wear and tear and lost cartilage in a joint.[22] In general, management of OA has been relegated to nonsteroidal anti-inflammatory drugs (NSAIDs). However, over-the-counter (OTC) supplements, such as glucosamine and chondroitin sulfate, omega-3 fatty acids, vitamin D, and cannabinoids (medical marijuana), have been promoted as alternatives to prescription anti-inflammatory medication.

Glucosamine and Chondroitin Sulfate

Glucosamine and chondroitin sulfate are endogenous chondroprotectors that are natural components of cartilage and synovial fluid.[22] These substances are considered symptomatic slow-acting drugs for osteoarthritis. Clinical trials, in vitro research, and meta-analyses have been inconsistent regarding the benefits of glucosamine and chondroitin sulfate in treating OA. However, there is appreciable published evidence that supports the potential of these supplements for the treatment of OA.[19]

Glucosamine inhibits the inflammatory process and increases synovial concentration of hyaluronic acid, another chondroprotector. Data has been equivocal. Clinical trials comparing a placebo to glucosamine 1,500 mg/day concluded that long-term glucosamine supplementation improved joint mobility and reduced pain, OA progression, and the risk of joint replacement.[22] Conversely, a meta-analysis revealed that glucosamine was ineffective in reducing joint pain.[19] When incorporating glucosamine with strength training for OA knee patients, a 13% reduction of serum cartilage oligomeric matrix protein (COMP) was found. Use of *ibuprofen* or a placebo with strength training over the same period of time showed no significant change in COMP.[31]

Chondroitin sulfate inhibits cartilage degradation and stimulates the anabolic process for forming new cartilage.[22] Randomized controlled trials validated the efficacy of chondroitin sulfate as a disease-modifying agent with secondary pain relief to 1,200 mg/day as a single dose or divided into 3 doses of 400 mg over the course of the day. Additionally, a 2-year study that combined chondroitin sulfate with glucosamine resulted in a reduction of joint space narrowing compared to use of a placebo or of either supplement alone.[19] Glucosamine and chondroitin sulfate are viable alternatives to NSAIDs and pain-relieving medication for patients with OA. Decisions on supplementation should consider the extent of the pathology, existing comorbidities, and the patient's preferences.

Omega-3-Fatty Acids

Omega-3 fatty acids also play a role in joint health. In vitro studies demonstrated increased collagen synthesis and decreased inflammation mediators, such as prostaglandin E_2 (PGE_2), whereas clinical studies concluded success in the treatment of rheumatoid arthritis. A study that combined glucosamine with the omega-3 fatty acids and docosahexaenoic acid (DHA) reduced pain in patients with hip or knee OA. Adding vitamins A, D, and E to the combination of glucosamine and omega-3 fatty acids resulted in an even greater improvement in pain with these groups.[22]

Vitamin D

Vitamin D's role in bone health is well known, but it functions beyond bone metabolism by controlling genes associated with immune and inflammatory modulation that could affect immune system function.[39] Vitamin D receptors have been located in virtually every tissue within the body, including bone, muscle, and immune system cells.[27,39] Sunshine is the most plentiful source of vitamin D, but certain factors impede this form of vitamin D production, including pollution, sunblock use, and pigmentation; dietary sources of vitamin D include egg yolks, fatty fish, and fortified milk.[27] Inadequate vitamin D levels can have deleterious effects, particularly for bone health. Vitamin D supplementation is a standard component of bone health. Vitamin D_3 (cholecalciferol) is more potent and longer acting than vitamin D_2 (ergocalciferol), as measured by the active form of vitamin D (25-hydroxyvitamin D, or 25(OH)D) in the blood. Vitamin D_3, which can be obtained OTC, is frequently used in daily doses of 1,000 to 5,000 IU (international units). Vitamin D_2 is available by prescription only as 50,000 IU capsules or OTC as an 8,000 IU/mL liquid.

Appropriate levels for vitamin D supplementation seem to vary. Observed vitamin D levels for professional basketball players have been defined as deficient at <20 ng/mL, insufficient at 20-32 ng/mL, and sufficient at >32 ng/mL.[11] See the Evidence in Pharmacology sidebar for additional details about vitamin D supplementation.

Evidence in Pharmacology

Vitamin D Supplementation

When vitamin D level is below 32 ng/mL, parathyroid hormone levels increase, leading to bone resorption to meet the body's need for calcium, which in turn increases the risk of stress fracture.[27] Insufficient vitamin D may be linked to inflammatory biomarkers that influence immune system function.[39] Cognitive functioning is also affected by insufficient vitamin D levels.[31] The connection between vitamin D and athletic performance is inconsistent. Gains in sprint times and vertical jump were found with vitamin D supplementation of 5,000 IU/day, but it was surmised that 25(OH)D levels >40 ng/mL may be required to achieve sufficient strength gains.[27]

Cannabinoids

Cannabidiol (CBD) and *tetrahydrocannabinol* (THC), the most common cannabinoids incorporated into medical preparations, are derived from the *Cannabis sativa* L. plant.[30] Medical *cannabis* is reviewed in detail in chapter 20. However, osteoarthritis patients may also benefit from medical *cannabis*, in part due to the presence of cannabinoid receptors in synovial tissue. The Cannabinoid Profile Investigation of Vaporized Cannabis in Patients with Osteoarthritis of the Knee (CAPRI) study researched the effect of THC on osteoarthritis pain. The research confirmed that neuropathic pain patients who smoked THC reported decreased pain intensity and improved sleep.[26]

Manipulation of Approved Medications to Enhance Performance

Medications that are approved for treating medical conditions have found their way into competitive sports. **Doping** is the use of banned athletic performance-enhancing drugs by athletic competitors. The term *doping* is widely used by organizations that regulate sporting competitions. The use of drugs to enhance performance is considered unethical, and therefore prohibited, by most international sports organizations, including the International Olympic Committee (IOC). Furthermore, athletes (or athletic programs) taking explicit measures to evade detection exacerbate the ethical violation with overt deception and cheating.[38] Similarly, blood doping is the misuse of certain techniques or substances to increase an athlete's red blood cell volume (RBCV), allowing the body to transport more oxygen to muscles and therefore increase stamina and performance.[41] Many PEDs are used for doping; this section focuses on common banned drugs: erythropoietin, beta-blockers, deer antler velvet, and the stimulants *ephedra*, *ephedrine*, and *pseudoephedrine*. Supplementation with these drugs is an accepted medical practice; however, each of these substances is subject to manipulation by those seeking enhanced performance through clandestine means.

Blood Doping and Erythropoietin

Blood doping is the practice of misusing certain techniques and substances to increase RBCV.

Since red blood cells (erythrocytes) carry oxygen to muscles, with blood doping, more erythrocytes are available to transport oxygen, thereby increasing aerobic capacity and endurance. Three widely known substances or methods are used for blood doping: erythropoietin (EPO), synthetic oxygen carriers, and blood transfusions. The primary uses of blood transfusions and synthetic oxygen carriers are for patients who have suffered massive blood loss, either during a major surgical procedure or due to major trauma. Erythropoietin is used in the treatment of anemia related to kidney disease or cancer. Misuse of these substances and techniques could lead to serious side effects, including the following:[40]

- Increased stress on the heart
- Blood clotting
- Stroke

EPO is a peptide hormone produced by the kidneys that increases RBCV by stimulating erythrocyte formation in bone marrow and enhancing the oxygen-carrying capacity of blood.[41] Recombinant EPO (rhEpo) is used to treat anemia associated with chronic kidney insufficiency, chemotherapy, and HIV-related infection by increasing the number of red blood cells in the circulation.[5] The medication Epogen is self-administered subcutaneously, although an intravenous option exists as well.[8] EPO supplementation causes increased RBCV over an 8-week period.[25] EPO use by athletes in competition was banned by WADA in the 1990s, and testing for its use was introduced during the 2000 Olympics in Sydney.[41]

Beta-Blockers

As described in chapter 12, the primary medical use of beta-blockers is to control hypertension, cardiac arrhythmias, angina pectoris (severe chest pain), migraine, and nervous or anxiety-related conditions. Common side effects include hypotension, bradycardia, sleep disorders, and spasm of the airways.[10,38] Beta-blockers are on the WADA list of banned substances.[42] Athletes in international shooting sports (e.g., pistol, rifle, and archery) see the beta-blocker's adverse effects of bradycardia and hypotension as benefits for their sport.[16] Although beta-blockers are not approved by the FDA for treating anxiety,[10] shooting athletes use them to ease tremors that could interfere with shooting the weapon and to reduce participation anxiety.[29]

Deer Antler Velvet

Deer antler velvet is one of many supplements sold through vendors and the Internet and marketed with claims of improved athletic performance, strength, or testosterone levels. Assessment of New Zealand deer antlers indicated them as a source of insulin-like growth factors I and II (in the antler tips), free fatty acids, and the minerals calcium, copper, iron, magnesium, manganese, phosphorous, potassium, selenium, sodium, sulfur, and zinc. Supporting these notions is literature from Russian, Chinese, and Korean sources that describes the tonic effect of deer antler velvet. A double-blind study of subjects using deer velvet extract (300 mg/day), deer velvet powder (1.5 g/day), or a placebo determined that subjects in the deer velvet powder group experienced improved isokinetic strength and endurance, but no improvements in testosterone, aerobic performance, RBCV, or measured blood volume. In general, no evidence exists that deer velvet powder and extract enhance testosterone, erythropoietic properties, or maximum oxygen consumption in people participating in aerobic training.[37]

Stimulants (*Ephedra, Ephedrine,* and *Pseudoephedrine*)

Athletes drawn to products that enhance energy and improve body composition may consume nutritional supplements containing the Asian herb *ma huang*, also known as *ephedra*. *Ma huang* has been associated with various medical remedies in Asia. It consists of *ephedrine* and *pseudoephedrine*, sympathomimetic alkaloids that are commonly found in nasal decongestants (discussed in chapter 11).[32] *Ephedra* was one of a plethora of nutritional supplements marketed to people attempting to lose weight and athletes hoping to enhance performance. The FDA issued a warning about its use in 1996[33] and, by 2003, reported >16,000 adverse events secondary to *ephedra* use, including heart attacks, strokes, seizures, and sudden death.[17] In 2003, the FDA announced that it was banning the sale of *ephedra* after it was linked to the deaths of multiple high-profile athletes.[33]

Pseudoephedrine is a popular OTC decongestant that is commonly available at drug stores. Since it can be used to manufacture illicit drugs (i.e., crystal methamphetamine), proper identification is required at the pharmacy for purchase and a limited monthly purchase amount has been set. Professional hockey players claim to use *pseudoephedrine* products for their primary purpose, as a decongestant, noting that their competitive season occurs during the cold and flu season of winter.[2] However, research published in 2006 indicated that 26.8% of intercollegiate hockey players had taken *pseudoephedrine* under the auspices of enhancing performance within the last 30 days.[1] A recent meta-analysis of the effect of *pseudoephedrine* on athletic performance indicated that any performance benefit was marginal at best and less than what could be achieved with *caffeine*.[12]

Summary

Athletes have incorporated nutritional supplements into their training regimens since the origin of competitions. Medications and supplements have been used inappropriately with the hope of gaining a competitive edge. This chapter describes several supplements commonly taken in this way that have limited evidence supporting their clinical use in treating neurological and skeletal conditions. Unfortunately, some medications and supplements intended for patients with medical conditions have been used to enhance athletic performance. Athletes need to be aware of which supplements are banned for athletic competition. Additionally, consumers should be aware that the claims listed on some supplements may not be based on human science. The next chapters focus on policies for drug use and abuse and drug testing procedures.

Case Studies

Case Study 1

Helen and Sylvia are sisters who have played recreational tennis for many years. Sylvia has a history of lower back dysfunction secondary to lumbar disc surgery. She has managed her chronic lumbosacral inflammation with 800 mg glucosamine chondroitin daily for several months. Recently, Helen felt a pop in her right elbow after making a serve. The next day, her lateral epicondyle presented with mild tenderness and swelling. At Sylvia's suggestion, Helen tried taking glucosamine rather than an OTC NSAID. After 5 days, Helen felt only minimal improvement and Sylvia suggested 1,200 mg/day rather than 800 mg. Helen tried the higher dose of glucosamine but opted for the NSAID after 2 days of no change.

Questions for Analysis

1. What is one possible reason that the glucosamine worked better for Sylvia than Helen?
2. Is the 800 mg daily use of glucosamine sufficient?

Case Study 2

Bobby is a 16-year-old star of a high school football team who sustained a concussion in the first half of the game just before the big homecoming game. The team physician examined him and withheld him from the remainder of the game; Bobby began the school's concussion protocol. His parents approached the AT and demanded that she start Bobby on a course of creatine monohydrate to accelerate his recovery so he could play for homecoming. When the AT said that this was not a viable approach, the parents stormed off and demanded to speak to the school's athletic director and principal.

Questions for Analysis

1. What might the AT have been considering when she said that creatine monohydrate was not a viable approach?
2. The principal met with the AT and reported that Bobby's parents had discussed the results of animal research that they believed proved their theory that Bobby should receive creatine monohydrate. Could this research validate that use of creatine monohydrate is appropriate in this case?

Summary of Selected Supplements and Performance-Enhancing Drugs

	ANABOLIC-ANDROGENIC STEROIDS (AAS; INCLUDES TESTOSTERONE)
Summary	The primary medical use of these compounds is to treat delayed puberty, some types of impotence, and wasting of the body caused by HIV infection or other muscle-wasting diseases. Physiological and psychological side effects of anabolic steroid abuse have the potential to affect any user, while other side effects are gender specific.
Side effects	*Physiological:* Acne; male pattern baldness; liver damage;* premature closure of the growth centers of long bones in adolescents, which may result in stunted growth;* stunted growth and disruption of puberty in children *Psychological:* Increased aggressiveness and sexual appetite, abnormal sexual and criminal behavior, and roid rage. Withdrawal can be associated with depression and, in some cases, suicide.
Sex-specific effects	*Males:* Breast tissue development,* shrinking of the testicles,* impotence, reduction in sperm production *Females:* Deepening of the voice;* cessation of breast development; growth of hair on the face, stomach, and upper back;* enlarged clitoris*
	HUMAN GROWTH HORMONE (HGH)
Summary	Abnormal concentration of hGH, its metabolites, or relevant ratios or markers in the urine sample will flag drug test levels for prohibited substances unless the athlete can demonstrate that the concentration was due to a physiological or pathological condition. Other examples of endogenous hormones include insulin, human chorionic gonadotropin (HCG), and adrenocorticotropin (ACTH).
Side effects	Severe headaches, loss of vision, acromegaly (protruding or enlarged jaw, brow, skull, hands and feet), high blood pressure and heart failure, diabetes and tumors, crippling arthritis
	CANNABINOIDS (MARIJUANA)
Summary	Schedule I drug under the Controlled Substances Act (CSA) considered to have high potential for abuse. It is accepted for medical use in many states but lacks accepted safety data for use under medical supervision.
Side effects	Increased heart rate, impaired short-term memory, slowed coordination and reaction of reflexes, diminished ability to concentrate, distorted sense of time and space, respiratory diseases, psychosis, hallucinations, hyperemesis syndrome
	BLOOD DOPING
Summary	Blood doping consists of administration of erythropoietin (EPO) or synthetic oxygen carriers and blood transfusions. EPO is used in the treatment of anemia related to kidney disease.
Side effects	Increased stress on the heart, heart attack, blood clotting, stroke, pulmonary embolism, hypertension, blood cancers or leukemia, and anemia. Blood transfusions increase the risk of acquiring infectious diseases, such as AIDS or hepatitis.
	BETA-BLOCKERS
Summary	The primary medical use of beta-blockers is to control hypertension, cardiac arrhythmias, angina pectoris (severe chest pain), migraine, and nervous or anxiety-related conditions.
Side effects	Lowered blood pressure, slow heart rate, sleep disorders, spasm of the airways
	STIMULANTS
Summary	Products used to enhance energy and improve body composition include *ma huang*, *ephedra*, *ephedrine*, and *pseudoephedrine*. Stimulants and sympathomimetic alkaloids are commonly found in nasal decongestants.
Side effects	Insomnia, anxiety, weight loss, dependence and addiction, dehydration, tremors, increased heart rate and blood pressure, increased risk of stroke, heart attack, and cardiac arrhythmia

*Effects may be permanent and can vary by person.
This list provides examples and is not intended to be comprehensive.

20

Cannabis and Cannabinoids

OBJECTIVES

After reading this chapter, you will be able to do the following:

- Summarize the acute and chronic effects of *cannabis* use
- Differentiate between the effects of *tetrahydrocannabinol* (THC) and *cannabidiol* (CBD)
- Explain the dangers of vaping synthetic cannabinoids
- Discuss the advantages and disadvantages of cannabinoid-based medicines
- Describe the regulations of *cannabis* and cannabinoid-based medicines for sport and athletics
- Implement clinical recommendations for advising patients who are prescribed *cannabis*-based medicine

Drugs Discussed in This Chapter

Drug class	Generic name	Trade name
Cannabinoids	*tetrahydrocannabinol* (THC)	Generic only
	cannabidiol (CBD)	Epidiolex
	dronabinol	Marinol, Syndros
	nabilone	Cesamet
	nabiximols	Sativex

This list is not exhaustive, but rather contains drugs commonly encountered in the athletic training setting. Always consult up-to-date information, confirm with a pharmacist, or discuss the use of therapeutic medications with the prescriber of the medication.

Marijuana, or *cannabis*, is the most commonly used non-pharmaceutical drug in the world, with 183 million users according to the 2017 *United Nations World Drug Report*.[43] Its use for medical purposes has recently increased[6,7] as there is considerable interest in the possible therapeutic uses of marijuana and its constituent compounds. Changes in marijuana policies across U.S. states, many of which have legalized marijuana for medical or recreational use, suggest that marijuana is gaining greater societal acceptance. Thus, it is particularly important for athletic trainers (ATs) to understand what is known about both the adverse health effects and the potential therapeutic benefits linked to marijuana.[34]

Cannabis

Cannabis is a plant of the Cannabaceae family and contains >80 biologically active chemical compounds. One type of *cannabis* plant is marijuana, which contains the chemical components responsible for the high feeling that is often associated with marijuana; these compounds are called **cannabinoids**.[18] *Cannabis* contains varying levels of the cannabinoids **delta-9-tetrahydrocannabinol** (THC), the component responsible for euphoria and intoxication, and **cannabidiol (CBD)**. *Cannabis* and its related products are widely available in multiple forms that can be eaten, drunk, smoked, and vaporized. *Cannabis* that is sold for both recreational and medical purposes contains varying levels of cannabinoids, and products may have inconsistent and uncertain purity.[33] Although anecdotal reports have sparked interest in treatment with *cannabis*, at present there is not enough evidence from randomized control trials to draw concrete conclusions with certainty about its safety or efficacy.

An example of the interest in *cannabis* as a treatment for a variety of disorders is the story of Charlotte Figi, who is described as "the girl who is changing medical marijuana laws across America."[37] Her parents and physicians say that Charlotte experienced a reduction of her epileptic seizures, which were brought on by Dravet syndrome, after her first dose of medical marijuana at 5 years of age. Dravet syndrome is a complex childhood epilepsy disorder that is associated with drug-resistant seizures and a high mortality rate. Among patients with Dravet syndrome, medications based on CBD are reported to have a greater reduction in convulsive-seizure frequency and higher rates of adverse events compared to a placebo.[11] Media coverage increased demand for Charlotte's Web, the product line named after Figi, and similar products high in CBD, which has been used to treat epilepsy in toddlers and children.[30,37]

Properties of *Cannabis* Strains

Cannabis Sativa Properties and Effects

- Higher THC levels, but also contains CBD
- Best to use during the day
- Energetic and uplifting
- Spacey, cerebral, or hallucinogenic high
- Stimulates appetite

Cannabis Indica Properties and Effects

- Higher CBD levels, but also contains THC
- Best to use during the night
- Calming, sedating, and relaxing
- Stimulates appetite
- Reduces anxiety and pain

Types of Cannabis

Three distinct types of *cannabis* plants exist that are categorized on morphology, native range, aroma, and subjective psychoactive characteristics.

1. *Cannabis sativa* (*C. sativa*) is the most widespread variety. It is usually tall and laxly branched and is found in warm lowland regions.
2. *Cannabis indica* are shorter, bushier plants adapted to cooler climates and highland environments.
3. *Cannabis ruderalis* is the informal name for the short plants that grow wild in Europe and Central Asia.

Breeders, seed companies, and cultivators of drug type *cannabis* often describe the characteristics of cultivars by categorizing them as "pure indica," "mostly indica," "indica/sativa," "mostly sativa," or "pure sativa." Another type of *cannabis* plant is *hemp*, which is derived from the *Cannabis sativa* family. By law, a plant must contain <0.3% cannabinoids to be considered *hemp*; otherwise, growers are at risk of prosecution under federal law.[14,20]

The National Institutes of Health (NIH) supports a broad portfolio of research on cannabinoids and the endocannabinoid system. This research portfolio includes some studies using the whole marijuana plant (*Cannabis sativa*), but most studies focus on individual cannabinoid compounds, including CBD. Individual cannabinoid chemicals may be isolated and purified from the marijuana plant or synthesized in the laboratory, or they may be naturally occurring (endogenous) cannabinoids found in the body.[33]

Endocannabinoid System

Cannabis acts on the brain by binding to cannabinoid receptors to produce a variety of effects, including euphoria, intoxication, and memory and motor impairments. These receptors are part of the **endocannabinoid system**, which affects the formation of brain circuits important for decision making, mood, and stress response.[6] The endocannabinoid system consists of the endocannabinoids, cannabinoid receptors, and the enzymes that synthesize and degrade endocannabinoids. Many of the effects of cannabinoids and endocannabinoids are mediated by 2 G protein–coupled cannabinoid receptors, CB1 and CB2, although additional receptors may be involved.[29] The CB1 receptor is the most abundant G protein–coupled receptor subtype in the central nervous system (CNS). These receptors bind with THC and mediate many of the psychoactive effects of cannabinoids. There is particularly high density of CB1 receptors in the basal ganglia, as well as in brain regions that are key components of the descending pain pathway and the circuitry for stress, fear, and anxiety. CB1 receptors are also expressed in most other tissues and organs of the body.[23] The CB2 receptor, which binds with CBD, is found in the CNS but is mainly distributed in the periphery, with particularly high density on cells and tissues of the immune system.[23] Both CB1 and CB2 couple primarily to inhibitory G proteins and are subject to the same pharmacological influences as other G protein–coupled receptors. Thus, partial agonism, **functional selectivity**, and inverse agonism all play important roles in determining the cellular response to specific cannabinoid receptor ligands.[17,29]

The analgesic effects of cannabinoids are facilitated via the endocannabinoid system to the pain pathways of the central and peripheral nervous systems.[35] Preclinical data support an influence of cannabinoids and modulators of the body's own **endogenous cannabinoids** (endocannabinoids) on nociception.[17]

With respect to pain, the components of the endocannabinoid system are expressed throughout nociceptive pathways (for more information on nociception, refer to chapter 7). Endocannabinoids are generated on demand in response to pain or stress and produce short-term antinociceptive effects via their actions as retrograde transmitters at presynaptic inhibitory CB1 receptors. Endocannabinoids play a key role in the resolution of acute pain states and in mediating stress-induced analgesia, and they are elevated at various sites in nociceptive pathways in chronic pain states, highlighting their role as endogenous analgesics.[23]

Cannabinoids

Cannabinoids are the biologically active constituents of *cannabis*, or synthetic compounds, usually having affinity for and activity at cannabinoid receptors. Herbal *cannabis* plant material typically contains >450 different compounds; >100 of these are classified as **phytocannabinoids**, which are purified or extracted from plant material.[23] Because of the potential for abuse and the widespread political stigmatization of *cannabis* as a street drug, a rational public debate on the use of medical *cannabis* and *cannabis*-based medicines is hampered by erroneous beliefs and inaccurate and inconsistent terminology. It is important to distinguish *cannabis* from *cannabis*-derived (or *cannabis*-based) medicines or pharmacological modulators of the endocannabinoid system. Unfortunately, the *cannabis* involved in illicit street trading or abuse is often confused with the therapeutic use of medical *cannabis* and *cannabis*-based medicines (see table 20.1). The discussion is further confused by the fact that CBD-containing oils and extracts of low or even unclear CBD content are freely sold as nutritional supplements (e.g., *cannabis* oils, topical ointments, gummies, edibles).[23]

The THC concentrations in available medical *cannabis* strains vary from 1% to 22%, and CBD concentrations vary from 0.05% to 9%. Very little evidence exists for determining which THC concentration and ratio of THC to CBD is best in terms of efficacy and safety.[23]

Pharmacokinetics (ADME) of Delta-9-Tetrahydrocannabinol

The primary psychoactive component of *cannabis*, THC, is rapidly absorbed into the bloodstream following inhalation and extensively metabolized in the liver into multiple metabolites. The equipotent THC metabolite 11-hydroxy-THC (11-OH-THC) is further oxidized to THCCOOH and other metabolites. THC is extensively metabolized to multiple other alcohols and acids, but THCCOOH was selected as the analyte monitored in urine for virtually all drug-testing programs, including those for intercollegiate and professional sports, the workplace, military, criminal justice, and drug treatment programs.

THC is distributed initially to the highly perfused organs, including the brain, heart, liver, and kidneys, with secondary distribution into adipose tissue because of its high lipophilicity. With chronic daily THC exposure, because of its lipophilicity, the THC storage in fat is large; the rate-limiting step in THC elimination is the slow release of stored drug from the tissues, especially adipose.[26] Cannabinoid concentrations in body fluids depend on the potency of the *cannabis*, smoking topography, frequency of *cannabis* use, and amount of time since last use. For example, in people who smoked *cannabis* less frequently than daily, THC was detected in their plasma for 6 to 27 hours after smoking a single *cannabis* joint containing approximately 34 mg THC. Among *cannabis* users who smoke less frequently than daily, a urine cannabinoid test would likely be positive for up to 4 days. However, among people who smoke *cannabis* daily for an extended period of time, use of that same joint could result in a positive urine specimen for up to 4 weeks.[26]

TABLE 20.1 Classifications of Cannabinoids

Term	Definition	Examples and typical products
(Herbal) *cannabis*, raw *cannabis*, marijuana, or flower	The whole plant or parts or material from the *Cannabis sativa* plant (e.g., flowers, buds, resin, and leaves)	*Cannabis sativa* and hashish*
Naturally occurring cannabinoids	Purified from plant sources	Cannabidiol (CBD) and delta-9-tetrahydrocannabinol (THC)
Phytocannabinoids	Cannabinoids found in leaves, flowers, stems, and seeds collected from the *C. sativa* plant	THC and CBD
Endocannabinoid or endogenous cannabinoids	Cannabinoids made by the body with an affinity for and activity at cannabinoid receptors	N-arachidonoyl-ethanolamine (AE), anandamide, or 2-arachidonoylglycerol (2-AG)
Cannabinoids	Biologically active constituents of *cannabis* or synthetic compounds, usually having affinity for and activity at cannabinoid receptors	THC; CBD; CP55,940; WIN55,212-2; and HU210
Synthetic cannabinoids	Synthesized in a laboratory	CB1 agonists, CB2 agonists, CB1/CB2 nonselective agonists, ajulemic acid (AJA), *nabilone*, and *dronabinol*
Medical or medicinal *cannabis* (or medical or medicinal marijuana)	*Cannabis* plant and plant material (e.g., flower, marijuana, hashish, buds, leaves, or full plant extracts) used for medical reasons	Bedrocan, Bedrobinol, and Tilray 10:10 Balance
Cannabinoid-based (or *cannabis*-derived) medicines	Medicinal *cannabis* extracts approved by a registered regulatory body with defined and standardized phytocannabinoid content, particularly THC and THC/CBD	*cannabidiol* (Epidiolex), *nabiximols* (Sativex), *dronabinol* (Marinol), and *nabilone* (Cesamet)

*Hashish, or hash, is an extract of the *Cannabis (C.) sativa* plant that contains concentrations of the psychoactive resins.

Based on Fisher et al. (2019); Häuse et al. (2018); National Institute on Drug Abuse (2018)

Evidence in Pharmacology

Secondhand *Cannabis* Exposure

People who do not smoke marijuana have expressed concerns about being around *cannabis* smokers similar to the way nontobacco users are concerned about secondhand smoke exposure. Passive *cannabis* absorption depends on different factors, such as the THC potency of the *cannabis*, the amount of *cannabis* smoked, and the duration and exposure of the amount that was smoked.[9] A study to produce secondhand exposure[25] placed *cannabis* smokers in close proximity to nonsmokers in an unventilated room to produce a high-intensity, short-term *cannabis* smoke environment. These results indicated that this extreme exposure could produce a positive test in nonsmokers, but at generally lower cutoff levels than those used in federal workplace drug-testing programs.[9]

Acute Effects of Cannabis Use

The behavioral and subjective effects of *cannabis* are highly dose dependent; they include euphoria, enhancement of sensory perception, sedation, relaxation, altered perceptions of time, lack of concentration, impairment of learning and memory, mood changes, panic reaction, paranoia, and impaired psychomotor activity (figure 20.1). Well-described physiological effects include tachycardia, conjunctival injection, dry mouth and throat, increased appetite, vasodilation, bronchodilation, increased sleep, and analgesia. This spectrum of behavioral effects is unique, preventing classification of the drug as a stimulant, sedative, tranquilizer, and hallucinogen. Subjective and physiological effects of *cannabis* appear after the first puff of a THC-containing product. Although *cannabis* smoking produces rapid changes in heart rate, pronounced hypotension and dizziness is observed in approximately 25% of people approximately 10 minutes after smoking.[26,36]

Marijuana impairs short-term memory and judgment and distorts perception. Concentration, sense of time, fine coordination, depth perception, tracking, and reaction time can be impaired for up to 24 hours—all of which can be hazardous in certain situations (e.g., driving, participating in contact sports).[36] Marijuana also affects brain systems that are still maturing throughout young adulthood, so regular use by teens may have negative and long-lasting effects on their cognitive development, putting them at a competitive disadvantage and possibly interfering with their well-being in other ways. Also, contrary to popular belief, marijuana can be addictive, and its use during adolescence may make other forms of problem use or addiction more likely.[34]

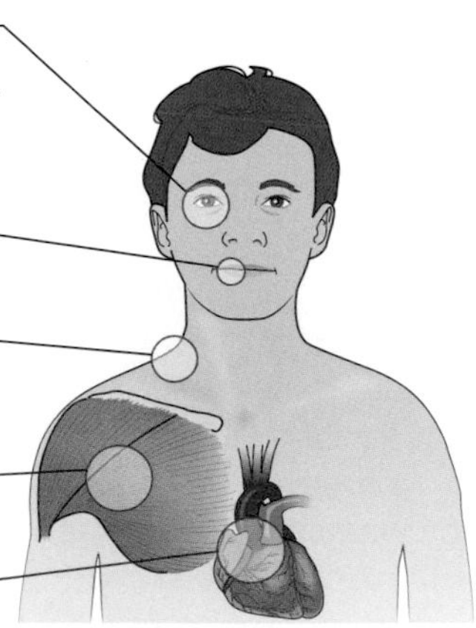

FIGURE 20.1 Short-term effects of *cannabis*.

Chronic Effects of Cannabis Use

Long-term users of marijuana report a sense of diminished ambition and energy. High-dose smokers can develop pulmonary symptoms (episodes of acute bronchitis, wheezing, coughing, and increased phlegm), and pulmonary function may be altered, manifested as large airway changes of unknown significance. Recent data suggest that heavy marijuana use is associated with significant cognitive impairment and anatomic changes in the hippocampus, particularly if marijuana use begins in adolescence.[36] When someone ingests CBD regularly over a long period of time, the chronic effects could include toxicity to the liver. During the U.S. Food and Drug Administration (FDA) review of Epidiolex—a purified form of CBD that the FDA approved in 2018 for use in the treatment of certain seizure disorders—the organization identified certain safety risks, including the potential for liver injury. These are serious risks that can be managed when an FDA-approved CBD drug product is taken under medical supervision, but it is less clear how these risks might be managed when CBD is used far more widely, without medical supervision, and not in accordance with FDA-approved labeling (additional details in the Medical Cannabinoids section).[44]

An extensive review of marijuana use[31] found only 1 study[42] that examined dependency and was limited to examining only self-reported surveys; however, this review provides important information for clinicians. This review reported that 10% of users meet the criteria for marijuana dependency. In those more likely to be dependent, moderate effects of genetics on dependency were reported. Other factors for dependency included tobacco use, start of marijuana use before the age of 17, and weekly marijuana use. Other reviews noted that those who were dependent on marijuana were more likely to develop psychosis, especially in those already at high risk for mental illness, and users with anxiety were more likely to develop marijuana dependency.[31] It is important for ATs to educate their patients that marijuana is not a harmless, recreational substance, particularly for members of certain at-risk groups.

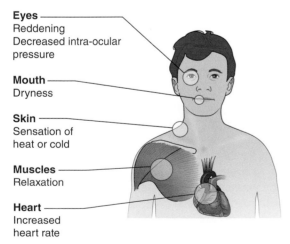

Adverse Effects of Cannabis

Advocates cite the safety profile of marijuana in the short term may have overshadowed some of the longer-term health risks that appear to be associated with even moderate use.[31] Negative health and adverse effects (AEs) are associated with marijuana use. Because of the nature of how marijuana functions in the brain, death due to overdose is not possible. However, harm from *cannabis* use has been reported for multiple mental health outcomes, including psychosis, mania, and suicide. There is evidence of structural, functional, and chemical brain changes that may underlie some of the associated risk for mental illness.

None of this evidence is causal; only associative evidence is available. The study designs available within humans are limited to observational cohorts because sufficiently powered randomized controlled trials would not be feasible or ethical. Nonetheless, ATs should be aware that a variety of health harms are associated with marijuana use and that serious symptoms or AEs could arise. Clinicians should consider additional preventive measures for their patients, such as referral to their directing physician or behavioral counselling specialists in addiction or dependency treatment.[31]

Synthetic Cannabinoids (K2/Spice)

Synthetic cannabinoids are part of a group of drugs called new psychoactive substances (NPS). NPS are unregulated mind-altering substances that have become newly available on the market and are intended to produce the same effects as illegal drugs.[2,32] Hundreds of brands now contain synthetic cannabinoids; common street names are K2, Spice, Joker, Black Mamba, Kush, and Kronic. Synthetic cannabinoids are sometimes incorrectly called synthetic marijuana (or fake weed) and are often promoted as safe or legal substitutes to natural marijuana. The liquid can contain nicotine, THC, CBD oils, and other substances and additives. Synthetic cannabinoids can produce very different actions from smoking natural marijuana. Some users report psychotic effects like extreme anxiety, paranoia, and hallucinations.[2] The effects can be much more intense, unpleasant, and sometimes dangerous compared to naturally grown marijuana.[2,32]

Synthetic cannabinoids are human-made mind-altering chemicals that are either sprayed on dried, shredded plant material (not actual marijuana) so they can be smoked or sold as liquids to be vaporized and inhaled in e-cigarettes and other devices.[32] Electronic cigarettes—or e-cigarettes—are also called vapes, e-hookahs, vape pens, tank systems, mods, and electronic nicotine delivery systems (ENDS). E-cigarettes work by heating a liquid to produce an aerosol that users inhale into their lungs as vapor.[41] Vaping products can be easily purchased from convenience stores and smoke shops and online. However, since 2012, synthetic cannabinoids are illegal in the United States, although the products are still sold illegally on the streets.[2,32] The Drug Enforcement Administration (DEA) has designated many active chemicals found most frequently in synthetic cannabinoids as Schedule I controlled substances because these products have a high potential for abuse and no medical benefit. Manufacturers attempt to evade these legal restrictions by substituting different chemicals in their mixtures, while the DEA continues to monitor and update the list of banned cannabinoid derivatives.[2,32]

As of late 2019, 1,888 cases of e-cigarette or vaping product use–associated lung injury (EVALI) have been reported to the CDC.[8] All EVALI patients have reported a history of using e-cigarette, or vaping, products. The latest national and state findings suggest that products containing THC, particularly those obtained off the street or from other informal sources (e.g., friends, family members, illicit dealers), are linked to most of the EVALI cases

RED FLAG

Marijuana Vaping

The use of e-cigarettes, or vaping, was introduced to the United States in 2007. Use is more popular among the 18- to 34-year-old age group than among older adults. Vaping concentrated marijuana (dabs) is called dabbing; this practice is reported by 31% of middle school and high school students and 75% of college age students who vape.[28] Many cases of vaping-related lung injury have been reported to the CDC; 91% of these cases required hospitalization, although the specific causes of this outbreak were unknown.[28] Most hospitalized patients reported using vaping products that contained THC, with and without nicotine. Based on this concern, the CDC recommends avoiding vaping THC and never manipulating or otherwise tampering with a packaged nicotine product.

and play a major role in the outbreak.[8] At this time, the FDA and CDC have not identified the cause or causes of the lung injuries in these cases, and the only commonality among all cases is that patients report the use of e-cigarette, or vaping, products.[8,28]

Cannabidiol

Marijuana is made from the dried leaves and buds of the *Cannabis sativa* plant. Cannabidiol (CBD) derived from the *Cannabis sativa* plant is the cannabinoid most commonly incorporated into medical preparations.[17,23,39] CBD was isolated from *cannabis* in 1940;[10] unlike THC, it does not cause a psychoactive effect.[39] Advocacy for CBD's therapeutic benefit emanated from medical application of the experiences of recreational marijuana users to a range of disorders, including pain, psychotic disorders, anxiety, depression, and inflammation.[7] Under the Controlled Substances Act (CSA), CBD is currently a Schedule I substance because it is a chemical component of the *cannabis* plant; however, nonclinical and clinical studies are currently being conducted to assess the abuse potential of CBD.[18] Other than approved prescription drugs, CBD products have not been evaluated or approved by the FDA for use as drug products. This means that for most CBD products available, the following are unknown:[19]

- If they are safe and effective to treat a particular disease
- What, if any, dosage may be considered safe
- How they could interact with other drugs or foods
- Whether they have dangerous side effects or other safety concerns

Pharmacokinetics and Pharmacodynamics of Cannabidiol

The 3 most popular routes of administration for CBD are topical, oral (edible), and sublingual.[10] The mechanism of action of CBD is an agonist for multiple cell-surface receptors linked to anti-inflammatory activity that promotes analgesia and opioid-sparing effects.[10] The pharmacokinetic and pharmacodynamic properties of CBD may lead to various adverse events and drug–drug interactions, and there is a lack of quality research in this area.[7] Almost 30% of medical users of CBD have reported side effects commonly associated with THC use, including red eyes, euphoria, and hunger.[10]

Medical Cannabinoids

Medical cannabinoids refer to the use of *cannabis* as medical therapy to treat disease or alleviate symptoms. Medical cannabinoids can be administered orally, sublingually, or topically; they can be smoked, inhaled, mixed with food, or made into tea.[13] The medicine can be taken in herbal form, extracted naturally from the plant, obtained by isomerization of cannabidiol, or manufactured synthetically.[24,46] Medical cannabinoids are typically used to treat chronic pain, muscle spasms, and nausea and vomiting associated with cancer treatment.[13] As previously mentioned, *cannabidiol* (CBD, Epidiolex) oral solution is FDA approved for the treatment of seizures associated with 2 rare and severe forms of epilepsy. This is the first FDA-approved drug that contains a purified drug substance derived from marijuana. The FDA has also approved 2 cannabidiol-based drugs, *dronabinol* (Marinol, Syndros) and *nabilone* (Cesamet), that are made from synthetic forms of compounds found in marijuana. They can be legally prescribed for the treatment of nausea and vomiting caused by chemotherapy when other treatments have failed.[12] Currently, a few cannabinoid-based medicines are available for marketing in different countries. Additional cannabinoid-based medicines are in different stages of development but have not yet been authorized for marketing.[1]

The content of THC and CBD in medical *cannabis* is highly variable, with typical ranges from 1% to 22% THC and 0.05% to 9% CBD.[17,23] By contrast, the THC and CBD concentrations in oromucosal spray, *nabiximols* (Sativex in Canada, the European Union, and other countries), and the THC content in plant-derived and synthetic THC are standardized.[17] It is not recommended to prescribe *cannabis* flowers with a high (>12.5%) THC content. A dose of no more than 1 inhalation 4 times per day is recommended for avoiding adverse effects and cognitive impairment.[23]

Many U.S. states now permit dispensing marijuana for medicinal purposes, and anecdotal evidence is mounting for the efficacy of marijuana-derived compounds. The discussion of the medical use of *cannabis* and cannabinoids must be clearly differentiated from the discussion of the legal status of recreational *cannabis*. Debate is ongoing in the medical and scientific communities as well as among social and political stakeholders regarding the medical use of *cannabis* and *cannabis*-based products, including cannabinoid-based medicines.[1] Despite the potential for negative consequences, there is support for the use of medical *cannabis* as an adjunct to or substitute for prescription medications such as opioids in the treatment of chronic pain, both in the prehospital and outpatient settings.[1,4,47] Prescribers of medical cannabinoids generally support patient choice or have personal experience with patients who were helped by the use of *cannabis*. Groups who oppose medicinal *cannabis* refer to the lack of evidence regarding treatment efficacy, the absence of an identified mechanism of action, inconsistency regarding dosage and THC levels in privately sold products, and concern about side effects.[47]

Contraindications to Medical Cannabinoid Use

A history of a hypersensitivity reaction to *cannabis* is an absolute contraindication to use of cannabinoid-based medicines.[23] Other absolute contraindications are for patients who are pregnant (or contemplating pregnancy), lactating, or of young age (i.e., children and adolescents), apart from in exceptional circumstances.[23] Current mental disorder or a history of mental disorders, especially substance abuse and dependence, and psychosis are relative contraindications. Seizures and severe cardiac disorders are relative contraindications.[23]

Evidence in Pharmacology

CBD for Treatment of Dravet Syndrome

Dravet syndrome is a catastrophic early-onset encephalopathic epilepsy with a high mortality rate. Currently, no antiepileptic drug is effective for this syndrome. A 2014 *Cochrane* review of all published randomized controlled trials involving the treatment of marijuana or 1 of marijuana's constituents in people with epilepsy concluded that no reliable conclusions can be drawn at present regarding the efficacy of cannabinoids as a treatment for epilepsy.[22] However, in 2017, the *New England Journal of Medicine*[11] reported that researchers used a randomized controlled trial to show that CBD use resulted in a greater reduction in convulsive-seizure frequency than placebo use among children and young adults with drug-resistant Dravet syndrome. Further trials are needed.

ATs working with patients who are prescribed cannabinoid-based medications should discuss any participation in contact sports with their prescriber. Patients should be advised not to drink alcohol or drive while under the influence of cannabinoid-based medicines.[23] Since cannabinoid-based medicines can have both pharmacokinetic and pharmacodynamic interactions with other drugs, it is recommended that prescribers reduce the dosage of other centrally acting drugs as far as possible before prescribing cannabinoid-based medicines. It is also recommended that prescribers advise patients not to smoke *cannabis* but instead to use topical medical *cannabis* ointments, such as oil extract, or a vaporizer with regulated and standardized inhalants. Patients should be advised by the prescriber to use only approved medical devices.[23]

Research on Cannabinoid-Based Medicines

Public interest in the use of *cannabis* products for medical purposes has been accelerated by advocacy and the legalization of marijuana for recreational and medical use. Many U.S. states have legalized herbal *cannabis* for medicinal use for a wide range of potential indications, including chronic pain management. Systematic reviews have come to partially divergent conclusions on the efficacy and safety of *cannabis*-based medicines for chronic pain. Some national guidelines and expert groups have given different recommendations on the role of *cannabis*-based medicines for some pain syndromes, such as neuropathic pain and fibromyalgia.[23]

The synthetic THC derivatives *dronabinol* (Marinol) and *nabilone* (Cesamet) were approved for treatment of nausea and vomiting secondary to chemotherapy and anorexia related to weight loss in HIV and AIDS patients. These medications were approved to treat other medical conditions as well; examples of the applications and efficacy of these medications include the following:[27,46]

- **Multiple sclerosis**—The medications improved spasticity, which resulted in improved mobility, with minimal safety concerns.
- **Chemotherapy-induced nausea and vomiting**—The absence of nausea was greater for combined *dronabinol* and *ondansetron* treatment compared to placebo use, but some adverse effects were experienced with use of *dronabinol* alone.

- **Pain management—***Dronabinol* reduced cancer pain, but it produced adverse effects; *nabilone* reduced diabetic neuropathy and was well tolerated despite some adverse effects.
- **Post-traumatic stress disorder—***Nabilone* decreased nightmares when compared to a placebo and produced no apparent adverse effects.

In perhaps one of the most comprehensive analyses of studies focusing on the effects of cannabinoids on pain reduction, researchers reviewed 42 studies and performed meta-analysis of 24 randomized control trials.[3] This analysis found moderate to high quality of evidence for the efficacy of cannabinoid-based medicines for treatment of chronic pain patients, especially for cancer pain. However, the studies on cancer pain were scarce and most were not from recent years; thus, chronic, noncancer pain and especially neuropathic pain were the most investigated and substantiated diagnoses suitable for cannabinoid-based medicine treatment. Conversely, postoperative pain studies showed an inverse result: Not only was there no pain reduction, in some cases, a placebo was more effective than cannabinoid-based medicine treatment. Although the primary analysis showed significant results favorable to the use of cannabinoid-based medicines over placebo, it is unclear whether the results represent any clinical significance.[3]

Performance Effects and Sport Regulation

The performance-enhancing effects of a substance are determined if the substance has "medical or other scientific evidence, pharmacological effect, or experience that the substance or method, alone or in combination with other substances or methods, has the potential to enhance or enhances sport performance."[26] Although *cannabis* does not have any overt performance-enhancing benefits, the 2021 World Anti-Doping Agency (WADA) prohibits its use during competition. According to WADA's Prohibited List (an international standard antidoping code; also discussed in chapter 19), substances of abuse are identified as such because they are frequently abused in society outside of the context of sport. The following are designated substances of abuse: *cocaine*, diamorphine (*heroin*), methylenedioxymethamphetamine (MDMA, or Ecstasy), and *tetrahydrocannabinol* (THC).[45,48] Players in the National Football League (NFL) have enlisted their management to lift the ban on CBD to avoid deterring individual players from using medical marijuana. An argument presented by the players is that when treating severe pain secondary to playing football their choice is either to use an opioid or marijuana; therefore, medical marijuana should be made an available option.[5] The league has taken a listening and learning posture of collection and analysis of scientific data.

The International Olympic Committee (IOC) consensus statement on pain in elite athletes concludes that further research and increased consistency in measures and methods across studies are needed. There is a need to better understand the incidence and prevalence of analgesic medication use in sport and the benefits and risks of various pharmacological and nonpharmacological treatments, and their combinations, for specific pain presentations. The IOC discussion about pain management in athletes does not include information about *cannabis*, although they do have protocols for use of steroid injections, anticonvulsants, antidepressants, and opioids. Due to the paucity of research into the efficacy of cannabinoid treatment for pain in athletes, the IOC consensus statement concluded that current evidence does not justify the use of cannabinoids for pain management in elite athletes.[49]

Cannabis use in athletes has been primarily studied in adolescent, elite, and collegiate athletes from an antidoping or antiabuse perspective. A review of *cannabis* use in elite athletes concluded that there was no evidence for use of *cannabis* as a performance-enhancing drug and that *cannabis* may play a role in pain management and concussion-related symptoms.[45,49] There is an apparent paradox in considering the effects of *cannabis* on athletic performance. Despite evidence that recreational *cannabis* use may acutely impair psychomotor skills and cognitive function, there is a perception among some athletes that *cannabis* use may have beneficial effects.[45] The literature is scant, and the illegal or prohibited status of *cannabis* worldwide has limited the ability to generate high-quality data on the patterns and prevalence of *cannabis* use among elite athletes.[45]

Sport-regulating agencies are endeavoring to use published scientific data to achieve the most objective judgment on the potential of substances or methods used for performance enhancement, doping practices, or unfair sportsmanship. When developing recommendations, athletics policymakers should assemble a diverse team of experts in the field of sports medicine, pharmacology, toxicology, doping, analytical chemistry, endocrinology, and hematology.[26] Historically, prohibition of recreational *cannabis* use has long been the dominant policy model for sport organizations. Consequently, a growing number of organizations have implemented *cannabis* policy reforms. As U.S. states and other countries continue to legalize and decriminalize approaches for the use and supply of *cannabis*,[16] athletics policies and recommendations must continue to evolve and be refined.

Regulation of Cannabis Use

Within the United States, different states have enacted independent laws, and most states currently allow the use of medical *cannabis* to some extent. In 1996, California became the first state to pass a law that permits the use of medical *cannabis*; many other states have authorized the use of medical *cannabis*, with wide variations among the individual laws.[1] Legalization of cannabinoid products began with the 2014 Farm Act, which approved legalization of CBD derived from 3 specific sources: industrial *hemp* cultivated in compliance with this legislation, imported nonpsychoactive *hemp*, and elements of *Cannabis sativa* that were not part of marijuana as defined in the Controlled Substance Act of 1970.[10,45]

Cannabis supplied through regulated dispensaries can provide herbal *cannabis*, *cannabis*-derived products (e.g., edibles, topicals), and *cannabis*-consumption devices. The methods of administration vary; widely used methods include oils, vaporizing, edibles, and capsules. Smoking *cannabis* for medical purposes is prohibited in many states; edible forms are also prohibited in some states.[1] In many U.S. states and European countries, there is a considerable gap between official authorizations for access of patients to medical *cannabis*.[1]

The business component of medical marijuana sales is significant. Sales of *hemp*-based CBD products, not including products derived from the *cannabis* plant, are projected to exceed $1 billion USD by 2023.[10] By 2027, the global estimate of overall medical marijuana is expected to approach $19 billion USD.[40] These products are available through an assortment of consumer sources, ranging from bakeries and gas stations to pharmacies and spas. Despite this seemingly ubiquitous availability, CBD products raise questions and concerns (see Red Flag sidebar). CBD is not regulated by the FDA in the United States; thus, there is the potential for discrepancies between the product's label and what is actually contained in the product. Independent scientific and industry analysis identified products that have higher CBD concentrations than labeled; whereas FDA tests revealed that 26% of the products examined in their study had less-than-optimal CBD levels, to the point that any potential clinical response was negated.[39] Also, >20% of tested CBD products contained significant levels of THC.[10]

RED FLAG

Concerns With CBD Products

The manufacturing process, proper dosage, potential side effects, and drug–drug interactions of CBD products have not been scrutinized by the FDA.[19] About 70% of these products have a CBD concentration that is mislabeled.[10] The FDA has concerns about therapeutic claims for CBD that may mislead the public. In 2019, the FDA issued a warning to a company that was illegally selling unapproved products containing CBD and making unsubstantiated claims that the products treated cancer, Alzheimer's disease, and opioid withdrawal pain.[19] Accurate information regarding CBD concentration is vital for consumer safety; although they are classified as food products, these products are often used for medically therapeutic purposes.[39]

In general, each U.S. state where medical or recreational *cannabis* is legal has certain criteria for permitted use. These requirements can vary widely and change quickly. In most states that have legalized *cannabis*, government regulations require producers to use an independent lab to measure the level of cannabinoid in dried *cannabis* flowers and oils so that the resulting products can be labelled appropriately. *Cannabis* analytical labs have had an evolution in the sophistication of the industry. Such labs are adopting standardized tests for potency and purity using gas chromatography and high-performance liquid chromatography. Producers must also test for contaminants, such as bacteria, mold, heavy metals, and 96 types of pesticide. Edible *cannabis* products have similarly stringent rules, and labels on such products must convey the same nutritional information as do those on any other food product.[38]

In various national, state, or provincial jurisdictions where *cannabis* is legal for medical purposes, *cannabis* can be authorized for medical purposes, rather than prescribed, because there may be no drug identification number or other such recognition by the relevant drug regulatory agencies. However, pharmaceutical cannabinoid agents that have been approved for clinical use by drug regulatory agencies, such as the FDA, are indeed prescribed.[21] Health insurance may cover the costs associated with the use of cannabinoids approved by the FDA, but not medical marijuana. Overall, additional studies are needed comparing the safety and efficacy of oral cannabinoids with various formulations of medical marijuana.[4]

Clinical Recommendations

Good-quality evidence indicates that substantial risk of adverse health outcomes may result from *cannabis* use. This risk may be reduced by informed behavioral choices among users and sound advice from ATs and other sports medicine practitioners. The evidence-based recommendations, education, and intervention tools inform patients about choices on the use of *cannabis*. However, it is important that institutions and athletics departments systematically communicate support in order for key recommendations to be effective. As legalization continues to evolve, policymakers must actively review and implement new recommendations toward reducing health risks related to *cannabis* use.[16] When working with patients who are considering using medical *cannabis* or *cannabis*-based medicines, ATs should have a thorough dialogue with the patient and in consultation with the prescriber and may consider a written treatment agreement (figure 20.2). Since ATs and other sports medicine clinicians may be placed in a position to advise on *cannabis* as a medicine, they should provide patients with information regarding the benefits and risks of use, as well as responsible medicinal use.

Evidence-based recommendations may reduce the risk of adverse health outcomes from *cannabis* use, especially in young users. Therefore, it is prudent to use good-quality evidence to develop recommendations to lower the risk of *cannabis* use. Based on a systematic review of current evidence, experts have developed 10 major recommendations for lower-risk *cannabis* use:[16,23]

1. The most effective way to avoid health risks related to *cannabis* use is abstinence.
2. Avoid early-age initiation of *cannabis* use (i.e., nothing before the age of 16 years).
3. Choose products with a low ratio (percentage) of THC or balanced THC:CBD ratio *cannabis* products.
4. Abstain from using synthetic cannabinoids (refer to section on Synthetic Cannabinoids).
5. Avoid combusted *cannabis* inhalation and give preference to nonsmoking use methods.
6. Avoid deep inhalation and other risky inhalation practices.
7. Avoid high-frequency (e.g., daily or near-daily) *cannabis* use.
8. Abstain from driving while under the influence of *cannabis*.
9. Members of populations at higher risk for health problems related to *cannabis* use should avoid use altogether.
10. Avoid combining previously mentioned risk behaviors (e.g., early initiation and high-frequency use).

Summary

Cannabis use is associated with a variety of health risks, including several for which the evidence is substantial. The primary challenge for sports medicine practitioners is to provide advice based on the best evidence available. Adolescent or young adults using *cannabis* may develop severe—that is, acute or chronic—health problems from use. With increases in the recognition of the analgesic effects of *cannabis* and cannabinoids and their potential utility for pain management, the legalization of *cannabis*, and the level of cannabinoids prescribed for medicinal purposes, there is a growing need to carefully evaluate the risk–benefit considerations of cannabinoids for the management of pain.[21] For patients who are prescribed and choose to take cannabinoid-based medicines, good clinical practice involves informing the patient on the potential benefits and risks.[23] The AT should review current literature and position statements because new evidence with cannabinoid-based medicines for chronic pain syndromes are continuously updated and revised. Additionally, the U.S. states and other countries that have moved toward authorization of medical *cannabis* or cannabinoid-based medicines for chronic pain may allow larger-scale empirical and population-level studies, which will further inform the evidence base. Therefore, the quantity and quality of evidence and the clinical experience of prescribers of medical *cannabis* and cannabinoid-based medicines will continue to improve.[23]

MEDICINAL *CANNABIS* AGREEMENT

Date: ___________________

I understand that ________________________ (clinician name) is helping me with the treatment of my chronic pain.

In considering the possibility of using medicinal *cannabis*, it is important to recognize that the risks of medicinal *cannabis* may be affected by specific medical conditions and patterns of use. I understand what has been explained to me and agree to the following conditions of treatment:

1. I must prevent children and adolescents from gaining access to medicinal *cannabis* because of the potential harm to their well-being. I will store *cannabis* in locked cabinets to prevent anyone else from using it.
2. I know that some people cannot control their use of *cannabis*. One example is using *cannabis* for reasons other than for the indication for which it was prescribed, such as getting high or stoned. This behavior may lead to not going to school, sports practice, or other obligations. I agree to discuss this with my doctor if this happens.
3. I realize that unless specifically recommended by my doctor, I should abstain from medicinal *cannabis* if any of the following conditions apply:
    - I am pregnant or considering pregnancy.
    - I am middle-aged or older and have a heart disease or heart rhythm problem.
    - I have a history of serious mental illness (e.g., schizophrenia, mania, or a history of hallucinations or delusions).
4. In order to reduce the risk of lung disease, I will avoid smoking *cannabis* with tobacco, avoid deep inhalation or breath-holding, and use a vaporizer rather than smoke or use a water pipe.
5. I will not drive a car or operate heavy machinery for 3-4 hours after use of medicinal *cannabis*, or longer if larger doses are used or the effects of impairment persist. I will use a designated driver for automobile transportation if I have to go out sooner than 3-4 hours after taking this medicine.
6. Since the potency of *cannabis* varies widely, I will use the minimum amount of medicinal *cannabis* needed to obtain relief from pain or other symptoms. When trying a new strain of *cannabis*, I will start with a very small amount and wait at least 10 minutes to see how it affects me before taking more.
7. If thought advisable by my health care provider, I might want to substitute one of the medicines containing THC-analogs that are approved by the U.S. Food and Drug Administration (FDA) rather than take natural *cannabis*.
8. I might notice a withdrawal syndrome for 2 weeks if I stop *cannabis* use abruptly. Trouble getting to sleep and angry outbursts might require that I withdraw from using *cannabis* slowly.
9. I understand that the course of treatment will have to be reevaluated regularly after I start the medicinal *cannabis*.
10. I will not use medicinal *cannabis* in public places unless the law specifically permits this.
11. I know that there is no legal precedent to help me if I am released from a sports team or if a urine toxicology screen is positive for *cannabis*.
12. I know that I may be asked to reduce or stop my intake of opioids (narcotics), sedative hypnotics (benzodiazepines), or alcohol. This will be done to reduce the risk of side effects from a combination of medications that affect the central nervous system.

Signed: ____

FIGURE 20.2 Sample written contract.

Adapted from Fischer et al. (2011); Fischer et al. (2017); Wilsey et al. (2015).

Case Studies

Case Study 1

Pedro sustained a lower back strain while working at a construction site. His colleague, Frank, recommended using CBD pills rather than conventional NSAIDs to manage the pain. Pedro bought a bottle of CBD pills at a local gas station market. After taking a dose of pills, he noticed that his eyes were starting to water and felt a sense of euphoria. Frank had told him that he would not experience anything unusual with the CBD, but Pedro had never felt anything similar to this when taking NSAIDs.

Questions for Analysis

1. What was Pedro likely experiencing?
2. Pedro looked over the ingredients list and did not see anything that indicated what could cause this. What might be the cause?

Case Study 2

Carolina was diagnosed with a melanoma on her forehead secondary to excessive suntanning as a young woman. She discussed trying medical marijuana with her dermatologist for her pain prior to having surgery to excise the melanoma. Her physician had concerns regarding dosing and frequency of medical marijuana and was unsure as to how Carolina could purchase it. Carolina consulted with a local naturopath who had appropriate dispensing credentials, and he met her request.

Questions for Analysis

1. What was the basis of Carolina's dermatologist's concern?
2. Is medical marijuana a viable option for Carolina's condition?

Cannabinoid-Based Medicines Discussed in This Chapter

generic (pronunciation) Trade name	Description	Indication
tetrahydrocannabinol (THC) (TET ra hye droe can NAB e nol) *cannabis*	Dose is adjusted per patient.	Medical application: analgesic, anticonvulsant, anti-inflammatory, appetite stimulant and antiemetic for AIDS patients with cancer. Because of its potential to cause positive drug test, it is banned at most competitive levels.
cannabidiol (CBD) (kan a bi DYE ol) Epidiolex	Oral solution contains 100 mg/mL (100 mL) CBD, alcohol, sesame oil, and strawberry flavor.	For seizures associated with Lennox-Gastaut syndrome or Dravet syndrome in patients 2 years of age and older
dronabinol (droe NAB i nol) Marinol, Syndros	Oral capsules or oral solution containing the plant-derived semisynthetic cannabinoid THC	For anorexia associated with weight loss in patients with AIDS and nausea and vomiting associated with cancer chemotherapy, mostly after the failure of previous treatments
nabilone (NA bi lone) Cesamet, Canemes	Oral capsules contain a synthetic cannabinoid similar to THC.	For nausea and vomiting due to chemotherapy, mostly after the failure of previous treatments
nabiximols (nab IX i mols) Sativex in Canada, EU, and other countries	Oromucosal spray is formulated from extracts of the *C. sativa* plant that contains the cannabinoids THC and CBD.	For multiple sclerosis–associated neuropathic pain and spasticity, mostly after the failure of previous treatments

Note: EU = European Union, AIDS = acquired immune deficiency syndrome

Based on Abuhasira, Shbiro, and Landschaft (2018); Badowski (2017); Drugs.com. *Cannabidiol* (2018); Drugs.com. *Cannabis* (2018); Häuser et al. (2018); Hazekamp et al. (2013); Whiting et al. (2015).

21

Drug Testing in Sport

OBJECTIVES

After reading this chapter, you will be able to do the following:

- Describe how drug education programs in sport developed and the evolution of modern drug-testing policies
- Define the role of the athletic trainer in the specimen collection protocol
- Outline the steps in the chain of custody of a sample specimen
- Describe the consequences of a positive drug test through various sport governing bodies
- Develop strategies for counseling an athlete about the unintended consequences of drug and supplement use in athletics

As described in chapter 19, athletes may go to extremes to gain a competitive edge, even to the point of being willing to sacrifice years from their lives to win. The herbs of the Roman Empire era have been replaced by contemporary designer drugs and inappropriate use of standard prescription medication. To ensure a level of fair play and competition integrity, many sport governing bodies have adopted drug screening programs to prevent the unacceptable use of drugs and supplements. This chapter describes drug education and testing protocols that have become common in many levels of sport. It provides details on how the athletic trainer (AT) can find information on drugs that are banned and reviews the general mechanics of specimen collection and testing, as well as penalties for violations. However, it must be emphasized here and throughout this chapter that the athlete alone is responsible for the drugs and supplements he ingests, injects, applies, or otherwise administers.

Drug Education

An overarching goal of sport governing bodies is to provide drug education seminars, lectures, and structured presentations pertaining to substance abuse.[2] For example, in professional basketball, all first-year players participate in a Rookie Transition Program that includes a drug prevention component.[36] Likewise, the National Collegiate Athletic Association (NCAA) is committed to the prevention of drug and alcohol abuse and deems student-athlete education as a best practice, providing resources that member institutions can use as needed. The general components of drug prevention recommended by the NCAA include the following:[27]

- Establishing a written policy
- Securing student-athlete written consent before drug testing
- Defining banned substances and the consequences of a positive test

Select Drugs Mentioned in This Chapter

Drug class	Generic name	Trade name
Beta-agonist and beta-2 agonist	*albuterol inhalation*	Ventolin HFA, ProAir
CNS stimulant	*amphetamine*	Adderall
Anticonvulsant, cannabinoid	*cannabidiol* (CBD)	Epidiolex
Antihypertensive, diuretic	*chlorothiazide*	Diuril
CNS stimulant	*ephedra*	Banned supplement
Alpha/beta agonist	*epinephrine*	Primatene
Masking agent	*finasteride*	Propecia, Proscar
Diuretic, masking agent	*furosemide*	Lasix
Beta-2 agonist	*levalbuterol inhalation*	Xopenex
CNS stimulant	*methamphetamine*	Desoxyn
Androgen	*metandienone*	Dianabol
Beta-blocker	*propranolol*	Inderal
Herbal supplement	*saw palmetto*	Generic
Masking agent	*tamoxifen*	Nolvadex
Androgen	*testosterone*	Depo-Testosterone, AndroGel
Anticonvulsant; cannabinoid	*tetrahydrocannabinol*	Cannabis (THC)
No therapeutic indication	*tetrahydrogestrinone*	None

This list is not exhaustive, but rather contains drugs commonly encountered in the athletic training setting. Always consult up-to-date information, confirm with a pharmacist, or discuss the use of therapeutic medications with the prescriber of the medication.

- Reviewing the rules of the institution and conference
- Recommending that all rules be presented annually at the start of each competitive season and as needed with midyear transfers
- Establishing defined punishments for positive drug tests

Drug education programs, historically, have focused more on the negative effect of drugs than on how to change athletes' attitudes and behaviors in relation to drug use. However, a group of head ATs in NCAA institutions indicated that their programs covered health-related topics regarding drug abuse and legal aspects of drug use and included programs pertaining to decision-making skills.[33] Early versions of intercollegiate athletic drug programs incorporated an education module, and many included a substance-abuse rehabilitation component for athletes who tested positive. Although education was considered a vital element of these programs, both ATs and athletes agreed that testing was a necessary deterrent to drug use.[35] Drug education can range in formality from structured team lectures from experts in the field to online resources from reputable sources.[25]

Clinical Application

Drug Education Resources

Athletic trainers should use as many high-quality resources as are available to provide drug education to athletes of all levels. Educational components available to ATs include printed materials, such as infographics and posters pertaining to banned drugs that could be strategically placed in common team areas. An excellent resource is a video from the NCAA that details the nature of banned substances, the testing protocol, and penalties associated with these substances.[27]

The Evolution of Drug Testing in Sport

Historically, the International Association of Athletic Federations (IAAF) relied on the honor system of athletes pledging that they were drug free. By the mid-20th century, athletes were doping with stimulants and anabolic steroids in order to run faster, throw farther, and jump higher.[9] During a 1960 Olympics race, a cyclist collapsed and died shortly thereafter. During the autopsy, amphetamines were identified as the cause of death. The 1960s experienced a proliferation of anabolic steroids in track and field, which prompted the European Athletic Federation to establish drug-testing protocols.[9] The International Olympic Committee (IOC) introduced drug testing for the 1968 Winter and Summer Olympic Games,[7] but the tests had poor analytical capacity and did little to deter drug use. These actions led other sport governing bodies to establish drug-testing protocols for both illicit drugs and performance-enhancing drugs (PEDs) for the purpose of preventing substance abuse. In conjunction with testing protocols, education and rehabilitation components were established.

Drug screening by individual collegiate athletics programs dates back to the mid-1980s. ATs were perceived as serving as the first line of detection for this type of program as a result of their proximity to the student-athletes as well as their frequent interactions with the medical community, coaches, and administrators.[35] A 1984 survey conducted by the National Athletic Trainers' Association (NATA) Drug Education Committee identified 21 schools with a drug-testing program, and 9 schools acknowledged conducting the testing on site.[23] An on-site testing system was often conducted by the AT staff in the athletic training facility. By 1985, an NCAA drug testing survey indicated that an additional 43 schools had some form of screening program. At that time, the following significant concerns were expressed to the NATA board of directors:[23]

- Philosophical perception that drug testing of student-athletes is discriminatory[35]
- Potential conflict of interest that could compromise an athlete's health and well-being[12]
- Questions regarding the vetting and approval of the testing program by the institution's medical and legal representatives[35]
- Concerns about the AT's role in imposing or enforcing sanctions for a positive test[12]
- Question of maintaining confidentiality of testing results[12]
- A general lack of the education and qualifications that an AT may have to properly assess the needs of an athlete with a substance abuse issue[35]

The **World Anti-Doping Agency (WADA)** was organized in 1999 following an IOC conference on doping. In 2004, WADA developed its code, which includes the following standards for organizing these areas:

- Testing (further described later)
- Laboratories
- Therapeutic use exemption
- Prohibited substances
- Methods
- Protection of personal information
- Signatories to the code

The **United States Anti-Doping Agency (USADA)** signed on to this code. These standards have been adopted by the NCAA and other various professional team organizations. They include substances that are banned year-round, for competition only, and for select sports. Various individual institutions and multiple professional sports leagues currently partner with Drug Free Sport to conduct their testing, in part because of its mission of working exclusively with athletes.[28] Their comprehensive approach determines the following:

- Who is to be tested
- How the specimen is collected
- Where the specimen is shipped for laboratory analysis

Athlete's Rights and Consent

The development of drug screening and testing programs generated diverse opinions within the athletic training community, with some ATs advocating for testing and others questioning the AT's role in these programs.[17,31] The legality of these programs was also controversial within general society. In 1994, a challenge by Stanford University student-athletes to their drug-testing program reached the California Supreme Court. In 1995, the U.S. Supreme

Court heard the case of an Oregon high school's drug-testing program. In both cases, the drug testing was ruled constitutional.[15] Professional athletes have a **collective bargaining agreement** with their governing body that incorporates their approval for testing. Intercollegiate student-athletes in an NCAA institution must grant consent to be tested as part of their participation in the university's athletic program. According to NCAA regulations,[24] each student-athlete is mandated to give annual consent to drug testing, and failure to do so at an appropriate time will result in the student being declared ineligible for participation.

Responsibility of the Sport Participant

One of the most important things the AT must consider is that the athlete alone is responsible for the drugs and supplements they ingest, inject, apply, or otherwise administer. It may be easy to presume that a product is safe from doping because it is purchased at a franchise nutritional supplement outlet or is marketed as being "all natural." Unlike the process for prescription medications, nutritional supplement manufacturers are not required to meet the same rigorous U.S. Food and Drug Administration (FDA) standards for product safety. Studies have revealed that a high percentage of products have been contaminated with a variety of substances. The FDA acknowledges that it is not authorized to review dietary supplement products for safety and effectiveness before a product is marketed.[14]

Using Supplements During Sport Participation

Competitive athletes subject to testing must exercise the utmost caution when selecting supplements. Reliable sources exist for determining whether a product runs the risk of yielding a positive drug test. The NCAA published a list of banned substances based on the categories noted in table 21.1.[26] Further, the athlete should not rely on this list to rule out any label ingredient. Conversely, the NCAA does not publish a list of approved supplements and drugs.[26] Other important resources for the AT are the National Center for Drug Free Sport and NSF International (originally branded as the National Sanitation Foundation in 1944, it's an organization that develops public health standards and provides certifications that help protect food, water, consumer products, and the environment).

Athletes commonly trust that their physician will not prescribe medications that would be problematic. One of the first incidents of an inadvertent positive drug test occurred in the 1972 Olympics. A young Team USA swimmer had his gold medal revoked because his postrace drug test identified 2 banned medications that masked PEDs.[30] The athlete claimed he had documented the medications prior to drug testing and that a mistake had been

TABLE 21.1 Categories and Examples of Substances Banned by the National Collegiate Athletics Association

Categories of banned substances	Common examples
Stimulants	*amphetamine* (Adderall), *caffeine* (guarana), *cocaine*, *ephedrine*, *methamphetamine*, *methylphenidate* (Ritalin)
Anabolic agents	*nandrolone*, *testosterone*
Alcohol and beta-blockers	Alcohol, *propranolol* (banned only for rifle shooters)
Diuretics and other masking agents	Diuril, Lasix, Microzide
Illicit drugs	*heroin*, synthetic cannabinoids (i.e., "spice")
Peptide hormones	colostrum, human growth hormone (hGH), IGF-1 (i.e., deer antler velvet) and related compounds
Antiestrogens	Arimidex, Nolvadex
Beta-2 agonists	Ventolin HFA, Xopenex, Proventil HFA, ProAir

Note: It is always the athlete's responsibility to check with the appropriate or designated athletics staff before using any substance.

made. Many years later, the United States Olympic Committee (USOC) acknowledged that the athlete had not cheated but rather was a victim of an administrative error.

Similarly, a highly ranked female tennis player was suspended by the International Tennis Federation (ITF) for 2 years due to a positive test for a PED, which was a medication she had used for many years following prescription from a medical doctor in her native country.[41] At the time of prescription, the medication had not been banned. However, after that medication was added to the banned substance list, she continued to take it and did not declare ingesting it on multiple occasions. The general consensus was that her positive test was accidental, and the athlete received a 2-year competition ban instead of the 4 years the ITF had sought.

Supplement Standards

To help athletes make safe decisions regarding supplement use, it is prudent to access independent testing standards and product certification programs that analyze and credential specific supplements. NSF International first developed standards for the manufacture and packaging of various food equipment. Eventually this program expanded into food and nutritional supplements. In 2004, NSF International established their banned substances certification program. The organization's certification through the Certified for Sports program consists of comprehensive laboratory testing and analysis of the manufacturing process of a supplement. This program certifies the accuracy of a supplement's label ingredients and verifies that the product does not contain unsafe levels of contaminants, prohibited substances, or masking agents. This program also screens supplements for a multitude of banned substances, including anabolic steroids, narcotics, stimulants, and masking agents. Products with the NSF certification have met a high standard; in order to be certified, each manufacturer has had the following verified through an NSF audit:[29]

- Ingredients on the product label are reviewed for accuracy and toxicology.
- Manufacturing facility is scrutinized and ingredients are analyzed.
- Annual laboratory analysis is conducted for banned substances and materials, such as heavy metals and pesticides or herbicides.

Clinical Application

Recommending or Providing Sport Supplements

The NSF International's Certified for Sport program helps athletes make safer decisions when choosing sport supplements. Several high-level sport governing bodies allow only products that are approved by Certified for Sport to be recommended or provided to the athletes. Products with NSF certification are recognized by several sporting agencies, including the National Football League, Major League Baseball, Professional Golf Association, Ladies Professional Golf Association, and the Canadian Centre for Ethics in Sports. Some manufacturers rely on a Certificate of Analysis (CoA) of a Drug or Formulation document, which provides the exact details relating to the quality control and specifications of the product; these are based on a sample from a specific batch and the material from which it was manufactured.[5]

The Drug Free Sport AXIS program is an online portal[11] available to athletes or administrators through a subscription service. An AT can forward information regarding a specific supplement or drug to the AXIS portal. Within a few days, Drug Free Sport will reply to the AT with information on the presence or absence of banned substances in that supplement. Individual supplement labels are reviewed by Drug Free Sport for the most accurate information; thus, an athlete can use this feedback as a risk assessment to make as informed a decision as possible regarding a specific supplement. Drug Free Sport regularly acknowledges that their information on the medication or supplement tested does not guarantee that it is safe; despite their best efforts, there is always a risk of the presence of an unreported banned substance.

The Drug-Testing Process

Typically, a drug-testing session can be scheduled with Drug Free Sport by the institution or the governing body during an athlete's competitive season or in the off-season. Drug Free Sport furnishes the names of the athletes to be tested on the scheduled day to the institution or team, which is then responsible for contacting the athletes. Many

Common Components of a Prototypical Intercollegiate Institutional Drug-Testing Program

Philosophy

- Provides for the well-being of student-athletes
- Enhances a level competitive playing field

Policy Overview

- The program is reviewed with student-athletes annually by the athletic department staff.
- Random testing is conducted during the academic year and possibly the summer.
- Student-athletes are mandated to give written consent to drug testing as a condition of their intercollegiate athletic participation.
- Medical exemption can be requested if a prescribed medication results in a positive drug test.

Notification and Specimen Collection

- Testing is facilitated by an outside agency.
- Commonly, the athletic training staff contacts the student-athletes at least 24 hours before they will be tested.
- Positive tests have penalties established by the individual institution.
- A positive test can be appealed by the student-athlete.

Drugs Tested

- Tests are analyzed at approved laboratories independent of the institution.
- Drugs tested for are in accordance with the NCAA list of banned substances.
- Consistency in testing protocols is followed.
- The organization is unbiased and free from conflicts of interest.

Adapted from McAlindon et al. (2014).

institutions have their own versions of drug-testing programs—for example, for violations of team rules or in anticipation of testing prior to an NCAA event. Once testing is scheduled, Drug Free Sport assigns a trained **doping control officer (DCO)** to the screening site, which can be a college campus, an event venue, or the athlete's home. The National Center for Drug Free Sport identifies approved laboratories for analysis and provides a consistent drug-testing program. This organization is unbiased and free of conflicts of interest with the institution or athlete involved in the screening. Selection for drug testing is random unless a specific athlete requires a follow-up test.

Drug-Testing Techniques

Current drug-testing techniques offer many advantages and some limitations. For example, urine specimens are relatively easy to obtain and are cost effective (table 21.2).[10,37,40] However, the presence of a witness during urine collection can be considered intrusive. Blood, hair, saliva, and sweat have also been used as drug-testing specimens in various settings, and each technique has advantages and drawbacks (table 21.3).[8,37] It is likely that mass drug screening conducted by the NCAA and U.S. professional sports leagues will continue to use urine specimens.

The AT's Responsibility for Drug Testing

An AT designated by the institution or team is usually the point-of-contact person with the athletes during the drug-testing process. If the screening is announced in advance, the AT contacts each athlete with the specific logistical information for the test, including time and location. If the testing is unannounced, the AT is usually the person responsible for informing athletes of their selection for testing when they arrive at the venue. The AT has a series of responsibilities prior to and during the drug-testing process:

TABLE 21.2 Urine Toxicology Detection Time of Banned Drugs

Banned drug or drug category	Typical urine detection time
Amphetamine	2-4 d
Methamphetamine	2-4 d
Cocaine	1-3 d
Cannabis • Casual use • Daily use • Chronic use	 1-3 d 5-10 d Up to 30 d
Opioids • *hydrocodone* • *hydromorphone* • *oxycodone* • *oxymorphone*	2-4 d
Anabolic steroids • *stanozolol*	3-4 d

TABLE 21.3 Comparison of Various Drug-Testing Techniques

Testing matrix	Drug detection time	Advantages	Limitations
Blood	12-24 hr	Accurate; use is increasing	Invasive and expensive; detects only short-term use
Hair	4-6 mo	Measures long-term use; accurate	Costly and time consuming; complicated by very short hair styles or hair dye
Saliva	12-24 hr	Easy to obtain	Very short detection time; oral cavity is easily contaminated
Sweat	1-4 wk	Tamper-proof patch; measures cumulative use	High potential for contamination

- Prior to drug testing, the AT secures the marshalling location, necessary restrooms, and the location where the Drug Free Sports representative will receive the specimen from the athlete and prepare it for shipment to the laboratory.
- During the drug-testing process, the AT may provide athletes with appropriate water or sports beverages in sealed individual containers to facilitate urination, if needed. This is particularly beneficial for dehydrated athletes. Individually wrapped snacks may also be provided if the urine is too dilute and the athlete has to produce another sample.
- The DCO, *not* the AT, accompanies the athlete to the restroom for specimen collection.
- Once drug testing is underway, the AT serves as the representative for the institution or team. The AT witnesses the documentation of the process and troubleshoots any problems that interfere with specimen collection.
- Occasionally, an athlete has trouble producing a specimen. In these instances, some light-intensity exercise may be beneficial. In these cases, the AT may escort and accompany the athlete to the necessary fitness equipment.
- After the athlete has produced a specimen, the AT accompanies him from the restroom to the specimen collection area to ensure there is no opportunity to introduce a masking agent or device into the specimen.

Ideally, ATs should not handle the specimen at any point during the collection process (table 21.4),[3,12,25] including specimen collection, analysis, or shipping to the testing laboratory. Testing at championship events is organized in a similar manner. Athletes are contacted at the first available time, such as once the event finishes, and they cannot leave the venue until the specimen is collected. In the event that an athlete is required to stay at the venue, the AT is usually the person who remains with the athlete. The steps of the NCAA drug-testing program specimen collection are similar to drug-testing protocols in other levels of international competition or professional sports.

RED FLAG

Paruresis: An Unintended Challenge to Specimen Collection

The discomfort of being witnessed during drug-testing collection can affect the process. Paruresis is the functional inability to urinate in the presence of others; it has been called "shy bladder" or "bashful bladder."[19] Research has identified that 3.8% of soldiers required to submit for drug testing have paruresis.[21] The Diagnostic and Statistical Manual of Mental Disorders (DSM-5) classifies paruresis as a social anxiety disorder (SAD). Others consider paruresis distinct from SAD because it is a condition in which normal physiological function is impaired without a physical cause. Paruresis has been associated with symptoms such as anxiety, depression, and poor quality of life.[20]

Laboratory Testing

In early drug-screening programs, some intercollegiate ATs conducted point-of-care tests in their athletic training facilities. These tests are subject to many variables and unreliable, which prompted the recommendation that ATs use an outside source and limit their involvement in collecting or packaging specimens.[12,23] Current recommendations are that drug testing in the United States should be conducted by Drug Free Sport or a WADA-approved laboratory for international competition. There are

TABLE 21.4 Sample Specimen Collection Protocol

Phase of the protocol	Description of phase
Collection station	Use of the exclusive marshalling area and restroom for specimen collection is limited to the collector, institutional representative, and selected athletes. Only food or drink provided by the institution is allowed in the area.
Specimen beaker	The athlete reports to the testing area with photo identification, signs in, selects a random beaker, and applies a specific barcode to the container.
Specimen collection	The collector must witness the athlete urinating in the specimen beaker. The use of the restroom must be exclusive to the testing area at all times during the testing process.
Viability of the specimen	To ensure that the specimen concentration has not been tampered with, a normal urine specimen should have the following characteristics: • Specific gravity ≥1.005; samples <1.005 are not sent for analysis. • Temperature: 90°F to 100°F (32°C to 37.7°C) within 4 min of voiding • pH: 4.5-8.0 • Urinary creatine ≥20 mg/dL
Dividing the sample	A viable specimen is split into A and B samples and poured into separate vials by the collector. It is then secured for shipping. The athlete witnesses the process of dividing the specimen and preparing the samples for shipment. If a specimen is unacceptable, the athlete must remain in the approved testing area until she provides a viable specimen.
Chain of custody	The chain of custody is maintained by providing the athlete with documentation regarding the testing logistics, including the specimen identification number and the DCO's name.
Shipment of sample	Signatures from athlete, collector, and the institutional witness certify the accuracy of the collection process. Samples are shipped to an approved laboratory for testing.

32 WADA-approved laboratories across the world, including in Africa, the Americas, Asia, Europe, and Oceania, with U.S. laboratories in Los Angeles, California, and Salt Lake City, Utah.[45]

Although ATs are not responsible for analyzing specimens for banned substances, they should have a general understanding of the testing techniques. The enzyme-multiplied immunoassay technique (EMIT) is an immunoassay testing modality that is generally used to screen the A sample of a specimen. The EMIT test employs visible spectroscopy to measure the presence of certain chemicals or molecules in a substance by evaluating the interaction of those chemicals with specific antibodies or antigens. A positive result from an EMIT test indicates that the test subject has been exposed to the tested drugs, but does not indicate the exact measure of drugs in the athlete's system. In most instances, when an EMIT test reveals possible drug use, the sample will then be followed by a more detailed confirmation test. An example of a substance that would merit a more detailed examination is poppy seeds, which contain morphine and may mimic the presence of an opioid; however, under normal circumstances, the amount present from eating a product with poppy seeds will be well below the level required for detection.

A positive test from sample A requires a separate confirmatory screening of sample B. In institutional testing by the National Center for Drug Free Sport and NCAA championship or year-round testing, the athlete can request that the B sample be tested. He can also personally request to witness the B sample test or have a representative witness it. This confirmation test is generally conducted via gas chromatograph–mass spectrophotometer (GC–MS), which can identify small quantities of a substance to confirm the presence of a specific drug. The gas chromatograph component separates the different drugs or metabolites in the specimen and the mass spectrophotometer component identifies the specific drugs or metabolites.[3] The GC–MS analysis is generally used for testing anabolic steroids and confirming a positive A sample test.[7] This technique is the most accurate and reliable testing method; however, it is the most time-consuming and expensive screening technique.

Testing for Marijuana

The U.S. federal government classifies marijuana as a Schedule I drug; however, various states and municipalities have decriminalized it in various ways. Although many states have legalized recreational and medicinal use of marijuana, most sport governing bodies still categorize marijuana and its derivatives as a banned substance. The NCAA does not recognize medical use as a viable defense for a positive test for marijuana[25] or consider marijuana a PED.[18] Although *cannabidiol* (CBD) products have a significant marketing presence, this drug component is also considered banned by the NCAA. As always, athletes use any drugs at their own risk. The penalties for a positive marijuana test are somewhat unique compared to sanctions for other drugs. Different programs vary regarding the quantitative level of tetrahydrocannabinol (THC) metabolites. For THC, the NCAA relies on a quantitative test rather than a simple positive test (the presence of the drug alone). As of July 2019, a marijuana test is positive if the sample is ≥35 ng/mL.[6]

Testing for Anabolic Steroids

In-season testing for anabolic steroids began in the 1970s and has evolved as athletes' methods of trying to cheat the test have become more sophisticated. Anabolic androgenic testing focuses on the conjugated steroid and steroid metabolites found in the urine sample.[1] As discussed in chapter 19, 2 general categories of anabolic androgenic steroids make up the focus of a drug test. Endogenous steroids, such as testosterone, are part of the natural human physiology; exogenous steroids, such as *stanozolol*, *metandienone*, and *oxandrolone*, are ingested by the athlete.[16] Endogenous steroids can affect the balance between testosterone and epitestosterone. Because testosterone is a naturally occurring substance and key to the fundamentals of doping with anabolic steroids, establishing an appropriate testosterone level presents a challenge to drug testing. In some cases of drug testing, the mere presence of a drug would constitute a positive test; however, anabolic steroid testing requires a quantitative test to determine if the **testosterone-to-epitestosterone (T/E) ratio** is acceptable.[4] Under normal conditions, the T/E ratio is 1:1; however, a T/E ratio exceeding 4:1 is the cutoff for a positive test for anabolic steroids.[43]

Masking Agents

A key component of the philosophy of drug testing is to maintain the integrity of the game. Despite this objective, inevitably, some athletes attempt to beat the system. A positive test can damage an athlete's reputation or have serious financial implications. It can be very tempting to cheat to pass a drug test when the likelihood of failing is significant. One common method of cheating is masking the banned substance with other drugs to manipulate the results; a more advanced approach to this method is opting for designer drugs that may be undetectable. A **masking agent** can reduce renal and urinary excretion of steroid conjugates, decrease urine concentration, or possibly inhibit endogenous steroid synthesis.[1] Although masking agents are banned, they have no direct performance-enhancing capacity. Examples of masking agents include the following:

- *probenecid*—A medication used to treat gout that can reduce urinary excretion of testosterone, epitestosterone, and norandrosterone.
- *finasteride*—Intended to treat benign prostatic hyperplasia or hair loss in men; masks use of *nandrolone*.
- Diuretics—Increase urine volume in general, which dilutes urine concentration of steroid metabolites.
- *ketoconazole*—An antifungal that can lower the T/E ratio for endogenous sources but not exogenous sources.

RED FLAG

Trying to Cheat on a Drug Test

Athletes who modify drug tests take the risk that they might still fail the test and face penalties for violating the testing policy. Commercial products are available with specific instructions and claims of detoxifying the system to prevent a positive drug test.[39] One mechanical device called the Whizzinator uses a prosthetic penis with a storage reservoir for borrowed urine.[22] The device also mimics natural urination and has a heating element to establish normal specimen temperature. ATs involved with drug testing should be aware of schemes athletes use to cheat during the testing process.

A different type of anabolic designer steroid was identified as part of the 2003 Bay Area Laboratory Co-operative (BALCO) case.[16] These substances produce a lesser concentration of the known analytes that are routinely subject to testing, and thus have no clinical background. One was identified as *tetrahydrogestrinone*. Between 2002 and 2008, 22 steroid compounds went undetected by WADA-accredited labs.[16]

Evidence in Pharmacology

The Cheating Challenge

The WADA code authorizes using "any reliable means" to meet the challenge of cheating, including witness statements, documentary evidence, or evaluation of longitudinal profiling.[45] In the United States, both the USADA and NCAA subscribe to the WADA code. At the international competition level, the **Athlete Biological Passport** established by WADA in 2014 assesses biomarkers over time in an indirect testing approach.[42] This system allows a personalization of tracking results by establishing upper and lower limits of an athlete's T/E ratio over time, long after the original substance was metabolized or excreted.

Assessing the specimen's specific gravity is the first-line defense against the prospect of a masking agent being used to alter a test. Diuretics are banned by many sport governing bodies to prevent masking. In 2018, a major league baseball player failed a drug test for taking a legally available diuretic. He said he had been prescribed the medication in his native country, where it is legal, and did not realize it was banned by his sport governing body. He was suspended for 80 games.[32]

Results of Drug Testing

In the event of a positive test, a designated contact person, such as the institution's administrator, is notified by Drug Free Sport. The NCAA will contact the institution with a report of negative tests in terms of a number, such as 19 athletes negative out of 20 athletes tested. Then they will contact the institution specifically regarding the positive tests. Essentially all screening programs have a penalty phase for a positive test that can vary from program to program or drug to drug. In most cases, punishment escalates with each successive positive test for an athlete. Penalties usually involve an individual punishment or temporary suspension from the team and generally include a rehabilitation component. In the IOC, NCAA, and professional major leagues, there are several stepwise sequential increases in the severity of the penalty incurred with each positive test. For example, an athlete may receive a lengthy ban after the third positive test of *cocaine* or PEDs. Drug-screening programs similar to these are found for professionals in auto racing, tennis, golf, boxing, and mixed martial arts.[34] At the conclusion of the 2019 season, Major League Baseball (MLB) modified their policy to add opioids and remove marijuana from its list of drugs of abuse and eliminated suspensions of minor league players for a positive marijuana test.[13]

Drug Exemptions

Divergences from standard drug-testing protocols are made for specific situations. A therapeutic use exemption (TUE) is allowed for a banned medication that is prescribed to an athlete by a physician.[25] In this case, documentation is necessary relative to the athlete's history, up-to-date diagnosis, and medication dosage. This is particularly true if the athlete is diagnosed with attention-deficit/hyperactivity disorder (ADHD) and treated with a restricted-use medication, such as Adderall or Ritalin. In this case, if the result of the sample A test is positive, prior to testing sample B, the institution can request medical exemption based on the athlete's history and physical exam; the AT should have the medical exception information on file in the event of a positive test. This is particularly important during the championship season if information is needed immediately for a medical exceptions appeal. The AT should provide the specific ADHD documentation to the NCAA. Other deviations from the routine protocol can be made on a case-by-case basis. In these cases, the DCO from Drug Free Sport can arrange for an alternate time for testing. These situations might include the following:[25]

- Time conflict due to academic reasons
- Illness or injury that precludes the athlete from being tested
- Need to return to competition

The TUE acknowledges that some banned substances have a legitimate medical purpose. One example is testosterone for the patient with testicular failure.[1] Granting this exemption would be based on the following conditions:

- The athlete's health would be impaired if the banned drug were withheld.
- The drug is not likely to enhance the athlete's performance.
- No reasonable or viable alternative to the banned drug exists.
- The necessity of using the prohibited substance is not secondary to any prior use.

Of note, there is no exemption for testosterone being given for female athletes because the FDA approves testosterone only for men. However, WADA grants a testosterone TUE to female-to-male (FTM) transgender athletes who require androgens. Testosterone is generally administered via intermuscular or topical routes at doses consistent with androgen-deficient men as per the prescribing endocrinologist.[44] As noted previously, there is a link between poppy seeds and opioids. In tests, commercially available poppy seeds paralleled morphine concentrations that could exceed the threshold for a positive drug test. Results of a study indicated that subjects had positive tests at a 24-hour test and at 48-hour intervals.[38] The recommendation is for athletes to avoid food with poppy seeds during time spans when they could be tested.

Summary

Nutritional supplements and prescription drug use for performance enhancement has occurred for centuries, leading to the development of drug-screening protocols to protect the integrity of competition. Various resources and information outlets can help today's athletes screen their supplements for potential banned substances. A comprehensive drug-screening program includes education, testing, and intervention. A drug-testing protocol has many common components and is a routine exercise for intercollegiate, professional, and elite international athletes. Many athletes have invested tremendous time and money in their opportunity for success; thus, a positive test can detrimentally affect their future. Drug testing has evolved from workplace tests done in the athletic training facility to a structured process managed by trained professionals. The many steps in the process aim to minimize the opportunity of masking banned substances or tampering with the sample. Positive tests generally result in escalating sanctions, which enhance the role of testing as a deterrent. Caution should be exercised in administering medication, since even standard supplements and prescription medications may inadvertently cause a positive test. Finally, athletes are ultimately responsible for what they ingest, inject, apply, or otherwise administer into their bodies.

Case Studies

Case Study 1

Khalid was the team manager of an international track and field team whose responsibilities included managing the team's meals. Although he had specifically instructed the restaurant to not include anything with poppy seed in the menu, one morning, Khalid saw a tray of poppy seed bagels on the athletes' buffet table. That afternoon, there was a spontaneous drug test. Among those tested were 2 athletes who had eaten the poppy seed bagels. Khalid was quite anxious at the time of the test and for 3 days afterwards until he received the notification that there were no problems associated with the testing.

Questions for Analysis

1. Why was Khalid so concerned about the drug testing on that day?
2. What are the chances of a poppy seed pastry causing a problem with drug testing?

Case Study 2

Jimmy, an employee for a large aircraft manufacturing facility, was selected for drug testing. The DCO sensed that something was inappropriate about Jimmy's sample because the beaker felt cold. The specific gravity was measured at 0.995, the sample was rejected, and Jimmy was told he needed to resubmit his sample because it was diluted. Jimmy produced a second sample approximately 45 minutes later, and his specific gravity was 1.006. Jimmy acknowledged that he had added some cold water to his original specimen while he was in the rest room. The DCO made a note of the admitted tampering and Jimmy was deemed to have a positive test.

Questions for Analysis

1. What were the signs that the specimen had been tampered with?
2. What did the penalty of tampering involve?

22

Medications for Surgery

OBJECTIVES

After reading this chapter, you will be able to do the following:

- Describe the basic concepts of general anesthesia
- Describe the levels of sedation and the stages of anesthesia
- Differentiate the anesthetic options for sports medicine surgery: general, regional, spinal, and local
- Explain the preparation for surgery, including fasting prior to surgery
- List frequent adverse effects of anesthesia

Select Drugs Mentioned in This Chapter

Drug class	Generic Name	Trade name
Common inhaled anesthetic	*ketamine*	Ketalar
	propofol	Diprivan
	sevoflurane	Sevorane

This list is not exhaustive, but rather contains drugs commonly encountered in the athletic training setting. Always consult up-to-date information, confirm with a pharmacist, or discuss the use of therapeutic medications with the prescriber of the medication.

Although the selection and administration of surgical anesthesia are beyond the athletic trainer's (AT's) scope, he should have a basic understanding of anesthesia protocols and how they vary according to the proposed type of diagnostic, therapeutic, or surgical intervention. **General anesthesia** is essentially a medically induced coma with loss of protective reflexes that results from the administration of 1 or more general **anesthetic agents**. General anesthetics depress the central nervous system (CNS) to a sufficient degree that otherwise intolerably painful medical procedures are possible. In some cases, the patient must be asleep to permit the performance of surgery and unpleasant procedures. General anesthetics have low therapeutic indices and thus require great care in administration. The **anesthesiologist** must select specific drugs and routes of administration that will produce general anesthesia based on the pharmacokinetic properties and the secondary effects of the various drugs.[6] As part of an interprofessional health care team, the AT should have a working knowledge of the context of the proposed diagnostic or surgical procedure and be mindful of the patient's characteristics and associated medical conditions when discussing appropriate anesthetic agents.[24] The AT is an important resource to the surgical team who can relate the patient's medical history and monitor complications secondary to surgery. The AT can counsel patients prior to surgery on what to expect when having anesthesia. This chapter details the importance of inhaled versus intravenous (IV) anesthesia, various nerve blocks used for regional anesthesia, and valuable information for patient care prior to and after surgery.

Concepts of Anesthesia

For minor procedures, conscious **sedation** techniques combine IV agents with local anesthetics. These drugs can provide profound **analgesia** while retaining the patient's ability to maintain a patent airway and respond to verbal commands.[10,15] For more extensive surgical procedures, anesthesia protocols commonly include intravenous drugs to induce the anesthetic state. These drugs are often combined with inhaled anesthetics to maintain an anesthetic state and neuromuscular blocking agents to effect muscle relaxation. When monitoring patients during surgery, vital signs are the standard method of assessing depth of anesthesia. **Electroencephalography** (EEG) monitoring, an automated technique based on quantification of anesthetic effects, is also useful.[15] The neurophysiologic state produced by general anesthetics is characterized by 5 primary **anesthesia end points**:[10,20,24]

1. **Analgesia**—Loss of response to pain
2. **Amnesia**—Loss of memory
3. **Immobility**—Loss of motor reflexes
4. **Coma (hypnosis)**—State of being unconscious or unresponsive to stimulus
5. **Paralysis**—Skeletal muscle relaxation

None of the currently available anesthetic agents when used alone can achieve all 5 of these desired effects well. An ideal anesthetic drug would induce rapid and smooth loss of consciousness, be rapidly reversible on discontinuation, and possess a wide margin of safety.[10] In practice, anesthesiology (figure 22.1) relies on the use of combinations of

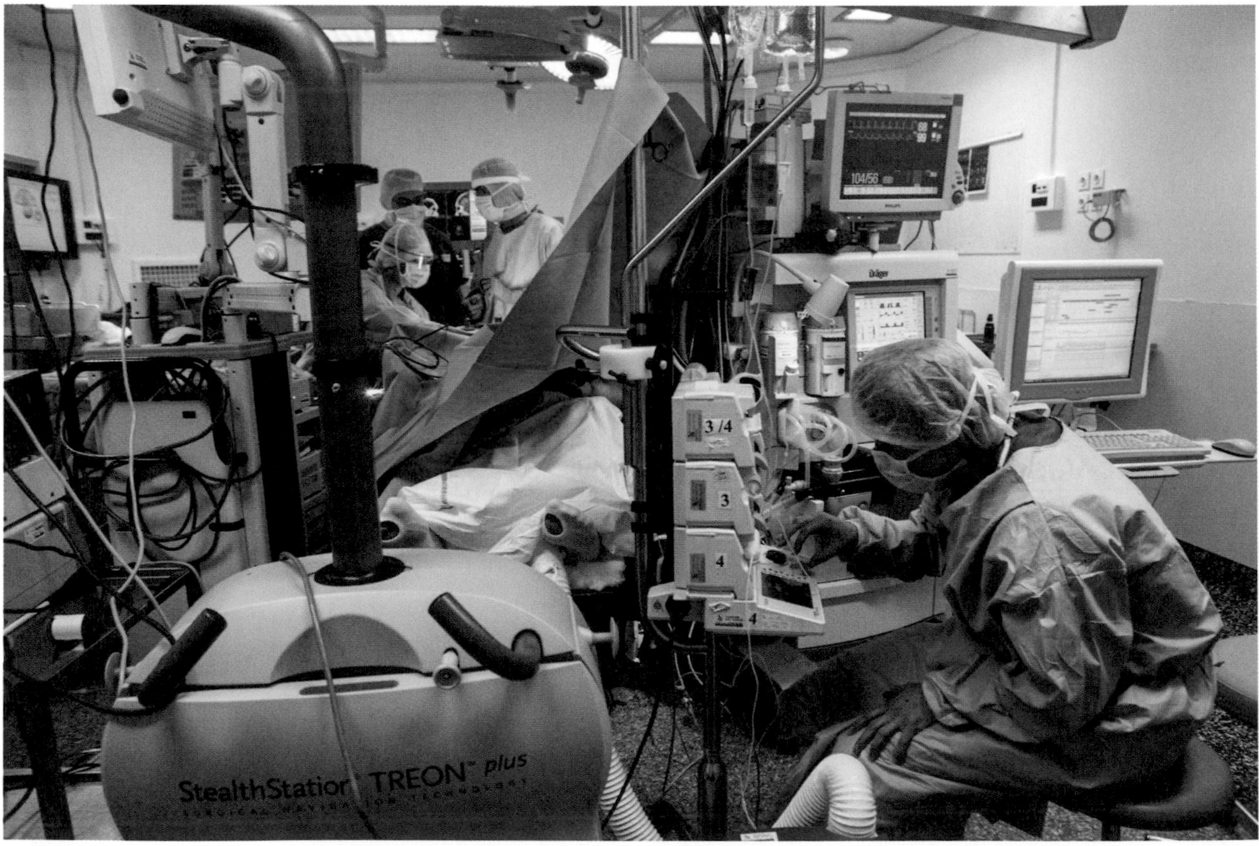

BSIP/Universal Images Group via Getty Images

FIGURE 22.1 Operating room with equipment for administering anesthesia with integrated systems for monitoring several vital parameters.

intravenous and inhaled drugs (balanced anesthesia techniques) to take advantage of the favorable properties of each agent while minimizing their adverse effects. Drugs are chosen to provide safe and efficient sedation based on the type and duration of the procedure and patient characteristics, such as organ function, medical conditions, and concurrent medications.[20,32] Different types of anesthesia affect the end points differently. For example, sedation, or twilight anesthesia, uses benzodiazepines to induce amnesia, while general anesthetics affect all end points. The goal of anesthesia is to achieve the end points required for the given surgical procedure with the least risk to the patient.[6]

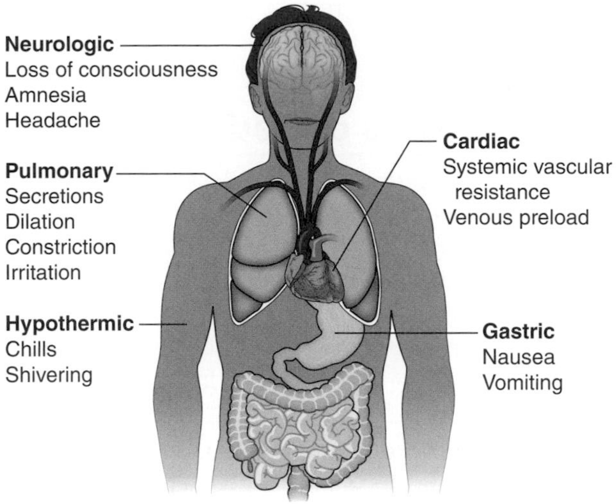

FIGURE 22.2 Effects of general anesthesia.

Effects of General Anesthesia

General anesthetics induce a generalized, reversible depression of the CNS. Under general anesthesia, there is a lack of perception of all sensations. The anesthetic state includes loss of consciousness, amnesia, and mobility (or a lack of response to noxious stimuli) but not necessarily complete analgesia. Other desirable effects provided by anesthetics or adjuvants during surgery may include muscle relaxation, loss of autonomic reflexes, analgesia, and light sedation (**anxiolysis**). All these effects facilitate safe and painless completion of the procedure; some effects are more important in certain types of surgery than others. For example, abdominal surgery necessitates near-complete relaxation of the abdominal muscles, whereas neurosurgery often requires light anesthesia that may be lifted rapidly when the neurosurgeon needs to judge the patient's ability to respond to commands.[32] The primary responses to general anesthesia are systemic vascular, pulmonary, hypothermic, and neurologic (figure 22.2).[24]

Systemic Vascular and Cardiac Effects

The hemodynamic effects produce a decrease in systemic arterial blood pressure. The causes of this hypotension include direct vasodilation, which in turn causes decreased vascular resistance and venous preload, myocardial depression, or both; a blunting of baroreceptor control; and a generalized decrease in central sympathetic tone.[24]

Pulmonary Effects

Nearly all general anesthetics reduce or eliminate both ventilatory drive and the reflexes that maintain airway patency. Therefore, ventilation generally must be assisted or controlled for at least some period during surgery. The gag reflex is lost and the stimulus to cough is blunted. Lower esophageal sphincter tone also is reduced, so both passive and active regurgitation may occur,[24] leading to undesirable outcomes such as **respiratory aspiration**. Reducing the potential of regurgitation and aspiration of the stomach contents into the lungs when a patient is under anesthesia is a major concern. An AT can help inform the patient of the importance of taking these precautions prior to surgery (see Preparation for a Surgical Procedure).

Hypothermic Effects

Patients commonly develop hypothermia (body temperature <36°C) during surgery. The reasons for this include low ambient temperature, exposed body cavities, cold intravenous fluids, altered thermoregulatory control, and reduced metabolic rate. Prevention of hypothermia is a major goal of the anesthesiologist during anesthetic care.[24]

Neurologic Effects

General anesthetics distribute well to all parts of the body, becoming most concentrated in the fatty tissues. The CNS is the primary site of action of anesthetics. Most likely, loss of consciousness and amnesia ensue from supraspinal action (i.e., action in the brain stem, midbrain, and cerebral cortex), while immobility in response to noxious stimuli is caused by depression of both supraspinal and spinal sensory and motor pathways. Different sites in the

CNS are observed differentially with increasing depth of anesthesia.[32]

Levels of Sedation

The levels of sedation occur in a dose-related continuum, which is variable and depends on individual patient response to various drugs. These artificial levels of sedation start with minimal or light sedation (anxiolysis), continues to moderate sedation, then deep sedation, and finally a state of general anesthesia. The hallmarks of escalation from 1 level to the next are recognized by changes in mentation, airway competency, respiratory competency, and cardiovascular effects (table 22.1).[1,10,20] This escalation in levels of sedation is often very subtle and unpredictable; therefore, the anesthesiologist must always be ready to manage the unanticipated next level of sedation.[20]

Stages of Anesthesia

The order of general anesthesia occurs through induction, maintenance, and recovery. **Induction** is the time from the administration of a potent anesthetic to the development of unconsciousness, while maintenance is the sustained period of general anesthesia. **Recovery** starts with the discontinuation of the anesthetic and continues until the return of consciousness and protective reflexes. Induction of anesthesia depends on how fast effective concentrations of the anesthetic reach the brain. Recovery is essentially the reverse of induction and depends on how fast the anesthetic diffuses from the brain. The depth of general anesthesia is the degree to which the CNS is depressed, which is evident in EEGs.[20]

Traditionally, anesthetic effects on the brain produce 4 stages or levels of increasing depth of CNS depression (figure 22.3; **Guedel's classification**). Modern anesthetics act very rapidly and achieve deep anesthesia quickly. The progressively greater depth of CNS depression is associated with increasing dose or time of exposure and is traditionally described as stages of anesthesia.[6,10,16,20,32]

Stage I: Analgesia or Induction

In stage I, the patient has decreased awareness of pain, sometimes with amnesia. Consciousness may be impaired, but it is not lost. The patient initially experiences analgesia without amnesia. Later in stage I, both analgesia and amnesia are produced. The analgesia of stage I is variable and depends on the specific anesthetic agent. With fast induction, the patient passes rapidly through the undesirable excitement phase (stage II).

TABLE 22.1 Levels of Sedation

Level of sedation	Minimal sedation anxiolysis	Moderate sedation or analgesia	Deep sedation or analgesia	General anesthesia
Responsiveness	Normal response to verbal stimulation	Purposeful* response to verbal or tactile stimulation	Purposeful* response following repeated or painful stimulation	Unarousable even with painful stimulus
Airway	Unaffected	No intervention required	Intervention may be required**	Intervention often required**
Spontaneous ventilation	Unaffected	Adequate	May be inadequate	Frequently inadequate
Cardiovascular function	Unaffected	Usually maintained	Usually maintained	May be impaired

*Reflex withdrawal from a painful stimulus is *not* considered a purposeful response.

**Intervention or rescue of a patient from a level of sedation that is deeper than intended must be performed by a practitioner who is proficient in airway management and advanced life support. The qualified practitioner corrects the adverse physiologic consequences of the deeper-than-intended level of sedation (such as hypoventilation, hypoxia, and hypotension) and returns the patient to the originally intended level of sedation. It is not appropriate to continue the procedure at an unintended level of sedation.

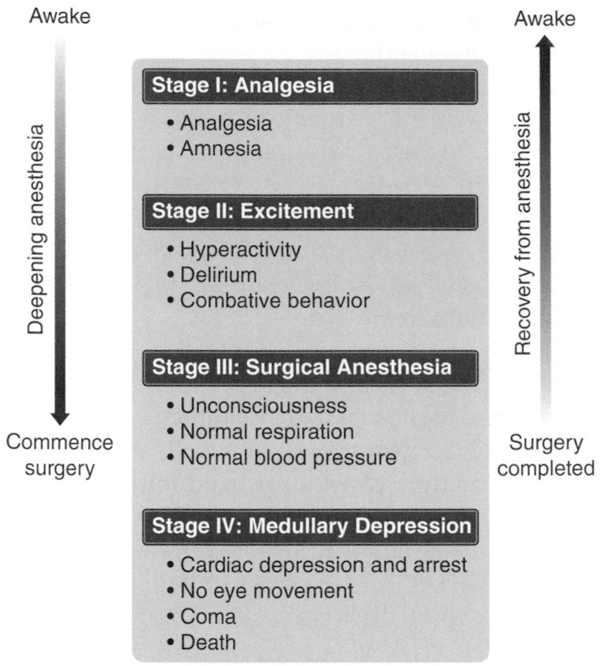

FIGURE 22.3 Stages of anesthesia.

Stage II: Disinhibition or Excitement

During this stage, the patient appears delirious and may vocalize but is completely amnesic. Respiration is rapid and heart rate and blood pressure increase. The patient appears to be delirious and excited. Amnesia occurs, reflexes are enhanced, and respiration is typically irregular. Retching and incontinence may occur.

Stage III: Surgical Anesthesia

This stage begins with slowing of respiration and heart rate and extends to complete cessation of spontaneous respiration (i.e., apnea). In this stage, the patient is unconscious and has no pain reflexes. The skeletal muscles relax, vomiting stops, and eye movements slow and then stop. The patient is unconscious and ready for surgery.

Stage IV: Medullary Depression or Overdose

This deep stage of anesthesia represents severe depression of the CNS, including the vasomotor center in the medulla and the respiratory center in the brain stem. Without circulatory and respiratory support, death would rapidly ensue in stage IV.[10] The anesthesiologist must take care to avoid stage IV, when the patient develops severe respiratory and cardiovascular depression that requires mechanical and pharmacologic support to prevent death.[16,32] This stage is lethal without cardiovascular and respiratory support.

Types of Anesthesia

Some surgeries often involve a singular choice of anesthesia, whereas others incorporate multiple options. Options for the anesthesiologist and surgeon include general anesthesia (inhaled and intravenous), neuromuscular blockade, and nerve blocks (central, peripheral, and local).

General Anesthesia

General anesthesia induces analgesia, sedation, amnesia, suppression of reflexes, and relaxation of muscles.[17] General anesthesia can be delivered by inhalation or intravenously and is well distributed to all parts of the body. The CNS is the primary site of action. Loss of consciousness and amnesia ensue from supraspinal action. Immobility is caused by depression of both supraspinal and spinal sensory and motor pathways. Different sites in the CNS are differentially affected by general anesthetics, giving rise to the classical stages observed with increasing anesthetic depth.[32]

Inhaled General Anesthesia

Inhaled anesthetics, such as *ketamine* (Ketalar), are gases delivered from a machine that is operated by an anesthesiologist. They work through gas exchange in the alveoli of the lungs. Uptake from the alveoli into the blood and distribution and partitioning into the compartments within the body are important determinants of the kinetics of these agents. The ideal anesthetic should have a rapid onset (induction) and offset (emergence).[8,10] Pharmacology of inhaled anesthetics relate to potency; an anesthetic that is more potent causes anesthesia at lower partial pressures. Typically, there is a tradeoff between fast induction and high potency. An anesthetic that has a rapid induction typically has a low potency. Conversely, a very potent anesthetic typically has a long induction time.[32]

Inhaled gases are used primarily for maintenance of anesthesia after administration of an IV drug. Depth of anesthesia can be rapidly altered by changing the concentration of the inhaled gas. Inhalational agents have steep dose–response curves with very narrow therapeutic indices, so the difference in concentrations from eliciting general anesthesia to cardiopulmonary collapse is small. No antagonists exist. To minimize waste, inhaled gases are delivered in a recirculation system that contains adsorbents to remove carbon dioxide and allow rebreathing of the gas.[20]

Intravenous General Anesthesia

Intravenous nonopioid anesthetics are used to facilitate rapid induction of anesthesia and have replaced inhalation as the preferred method of anesthesia induction in most settings. Intravenous agents are also commonly used to provide sedation during monitored anesthesia care. With the introduction of *propofol*, IV anesthesia also became a good option for the maintenance of anesthesia. These anesthetics do not produce all 5 desired effects of anesthesia (unconsciousness, amnesia, analgesia, inhibition of autonomic reflexes, and skeletal muscle relaxation), thus they are likely to be combined with multiple drugs to result in balanced anesthesia.[8]

Intravenous medications, commonly *propofol* or *midazolam*, are administered to establish a level of unconsciousness. In some cases, oxygen may be administered through a face mask to complement IV medication rather than incorporating an inhaled anesthetic.[9] This technique is referred to as **total intravenous anesthesia (TIVA)**. Intravenous anesthetics cause rapid induction of anesthesia, often occurring in ≤1 minute. Their use is the most common way to induce anesthesia before maintenance of anesthesia with an inhalation agent. IV anesthetics may be used as single agents for short procedures or administered as infusions (e.g., TIVA) to help maintain anesthesia during longer surgeries. In lower doses, they may be used solely for sedation.[20]

Balanced Anesthesia

No single drug achieves all desired goals of anesthesia. The ideal anesthetic drug would provide hypnosis, amnesia, analgesia, and muscle relaxation without undesirable changes in blood pressure, pulse, or breathing. In a method called **balanced anesthesia**, several inhaled or intravenous drugs are used in combination, each with a specific effect, to achieve analgesia, muscle relaxation, unconsciousness, and amnesia. Balanced anesthesia attempts to target each end point with a combination of drugs, thereby reducing the dose and toxicity of each.[6] The anesthetic effects of simultaneously administered general anesthetics are additive and offer a better risk profile to the person under anesthesia and rapid recovery.[32] For example, *propofol* (injection) might be used to start the anesthetic, *fentanyl* (injection) to blunt the stress response, *midazolam* (injection) to ensure amnesia, and *sevoflurane* (inhaled) during the procedure to maintain the effects.

Adjuvant (Adjunct) Drugs

Adjuvant drugs (also called **adjuncts**) are a critical part of the practice of anesthesia and include drugs that affect gastrointestinal motility, nausea and vomiting, anxiety, and analgesia. Adjuncts are used in collaboration to help make the anesthetic experience safe and pleasant.[20] Adjuvant drugs provide additional effects that are desirable during surgery but are not necessarily provided by the general anesthetics.[32] **Postoperative nausea and vomiting (PONV)** is the phenomenon of nausea, vomiting, or retching experienced by a patient in the postanesthesia care unit (PACU) or in the 24 hours following a surgical procedure. It is an unpleasant complication that affects about 10% of the population undergoing general anesthesia each year. Medications commonly used to prevent PONV are usually administered toward the end of surgery.[20]

Intravenous Local Anesthesia

Local anesthetics can be injected intravenously into a distal extremity to provide regional anesthesia

Evidence in Pharmacology

Postoperative Nausea and Vomiting

Postoperative nausea and vomiting following TIVA is the second most common postsurgical complaint aside from pain. Nausea and vomiting are controlled by the vomiting center, a neuroanatomical site in an ill-defined region within the reticular formation of the brain.[27] The first-line approach may include a serotonin antagonist such as the antiemetic *ondansetron* (Zofran), which inhibits serotonin and reduces nausea and vomiting.[31] *Ondansetron* can be administered as a postsurgical IV (4 mg) or oral (8 mg) medication for home care.[27]

Evidence in Pharmacology

General Anesthesia Versus Regional Nerve Blocks

A single center study compared general anesthesia to regional anesthesia for elderly patients with hip fractures based on the hypothesis that the regional approach would result in less morbidity and save costs. Benefits of regional anesthesia included perioperative pain control and postsurgical pain management with less reliance on opioids. The potential of postoperative hypotension was minimized with regional versus general anesthesia. Further, patients with regional anesthesia had less respiratory depression than those with general anesthesia, resulting in lower incidence of postoperative ventilator requirements that would necessitate intensive care admission. However, regional anesthesia did not reduce hospitalization costs or postoperative morbidity or mortality compared to general anesthesia.[19]

to that limb. Generally, practitioners encourage venous blood to drain from the limb by elevating the limb above the level of the heart before applying a proximal tourniquet and injecting the anesthetic into the vein. This approach allows high local concentrations of anesthetic to reach the nerves in the limb while limiting the redistribution of the anesthetic and thus preventing systemic toxicity. This type of local anesthesia, also called **Bier block**, is used for arm and hand surgery. Systemic intravenous *lidocaine* is used to reduce postoperative pain and is also administered for relief of chronic pain from injury or disease (e.g., diabetic neuropathy). Relief of chronic pain often lasts for weeks following a single, brief *lidocaine* infusion, even though the drug is cleared from the circulation within a few hours. The mechanism underlying this long duration of effect remains uncertain.[5]

Neuromuscular Blocks

Neuromuscular blocks (or blockades) are used to facilitate endotracheal intubation and provide muscle relaxation when needed for surgery. Their mechanism of action is via blockade of nicotinic acetylcholine receptors on the skeletal muscle cell membrane.[20] Paralysis, or temporary muscle relaxation with a neuromuscular blocker, is an integral part of modern anesthesia. The first drug used for this purpose was ***curare***, introduced in the 1940s, which has now been superseded by drugs with fewer side effects and, generally, shorter duration of action. Muscle relaxation allows surgery within major body cavities, such as the abdomen and thorax, without the need for very deep anesthesia.[12,20] A variety of techniques (central, peripheral, and local) for blocking neuromuscular function are crucial to the practice of anesthesia.

Central Nerve Block

Central nerve blocks include a variety of techniques (e.g., spinal anesthesia, also called spinal block or **neuraxial blockade**) that involve administration of drugs near the spinal cord by delivery into the epidural or **intrathecal space** (see figure 6.3).[17] Central nerve blocks include both epidural and intrathecal (spinal) anesthesia. The early effects of these procedures result primarily from impulse blockade in spinal roots; in later phases, anesthetic drug penetrates and may act within the spinal cord. *Bupivacaine* is particularly useful as an epidural anesthetic during labor in childbirth because, at low concentrations, it provides adequate pain relief without significant motor block. Reports of *bupivacaine* cardiotoxicity have led to decreased use of this agent in high concentrations (>0.5% weight:volume), although the dilute solutions used in **obstetrics** are rarely toxic.[5]

An adverse event of the central nerve block process is a postdural puncture headache, which occurs if the dura is inadvertently punctured by either the epidural injection itself or the placement of an epidural catheter. This outcome may result in a leak of cerebrospinal fluid (CSF) and cause an extremely intense headache.[28] This event is not common, and risk factors include needle diameter size, female patient <60 years old, and the experience of the personnel administering the injection.[28,29] The patient is likely to experience the headache within 72 hours after the injection, and pain is exacerbated by standing and head motion and possibly accompanied by nausea, blurred vision, and dizziness.[28,29] The most prompt resolution of this condition is the epidural blood patch, an injection of autologous blood (i.e., blood taken from the patient) into the epidural space to stop the CSF leak; this technique has an 85% success rate with 1 injection.[28] Typically, the source of the blood for the patch is the antecubital vein. Without use of the blood patch, the headache is likely to resolve in 7 to 10 days.

Peripheral Nerve Block

Peripheral nerve blocks are increasingly used for pain control associated with trauma and surgery. A peripheral nerve block has many patient-centered benefits relative to pain control, more prompt recovery, and shorter stay in the surgical facility.[14] Generally, local anesthetics are injected percutaneously using anatomic landmarks, ultrasound guidance, or fluoroscopic techniques to safely deliver the anesthetic near the specific targeted nerve. Anesthetics can be delivered as **bolus injections** (single shot or, occasionally, repeated nerve block) or as **continuous infusions** via catheters that are inserted near the target nerve. Single-shot injections may be used to provide short-term anesthesia for a procedure. For example, femoral nerve blocks often use continuous infusions of local anesthetics to control pain from a hip fracture, both prior to and for days after surgery.

Peripheral nerve blocks are also used in the management of trauma. Intercostal nerve blocks can reduce pain after rib fracture, possibly improving lung mechanics and reducing rates of pulmonary complications such as pneumonia. Examples of other useful peripheral blocks include transversus abdominis plane (TAP) block for the anterior abdominal wall; interscalene, cervical plexus, and brachial plexus blocks for shoulder and arm surgery; and femoral and popliteal blocks for the distal lower limb.[5]

Local Field Block

A local field block is used for smaller areas such as the wrist, fingers, and toes. This approach is more viable if the surgery is <60 minutes. To create a **bloodless field**, a pneumatic tourniquet is used that restricts blood flow and minimizes blood loss by obstructing arterial supply to the limb. With the limb elevated, a soft rubber bandage (Esmarch's bandage) is systematically applied from the fingertips down toward the tourniquet to expel venous blood (exsanguination) from the limb so that the surgical procedure can be completed.[21]

Common Applications of Anesthesia in Sports Medicine

Anesthesia is commonly administered in the sports medicine setting to prevent pain from an incision, tissue manipulation, and suturing. Based on the procedure, anesthesia may be provided locally or as general anesthesia. Spinal anesthesia may be used when the surgical site is too large or deep for a local block, but general anesthesia may not be desirable. With local and spinal anesthesia, the surgical site is anesthetized, but the patient can remain conscious or minimally sedated. In contrast, general anesthesia renders the patient unconscious and paralyzed during surgery. The patient is intubated and placed on a mechanical ventilator, and anesthesia is produced by a combination of injected and inhaled agents. Choice of surgical method and anesthetic technique aims to reduce the risk of complications, shorten the time needed for recovery, and minimize the surgical stress response. General anesthesia such as *propofol* and *sevoflurane* has been used for knee arthroscopy, although there may be an increase in incidence of nausea and vomiting associated with *sevoflurane*. The combination of *propofol* and *sevoflurane* requires less recovery time in the PACU compared to epidural and spinal techniques. Spinal or epidural anesthesia for the lower extremity using *bupivacaine* or *lidocaine* is considered reliable and can be accomplished with 1 injection to the spine.[22]

Lower-Extremity Surgery

Nerve blocks are commonly used for hip, knee, and ankle surgery (table 22.2).[14,21] For example, a femoral nerve block is frequently used for outpatient knee arthroscopy. For open reduction with internal fixation of an ankle fracture, a popliteal nerve block with *ropivacaine* may be used and possibly be complemented by a saphenous nerve block. The popliteal block is a relatively comfortable anesthesia for the patient to tolerate.[14]

TABLE 22.2 Common Lower-Extremity Peripheral Nerve Blocks

Category of block	Target or application
Femoral neve	Patella, knee, procedures involving the anterior thigh
3-in-1	Femoral, obturator, lateral cutaneous nerve
Saphenous nerve	Distal to the knee; available for ankle if combined with a popliteal block
Sciatic nerve	Surgery distal to the knee
Popliteal	Foot or ankle surgery
Ankle	Foot procedures
Digital	Minor toe procedures

In the case of an anterior cruciate ligament (ACL) reconstruction, the femoral block is a traditional and commonly used regional anesthesia. A femoral block with 30 mL of 0.5% *ropivacaine* is viable for 12 to 18 hours.[4] This medication can be complemented with the IV administration of *midazolam* or *propofol* prior to surgery and *bupivacaine* administered as a spinal injection.[12] However, there is a concern of quadriceps muscle weakness 6 months after surgery.[26] To minimize this risk, an adductor canal block has been advocated in lieu of the femoral block with the consideration that anesthesia of the adductor canal promotes a sensory blockade of the quadriceps muscles without compromising the motor fibers of the femoral nerve that innervate the quadriceps. Results of a study comparing outcomes of ACL reconstructions using the femoral nerve block or adductor canal blocks indicated comparable ability to complete an immediate postoperative straight-leg raise and isokinetic knee extension strength at 3 or 6 months after surgery. However, the adductor canal group demonstrated better proprioception soon after surgery;[26] thus, this approach may have benefits relative to athletic performance.

Upper-Extremity Surgery

General anesthesia is commonly used for upper-extremity surgery—for example, rotator cuff surgery. However, the interscalene block and subscapular block are options, either used alone or as an adjunct (table 22.3) to general anesthesia in upper-extremity surgery.[21,23] The medications *ropivacaine* or *bupivacaine* are appropriate choices for these blocks. Both interscalene and suprascapular blocks are easy to administer and comfortable for the patient. Injury to the elbow medial collateral ligament in throwing and overhead athletes responds well to an axillary, interscalene, or Bier block in conjunction with intravenous sedation.[23] The regional nerve blocks result in less nausea and vomiting in the PACU, whereas general anesthesia may allow more complete relaxation of the upper body and trunk.

TABLE 22.3 Common Upper-Extremity Peripheral Nerve Blocks

Category of block	Target or application
Interscalene	Proximal procedure of the arm; need ulnar nerve block for hand or forearm procedures
Supraclavicular	Arm, elbow, forearm
Infraclavicular	Elbow, forearm, hand
Axillary	Radian, median, ulnar nerves; procedures of elbow, forearm, or hand
Elbow	Hand specific to ulnar, median, and radial nerves or musculoskeletal nerve
Wrist	General hand or site specific
Digital	Fingers; minor procedures

Preparation for a Surgical Procedure

Preparation for surgery includes specific patient instructions, including having the patient remove personal items such as contact lenses and jewelry. The anesthesiologist will review the patient's pertinent medical history for conditions such as diabetes or sickle cell trait that may predispose her to regurgitation and respiratory aspiration.[2]

RED FLAG

Sickle Cell Trait and Surgical Complications

Literature is lacking relative to people with the sickle cell trait who experience complications secondary to surgery. Despite a scarcity of evidence-based guidelines, management of anesthesia for the sickle cell patient is left to the surgeon and anesthesiologist, who base decisions on their personal experiences.[25] To be prudent, the AT working with an athlete with the sickle cell trait who needs surgery should alert the surgeon prior to the procedure to ensure that risk management procedures are undertaken.

As described in the Adverse Effects of Anesthesia section, ATs can consistently recommend that patients follow the principle of no eating after midnight the night before surgery. Fasting prior to surgery is intended to prevent regurgitation, which could cause aspiration during surgery. The American Society of Anesthesiologists recommends that patients follow these fasting timelines prior to receiving general or regional anesthesia:[2]

- **2 hours before:** Consume nothing.
- **2-6 hours before:** Clear liquids (excluding alcohol) permitted.
- **6-8 hours before:** Milk, juice, or light food such as cereal or toast permitted.
- **8 hours before:** From this point on, avoid heavy foods, such as fried food, fatty foods, and meats.

During the procedure, the anesthesiologist monitors the airway, pulse, and respiration rate for the anesthesia.

Recovery From a Surgical Procedure

Recovery from general anesthesia should proceed quickly so that patients can maintain their own airways as soon as possible following surgery. In general, the stages of recovery from anesthesia occur in the opposite sequence from those of anesthesia induction, including the unpleasant excitement stage.[32] Postsurgical pain can be treated in multiple ways, including an intravenous administration of *ibuprofen* prior to the start of surgery or *ketorolac* as surgery concludes.[30] An additional nerve block can be used for the lower extremity. For rotator cuff surgery, an indwelling perineural catheter can be used to manage postsurgical pain, delivering local anesthetic for 48 to 72 hours.[21]

Complementing anesthesia is postoperative pain management, which may include a separate peripheral nerve block, analgesic administered through a catheter, or an intravenous NSAID. An analgesic such as *bupivacaine* or *ropivacaine* can be administered with an intraarticular injection to extend the anesthetic effect for several hours. Another postsurgical option is the multimodal regimen, which uses *acetaminophen*, an NSAID, or oral opioid that minimizes parenteral opioid use. Anesthesiologists and surgeons are advised to avoid prescribing opioids as much possible during the postsurgical period.[14]

Adverse Effects of Anesthesia

Adverse effects of anesthesia manifest themselves in a variety of ways. The most common effect of anesthesia is PONV; however, inhaled anesthetics, which resolve faster, minimize the prospects of this occurring. Severe or catastrophic outcomes, such as the incidence of an embolism, are statistically rare but still of significant concern. In a study of >700 adolescent patients who underwent knee arthroscopy, 0.67% reported either a deep vein thrombosis (DVT) or pulmonary embolism (PE), while 0.27% sustained a venous thromboembolism (VTE).[18] In a study of nearly 5,000 ACL reconstruction patients, 0.55% required treatment for a DVT and 0.12% presented with a postsurgical PE. Although these adverse outcomes are rare, the AT and surgeon should be cognizant of the patient that presents with deep posterior lower leg pain, swelling, and heat secondary to surgery.

There is also concern for an adverse effect associated with the use of a nerve block for ACL reconstruction. In 2018, a professional football player initiated a malpractice claim against his surgical team and anesthesiologist for an adductor canal block that was improperly administered several years prior. The block in this case was administered once the arthroscopy began after the surgeons realized a more advanced surgical procedure was necessary. As a result of the misplaced injection, it was claimed that the player's femoral and saphenous nerves were damaged and argued that this nerve damage compromised his quadriceps musculature intervention and function as a skilled football player.[7]

RED FLAG

Risk of Extended Tourniquet Times

Tourniquet time >120 minutes increases the risk of developing a DVT and other VTEs.[3] The postsurgical complication rate of VTE is estimated to be low (1% to 2%) following arthroscopic knee surgery, but rises to 7% to 30% following total knee arthroplasty.[13] Also, people with the sickle cell trait have an approximately 1.5-fold increased risk for VTE in general, and this risk extends to postsurgical conditions.[11] There is no direct concern of anesthesia for the patient with the sickle cell trait. However, it may be beneficial for the AT to alert the surgeon prior to surgery on a patient with the sickle cell trait, considering this population's VTE risks.

Summary

As an important member of the interprofessional health care team, the AT should be aware of anesthesia options or a surgeon's preferences. The AT can assist with providing the patient with preoperative information and must be cognizant of presurgical preparation as well as postsurgical complications commonly associated with anesthesia. Inhaled and intravenous anesthetics are used to produce the clinical features of general anesthesia, including unconsciousness, immobility, and amnesia. Currently, the combined use of adjuvants and balanced anesthesia with multiple inhaled or intravenous anesthetics achieves all of the goals of general anesthesia, including fast induction and a state of analgesia, amnesia, and muscle relaxation.[32]

Case Studies

Case Study 1

Bobby is a professional basketball player who was cleared for return to play 4 weeks after a left knee arthroscopy. The arthroscopy required 30 minutes of general anesthesia. On his third day of practice after returning to play, he reported calf pain in his left leg. Evaluation indicated mild palpable tenderness, associated with a dynamic overload of the leg that likely occurred while Bobby was sprinting at practice the previous day. The differential diagnosis was triceps surae muscle strain; however, the athletic trainer spoke to Bobby's surgeon about the prospect of deep vein thrombosis (DVT). Although the physician thought the risk of DVT was minimal, a Doppler ultrasound was ordered. The results were negative.

Questions for Analysis

1. What is the possible relationship between tourniquet time and DVT development?
2. How common is a DVT secondary to knee arthroscopy?

Case Study 2

Sandy is a novice fitness instructor who strained her lower back while demonstrating squat techniques. She was diagnosed with a L5-S1 disc bulge by an orthopedic physician, who prescribed 3 weeks of rehabilitation. At follow-up, Sandy had not progressed as the physician had anticipated; therefore, he ordered an epidural steroid injection. One hour after the injection, Sandy had a mild headache. At 11:00 a.m. the next day, she called her physician with a severe headache. The physician made arrangements to have an anesthesiologist administer an epidural blood patch of Sandy's own blood that evening, which resolved her headache completely.

Questions for Analysis

1. What is a blood patch?
2. What happened to cause the headache?

Drugs Described in This Chapter

Drug class	*generic* (pronunciation) Trade name	Clinical application
Common anesthetic	*ketamine** (KEET a meen) Ketalar	Used for starting and maintaining anesthesia. Induces a dissociative, trancelike state while providing pain relief, sedation, and memory loss. Also used for chronic pain and sedation.
	midazolam (MID aye zoe lam) Versed (benzodiazepine; refer to chapter 18 for details)	Medication used for anesthesia and procedural sedation. When administered intravenously, it begins to work within 5 min; when injected intramuscularly, it works within 15 min. Effects last for between 1 and 6 hr.
	*propofol** (PRO-puh-fol) Diprivan	IV sedative or hypnotic that is the first choice for induction or maintenance of anesthesia.
	sevoflurane (see-voe-FLOOR-ane) Sevorane	Commonly used for induction and maintenance of general anesthesia, especially in the outpatient setting. Often administered as an inhaled mixture of nitrous oxide and oxygen. Often used to put children to sleep for surgery.

*This drug is on the World Health Organization's list of essential medicines, which covers the safest and most effective medicines needed in a health system.

Glossary

absolute risk—Written as a percentage, the number of people who actually experience a medical event compared to the total number of people who could experience this event.

absorption—Movement of a drug from the site of administration to the bloodstream.

acne vulgaris—Formation of comedones, papules, pustules, nodules, or cysts as a result of obstruction and inflammation of hair follicles and their accompanying sebaceous gland.

acromegaly—Abnormal growth of the hands, feet, and face, caused by overproduction of growth hormone by the pituitary gland.

active ingredient—Component of a drug product intended to provide pharmacological activity or another direct effect in the diagnosis, cure, mitigation, treatment, or prevention of disease.

acute adrenal insufficiency—Disorder in which the adrenal glands do not make enough cortisol; also called Addison's disease.

acute infectious (septic) arthritis—Joint infection that is usually bacterial, evolves over hours or days, resides in synovial or periarticular tissues, and can rapidly destroy joint structures.

acute pain—Pain with a sudden onset that is expected to last a short time (i.e., <6 months).

acute pyelonephritis—Sudden and severe kidney infection that causes the kidneys to swell and may permanently damage them; can be life threatening.

acute stress disorder (ASD)—Symptoms lasting for 3 days to 1 month following exposure to 1 or more traumatic events. Symptoms develop after someone either personally experiences or witnesses someone else going through one of the following events: threat of death or actual death, serious injury, or physical violation.

additive effect—Occurs when 2 or more drugs combine to produce an effect greater than the effect of either drug taken alone.

adjuvant drug—An agent that modifies the effect of other agents; also called an adjunct.

adjuvants—Generic term for a medication (e.g., antidepressant, anticonvulsant) that is not designed to manage pain but has effects that can help reduce the need for designated analgesics.

administration—The direct application or furnishing of a single dose of a drug.

adrenal crisis—Life-threatening state caused by insufficient levels of cortisol, which is a hormone produced and released by the adrenal gland.

adrenergic receptor—Class of G protein–coupled receptors that are targets of many catecholamines, such as norepinephrine (noradrenaline) and epinephrine (adrenaline); also called adrenoceptors.

adrenocorticotropic hormone (ACTH)—Hormone produced by the anterior pituitary gland that encourages growth of the adrenal cortex and stimulates corticosteroid secretion.

adverse drug effect/event (ADE)—Injury or harm that results from medication use. Some ADEs are caused by preventable errors.

adverse drug reaction (ADR)—An unwanted, undesirable effect of a medication that occurs during usual clinical use.

adverse effect—Harmful or abnormal result such as illness or death that is caused by administration of a medication.

affinity—Probability of the drug occupying a receptor at any given instant.

agonist—Compound that binds to a receptor and produces the biological response.

allergy—Misguided reaction to foreign substances by the immune system, particularly pathogens.

allodynia—Pain resulting from a stimulus that would not normally provoke pain (e.g., light touch to the skin); also, a condition marked by such pain.

allosteric—Relating to or denoting the alteration of the activity of a protein through the binding of an effector molecule at a specific site.

alopecia—Hair loss that may either occur naturally or be related to disease or the use of certain medications.

amenorrhea—Abnormal absence or suppression of menstruation.

anabolic-androgenic steroids (AAS)—Any of a group of synthetic steroid hormones that promotes the storage of protein and the growth of tissue, sometimes used by athletes to increase muscle size and strength.

analgesia—A state of decreased awareness of pain, sometimes with amnesia.

analgesic drug—Any member of the group of drugs used to achieve analgesia, or relief from pain; also called painkiller.

anaphylaxis—Severe, rapid-onset allergic reaction that affects many body systems due to the release of inflammatory mediators and cytokines from mast cells and basophils; typically due to an immunologic reaction but sometimes also a nonimmunologic mechanism.

anesthesia end point—Goal to be achieved for the given surgical procedure with the least risk to the patient.

anesthesiologist—A physician with specialized training in anesthesiology. This medical specialty is concerned with the total perioperative care of patients before, during, and after surgery.

anesthetic—Drug that produces a temporary loss of sensation or awareness. May be divided into two broad classes: general anesthetics, which cause a reversible loss of consciousness, and local anesthetics, which cause a reversible loss of sensation for a limited region of the body without necessarily affecting consciousness.

anesthetic agents—A drug used to induce a temporary loss of sensation or awareness.

angioedema—Swelling of the lower layer of skin and tissue just under the skin or mucous membranes.

angiotensin-converting enzyme (ACE)—A central component of the renin–angiotensin system that controls blood pressure by regulating the volume of fluids in the body.

anorexia nervosa—Psychiatric disorder characterized by an unrealistic fear of weight gain, self-starvation, and conspicuous distortion of body image.

antagonist—Agent that prevents an agonist from binding to a receptor and thus either blocks or reverses the effect of agonists. They have no effect of their own.

antibacterial—Substance that destroys bacteria or suppresses their growth or their ability to reproduce.

antibiotic—Medicines that treat infections by killing bacteria. They don't work on viruses, such as the flu.

antibiotic resistance—Ability of bacteria and other microorganisms to resist the effects of an antibiotic to which they were once sensitive.

anticoagulant—Agent that slows down clotting, thereby reducing fibrin formation and preventing clots from forming and growing.

antiemetic—Drug that prevents or treats nausea and vomiting.

antimicrobial—Destructive to or inhibiting the growth of microorganisms, including bacteria, viruses, and fungi.

antiplatelet—Agent that prevents platelets from forming, growing, and clumping.

antipyretic—Drug that reduces fever.

antithrombotic—Agent that reduces the formation of blood clots and is used therapeutically for prevention or treatment of a dangerous blood clot.

antitussive—Medicine used to suppress or relieve coughing.

anxiety—A feeling of worry, nervousness, or unease, typically about an imminent event or something with an uncertain outcome.

anxiolysis—A medication or other intervention that inhibits anxiety; also called antipanic or antianxiety agent.

anxiolytics—A medication or other intervention that inhibits anxiety; also called sedatives, antipanic or antianxiety agent.

apathy—Lack of interest, enthusiasm, or concern.

appendicitis—Inflammation of the appendix, usually associated with infection of the appendix causing fever, loss of appetite, and pain.

arachidonic acid cascade—Physiologic pathway responsible for the formation of prostaglandins from the substrate arachidonic acid that is released when cell membrane damage occurs.

area under the curve (AUC)—In the plasma level curve, the total amount of a drug absorbed by the body is proportional to the area under the curve, assuming linear pharmacodynamics with elimination rate constant.

arthralgia—Pain that originates within a joint.

arthritis—Inflammation, swelling, and tenderness of 1 or more joints that typically worsen with age.

asthenia—Abnormal physical weakness or lack of energy.

Athlete Biological Passport—Method of intra-athlete monitoring of performance enhancement drug test results; results are monitored serially over a period of time in order to verify that the athlete is not involved in illicit doping.

atopy—Predisposition toward developing certain allergic hypersensitivity reactions after exposure to an environmental antigen, especially one that is inhaled or ingested.

atrophic gastritis—Process of chronic inflammation of the gastric mucosa of the stomach, leading to a loss of gastric glandular cells and their eventual replacement by intestinal and fibrous tissues.

aura—Sensation perceived by a patient that precedes a condition affecting the brain.

avascular necrosis—Death of bone tissue due to a lack of blood supply, leading to tiny breaks in the bone and the bone's eventual collapse; also called osteonecrosis.

bacteremia—Presence of viable bacteria in the circulating blood.

bactericidal—Agents that kill bacteria.

bacteriostatic—Agents that slow down or stall the growth of bacteria.

balanced anesthesia—Anesthesia produced by a mixture of drugs; often includes both inhaled and intravenous agents.

basal state—State of the body early in the morning, approximately 12 hours after the last ingestion of food or other nutrition; during this time, fasting blood work is drawn.

benzodiazepines—A class of drugs that act as tranquilizers; commonly used in the treatment of anxiety.

Bier block—Regional anesthesia by intravenous injection that is used for surgical procedures on the forearm or the lower leg; performed in a bloodless field maintained by a pneumatic tourniquet that also prevents anesthetic from entering the systemic circulation.

binding site—Region on a macromolecule such as a protein that binds to another molecule with specificity. The binding partner of the macromolecule is referred to as a *ligand*.

bioavailability—Percentage of an administered dose that reaches the systemic circulation.

bioequivalence—FDA requirement that generic medications meet the same standards for safety and efficacy as their brand-name counterparts.

biopharmaceutics—Study of the chemical and physical properties of drugs and the biological effects they produce.

biopsychosocial model—A framework that accounts for the biological, psychological, and social dimensions of illness and disease; provides a basis for the understanding and treatment of disease, taking into account the patient, his social context, and the effect of illness on that person from a societal perspective. The model states that ill health and disease are the result of interactions among biological, psychological, and social factors.

biotransformation—Chemical alteration of drugs in the body. *See also* metabolism.

black box warning (BBW)—Medication packaging required by the FDA to be included in all print and broadcast advertisements; informational text surrounded by a black box that acknowledges the risks of the medication, outlines practice guidelines, and provides warnings and updated information regarding practice guidelines or specific at-risk populations.

blood-brain barrier (BBB)—Layer of tightly packed cells in the walls of brain capillaries that prevent substances in the blood from diffusing freely into the brain.

bloodless field—Surgical procedures performed without blood flow to the limb; maintained by a pneumatic tourniquet that also prevents anesthetic from entering the systemic circulation.

bolus—A discrete amount of medication, drug, or other compound administered within a specific time, generally within 30 minutes, in order to raise its concentration in the blood to an effective level; from the Latin *bolus*, meaning "ball."

bolus injections—A large dose of a medication administered by injection for the purpose of rapidly achieving the needed therapeutic concentration in the bloodstream.

breakthrough bleeding—Abnormal flow of blood from the uterus that occurs between menstrual periods; especially due to irregular sloughing of the endometrium in women taking contraceptive hormones.

breakthrough pain—Brief, transitory exacerbation of moderate to severe pain; typically occurs in patients with underlying persistent pain that may otherwise be controlled.

broad spectrum—Antibiotic that acts on both Gram-positive and Gram-negative bacteria or any antibiotic that acts against a wide range of disease-causing bacteria.

bulimia nervosa—A serious, potentially life-threatening eating disorder in which patients eat large amounts of food with a sense of loss of control and then purge.

cannabidiol (CBD)—A phytocannabinoid found in *cannabis* that is devoid of psychoactive activity, with analgesic, anti-inflammatory, antineoplastic, and chemopreventive activities.

cannabinoids—Class of diverse chemical compounds that act on cannabinoid receptors, which are part of the endocannabinoid system found in cells that alters neurotransmitter release in the brain.

cerebral vascular accident (CVA)—Stroke; a sudden interruption of the blood supply to the brain caused by rupture of an artery in the brain (cerebral hemorrhage) or the blocking of a blood vessel, as by a clot of blood (cerebral occlusion).

chemokines—Family of small cytokines, or signaling proteins, secreted by cells.

chemotactic—Movement of a cell in a particular direction as a result of attraction by an increasing concentration of a chemical (chemotactic) substance; also called chemotaxis.

cholecystitis—Inflammation of the gallbladder that occurs most commonly because of an obstruction of the cystic duct from cholelithiasis (gall stones).

chronic pain—Pain that lasts longer than several months or for longer than the typical healing time.

clearance (CL)—Volume of fluid in the body that is cleared of a drug per unit of time.

clinical trials—Research studies to evaluate the effect of an intervention on health outcomes in humans.

clinically meaningful improvement—Practical importance of a treatment effect, or whether it has a genuine, palpable, and noticeable effect on daily life; also called end points. End points can in themselves represent or characterize the clinical outcome of interest.

collective bargaining agreement—A binding contract between labor and management that stipulates various work conditions that the employees abide by.

commensal—Association between two organisms in which one benefits and the other derives neither benefit nor harm.

compartment—A defined volume of body fluids in which the concentration of a drug is determined in the central compartment (plasma) and the peripheral compartment (extravascular cells and tissues).

competitive antagonist—Makes the agonist look less potent by shifting the dose–response curve to the right.

conformational—A change in the shape of a macromolecule, often induced by environmental factors.

congener—Closely related to or derived from the same source.

continuous infusion—A controlled method of intravenous administration of drugs, fluids, or nutrients that is given without interruption instead of by bolus.

contraception—Deliberate prevention of conception or impregnation.

controlled substances—Medications that are strictly regulated by a governmental agency due to their potential for abuse or addiction or have no medical use.

coronary artery disease (CAD)—Impedance or blockage of 1 or more arteries that supply blood to the heart, usually due to atherosclerosis (hardening of the arteries).

corticosteroid—Steroid hormones produced from cholesterol by the adrenal cortex that are involved in a wide range of physiological processes, including stress response, immune response, and regulation of inflammation.

corticotropin-releasing hormone (CRH)—A hormone synthesized in the hypothalamus as part of the stress response; regulates the secretion of adrenocorticotropic hormone (ACTH).

cortisol—Anti-inflammatory and immunosuppressive glucocorticoid produced by the adrenal cortex that may become elevated in response to physical or psychological stress.

coryza—Inflammation of the mucous membranes lining the nasal cavity, usually causing a running nose, nasal congestion, and loss of smell.

C-reactive protein (CRP)—A plasma protein that rises in the blood with the inflammation from certain conditions.

cultural competence—Ability of health care providers to effectively deliver services that meet the social, cultural, and linguistic needs of patients.

curare—Plant extract alkaloid used for arrow poisons in Central and South America that causes weakness of the skeletal muscles and, when administered in a sufficient dose, eventual death by asphyxiation due to paralysis of the diaphragm.

curettage—Removal of tissue, growths, or other material from the wall of a cavity or other surface with a curette (scoop-shaped surgical instrument for scraping and removing tissue).

Cushing's syndrome—Disorder caused by the body's long-term exposure to an excess of the hormone cortisol; also called hypercortisolism.

cyclooxygenase (COX)—The enzyme responsible for prostaglandin (COX) synthesis.

cytochrome P450 (CYP) enzyme system—Group of enzymes involved in drug metabolism and found in high levels in the liver that change many drugs into less toxic forms that are easier for the body to excrete.

cytokines—Broad and loose category of small proteins important in cell signaling. Cytokines are peptides and cannot cross the lipid bilayer of cells to enter the cytoplasm.

debridement—Procedure involving thorough cleaning and removal of infected and nonviable (necrotic or dead) tissue, foreign debris, and residual material from an area.

delta-9-tetrahydrocannabinol (THC)—Component of marijuana; binds to receptors in the brain, producing euphoria and a variety of potentially harmful effects, including intoxication and memory and motor impairments.

depression—Mood disorder that causes a persistent feeling of sadness and loss of interest; also called major depressive disorder or clinical depression.

depressive disorders—Characterized by sadness severe or persistent enough to interfere with function; often marked by decreased interest or pleasure in activities.

dermatologic reactions—*See* drug hypersensitivity reactions (DHR).

dermatophytes—Group of fungi that infect keratinous tissue and invade the hair, skin, and nails of a living host; also called dermatophytosis.

desquamation—Loss of bits of outer skin by peeling, shedding, or coming off in scales.

diabetes—Chronic, metabolic disease characterized by elevated levels of blood glucose (or blood sugar), which leads over time to serious damage to the heart, blood vessels, eyes, kidneys and nerves; also called diabetes mellitus.

diapedesis—Passage of blood cells through capillary walls into the tissues.

diaphoresis—Sweating, especially to an unusual degree as a symptom of disease or a side effect of a drug.

discontinuation syndrome—Set of symptoms occurring with the discontinuation or dosage reduction of some types of medications and recreational drugs; also called withdrawal syndrome.

disease-modifying antirheumatic drugs (DMARDs)—Diverse group of drugs that modify the inflammatory processes underlying rheumatoid arthritis and similar autoimmune conditions.

disintegration—Time required for a dosage form to break up into granules of a certain size (or smaller) under carefully specified conditions.

dispensing—Preparing, packaging, and labeling a prescription drug or device for subsequent use by a patient.

disposition—Refers to all processes involved in the absorption, distribution, metabolism, and excretion of drugs in a living organism.

dissolution—Dissolve or mix into a liquid.

diuretic—Any substance that promotes diuresis, or the increased production of urine.

doping—Colloquial term associated with an athlete's use of performance-enhancing drugs for the purpose of gaining a competitive advantage.

doping control officer (DCO)—A professional designated by Drug Free Sport to collect urine specimens for testing for banned substances.

dosage form—Pharmaceutical drug products in the form in which they are marketed for use, with a specific mixture of active ingredients and inactive components (excipients), in a particular configuration (e.g., capsule shell), and portioned into a particular dose; also called unit doses.

drug—Any substance (other than food and water) that is consumed, inhaled, injected, smoked, absorbed via the skin, or dissolved under the tongue to create a physiological or psychological change within the body.

drug allergies—Immune response that occurs soon after a drug is taken but generally does not occur after the first dose; typically, the response occurs when the drug is given after an initial exposure. *See also* drug hypersensitivity reactions (DHR).

drug class—Classification of medications and other compounds based on similar characteristics, such as mode of action, mechanism of action, chemical structures, or therapeutic indications.

drug delivery—Integration of drug release formulations, dosage form, and route of administration.

drug hypersensitivity reactions (DHR)—Immune-mediated reaction to a drug. Symptoms range from mild to severe and include rash, anaphylaxis, and serum sickness.

drug receptor—Specific proteins, situated either in cell membranes or, in some cases, in the cellular cytoplasm.

drug–receptor complex—A complex made up of a protein located on a cell membrane that is capable of being stimulated by drugs in the extracellular fluid and translating that stimulation into an intracellular response.

drug target—Biological target of a pharmacologically active drug compound, most commonly proteins such as enzymes, ion channels, and receptors.

dysesthesia—Condition in which a disagreeable sensation is produced by ordinary stimuli; caused by lesions of the peripheral or central sensory pathways. Dysesthesia involves sensations, whether spontaneous or evoked, such as burning, wetness, itching, electric shock, and pins and needles.

dysfunctional pain—Maladaptive pain that neither protects nor supports healing and repair; caused by a malfunction of the somatosensory apparatus itself. Dysfunctional pain can be considered a disease in its own right.

dyslipidemia—Disorder of lipoprotein metabolism, including lipoprotein overproduction or deficiency.

dyspareunia—Genital pain experienced before, during, or after sexual intercourse.

dyspepsia—Indigestion, stomach upset, or difficult or disturbed digestion; may be accompanied by symptoms such as nausea and vomiting, heartburn, bloating, and stomach discomfort.

dyspnea—Difficult or labored breathing.

dysuria—Painful or difficult urination.

effective dose (ED_{50})—Dose required to produce the desired effect in 50% of subjects.

effectiveness—Differs from *efficacy* in that it takes into account how well a drug works in real-world use.

efficacy—Maximal response a drug can produce, regardless of dose.

eicosanoids—Signaling hormones made by the enzymatic or nonenzymatic oxidation of arachidonic acid, including prostaglandins, prostacyclins, thromboxanes, and leukotrienes. *See also* prostaglandins.

electroencephalography (EEG)—Twenty electrodes are distributed over the scalp to detect electric brain changes during unconsciousness.

E_{max}—Maximal response produced by the drug; all receptors are occupied and no additional drug will produce an additional response.

embolus—Blood clot, fat globule, bubble of air or other gas, or foreign material.

emergency contraception—Forms of contraception, especially contraceptive pills (i.e., morning-after pills), that are effective at preventing pregnancy if administered within a specified period of time after sexual intercourse.

emesis—Involuntary, forceful expulsion of the stomach contents through the mouth and sometimes the nose; vomiting.

emollient—Thick liquid or cream that softens skin or reduces pain.

endocannabinoid system—Biological system composed of endocannabinoids and cannabinoid receptor proteins that are expressed throughout the central nervous system (including the brain) and peripheral nervous system.

endogenous cannabinoids—Endogenous lipid-based retrograde neurotransmitters that bind to cannabinoid receptors; also called endocannabinoids.

endogenous hormones—Substances secreted in the body, with different biological roles and functions.

endogenous—Originating or produced within an organism, tissue, or cell.

endometritis—Inflammatory condition of the lining of the uterus; usually due to an infection.

endorphin—Peptide hormones secreted within the brain and nervous system that activate the body's opiate receptors, causing an analgesic effect; also called beta-endorphin.

enema—Injection of fluid into the lower bowel by way of the rectum.

enteral—Drug administered through the digestive tract, including oral, sublingual, and rectal routes.

enteric coating—Coated with a material that permits transit through the stomach to the small intestine before the medication is released.

equianalgesic—Equivalent doses of analgesics, usually compared to *morphine*; also called morphine equivalent.

equipotent—Having equal effect or capacity.

ergogenic—Technique or substance used for the purpose of enhancing athletic performance.

euglycemia—Condition of having a normal concentration of glucose in the blood; good glycemia regulation or good glycemia.

euphoria—Feeling or state of intense excitement, happiness, well-being, or elation.

exclusivity—Delays and prohibitions on approval of competitor drugs; promotes a balance between new drug innovation and greater public access to drugs that result from generic drug competition.

excoriation—Injury to a surface of the body caused by trauma, such as scratching, abrasion, or a chemical or thermal burn.

excretion—Process of eliminating metabolic waste, which primarily exits the body through the urine, tears, saliva, and sweat.

exogenous—Caused by something outside the body.

expectorant—Medicine that promotes the secretion of sputum by the air passages; used to treat coughs.

extravascular—Drug administered through enteral, inhalation, or other routes outside of the vascular system.

fasting blood glucose level—How much glucose (sugar) is in the blood after an overnight fast or after no caloric intake for ≥8 hours.

fermentable oligo-di-monosaccharides and polyols (FODMAPs)—Short chain carbohydrates that are poorly absorbed in the small intestine and are prone to absorb water and ferment in the colon causing digestive discomfort in some people.

fibrinolytic—Any agent that is capable of stimulating the dissolution of a blood clot; also called clot-buster.

fibrosis—Excessive deposition of fibrous tissue that can interfere with normal tissue function.

first-pass metabolism (first-pass effect)—Process in which a drug that is administered by mouth, absorbed from the GI tract, transported via the portal vein to the liver, and metabolized such that only a small proportion of the active drug reaches the systemic circulation and its intended target tissue.

fluctuant—Movable and compressible; property of yielding to alternate pressure by palpating fingers so as to suggest that the area being felt contains fluid. Fluctuation is often exhibited by a swelling.

fluoroscopy—Imaging technique that uses X-rays to obtain real-time moving images of the internal structure and function of a patient; for example, the pumping action of the heart or the motion of the ankle can be watched.

fomite—Object (e.g., a towel or clothing) that can transmit infectious agents from 1 person to another.

formulary—List of details of medicines that may be prescribed.

formulation—Process of preparing a drug in a particular way or in a specific form, such as a tablet, capsule, linctus, ointment, or for 1 of the various forms of injection.

functional selectivity—Ligand-dependent selectivity for certain signal transduction pathways at the same receptor.

general anesthesia—State of unconsciousness, analgesia, and amnesia, with skeletal muscle relaxation and loss of reflexes.

generic name—Drug that contains the same chemical substance as a drug that was originally protected by patents. Generic drugs are allowed for sale after the patents on the original drugs expire. Because the active chemical substance is the same, the medical profile of generics is considered to be equivalent in performance.

gestational diabetes—State of hyperglycemia that develops during pregnancy.

glomerular filtration rate (GFR)—Expression of the quantity of glomerular filtrate formed each minute in the nephrons of both kidneys, usually measured by the rate of clearance of creatinine; also, a test used to check the functioning levels of the kidneys.

glucocorticoids—Group of corticosteroids involved in the metabolism of carbohydrates, proteins, and fats that have anti-inflammatory activity. *See also* cortisol.

glycation—Reaction that takes place when glucose becomes attached to proteins or lipids without the moderation of an enzyme. This results in the formation of rogue molecules known as *advanced glycation end products (AGEs)*.

glycemic control—The delicate balancing act in which the diabetic patient must maintain euglycemic blood glucose levels, this goal requires education, decision strategies, volitional control, and the wisdom to avoid hyper- and hypoglycemia (plasma glucose <60 mg/dL).

gout—Form of inflammatory arthritis in which high levels of uric acid result in needlelike crystals in a joint that cause sudden, severe episodes of pain, tenderness, redness, warmth, and swelling.

gradient—Difference in concentration of a dissolved substance in a solution between a region of high density and 1 of lower density.

Gram stain—Method of staining used to distinguish and classify bacterial species into Gram-positive and Gram-negative groups.

Gram-negative bacteria—In Gram's method of staining, the crystal violet stain is lost (and takes the color of the red counterstain). This is characteristic of bacteria that have a cell wall composed of a thin layer of peptidoglycan.

Gram-positive bacteria—Gram staining appears as purple colored because the thick peptidoglycan layer in the bacterial cell wall retains the stain after it is washed away from the rest of the sample.

granulomas—In chronic inflammation, formation of a mass of cells consisting of activated macrophages surrounded by activated lymphocytes.

Guedel's classification—A means of assessing depth of general anesthesia.

gynecologist—Physician who specializes in the care, diagnosis, and treatment of disorders of the female reproductive system.

gynecomastia—An endocrine system disorder in which a noncancerous increase in the size of male breast tissue occurs.

half-life ($t_{1/2}$)—The time it takes for half of the drug to be eliminated from the body; also called elimination half-life.

half-maximal effective concentration (EC_{50})—The concentration required to obtain a 50% effect or a response halfway between the baseline and maximum after a specified exposure time.

HbA1c—Form of hemoglobin (Hb) that is chemically linked to a sugar; also called A1c.

health-related quality of life (HRQOL)—A multidimensional concept that includes domains related to physical, mental, emotional, and social functioning and focuses on the effect that health status has on quality of life.

hematuria—Discharge of blood in the urine, making the urine either slightly blood tinged, grossly bloody, or a smoky brown color.

hepatotoxicity—Drug-induced liver injury; a cause of acute and chronic liver disease; also called hepatic toxicity.

high-alert medication—Drug that is likely to cause significant harm when used in error.

histamine—Compound released by cells in response to injury and in allergic and inflammatory reactions, causing contraction of smooth muscle and dilation of capillaries.

histamine-1 receptor—Receptor for histamine on cell membranes that modulates the dilation of blood vessels and the contraction of smooth muscle.

hydrophilic (water-soluble)—Molecule or drug that is attracted to water molecules and is dissolved by water.

hydrophobic—Molecules that are not attracted to water and are repelled by it.

hyperemesis—Persistent severe vomiting leading to weight loss and dehydration; condition common with pregnancy.

hyperemia—Increase in amount of blood in a body part, as from an increased flow of blood due to vasodilation.

hyperglycemia—Excessive amount of glucose circulating in blood plasma >200 mg/dL, but symptoms may not start to become noticeable until even higher ~250-300 mg/dL.

hyperhidrosis—Extreme and excessive sweating.

hypersensitivity disorders—Undesirable reactions produced by the normal immune system, including allergies and autoimmunity; also called hypersensitivity reaction or intolerance.

hyperuricemia—Condition in which there is too much uric acid in the blood, leading to several diseases, including a painful type of arthritis called gout.

hypnotics—Commonly known as *sleeping pills*; class of psychoactive drugs whose primary function is to induce sleep; used in the treatment of insomnia (sleeplessness) or for surgical anesthesia.

hypochloremia—Serum chloride level <95 mEq/L (normal is 101 to 112 mEq/L).

hypoglycemia—Blood plasma glucose levels are generally maintained between 72 and 144 mg/dL; although 70 mg/dL is commonly cited as the lower limit of normal glucose, symptoms of hypoglycemia often do not occur until 50 to 54 mg/dL.

hypokalemia—Condition of below-normal levels of potassium in the blood serum.

hyponatremia—Low sodium concentration in the blood, generally defined as a sodium concentration <135 mmol/L (135 mEq/L), with severe hyponatremia being <120 mEq/L.

hypothalamic-pituitary-adrenal (HPA) axis—Feedback response between the hypothalamus, pituitary, and adrenal glands that assists in regulating body temperature, digestion, immune system, mood, sexuality, and overall energy.

idiosyncrasy—Drug reaction that occurs rarely and unpredictably among the population; also called idiosyncratic drug reaction. Not to be mistaken with *idiopathic*, which implies that the cause is not known.

ileus—Painful temporary arrest of intestinal peristalsis of the ileum or other part of the intestine.

immunosuppression—Suppression of the immune system and its ability to fight infection.

impetigo—Superficial skin infection with crusting or bullae caused by streptococci, staphylococci, or both.

implants—Sterile device placed under the skin or other tissues that releases a drug either locally to a specific part of the body or systemically by slowly dissolving to release the drug into the bloodstream.

in vitro—Process taking place in a test tube, culture dish, or elsewhere outside a living organism.

in vivo—Process taking place in a living organism.

incompetence—Incomplete closing of the lower esophageal sphincter that allows reflux of gastric contents into the esophagus, causing burning pain.

induction—The time from administration of an anesthetic to development of unconsciousness.

infection—Invasion of a host organism's bodily tissues by disease-causing organisms.

inflammation—Localized physical condition in which part of the body becomes reddened, swollen, hot, and often painful, especially as a reaction to injury or infection.

infusion—Administration of medication through a needle or catheter with a pump that delivers fluids into a patient's body in controlled amounts.

insulin—Hormone made by the pancreas that controls the level of the sugar glucose in the blood by allowing cells to use glucose for energy.

insulin resistance—Diminished ability of cells to respond to the action of insulin in transporting glucose from the bloodstream into muscle and other tissues.

intent to harm—Desire to commit an act with destructive consequences.

interleukin-1 (IL-1)—Cytokines that participate in the regulation of immune responses, inflammatory reactions, and hematopoiesis.

interleukin-6 (IL-6)—Cytokine involved in a wide variety of biological functions essential in the final differentiation of B cells into immunoglobulin-secreting cells, as well as for inducing myeloma and plasmacytoma growth, nerve cell differentiation, and, in hepatocytes, acute-phase reactants. Also known as B-cell stimulatory factor-2 (BSF-2) and interferon beta-2.

interprofessional health care team—A group of professionals with the common goal of improving patient outcomes who use a process in which communication and decision making is encouraged, enabling a synergistic influence of grouped knowledge and skills; also called collaborative practice.

intertriginous areas—Between the toes or folds of skin. *See also* intertrigo.

intertrigo—Superficial skin disorder involving any area of the body where opposing skin surfaces may touch and rub.

intestinal metaplasia—Occurs when cells in the tissues of the upper digestive tract, often in the stomach or esophagus, change and become more like cells from the intestines.

intrathecal—Introduced into the CSF in the space under the arachnoid membrane of the brain or spinal cord.

intrathecal space—Route of administration for drugs via an injection into the spinal canal or the subarachnoid space so that it reaches the cerebrospinal fluid (CSF). Often used in implantable pain management treatments such as implanted drug pumps, also known as pain pumps or morphine pumps.

intrinsic activity—Measure of a drug's effectiveness in generating the intended change of cellular activity.

inverse agonist—An agent that binds to the same receptor as an agonist but induces a pharmacological response opposite to that of the agonist.

irreversible antagonist—Pharmacologic antagonist that cannot be overcome by increasing the dose of the agonist.

isotonic saline—Mixture of sodium chloride in water that has a number of uses in medicine, such as wound cleansing, contact lenses removal, and relief for dry eyes; also called saline solution.

keloids—Abnormal healing response causing scars that are markedly overgrown, thickened, and disfiguring.

keratinolytic—Treatment to remove warts and other lesions in which the epidermis produces excess skin; also called keratolysis.

ketoacidosis—A feature of uncontrolled diabetes mellitus characterized by a combination of ketosis and acidosis. Symptoms include slow, deep breathing with a fruity odor to the breath; confusion; frequent urination (polyuria); poor appetite; and eventually loss of consciousness.

ketosis—Accumulation of ketones, a type of acid that forms when the body breaks down fat for energy.

lassitude—Weariness of body or mind from strain or oppressive climate; lack of energy; listlessness or languor.

lavage—Washing out of a body cavity with water or a medicated solution.

LD_{50}—Dose that is lethal to 50% of a tested population after a specified test duration. Used as a general indicator of a drug's acute toxicity. A lower LD_{50} is indicative of increased toxicity.

liberation—Release of the drug from its dosage form.

lichenification—Thick, leathery skin; usually the result of constant scratching and rubbing.

ligand—Molecule that binds to a receptor and produces a biological response.

lipophilic (lipid-soluble)—Ability of a molecule or drug to dissolve in fats, oils, and lipids.

local anesthetic systemic toxicity (LAST)—A life-threatening adverse event that occurs after administration of local anesthetic drugs through a variety of routes.

locally acting—Drug applied to the skin or mucous membranes to achieve high concentration at the site of application.

loculation—Having, formed of, or divided into small cavities or compartments.

maceration—Moisture-damaged skin poses a risk of infection.

malaise—General feeling of discomfort, illness, or uneasiness whose exact cause is difficult to identify.

margin of safety—Difference between the usual effective dose and the dose that causes severe or life-threatening side effects.

masking agent—Medication or nutritional supplement taken with the express purpose of tampering with a drug test; the masking agent hides the presence of a banned substance in the blood and thus protects the athlete from failing the drug test.

mast cells—Cells filled with basophil granules, found in high numbers in connective tissue, that release histamine and other substances during inflammatory and allergic reactions.

maximum plasma concentration (C_{max})—Maximum (or peak) plasma concentration of a drug in a specific area of the body after the drug has been administered.

mechanism of action—Specific biochemical interaction including a specific molecular target where a drug binds to produce its pharmacological effect.

medical cannabinoids—Use of *cannabis* as medical therapy to treat disease or alleviate symptoms. Medical cannabinoids can be administered orally, sublingually, or topically; they can be smoked, inhaled, mixed with food, or made into tea.

medication—*See* prescription drug.

melena—Dark, sticky feces containing partly digested blood; appears following internal bleeding or the swallowing of blood.

mental disorder—Pattern of behavioral or psychological symptoms that affect multiple life areas and create distress for the person experiencing these symptoms; also called psychological disorder.

mental health condition—Problem with mental function that interferes with the ability to participate in productive activities, have fulfilling relationships with other people, adapt to change, and cope with adversity.

mentation—Mental activity.

metabolic acidosis—Acidosis resulting from excess acid due to abnormal metabolism, excessive acid intake, or renal retention or from excessive loss of bicarbonate (as in diarrhea).

metabolic alkalosis—Alkalosis caused by too much bicarbonate in the blood.

metabolism—Metabolic breakdown of drugs by the body, primarily occurring in the liver through specialized enzymatic systems, to make the drug more water-soluble and increase the rate of excretion in the urine. *See also* biotransformation.

metabolite—Product of metabolism.

microbiome—Collection of microorganisms that live on the skin and in saliva, the mouth, the eyes, and GI tract; also called human microbiota.

miliaria—An inflammatory disorder of the skin that is characterized by redness, eruptions (as of vesicles), and burning or itching due to blockage of sweat gland ducts; also called prickly heat.

minimal inhibitory concentration (MIC)—Lowest concentration of a chemical, usually a drug, that prevents visible growth of a bacterium or bacteria.

miscible—Property of 2 substances to fully dissolve in each other at any concentration, forming a homogeneous solution.

mollusca—Round, firm, painless bumps ranging in size from a pinhead to a pencil eraser; appear as a result of molluscum contagiosum, a relatively common viral infection of the skin.

mood disorder—Group of conditions where a disturbance in the person's mood is the main underlying feature; also known as mood affective disorders. The main types of mood disorders are major depressive disorder, bipolar disorder, and seasonal affective disorder (SAD).

motion sickness—Condition characterized by a disturbance of the inner ear, resulting in difficulties in spatial orientation as well as an impaired sense of balance and equilibrium. It is caused by a repetitive motion such as the movement of a vehicle, the motion of a plane in the air, or being on a boat.

mucocutaneous infection—Disorder characterized by persistent, debilitating, or recurrent infections of the skin, nails, and mucous membranes, mainly with the fungal pathogen *Candida albicans*.

multidrug-resistant organisms (MDROs)—Bacteria and other microorganisms that have developed resistance to antimicrobial drugs.

mu-opioid receptors (MOR)—Receptors of clinical importance that bind to opioids in the nervous system and other tissues; also called μ-opioid receptors.

myalgia—Muscle pain; a symptom that presents with a large variety of diseases.

myocardial infarction (MI)—A life-threatening condition that occurs when blood flow to the heart muscle is abruptly cut off, causing tissue damage; also called acute myocardial infarction (AMI) or heart attack. MI is usually the result of a blockage in 1 or more of the coronary arteries.

myopathy—General term referring to any disease of the muscles.

narcotic—Drug or other substance, often sold illegally, that affects mood or behavior and is consumed for nonmedical purposes.

narrow spectrum—Antibiotic drug that is effective against only a specific group of bacteria.

nasal decongestants—Drug that shrinks swollen membranes in the nose, making it easier to breathe.

nasal insufflation—Local application of a drug to the mucous membranes of the nose to achieve a systemic action; also called nasal inhalation.

nephropathy—Kidney damage leading to renal failure.

neuralgia—*See* neuropathic pain.

neuraxial blockade—Anesthetic that is placed around the nerves of the central nervous system, such as in subarachnoid anesthesia, and epidural anesthesia; also called spinal anesthesia.

neuropathic pain—Pain caused by damage or disease affecting the somatosensory nervous system that may be associated with abnormal sensations (*dysesthesia*) or pain from normally unpainful stimuli (*allodynia*). It may be continuous or episodic (paroxysmal), and is often described as burning, stabbing, shooting, aching, or like an electric shock.

neuropathy—In diabetics, nerve damage that causes impotence and foot disorders that may lead to amputation.

noncompetitive antagonist—Reduces the maximal response that an agonist can produce.

noncontrolled substances—Prescription medications with less risk of abuse or addiction whose purpose covers various medical conditions.

nonsteroidal anti-inflammatory drugs (NSAIDs)—Inhibitors of cyclooxygenase; the term *nonsteroidal* differentiates NSAIDs from corticosteroid drugs.

normal saline—A sterile solution of 0.85% sodium chloride that is isotonic to body fluids; used to temporarily maintain living tissue and as a solvent for parenterally administered drugs.

noxious stimulus—Anything that is perceived as painful or harmful.

number needed to harm (NNH)—Epidemiological measure indicating how many people on average need to be exposed to a risk factor over a specific period to cause harm in an average of 1 person who would not otherwise have been harmed.

number needed to treat (NNT)—Average number of patients who need to be treated to prevent 1 additional bad outcome. The inverse of the absolute risk reduction.

obstetrics—Field of medicine concentrated on pregnancy, childbirth, and the postpartum period.

opioid-induced constipation (OIC)—Condition in which bowel movements are infrequent or incomplete (fewer than 3 per week); cited as a side effect of opioid medications.

opioid receptors—Any of the several receptors to which opiates bind. *See also* mu-opioid receptors.

opioids—Drugs possessing some properties characteristic of opiate narcotics but not derived from opium.

osteomyelitis—Infection in a bone caused by bacteria traveling through the bloodstream or spreading from nearby tissue; may also result from an injury that exposes the bone.

osteonecrosis—*See* avascular necrosis.

osteopenia—Reduction in bone volume to below-normal levels, especially due to inadequate replacement of the bone lost to normal lysis.

osteoporosis—Disorder in which the bones become increasingly porous, brittle, and subject to fracture due to loss of calcium and other mineral components; sometimes results in pain, decreased height, and skeletal deformities.

over-the-counter (OTC) drugs—Medications that are available to the public without a prescription.

pain—Unpleasant sensory and emotional experience associated with actual or potential tissue damage or described in terms of such damage.

pandemic—An outbreak of disease prevalent over a whole country or the world.

paralytic ileus—Obstruction of the intestine due to paralysis of the intestinal muscles.

parenteral—Drug administration from routes outside the GI tract, such as intravenous routes.

paronychia—Infection of the periungual (around the nail) tissues causing redness, warmth, and pain along the nail margin.

partial agonists—Drugs that bind to and activate a given receptor but have only partial efficacy relative to a full agonist.

patch—Medicated adhesive patch placed on the skin to deliver a specific dose of medication through the skin and into the bloodstream; also called transdermal patch.

patent—Property rights granted during the development of a drug.

patient-reported outcome (PRO)—Measure that is directly reported by the patient (i.e., without an interpretation of the patient's response by a clinician or anyone else); pertains to the patient's health, quality of life, or functional status associated with health care or treatment. These outcomes may be measured in absolute terms, such as a patient's rating of the severity of pain.

peak expiratory flow (PEF)—Maximum airflow during a forced expiration, beginning with the lungs fully inflated; also called peak expiratory flow rate (PEFR). Measured with a peak flow meter.

peak flow meter—Small handheld device used to monitor a person's ability to breathe out air; also called spirometer. It measures the airflow through the bronchi and thus the degree of obstruction in the airways.

perennial rhinitis—Inflammatory condition of the nose characterized by nasal obstruction, sneezing, itching, or rhinorrhea that occurs for ≥1 hour on most days throughout the year.

performance-enhancing drugs (PEDs)—Substance (such as an anabolic steroid, human growth hormone, or erythropoietin) that is used illicitly to improve athletic performance.

peripherally inserted central catheter (PICC line)—Catheter that enters the body through the skin at a peripheral site, extending into the superior vena cava; stays in place for days or weeks.

peritonitis—Inflammation of the peritoneum, typically caused by bacterial infection either via the blood or after rupture of an abdominal organ.

petechiae—Small reddish or purplish spot containing blood that appears on the skin or mucous membrane as a result of localized hemorrhage.

petrolatum—Semisolid mixture of hydrocarbons used as a topical ointment for its healing properties.

pharmacodynamics—Study of what a medication does to the body.

pharmacokinetics—Branch of pharmacology concerned with the movement of drugs within the body and the actions of the body on the drug.

pharmacotherapy—Treatment of disease through the administration of drugs.

pharmacy health literacy—Degree to which a health care provider can obtain, process, and understand basic health and medication information and pharmacy services needed to make appropriate health decisions.

phocomelia—Rare congenital deformity in which the hands or feet are attached close to the trunk and the limbs are grossly underdeveloped or absent. This condition was a side effect of the drug *thalidomide* taken during early pregnancy.

phytocannabinoids—Any plant-derived natural product capable of directly interacting with cannabinoid receptors, sharing chemical similarity with cannabinoids, or both.

polarity—Separation of an electric charge, leading to a molecule having a negatively charged end and a positively charged end.

polypharmacy—Simultaneous use of multiple drugs to treat a single ailment or condition or simultaneous use of multiple drugs by 1 patient.

postoperative nausea and vomiting (PONV)—Nausea, vomiting, or retching experienced by a patient up to 24 hours following a surgical procedure.

postprandial—After a meal, especially after dinner.

post-traumatic stress disorder (PTSD)—A mental health condition triggered by either experiencing or witnessing a terrifying event. Symptoms may include flashbacks, nightmares, severe anxiety, and uncontrollable thoughts about the event.

potency—Measure of the dose that is required to produce a response.

prandial—Referring to a meal or to the effects of a meal.

prediabetes—Fasting blood glucose level of 100-125 mg/dL or a 2-hour post-oral glucose tolerance test of 140-200 mg/dL; individual with prediabetes are at increased risk for macrovascular disease, as well as diabetes.

prescribers—Health care practitioners who are legally approved to prescribe medication (e.g., medical doctor, doctor of osteopathy, nurse practitioner, physician assistant).

prescription drug—Pharmaceutical that requires a physician's prescription in order to be dispensed.

priapism—Persistent and painful erection of the penis.

prodrug—Medication or compound that is metabolized into a pharmacologically active drug.

prostaglandins—Hormone-like substance formed as cyclooxygenase metabolizes from arachidonic acid; perform a variety of functions, such as the contraction and relaxation of smooth muscle, the dilation and constriction of blood vessels, control of blood pressure, and modulation of inflammation.

protocol—Preestablished written procedures or guidelines for medical care of a specified clinical situation that are physician authorized and based on patient presentation.

pruritus—Intense itching sensation that can have various causes (e.g., allergies or infection).

pseudoallergic reaction—Condition with similar presentation to a true allergy, although due to different causes.

psychogenic vomiting—Emesis without any obvious organic pathology; associated with emotional distress and anxiety.

psychotherapy—Use of psychological methods to improve a person's well-being and mental health, relationships, and social skills and to resolve or mitigate troublesome behaviors, beliefs, compulsions, thoughts, or emotions.

pulsus paradoxus—Inspiratory decrease in blood pressure of >10 mmHg or more during normal breathing.

purulent—Consisting of, containing, or discharging pus.

radiculopathy—Irritation of or injury to a nerve root (as from being compressed) that typically causes pain, numbness, or weakness in the part of the body that is supplied with nerves from that root.

rate-limiting step—Slowest step in a metabolic pathway; determines the overall rate of the other reactions in the pathway.

recombinant human analogs—Recombinant human insulin, a form of insulin made from recombinant DNA that is identical to human insulin; used to treat diabetics who are allergic to preparations made from bovine (beef) or porcine (pork) insulin.

recovery—After receiving anesthesia, the time period from when the anesthetic is discontinued until the return of consciousness and protective reflexes.

referred pain—Pain perceived at a site different from the location of the injured or diseased part of the body; due to nerve signals from several areas of the body that travel on the same nerve pathway leading to the spinal cord and brain.

relative risk—Ratio of the chance of a disease developing among members of a population who are exposed to a factor compared with members of a similar population not exposed to the factor.

renin–angiotensin system—A hormone system that regulates blood pressure and fluid and electrolyte balance, as well as systemic vascular resistance.

reproductive health—Diseases, disorders, and conditions that affect the functioning of the male and female reproductive systems during all stages of life.

resident flora—*See* microbiome.

respiratory aspiration—Inhaling toxic substances, usually gastric contents, into the lungs.

retinopathy—Damage to eyes that leads to blindness.

reverse distributor—An alternative for disposal of controlled substances is to surrender the substances to an approved independent company; also called surrender to independent companies. Companies must be licensed by the Department of Health and Human Services to receive such substances and registered with the DEA.

reversible antagonist—A pharmacological antagonist whose effect can be countered by increasing the concentration of agonist.

Reye's syndrome—A rare but serious condition that causes swelling in the liver and brain; most often affects children and teenagers recovering from a viral infection, such as the flu or chicken pox. *Aspirin* (salicylate) is the major preventable risk factor for Reye's syndrome.

rhabdomyolysis—Serious syndrome of muscle injury that causes release of intramuscular proteins, especially creatine kinase (CK) and myoglobin into the bloodstream. If untreated, leads to myoglobinuria (urine is dark-tea or rust colored) and causes severe kidney damage.

rheumatic diseases—Inflammatory conditions that chiefly affect the joints, tendons, ligaments, muscles, and bones; characterized by pain, stiffness, and swelling.

rhinorrhea—Excessive discharge of mucus from the nose.

salpingitis—Infection and inflammation in the fallopian tubes; the term is often used synonymously with *pelvic inflammatory disease*.

seasonal allergic rhinitis—Allergic symptoms that typically occur at a particular time of the year; also called hay fever.

secretagogue—A substance that prompts secretion of another substance.

sedation—Reduction of anxiety or irritability by administering sedative drugs, usually to facilitate a medical procedure or diagnostic procedure.

sedatives—*See* anxiolytics.

selection pressure—The influence exerted by some factor (such as an antibiotic) on natural selection to promote one group of organisms over another. In the case of antibiotic resistance, antibiotics cause a selective pressure by killing susceptible bacteria, allowing antibiotic-resistant bacteria to survive and multiply.

selectivity—Degree to which a drug acts on a given receptor relative to other available cellular receptors.

self-neglect—Behavioral condition in which a person neglects to attend to her basic needs, such as personal hygiene, appropriate clothing, feeding, or tending appropriately to any medical conditions she has.

septic shock—Bacterial toxins, and the immune system response to them, that cause a dramatic drop in blood pressure, preventing the delivery of blood to the organs.

serotonin syndrome—Group of symptoms that may occur with the use of certain serotonergic medications or drugs.

sexual health—State of physical, emotional, mental, and social well-being in relation to sexuality; not merely the absence of disease, dysfunction, or infirmity.

short-acting rescue drugs—Bronchodilators that relieve acute asthma symptoms or attacks very quickly by opening the airways; also called quick-acting medication, reliever medications, or rescue medications.

side effect—Undesirable secondary effect that occurs in addition to the desired therapeutic effect of a drug or medication. Side effects may vary for each patient depending on the person's disease state, age, weight, gender, ethnicity, genetics, and general health.

signal transduction—Process by which an intracellular response is triggered by a chemical or physical signal that is transmitted through a cell as a series of molecular events, most commonly protein phosphorylation catalyzed by protein kinases.

solubility—Degree to which a substance dissolves in a solvent to make a solution.

somatic—Coming from or related to tissues such as the skin, soft tissues, muscle, and bone structures.

somnolence—Having a strong desire for sleep or sleeping for unusually long periods of time; also called sleepiness or drowsiness.

specificity—Binding site or receptor that is activated only by a single molecule or class of molecules.

standing orders—Prewritten medication order and specific instructions from the licensed independent practitioner to administer a medication to a person in clearly defined circumstances.

steady-state concentration (Css)—Drug dosing that is in dynamic equilibrium with its elimination.

striae—Broad, purplish, shiny, or whitish lines of atrophy on the skin, most commonly affecting pregnant women and occurring on the abdomen, breasts, or thighs.

superimposed bacterial infection—Infection occurring after or on top of an earlier infection, especially following treatment with broad-spectrum antibiotics.

suppository—Solid dosage form used to deliver medications that is inserted into the rectum, vagina, or urethra, where it dissolves or melts and exerts local or systemic effects.

suppuration—Discharging of pus from a wound.

suspension—Liquid with small pieces of drug that are not completely dissolved; must always be shaken (or stirred) before administration so that the right amount of drug is delivered.

synovitis—Inflammatory condition of the synovial membrane of a joint as the result of an aseptic wound or a traumatic injury, such as a sprain or severe strain.

systemic inflammatory response syndrome (SIRS)—Inflammatory state affecting the whole body. It is the body's response to an infectious or noninfectious insult.

targeted peripheral analgesia—Pain relief with a mechanism of action primarily through reducing pain transmission within the peripheral nervous system.

teratogenic drug—Drug that can interfere with fetal development, potentially causing birth defects.

testosterone-to-epitestosterone (T/E) ratio—Ratio between testosterone and epitestosterone; determines if the urine specimen is positive for anabolic steroid use.

therapeutic equivalence—Drug that has the same active ingredients in the same form and has the same actions within the body.

therapeutic index (TI)—Ratio between the lethal dose and the therapeutic dose of a drug; used as a measure of the relative safety of the drug for a particular treatment.

therapeutic level—Level of drug in the bloodstream in which that drug is expected to be effective without causing any serious problems to the patient.

therapeutic range—Range of drug dosage or concentration in a bodily system that provides safe effective therapy.

therapeutic response—Response after a treatment of any kind, the results of which are judged to be useful or favorable.

therapeutic window—*See* therapeutic index (TI).

thromboembolism—Formation of a blood clot inside a blood vessel, obstructing the flow of blood through the circulatory system.

thrombosis—Vascular disease caused by the formation of a blood clot (thrombus) inside a blood vessel, obstructing the flow of blood through the circulatory system.

thrombotic—Formation or presence of a blood clot in a vein or artery.

thrombus—A blood clot that forms in a vessel and remains there.

topical delivery system (vehicle)—Substance that carries a specific drug into contact with and through the skin. The challenge to topical drug delivery is the transport across the skin barrier.

total intravenous anesthesia (TIVA)—A technique involving the use of intravenous drugs to anesthetize the patient without the use of inhalational agents.

toxic megacolon—Potentially lethal complication of inflammatory bowel disease or infectious colitis that is characterized by total or segmental nonobstructive colonic dilatation plus systemic toxicity.

toxicity—The degree to which a substance (a toxin or poison) can produce harm.

trade name—Brand name of a drug that is developed by the company requesting approval for the drug; identifies the medication as the exclusive property of that company.

transient ischemic attack (TIA)—A temporary blockage of blood flow to the brain that does not cause permanent damage but may signal a full-blown stroke ahead; also called a mini-stroke.

traveler's diarrhea—Digestive tract disorder commonly caused by eating contaminated food or drinking contaminated water, resulting in loose stools and abdominal cramps.

trocar—Sharp, pointed surgical instrument fitted with a cannula; used especially to insert the cannula into a body cavity as a drainage outlet.

troche—Small medicated hard lozenge (e.g., cough drop) or a soft gelatin (e.g., a gummy) meant to dissolve slowly in the mouth.

tumor necrosis factor-alpha (TNF-α)—Signaling protein (cytokine) involved in systemic inflammation and acute phase reaction.

United States Anti-Doping Agency (USADA)—The United States agency that subscribes to the WADA code in order to apply similar standards of drug-free participation for various competitive U.S. athletes.

United States Pharmacopeia–National Formulary (USP–NF)—Combination of 2 compendia: the United States Pharmacopeia (USP) and the National Formulary (NF). It contains standards for medicines, dosage forms, drug substances, excipients, biologics, compounded preparations, medical devices, dietary supplements, and other therapeutics.

upper respiratory infection (URI)—Illness caused by an acute infection that involves the upper respiratory tract, including the nose, sinuses, pharynx, or larynx; also called upper respiratory tract infection (URTI).

urticaria—Rash of round, red welts on the skin that itch intensely, sometimes with dangerous swelling; caused by an allergic reaction, typically to a drug or specific foods.

vertigo—Whirling sensation and loss of balance, particularly when looking down from a great height; caused by disease affecting the inner ear or the vestibular nerve.

virulence—Ability of an organism to infect the host and cause a disease.

visceral pain—Pain that involves organ systems such as the heart, lungs, or gastrointestinal and genitourinary tracts; also called organ pain.

volume of distribution (V_d)—Concentration of a drug in the peripheral tissue compartment compared to the concentration in the plasma within the central compartment.

withdrawal bleeding—The monthly bleeding women experience while using a hormonal birth control method, such as the pill, the patch, or the NuvaRing; also called hormonal period or fake period.

World Anti-Doping Agency (WADA)—An independent global agency with the mission of education, research, and facilitation of anti-doping athletic participation. The WADA code has been accepted by nations that share the mission of creating a drug-free competitive environment.

References

Chapter 1

1. Asperheim MK. *Introduction to Pharmacology.* 12th ed. St. Louis, MO: Saunders Elsevier; 2012.
2. BOC Standards of Professional Practice 2019. Board of Certification website. http://bocatc.org/system/document_versions/versions/171/original/boc-standards-of-professional-practice-2019-20181207.pdf?1544218543. Accessed February 7, 2019.
3. Carlson C. Traveling with medication. NCAA website. www.ncaa.org/sport-science-institute/traveling-medication. Published March 17, 2015. Accessed September 20, 2018.
4. Chang CJ, Weston T, Higgs JD, et al. Inter-Association Consensus Statement: The management of medications by the sports medicine team. *J Athl Train.* 2018;53(11):1103-1112.
5. Commission on Accreditation of Athletic Training Education. CAATE 2020 Standards for Accreditation of Professional Athletic Training Programs. https://caate.net/wp-content/uploads/2018/02/2020-Standards-for-Professional-Programs-copyedited-clean.pdf. Accessed September 10, 2018.
6. The Controlled Substances Act. U.S. Drug Enforcement Administration website. www.dea.gov/controlled-substances-act. Published 1970. Accessed February 10, 2019.
7. Drug scheduling. U.S. Drug Enforcement Administration website. www.dea.gov/drug-scheduling. Published 2018. Accessed February 6, 2019.
8. Cortisone. Drugs.com. www.drugs.com/ppa/cortisone.html. Published 2019. Accessed July 23, 2019.
9. The FDA's drug review process: Ensuring drugs are safe and effective. U.S. Food and Drug Administration website. www.fda.gov/Drugs/ResourcesForYou/Consumers/ucm143534.htm. Updated November 24, 2017. Accessed February 8, 2019.
10. Kaeding CC, Borchers J. Issues for the traveling team physician. *J Knee Surg.* 2016;29(5):364-369.
11. Katzung BG. Introduction: The nature of drugs and drug development and regulation. In: Katzung BG, ed. *Basic and Clinical Pharmacology.* 14th ed. New York, NY: McGraw-Hill Education; 2017:1-19.
12. Koller DL. Team physicians, sports medicine, and the law. An update. *Clin Sports Med.* 2016;35(2):245-255.
13. National Collegiate Athletic Association. *2017-2018 NCAA Sports Medicine Handbook.* 26th ed. 2017. Accessed February 10, 2019.
14. The Controlled Substances Act. The United States Department of Justice website. www.justice.gov/jm/jm-9-100000-controlled-substances-act. Published 1970. Accessed July 20, 2020.
15. Cleary MA, Flanagan KW. *Acute and Emergency Care in Athletic Training.* Champaign, IL: Human Kinetics; 2019.

Chapter 2

1. Alaranta A, Alaranta H, Helenius I. Use of prescription drugs in athletes. *Sports Med.* 2008;38(6):449-463.
2. Anderson L. Medical abbreviations on pharmacy prescriptions. Drugs.com. www.drugs.com/article/prescription-abbreviations.html. Published 2016. Accessed October 10, 2018.
3. Benjamin DM. Reducing medication errors and increasing patient safety: case studies in clinical pharmacology. *J Clin Pharmacol.* 2003;43(7):768-783.
4. Carlson C. Traveling with medication. NCAA website. www.ncaa.org/sport-science-institute/traveling-medication. Published March 17, 2015. Accessed September 20, 2018.
5. Chang CJ, Weston T, Higgs JD, et al. Inter-Association Consensus Statement: the management of medications by the sports medicine team. *J Athl Train.* 2018;53(11):1103-1112.
6. Commission on Accreditation of Athletic Training Education. CAATE 2020 Standards for Accreditation of Professional Athletic Training Programs. https://caate.net/wp-content/uploads/2018/02/2020-Standards-for-Professional-Programs-copyedited-clean.pdf. Published 2018. Accessed September 10, 2018.
7. Council on School Health. Policy statement—guidance for the administration of medication in school. *Pediatrics.* 2009;124(4):1244-1251.
8. Diehl J, Kinart C, Cohen R. *BOC Facility Principles.* Omaha, NE: Board of Certification; 2015.
9. Diehl J, Dean C, et al. *BOC Guiding Principles for AT Policy and Procedure Development.* www.bocatc.org/system/comfy/cms/files/files/000/000/529/original/Guiding_Principles_for_AT_Policies_and_Procedures.pdf. Published 2017. Accessed February 6, 2019.
10. The Controlled Substances Act. The U.S. Drug Enforcement Administration website. www.dea.gov/controlled-substances-act. Published 1970. Accessed February 10, 2019.
11. Dunne EM, Striley CW, Mannes ZL, Asken BM, Ennis N, Cottler LB. Reasons for prescription opioid use while playing in the national football league as risk factors for current use and misuse among former players. *Clin J Sport Med.* 2020:30(6):544-549.

12. Edmunds MW. *Introduction to Clinical Pharmacology.* 8th ed. St. Louis, MO: Elsevier; 2016.
13. Garrett SD, Zapantis A. Institutional pharmacy practice. In: Nemire RE, Kier KL, Assa-Eley M, eds. *Pharmacy Student Survival Guide.* 3rd ed. New York, NY: McGraw-Hill Education; 2014:461-511.
14. Hollingsworth JC, Fox BI. Pharmacy informatics: enabling safe and efficacious medication use. In: Malone PM, Malone MJ, Park SK, eds. *Drug Information: A Guide for Pharmacists.* 6th ed. New York, NY: McGraw-Hill Education; 2017:1115-1152.
15. Huff P. Drug distribution in the athletic training room. *Clin Sports Med.* 1998;17(2):211-228.
16. Hughes R. *Patient safety and quality: an evidence-based handbook for nurses.* Rockville, MD: Agency for Healthcare Research and Quality; 2008.
17. Federico, F. The five rights of medication improvement. Institute for Healthcare Improvement website. www.ihi.org/resources/Pages/ImprovementStories/FiveRightsofMedicationAdministration.aspx. Published 2018. Accessed October 1, 2018.
18. List of error-prone abbreviations. Institute for Safe Medication Practices website. www.ismp.org/recommendations/error-prone-abbreviations-list. Published October 2, 2017. Accessed October 9, 2020.
19. Jaffe TA. Taking a seat at the table: what is a radiologist doing on the hospital formulary committee? *Acad Radiol.* 2012;19(12):1581-1582.
20. Kaeding CC, Borchers J. Issues for the traveling team physician. *J Knee Surg.* 2016;29(5):364-369.
21. Kahanov L, Roberts J, Wughalter EM. Adherence to drug-dispensation and drug-administration laws and guidelines in collegiate athletic training rooms: a 5-year review. *J Athl Train.* 2010;45(3):299-305.
22. Kahanov L, Furst D, Johnson S, Roberts J. Adherence to drug-dispensation and drug-administration laws and guidelines in collegiate athletic training rooms. *J Athl Train.* 2003;38(3):252-258.
23. Kahanov L, Abdenour T, Faulstick J, Pavlovich M, Swann E, Walters D. Consensus statement: Managing prescription and non-prescription medications in the athletic training facility. www.nata.org/sites/default/files/managingmedication.pdf. Published 2009. Accessed September 30, 2018.
24. Klafs CE, Arnheim DD. *Modern principles of athletic training: The science of injury prevention and care.* 3rd ed. Saint Louis, MO: Mosby; 1973.
25. Magnus B, Miller M. *Pharmacology application in athletic training.* Philadelphia, PA: FA Davis; 2005.
26. About medication errors. What is a medication error? National Coordinating Council for Medication Error Reporting and Prevention (NCC MERP) website. www.nccmerp.org/about-medication-errors. Published 2019. Accessed June 19, 2019.
27. Nickell R. Eight principles for managing prescription medications in the athletic training room. *Athl Ther Today.* 2005;10(1):6-9.
28. Palmer KL. FDA issues final guidance addressing repackaging of certain human drug products and outsourcing facilities. *FDA Law Blog.* www.fdalawblog.net/2017/01/fda-issues-final-guidance-addressing-repackaging-of-certain-human-drug-products-by-pharmacies-and-ou/. Published January 18, 2017. Accessed September 28, 2018.
29. Parker C. Understanding the directions on prescription drug labels. www.drugsdb.com/blog/understanding-prescription-drug-labels.html. Published February 3, 2012. Accessed October 10, 2018.
30. Parrish RH. Lecture 2—What is a formulary, anyway? (Or the Cliff Notes Version of drug stewardship and expense control). *Pharmacy.* 2018;6(3):69.
31. St Mary EW. Legal and ethical dilemmas in drug management for team physicians and athletic trainers. *South Med J.* 1998;91(5):421-424.
32. Tscholl P, Alonso JM, Dolle G, Junge A, Dvorak J. The use of drugs and nutritional supplements in top-level track and field athletes. *Am J Sports Med.* 2010;38(1):133-140.
33. Tyreman C. How to avoid drug errors: the five "rights" of medicines administration. *Nursing Times.* www.nursingtimes.net/clinical-archive/medicine-management/five-rights-of-medication-administration/how-to-avoid-drug-errors-the-five-rights-of-medicines-administration/5018923.article. Published September 4, 2010. Accessed May 18, 2021.
34. Guidance for industry on repackaging of certain human drug products by pharmacies and outsourcing facilities. Regulations.gov. www.regulations.gov/document?D=FDA-2014-D-1524-0050. Accessed July 1, 2019.
35. Whitehill WR, Wright KE, Robinson JB. Guidelines for dispensing medications. *J Athl Train.* 1992;27(1):20-22.

Chapter 3

1. AHRQ Pharmacy Health Literacy Center. Agency for Healthcare Research and Quality website. www.ahrq.gov/professionals/quality-patient-safety/pharmhealthlit/index.html. Published July 2013. Accessed April 30, 2019.
2. ASHP guidelines on adverse drug reaction monitoring and reporting. *Am J Health Syst Pharm.* 1995;52(4):417-419.
3. Andrews EB, Gilsenan AW, Midkiff K, et al. The US postmarketing surveillance study of adult osteosarcoma and teriparatide: study design and findings from the first 7 years. *J Bone Miner Res.* 2012;27(12):2429-2437.
4. Baca QJ, Golan DE. Pharmacodynamics. In: Golan DE, Armstrong E, Armstrong A, eds. *Principles of Pharmacology: The Pathophysiologic Basis of Drug Therapy.* 4th ed. Philadelphia. PA: Wolters Kluwer; 2017.
5. Bushra R, Aslam N, Khan AY. Food-drug interactions. *Oman Med J.* 2011(2):77-83.
6. Buxton ILO. Principles of prescription order writing and patient compliance. In: Brunton LL, Hilal-Dandan

R, Knollmann BC, eds. *Goodman & Gilman's: The Pharmacological Basis of Therapeutics*. 13th ed. New York, NY: McGraw-Hill Education; 2017.

7. Cleary MA, Flanagan KW. *Acute and Emergency Care in Athletic Training*. Champaign, IL: Human Kinetics; 2020.
8. Sinha, S. Jardiance. www.drugs.com/jardiance.html. Published 2019. Accessed August 17, 2019.
9. Erickson MA, Penning TM. Drug toxicity and poisoning. In: Brunton LL, Hilal-Dandan R, Knollmann BC, eds. *Goodman & Gilman's: The Pharmacological Basis of Therapeutics*. 13th ed. New York, NY: McGraw-Hill Education; 2017.
10. Frequently asked questions on patents and exclusivity. U.S. Food and Drug Administration website. www.fda.gov/drugs/development-approval-process-drugs/frequently-asked-questions-patents-and-exclusivity#What_is_the_difference_between_patents_a. Published 2018. Accessed April 30, 2019.
11. Guy J. *Pharmacology for the Prehospital Professional*. Burlington, MA: Jones & Bartlett Learning; 2012.
12. Hollingsworth JC, Fox BI. Pharmacy informatics: enabling safe and efficacious medication use. In: Malone PM, Malone MJ, Park SK, eds. *Drug Information: A Guide for Pharmacists*. 6th ed. New York, NY: McGraw-Hill Education; 2018.
13. Hughes R. *Patient Safety and Quality: An Evidence-Based Handbook for Nurses*. Rockville, MD: Agency for Healthcare Research and Quality; 2008.
14. 'High-alert' medications and patient safety. *Int J Qual Health Care*. 2001;13(4):339-340.
15. Katzung BG. Introduction: The nature of drugs, drug development and regulation. In: Katzung BG, ed. *Basic & Clinical Pharmacology*. 14th ed. New York, NY: McGraw-Hill Education; 2017.
16. Katzung BG, Kruidering-Hall M, Trevor AJ. Immunopharmacology. In: *Katzung & Trevor's Pharmacology: Examination & Board Review*. 12th ed. New York, NY: McGraw-Hill Education; 2019.
17. Lieberman P, Nicklas RA, Oppenheimer J, et al. The diagnosis and management of anaphylaxis practice parameter: 2010 update. *J Allergy Clin Immunol*. 2010;126(3):477-480, e471-442.
18. Lynch SS. Drug efficacy and safety. Merck Manual Professional Version website. www.merckmanuals.com/professional/clinical-pharmacology/concepts-in-pharmacotherapy/drug-efficacy-and-safety. Accessed April 30, 2019.
19. Smith Marsh DE. Adverse drug reactions. Merck Manual Professional Version website. www.merckmanuals.com/professional/clinical-pharmacology/adverse-drug-reactions/adverse-drug-reactions. Updated August 2018. Accessed April 30, 2019.
20. About medication errors. National Coordinating Council for Medication Error Reporting and Prevention (NCC MERP) website. www.nccmerp.org/about-medication-errors. Published 2019. Accessed June 19, 2019.
21. Sheehan AH, Jordan JK. Formulating an effective response: a structured approach. In: Malone PM, Malone MJ, Park SK, eds. *Drug Information: A Guide for Pharmacists*. 6th ed. New York, NY: McGraw-Hill Education; 2018.
22. Shields KM, Park SK. Drug information resources. In: Malone PM, Malone MJ, Park SK, eds. *Drug Information: A Guide for Pharmacists*. 6th ed. New York, NY: McGraw-Hill Education; 2018.
23. Solotke MT, Dhruva SS, Downing NS, Shah ND, Ross JS. New and incremental FDA black box warnings from 2008 to 2015. *Expert Opin Drug Safety*. 2018;17:117-123.
24. Stringer JL. Where to start. In: Stringer JL. *Basic Concepts in Pharmacology: What You Need to Know for Each Drug Class*. 5th ed. New York, NY: McGraw-Hill Education; 2017:1-4.
25. Stringer JL. Receptor Theory. In: Stringer JL. *Basic Concepts in Pharmacology: What You Need to Know for Each Drug Class*. 5th ed. New York, NY: McGraw-Hill Education; 2017:5-10.
26. Sylvia LM. Allergic and pseudoallergic drug reactions. In: DiPiro JT, Talbert RL, Yee GC, Matzke GR, Wells BG, Posey LM, eds. *Pharmacotherapy: A Pathophysiologic Approach*. 9th ed. New York, NY: The McGraw-Hill Companies; 2014.
27. Tam VH. Application of pharmacokinetics to clinical situations. In: Shargel L, Yu ABC, eds. *Applied Biopharmaceutics & Pharmacokinetics*. 7th ed. New York, NY: McGraw-Hill Education; 2016.
28. Patient safety. The Joint Commission website. www.jointcommission.org/facts_about_patient_safety. Published 2019. Accessed June 19, 2019.
29. World Health Organization. *Introduction to Drug Utilization Research*. http://apps.who.int/medicinedocs/pdf/s4876e/s4876e.pdf. Geneva, Switzerland: Author; 2003. Accessed April 30, 2019.

Chapter 4

1. Baca QJ, Golan DE. Pharmacokinetics. In: Golan DE, Armstrong E, Armstrong A, eds. *Principles of Pharmacology: The Pathophysiologic Basis of Drug Therapy*. 4th ed. Philadelphia, PA: Wolters Kluwer; 2017:27-42.
2. Bauer LA. Clinical pharmacokinetics and pharmacodynamics. In: DiPiro JT, Talbert RL, Yee GC, Matzke GR, Wells BG, Posey LM, eds. *Pharmacotherapy: A Pathophysiologic Approach*. 10th ed. New York, NY: McGraw-Hill Education; 2017:7-8.
3. Coombes JS, van Rosendal SP. Use of intravenous rehydration in the National Football League. *Clin J Sport Med*. 2011;21(3):185-186.
4. Edmunds MW. *Introduction to Clinical Pharmacology*. 8th ed. St. Louis, MO: Elsevier; 2016.
5. Fitzsimmons S, Tucker A, Martins D. Seventy-five percent of National Football League teams use pregame hyperhydration with intravenous fluid. *Clin J Sport Med*. 2011;21(3):192-199.

6. Hilal-Dandan R, Brunton LL. *Goodman and Gilman's Manual of Pharmacology and Therapeutics.* 2nd ed. New York, NY: McGraw-Hill Education; 2013.

7. Hoekelman RA. Take two aspirin and call me in the morning: salicylate use and Reye's syndrome. *Arch Ped Adolescent Med.* 1982;136(11):973.

8. Katzung BG. *Basic & Clinical Pharmacology.* 14th ed. New York, NY: McGraw-Hill Education; 2018.

9. Katzung BG, Kruidering-Hall M, Trevor AJ. *Katzung & Trevor's Pharmacology: Examination and Board Review.* 12th ed. New York, NY: McGraw-Hill Education; 2018.

10. Khazaeinia T, Ramsey AA, Tam YK. The effects of exercise on the pharmacokinetics of drugs. *J Pharm Pharm Sci.* 2000;3(3):292-302.

11. Le J. Drug absorption. Merck Manual Professional Version website. www.merckmanuals.com/professional/clinical-pharmacology/pharmacokinetics/drug-absorption. Published 2019. Accessed February 21, 2019.

12. Lenz TL, Lenz NJ, Faulkner MA. Potential interactions between exercise and drug therapy. *Sports Med.* 2004;34(5):293-306.

13. Mobley WC. Introduction to biopharmaceutics. In: Amiji MM, Cook TJ, Mobley WC, eds. *Applied Physical Pharmacy.* 2nd ed. New York, NY: McGraw-Hill Education; 2013.

14. Pandit NK, Soltis R. *Introduction to the Pharmaceutical Sciences: An Integrated Approach* 2nd ed. Baltimore, MD: Lippincott Williams & Wilkins; 2012.

15. Pelletier-Dattu CE. *Lange Smart Charts: Pharmacology.* 2nd ed. New York, NY: McGraw-Hill Medical; 2017.

16. Rowland M, Thomas NT. *Clinical Pharmacokinetics: Concepts and Applications.* 4th ed. Baltimore, MD: Lippincott Williams & Wilkins; 2011.

17. Sandmann BJ, Amiji MM. Solubility, dissolution, and partitioning. In: Amiji MM, Cook TJ, Mobley WC, eds. *Applied Physical Pharmacy.* 2nd ed. New York, NY: McGraw-Hill Education; 2013.

18. Shargel L, Yu ABC. Introduction to biopharmaceutics and pharmacokinetics. In: Shargel L, Yu ABC, eds. *Applied Biopharmaceutics & Pharmacokinetics.* 7th ed. New York, NY: McGraw-Hill Education; 2016.

19. Shields KM, Park SK. Drug information resources. In: Malone PM, Malone MJ, Park SK, eds. *Drug Information: A Guide for Pharmacists.* 6th ed. New York, NY: McGraw-Hill Education; 2018: 59-112.

20. Stringer JL. *Basic Concepts in Pharmacology: What You Need to Know for Each Drug Class.* 5th ed. New York, NY: McGraw-Hill Education; 2017.

21. Tam VH. Application of pharmacokinetics to clinical situations. In: Shargel L, Yu ABC, eds. *Applied Biopharmaceutics & Pharmacokinetics.* 7th ed. New York, NY: McGraw-Hill Education; 2016:681-734.

22. Yellepeddi V. Pharmacokinetics. In: Whalen K, Radhakrishnan R, Feild C, eds. *Pharmacology.* 7th ed. Philadelphia, PA: Wolters Kluwer; 2019:1-22.

Chapter 5

1. Alenghat FJ, Golan DE. Drug-receptor interactions. In: Golan DE, Armstrong EJ, Armstrong AW, eds. *Principles of Pharmacology: The Pathophysiologic Basis of Drug Therapy.* 4th ed. Philadelphia, PA: Wolters Kluwer Health; 2017:2-16.

2. Ament PW, Bertolino JG, Liszewski JL. Clinically significant drug interactions. *Am Fam Physician.* 2000;61(6):1745-1754.

3. Aronson J. *Pharmacodynamics: How Drugs Work.* www.cebm.net/wp-content/uploads/2016/05/Pharmacodynamics-How-drugs-work.pdf. Published 2016. Accessed October 7, 2020.

4. Baca QJ, Golan DE. Pharmacodynamics. In: Golan DE, Armstrong E, Armstrong A, eds. *Principles of Pharmacology: The Pathophysiologic Basis of Drug Therapy.* 4th ed. Philadelphia. PA: Wolters Kluwer; 2017:17-26.

5. Blumenthal DK. Pharmacodynamics: Molecular mechanisms of drug action. In: Brunton LL, Hilal-Dandan R, Knollmann BC, eds. *Goodman & Gilman's: The Pharmacological Basis of Therapeutics.* 13th ed. New York, NY: McGraw-Hill Education; 2017:31-54.

6. Erickson MA, Penning TM. Drug toxicity and poisoning. In: Brunton LL, Hilal-Dandan R, Knollmann BC, eds. *Goodman & Gilman's: The Pharmacological Basis of Therapeutics.* 13th ed. New York, NY: McGraw-Hill Education; 2017:55-64.

7. Farinde A. Drug-receptor interactions. Merck Manual Professional Version website. www.merckmanuals.com/professional/clinical-pharmacology/pharmacodynamics/drug%E2%80%93receptor-interactions. Published 2016. Accessed May 19, 2019.

8. Guy J. *Pharmacology for the Prehospital Professional.* Burlington, MA: Jones & Bartlett Learning; 2012.

9. Katzung BG. Introduction: The nature of drugs and drug development and regulation. In: Katzung BG, ed. *Basic & Clinical Pharmacology.* 14th ed. New York, NY: McGraw-Hill Education; 2017:1-19.

10. Katzung BG, Kruidering-Hall M, Trevor AJ. *Katzung & Trevor's Pharmacology: Examination & Board Review.* 12th ed. New York, NY: McGraw-Hill Education; 2019.

11. Kuper K. Vancomycin dosing guidelines: What you need to know. DoseMeRx website. https://doseme-rx.com/news/20200330-vancomycin-dosing-guidelines-what-to-know. Published March 30, 2020. Accessed October 7, 2020.

12. Lorenzini KI, Daali Y, Dayer P, Desmeules J. Pharmacokinetic-pharmacodynamic modelling of opioids in healthy human volunteers. A minireview. *Basic Clin Pharmacol Toxicol.* 2012;110:219-226.

13. Lynch SS. Drug efficacy and safety. Merck Manual Professional Version website. www.merckmanuals.com/professional/clinical-pharmacology/concepts-in-pharmacotherapy/drug-efficacy-and-safety. Published 2016. Accessed April 30, 2019.

14. Marino M, Zito PM. *Pharmacodynamics*. Treasure Island, FL: StatPearls; 2019.
15. Peris J. Drug–receptor interactions and pharmacodynamics. In: Whalen K, Radhakrishnan R, Feild C, eds. *Pharmacology*. 7th ed. Philadelphia, PA: Wolters Kluwer 2019:23-36.
16. Rybak MJ, Le J, Lodise TP, et al. Executive summary: Therapeutic monitoring of vancomycin for serious *Methicillin*-resistant *Staphylococcus aureus* infections: A revised consensus guideline and review of the American Society of Health-System Pharmacists, the Infectious Diseases Society of America, the Pediatric Infectious Diseases Society, and the Society of Infectious Diseases Pharmacists. *Pharmacotherapy*. 2020;40(4):363-367.
17. Stringer JL. *Basic Concepts in Pharmacology: What You Need to Know for Each Drug Class*. 5th ed. New York, NY: McGraw-Hill Education; 2017.
18. Tam VH. Application of Pharmacokinetics to Clinical Situations. In: Shargel L, Yu ABC, eds. *Applied Biopharmaceutics & Pharmacokinetics*. 7th ed. New York, NY: McGraw-Hill Education; 2015:681-733.

Chapter 6

1. Arevalo-Rodriguez I, Munoz L, Godoy-Casasbuenas N, et al. Needle gauge and tip designs for preventing post-dural puncture headache (PDPH). *Cochrane Database Syst Rev*. 2017;4:CD010807.
2. Baca QJ, Golan DE. Pharmacokinetics. In: Golan DE, Armstrong E, Armstrong A, eds. *Principles of Pharmacology: The Pathophysiologic Basis of Drug Therapy*. 4th ed. Philadelphia, PA: Wolters Kluwer; 2017:27-42.
3. Bauer LA. Clinical pharmacokinetics and pharmacodynamics. In: DiPiro JT, Talbert RL, Yee GC, Matzke GR, Wells BG, Posey LM, eds. *Pharmacotherapy: A Pathophysiologic Approach*. 10th ed. New York, NY: McGraw-Hill Education; 2017:7-8.
4. Bertrand N, Leroux J-C. The journey of a drug-carrier in the body: An anatomo-physiological perspective. *J Control Release*. 2012;161(2):152-163.
5. Bicket MC, Chakravarthy K, Chang D, Cohen SP. Epidural steroid injections: an updated review on recent trends in safety and complications. *Pain Manag*. 2015;5(2):129-146.
6. Edmunds MW. *Introduction to Clinical Pharmacology*. 8th ed. St. Louis, MO: Elsevier; 2016.
7. Epstein NE. Neurological complications of lumbar and cervical dural punctures with a focus on epidural injections. *Surg Neurol Int*. 2017;8:60.
8. Givan GV, Diehl JJ. Intravenous fluid use in athletes. *Sports Health*. 2012;4(4):333-339.
9. Guy J. *Pharmacology for the Prehospital Professional*. Burlington, MA: Jones & Bartlett Learning; 2012.
10. Hilal-Dandan R, Brunton LL. *Goodman and Gilman's Manual of Pharmacology and Therapeutics*. 2nd ed. New York, NY: McGraw-Hill Education; 2013.
11. Holford NHG. Pharmacokinetics and pharmacodynamics: rational dosing and the time course of drug action. In: Katzung BG, ed. *Basic & Clinical Pharmacology*. 14th ed. New York, NY: McGraw-Hill Education; 2017:41-55.
12. Nursing skills. Preparing and administering oral tablet and liquid medications. JOVE website. www.jove.com/science-education/10258/preparing-and-administering-oral-tablet-and-liquid-medications. Published 2019. Accessed July 10, 2019.
13. Katzung BG, Kruidering-Hall M, Trevor AJ. *Katzung & Trevor's Pharmacology: Examination & Board Review*. 12th ed. New York, NY: McGraw-Hill Education; 2018.
14. Krohn A. Use of IVs to hydrate high school football players sparks controversial debate. *Atlanta Journal-Constitution*. November 29, 2018. www.ajc.com/blog/high-school-sports/use-ivs-hydrate-high-school-football-players-sparks-controversial-debate/ah8E7VpVq-FoP1GPe0sjcjL. Accessed July 11, 2019.
15. Le J. Drug absorption. Merck Manual Professional Version website. www.merckmanuals.com/professional/clinical-pharmacology/pharmacokinetics/drug-absorption. Published 2019. Accessed February 21, 2019.
16. The administration of medicines. *Nursing Times*. November 19, 2007. www.nursingtimes.net/clinical-archive/medicine-management/the-administration-of-medicines/288560.article. Accessed June 20, 2019.
17. Perrie Y. Controlling drug delivery. In: Perrie Y, Rades T, eds. *Pharmaceutics: Drug Delivery and Targeting*. London: Pharmaceutical Press; 2009.
18. Perron CE. Intraosseous infusion. Up-to-Date website. www-uptodate-com.libproxy.chapman.edu/contents/intraosseous-infusion. Published 2020. Accessed October 23, 2020.
19. Peterson C, Hodler J. Adverse events from diagnostic and therapeutic joint injections: a literature review. *Skeletal Radiol*. 2011;40(1):5-12.
20. Potter P, Perry A, Stockert P, Hall A. *Essentials for Nursing Practice*. 8th ed. St. Louis, MO: Elsevier; 2015.
21. Rochwerg B, Almenawer SA, Siemieniuk RAC, et al. Atraumatic (pencil-point) versus conventional needles for lumbar puncture: a clinical practice guideline. *BMJ*. 2018;361:k1920.
22. Shepherd M. Administration of drugs 1: oral route. *Nursing Times*. 2011;107(32-33):18.
23. Stephens MB, Beutler AI, O'Connor FG. Musculoskeletal injections: a review of the evidence. *Am Fam Physician*. 2008;78(8):971-976.
24. Stringer JL. *Basic Concepts in Pharmacology: What You Need to Know for Each Drug Class*. 5th ed. New York, NY: McGraw-Hill Education; 2017.
25. Suarez S, Marroum PJ, Hughes M. Biopharmaceutic considerations in drug product design and in vitro drug product performance. In: Shargel L, Yu ABC, eds. *Applied Biopharmaceutics & Pharmacokinetics*. 7th ed. New York, NY: McGraw-Hill Education; 2016:415.

26. Tam VH. Application of pharmacokinetics to clinical situations. In: Shargel L, Yu ABC, eds. *Applied Biopharmaceutics & Pharmacokinetics*. 7th ed. New York, NY: McGraw-Hill Education; 2016:681-734.
27. Urits I, Viswanath O, Petro J, Aner M. Management of dural puncture headache caused by caudal epidural steroid injection. *J Clin Anesth*. 2019;52:67-68.
28. Woo TM, Wynne AL. *Pharmacotherapeutics for Advanced Practice Nurse Prescribers*. 4th ed. Philadelphia, PA: F.A. Davis; 2016.
29. Xu C, Peng H, Li R, et al. Risk factors and clinical characteristics of deep knee infection in patients with intra-articular injections: A matched retrospective cohort analysis. *Semin Arthritis Rheum*. 2018;47(6):911-916.
30. Yellepeddi V. Pharmacokinetics. In: Whalen K, Radhakrishnan R, Feild C, eds. *Pharmacology*. 7th ed. Philadelphia, PA: Wolters Kluwer; 2019:1-22.

Chapter 7

1. Aminoshariae A, Khan A. Acetaminophen: old drug, new issues. *J Endod*. 2015;41(5):588-593.
2. Baca QJ, Schulman JM, Strichartz GR. Local anesthetic pharmacology. In: Golan DE, Armstrong E, Armstrong A, eds. *Principles of Pharmacology: The Pathophysiologic Basis of Drug Therapy*. 4th ed. Philadelphia, PA: Wolters Kluwer; 2017:167-182.
3. Benoist JL, Gammaitoni AR. The 5% Lidocaine patch reduces pain intensity in professional athletes with sports injury pain without significant systemic effects or cognitive and performance impairment. *Arch Phys Med Rehabil*. 2005(9):e34.
4. Catterall WA, Mackie K. Local anesthetics. In: Brunton LL, Hilal-Dandan R, Knollmann BC, eds. *Goodman & Gilman's: The Pharmacological Basis of Therapeutics*. 13th ed. New York, NY: McGraw-Hill Education; 2017:405-420.
5. CDC guideline for prescribing opioids for chronic pain. Centers for Disease Control and Prevention website. www.cdc.gov/drugoverdose/prescribing/guideline.html. Published 2016. Accessed January 26, 2021.
6. Chandrasekharan NV, Dai H, Roos KL, et al. COX-3, a cyclooxygenase-1 variant inhibited by acetaminophen and other analgesic/antipyretic drugs: cloning, structure, and expression. *Proc Natl Acad Sci U S A*. 2002;99(21):13926-13931.
7. Drahl C. How does acetaminophen work? *Chemical and Engineering News*. 2014;92(29):31-32. https://cen.acs.org/articles/92/i29/Does-Acetaminophen-Work-Researchers-Still.html. Accessed March 25, 2019.
8. Drakos M, Birmingham P, Delos D, et al. Corticosteroid and anesthetic injections for muscle strains and ligament sprains in the NFL. *HSS J*. 2014;10(2):136-142.
9. Acetaminophen. Drugs.com website. www.drugs.com/acetaminophen.html. Published 2018. Accessed November 6, 2019.
10. El-Boghdadly K, Pawa A, Chin KJ. Local anesthetic systemic toxicity: current perspectives. *Local Reg Anesth*. 2018;11:35-44.
11. Galeotti N, Di Cesare Mannelli L, Mazzanti G, Bartolini A, Ghelardini C. Menthol: a natural analgesic compound. *Neurosci Lett*. 2002;322(3):145-148.
12. Hashmi JA, Baliki MN, Huang L, et al. Lidocaine patch (5%) is no more potent than placebo in treating chronic back pain when tested in a randomised double blind placebo controlled brain imaging study. *Mol Pain*. 2012;8:29.
13. How to apply a transdermal patch. Healthline website. www.healthline.com/health/general-use/how-to-use-transdermal-patch#troubleshooting. Published 2019. Accessed November 8, 2019.
14. Herndon CM, Strickland JM, Ray JB. Pain management. In: DiPiro JT, Talbert RL, Yee GC, Matzke GR, Wells BG, Posey LM, eds. *Pharmacotherapy: A Pathophysiologic Approach*. 10th ed. New York, NY: McGraw-Hill Education; 2017:909-926.
15. Hines R, Keaney D, Moskowitz MH, Prakken S. Use of lidocaine patch 5% for chronic low back pain: a report of four cases *Pain Manag*. 2002(4):361.
16. Tylenol dosage for adults. Tylenol website. www.tylenol.com/safety-dosing/usage/dosage-for-adults. Published 2016. Accessed March 1, 2019.
17. Jones DM, Saltzman CL, El-Khoury G. The diagnosis of the os trigonum syndrome with a fluoroscopically controlled injection of local anesthetic. *Iowa Orthop J*. 1999;19:122-126.
18. Katz NP, Gammaitoni AR, Davis MW, Dworkin RH, Lidoderm Patch Study Group. Lidocaine patch 5% reduces pain intensity and interference with quality of life in patients with postherpetic neuralgia: an effectiveness trial. *Pain Med*. 2002;3(4):324-332.
19. Khanna M, Peters C, Singh JR. Treating pain with the lidocaine patch 5% after total knee arthroplasty. *PM&R*. 2012;4:642-646.
20. Kivitz A, Fairfax M, Sheldon EA, et al. Comparison of the effectiveness and tolerability of lidocaine patch 5% versus celecoxib for osteoarthritis-related knee pain: post hoc analysis of a 12 week, prospective, randomized, active-controlled, open-label, parallel-group trial in adults. *Clin Ther*. 2008;30(12):2366-2377.
21. Kolasinski SL, Neogi T, Hochberg MC, et al. 2019 American College of Rheumatology/Arthritis Foundation Guideline for the Management of Osteoarthritis of the Hand, Hip, and Knee. *Arthritis Care Res*. 2020;72(2):149-162.
22. Lee WM. Acetaminophen (APAP) hepatotoxicity—Isn't it time for APAP to go away? *J Hepatol*. 2017;67(6):1324-1331.
23. Marmura MJ, Silberstein SD, Schwedt TJ. The acute treatment of migraine in adults: The American Headache Society evidence assessment of migraine pharmacotherapies. *Headache*. 2015;55(1):3-20.
24. Fentanyl (transdermal route). Mayo Clinic website. www.mayoclinic.org/drugs-supplements/fentanyl-transdermal-route/proper-use/drg-20068152. Published 2019. Accessed November 8, 2019.

25. McGill MR, Jaeschke H. Metabolism and disposition of acetaminophen: recent advances in relation to hepatotoxicity and diagnosis. *Pharm Res.* 2013;30(9):2174-2187.

26. Nalamachu S, Crockett RS, Gammaitoni AR, Gould EM. A comparison of the lidocaine patch 5% vs naproxen 500 mg twice daily for the relief of pain associated with carpal tunnel syndrome: a 6-week, randomized, parallel-group study. *MedGenMed.* 2006;8(3):33.

27. Neal DR, Jackson KC. Pain management. In: Stein SM, ed. *Boh's Pharmacy Practice Manual: A Guide to the Clinical Experience.* 4th ed. Baltimore, MD: Wolters Kluwer Health; 2014.

28. Ouellet M, Percival MD. Mechanism of acetaminophen inhibition of cyclooxygenase isoforms. *Arch Biochem Biophys.* 2001;387(2):273-280.

29. Pasero C. Lidocaine patch 5% for acute pain management. *J Perianesth Nurs.* 2013;28(3):169-173.

30. Patel HH, Pearn ML, Patel PM, Roth DM. General anesthetics and therapeutic gases. In: Brunton LL, Hilal-Dandan R, Knollmann BC, eds. *Goodman & Gilman's: The Pharmacological Basis of Therapeutics.* 13th ed. New York, NY: McGraw-Hill Education; 2017:387-404.

31. Pergolizzi JV, Jr., Taylor R, Jr., LeQuang JA, Raffa RB, NEMA research group. The role and mechanism of action of menthol in topical analgesic products. *J Clin Pharm Ther.* 2018;43(3):313-319.

32. Acetaminophen: drug summary. Prescribers' Digital Reference. www.pdr.net/drug-summary/Ofirmev-acetaminophen-1346#:~:text=Maximum%20Dosage&text=The%20total%20daily%20maximum%20dose,of%20acetaminophen%20from%20all%20sources.&text=1%2C000%20mg%2Fdose%20PO%2FPR,max%20doses%2C%20see%20individual%20products. Published 2021. Accessed January 26, 2021.

33. SchiØDt FV, Rochling FA, Casey DL, Lee WM. Acetaminophen toxicity in an urban county hospital. *N Engl J Med.* 1997;337(16):1112-1117.

34. Sebak S, Orchard JW, Golding LD, Steet E, Brennan SA, Ibrahim A. Long-term safety of using local anesthetic injections in professional rugby league for modified indications. *Clin J Sport Med.* 2018;28(5):435-442.

35. Stanos SP. Special article: topical agents for the management of musculoskeletal pain. *J Pain Symptom Manag.* 2007;33:342-355.

36. Warren L, Pak A. Local anesthetic systemic toxicity. Up-to-Date website. www-uptodate-com.libproxy.chapman.edu/contents/local-anesthetic-systemic-toxicity?search=local-anesthetic%20systemic%20toxicity%20(LAST)&source=search_result&selectedTitle=1~150&usage_type=default&display_rank=1. Published 2020. Accessed January 26, 2021.

37. Washington State Agency Medical Directors' Group. *Interagency Guideline on Prescribing Opioids for Pain.* www.agencymeddirectors.wa.gov/Files/2015AMDGOpioidGuideline.pdf. Published June 2015. Accessed February 11, 2021.

38. Wells BG, DiPiro JT, Schwinghammer TL, DiPiro CV. *Pharmacotherapy Quick Guide.* New York, NY: McGraw-Hill Education; 2017.

39. Woolf CJ. What is this thing called pain? *J Clin Invest.* 2010;120(11):3742-3744.

40. Headache disorders. World Health Organization website. www.who.int/en/news-room/fact-sheets/detail/headache-disorders. Published April 8, 2016. Accessed October 6, 2019.

41. World Health Organization. *WHO Model List of Essential Medicines.* 20th ed. www.who.int/medicines/publications/essentialmedicines/en. Published 2017. Accessed November 26, 2018.

42. WHO's cancer pain ladder for adults. World Health Organization website. www.who.int/cancer/palliative/painladder/en. Published 2019. Accessed March 25, 2019.

43. Yaksh T, Wallace M. Opioids, analgesia, and pain management. In: Brunton LL, Hilal-Dandan R, Knollmann BC, eds. *Goodman & Gilman's: The Pharmacological Basis of Therapeutics.* 13th ed. New York, NY: McGraw-Hill Education; 2017:355-386.

Chapter 8

1. CDC guideline for prescribing opioids for chronic pain. Centers for Disease Control and Prevention website. www.cdc.gov/drugoverdose/prescribing/guideline.html. Published 2019. Accessed May 6, 2019.

2. Norco dosage. Drugs.com website. www.drugs.com/dosage/norco.html. Updated November 28, 2019. Accessed December 26, 2019.

3. Tramadol. Drugs.com website. www.drugs.com/tramadol.html. Published 2019. Accessed December 26, 2019.

4. Fookes C. Narcotic analgesics. Drugs.com website. www.drugs.com/drug-class/narcotic-analgesics.html. Updated February 28, 2018. Accessed November 8, 2019.

5. Griffin RS, Woolf CJ. Pharmacology of analgesia. In: Golan DE, Armstrong E, Armstrong A, eds. *Principles of Pharmacology: The Pathophysiologic Basis of Drug Therapy.* 4th ed. Philadelphia, PA: Wolters Kluwer; 2017:288-307.

6. Herndon CM, Strickland JM, Ray JB. Pain management. In: DiPiro JT, Talbert RL, Yee GC, Matzke GR, Wells BG, Posey LM, eds. *Pharmacotherapy: A Pathophysiologic Approach.* 10th ed. New York, NY: McGraw-Hill Education; 2017:909-926.

7. Hill M, Strain EC. Opiods: what you should know. Johns Hopkins Medicine website. www.hopkinsmedicine.org/opioids/index.html. Published 2020. Accessed October 26, 2020.

8. Huecker M, Azadfard M, Leaming J. Opioid addiction. *Stat Pearls.* www.ncbi.nlm.nih.gov/books/NBK448203. Published 2019. Accessed December 26, 2019.

9. Signs of opioid abuse. Johns Hopkins Medicine website. www.hopkinsmedicine.org/opioids/signs-of-opioid-abuse.html. Published 2020. Accessed October 26, 2020.

10. Munzing T. Physician guide to appropriate opioid prescribing for noncancer pain. *Perm J.* 2017;21:16-169.
11. 2018 annual surveillance report of drug-related risks and outcomes—United States. Centers for Disease Control and Prevention website. www.cdc.gov/drugoverdose/pdf/pubs/2018-cdc-drug-surveillance-report.pdf. Published 2018. Accessed May 5, 2019.
12. Scholl L, Seth P, Kariisa M, Wilson N, Baldwin G. Drug and opioid-involved overdose deaths—United States, 2013-2017. *MMWR.* 2019;67(51/52):1419-1427.
13. Schumacher MA, Basbaum AI, Naidu RK. Opioid agonists & antagonists. In: Katzung BG, ed. *Basic & Clinical Pharmacology.* 14th ed. New York, NY: McGraw-Hill Education; 2017.
14. Shelton KN, Clements JN. Naloxegol for managing opioid-induced constipation. *JAAPA.* 2017;30(9):51-53.
15. Smith HS. Opioid metabolism. *Mayo Clin Proc.* 2009;84(7):613-624.
16. Uritsky TJ. Methylnaltrexone: peripherally acting micro-opioid receptor antagonist. *J Adv Pract Oncol.* 2019;10(1):62-67.
17. CDC Wonder. Centers for Disease Control and Prevention website. https://wonder.cdc.gov. Published 2018. Accessed January 28, 2021.
18. van Steenbergen H, Eikemo M, Leknes S. The role of the opioid system in decision making and cognitive control: A review. *Cogn Affect Behav Neurosci.* 2019;19(3):435-458.
19. Washington State Agency Medical Directors' Group. *Interagency Guideline on Prescribing Opioids for Pain.* www.agencymeddirectors.wa.gov/Files/2015AMDGOpioidGuideline.pdf. Published June 2015. Accessed February 11, 2021.
20. WHO's cancer pain ladder for adults. World Health Organization website. www.who.int/cancer/palliative/painladder/en/. Published 2019. Accessed March 25, 2019.
21. Yaksh T, Wallace M. Opioids, analgesia, and pain management. In: Brunton LL, Hilal-Dandan R, Knollmann BC, eds. *Goodman & Gilman's: The Pharmacological Basis of Therapeutics.* 13th ed. New York, NY: McGraw-Hill Education; 2017:355-386.

Chapter 9

1. Almond E. Medication can be bitter pill: The Easley case is an example of the abuse of over-the-counter products. The danger is that such abuse can have unknowing victims. *Los Angeles Times.* August 12, 1990. www.latimes.com/archives/la-xpm-1990-08-12-sp-1106-story.html. Accessed July 28, 2019.
2. Antman EM. Evaluating the cardiovascular safety of nonsteroidal anti-inflammatory drugs. *Circulation.* 2017;135(21):2062-2072.
3. Bandoli G, Palmsten K, Forbess Smith CJ, Chambers CD. A review of systemic corticosteroid use in pregnancy and the risk of select pregnancy and birth outcomes. *Rheum Dis Clin North Am.* 2017;43(3):489-502.
4. Becker DE. Basic and clinical pharmacology of glucocorticosteroids. *Anesth Prog.* 2013;60(1):25-31.
5. Bhala N, Emberson J, Merhi A, et al. Vascular and upper gastrointestinal effects of non-steroidal anti-inflammatory drugs: meta-analyses of individual participant data from randomised trials. *Lancet.* 2013;382(9894):769-779.
6. Davies NM, Skjodt NM. Choosing the right nonsteroidal anti-inflammatory drug for the right patient: a pharmacokinetic approach. *Clin Pharmacokinet.* 2000;38(5):377-392.
7. Dean L. Comparing NSAIDs. *PubMed Clinical Q&A.* 2011;2008-2013.
8. Dilisio MF. Osteonecrosis following short-term, low-dose oral corticosteroids: a population-based study of 24 million patients. *Orthopedics.* 2014;37(7):e631-636.
9. Dixit M, Doan T, Kirschner R, Dixit N. Significant acute kidney injury due to non-steroidal anti-inflammatory drugs: inpatient setting. *Pharmaceuticals (Basel).* 2010;3(4):1279-1285.
10. Mayo Clinic staff. Avascular necrosis. Drugs.com website. www.drugs.com/mcd/avascular-necrosis. Published 2018. Accessed November 5, 2019.
11. Fares-Frederickson N, David M. Introduction to immunity and inflammation. In: Brunton LL, Hilal-Dandan R, Knollmann BC, eds. *Goodman & Gilman's: The Pharmacological Basis of Therapeutics.* 13th ed. New York, NY: McGraw-Hill Education; 2017:621-636.
12. Fookes C. Glucocorticoids. Drugs.com website. www.drugs.com/drug-class/glucocorticoids.html. Published 2018. Accessed July 23, 2019.
13. Griffin RS, Woolf CJ. Pharmacology of analgesia. In: Golan DE, Armstrong E, Armstrong A, eds. *Principles of Pharmacology: The Pathophysiologic Basis of Drug Therapy.* 4th ed. Philadelphia, PA: Wolters Kluwer; 2016:288-307.
14. Grosser T, Smyth E, FitzGerald G. Pharmacotherapy of inflammation, fever, pain, and gout. In: Brunton LL, Hilal-Dandan R, Knollmann BC, eds. *Goodman & Gilman's: The Pharmacological Basis of Therapeutics.* 13th ed. New York, NY: McGraw-Hill Education; 2017:685-710.
15. Harirforoosh S, Asghar W, Jamali F. Adverse effects of nonsteroidal antiinflammatory drugs: an update of gastrointestinal, cardiovascular and renal complications. *J Pharm Pharm Sci.* 2013;16(5):821-847.
16. Treating lupus with steroids. Johns Hopkins Lupus Center website. www.hopkinslupus.org/lupus-treatment/lupus-medications/steroids. Published 2019. Accessed July 26, 2019.
17. Katzung BG, Kruidering-Hall M, Trevor AJ. NSAIDs, acetaminophen, & drugs used in rheumatoid arthritis & gout. In: *Katzung & Trevor's Pharmacology: Examination & Board Review.* 12th ed. New York, NY: McGraw-Hill Education; 2018: 304-314.
18. Li J, Zhang N, Ye B, et al. Non-steroidal anti-inflammatory drugs increase insulin release from beta cells

by inhibiting ATP-sensitive potassium channels. *Br J Pharmacol.* 2007;151(4):483-493.

19. Liu LH, Zhang QY, Sun W, Li ZR, Gao FQ. Corticosteroid-induced osteonecrosis of the femoral head: detection, diagnosis, and treatment in earlier stages. *Chin Med J (Engl).* 2017;130(21):2601-2607.
20. Mont MA, Pivec R, Banerjee S, Issa K, Elmallah RK, Jones LC. High-dose corticosteroid use and risk of hip osteonecrosis: meta-analysis and systematic literature review. *J Arthroplasty.* 2015;30(9):1506-1512, e1505.
21. Myrex P, Harper L, Gould S. Corticosteroid injection for an orthopedic complaint in a female with gestational diabetes. *Sports Med Open.* 2018;4(1):3.
22. Adrenal insufficiency & Addison's disease. Health Information. National Institute of Diabetes and Digestive and Kidney Diseases website. www.niddk.nih.gov/health-information/endocrine-diseases/adrenal-insufficiency-addisons-disease. Published 2019. Accessed November 5, 2019.
23. Negm AA, Furst DE. Nonsteroidal anti-inflammatory drugs, disease-modifying antirheumatic drugs, nonopioid analgesics, & drugs used in gout. In: Katzung BG, ed. *Basic & Clinical Pharmacology.* 14th ed. New York, NY: McGraw-Hill Education; 2017.
24. Nelson DA, Marks ES, Deuster PA, O'Connor FG, Kurina LM. Association of nonsteroidal anti-inflammatory drug prescriptions with kidney disease among active young and middle-aged adults. *JAMA Netw Open.* 2019;2(2):e187896.
25. Ong CK, Lirk P, Tan CH, Seymour RA. An evidence-based update on nonsteroidal anti-inflammatory drugs. *Clin Med Res.* 2007;5(1):19-34.
26. Pai AB. Keeping kidneys safe: the pharmacist's role in NSAID avoidance in high-risk patients. *J Am Pharm Assoc.* 2015;55(1):e15-23; quiz e24-15.
27. Pai AB, Divine H, Marciniak M, et al. Need for a judicious use of nonsteroidal anti-inflammatory drugs to avoid community-acquired acute kidney injury. *Ann Pharmacother.* 2019;53(1):95-100.
28. Raab CP. Reye syndrome (Reye's syndrome). Merck Manual Professional Version website. www.merckmanuals.com/professional/pediatrics/miscellaneous-disorders-in-infants-and-children/reye-syndrome?query=Reye%E2%80%99s%20Syndrome. Published 2019. Accessed August 29, 2019.
29. Reed GW, Abdallah MS, Shao M, et al. Effect of aspirin coadministration on the safety of celecoxib, naproxen, or ibuprofen. *J Am Coll Cardiol* 2018;71(16):1741.
30. Ruszniewski P, Soufflet C, Barthelemy P. Nonsteroidal anti-inflammatory drug use as a risk factor for gastro-oesophageal reflux disease: an observational study. *Aliment Pharmacol Ther.* 2008;28(9):1134-1139.
31. Schimmer BP, Funder JW. Adrenocorticotropic hormone, adrenal steroids, and the adrenal cortex. In: Brunton LL, Hilal-Dandan R, Knollmann BC, eds. *Goodman & Gilman's: The Pharmacological Basis of Therapeutics.* 13th ed. New York, NY: McGraw-Hill Education; 2017: 845-862.
32. Solomon DH. NSAIDs: Therapeutic use and variability of response in adults. Up-to-Date website. www-uptodate-com.libproxy.chapman.edu/contents/nsaids-therapeutic-use-and-variability-of-response-in-adults?search=antiinflammatory%20medications&source=search_result&selectedTitle=1~150&usage_type=default&display_rank=1. Published 2019. Accessed July 21, 2019.
33. Stringer JL. *Basic Concepts in Pharmacology: What You Need to Know for Each Drug Class.* 5th ed. New York, NY: McGraw-Hill Education; 2017.
34. Stringer JL. *Basic Concepts in Pharmacology: What You Need to Know for Each Drug Class.* 5th ed. New York, NY: McGraw-Hill Education; 2017.
35. Addison disease. MedlinePlus website. https://medlineplus.gov/addisondisease.html. Published 2019. Accessed November 5, 2019.
36. Wongrakpanich S, Wongrakpanich A, Melhado K, Rangaswami J. A comprehensive review of non-steroidal anti-inflammatory drug use in the elderly. *Aging Dis.* 2018;9(1):143-150.
37. World Health Organization. *WHO Model List of Essential Medicines.* 20th ed. www.who.int/medicines/publications/essentialmedicines/en. Published 2017. Accessed November 26, 2018.

Chapter 10

1. Bartlett JG. Clinical practice. Antibiotic-associated diarrhea. *N Engl J Med.* 2002;346(5):334-339.
2. Batchelder N, So TY. Transitioning antimicrobials from intravenous to oral in pediatric acute uncomplicated osteomyelitis. *World J Clin Pediatr.* 2016;5(3):244-250.
3. Beauduy CE, Winston LG. Beta-lactam and other cell wall- and membrane-active antibiotics. In: Katzung BG, ed. *Basic & Clinical Pharmacology.* 14th ed. New York, NY: McGraw-Hill Education; 2017:795-814.
4. Bush LM. Overview of bacteria. Merck Manual Consumer Version website. www.merckmanuals.com/home/infections/bacterial-infections-overview/overview-of-bacteria. Published 2018. Accessed July 14, 2019.
5. Bush LM, Vazquez-Pertejo MT. Staphylococcal infections. Merck Manual Professional Version website. www.merckmanuals.com/professional/infectious-diseases/gram-positive-cocci/staphylococcal-infections?query=MRSA. Updated June 2019. Accessed August 20, 2019.
6. Amoxicillin. Drugs.com. www.drugs.com/ppa/amoxicillin.html. Published 2019. Accessed July 24, 2019.
7. Macrolide derivatives. Drugs.com. www.drugs.com/drug-class/macrolide-derivatives.html. Published 2019. Accessed July 24, 2019.
8. Tetracycline (systemic). Drugs.com. www.drugs.com/ppa/tetracycline-systemic.html. Published 2019. Accessed July 24, 2019.
9. Using antibiotics responsibly: Factsheet for experts. European Centre for Disease Prevention and Control website. http://ecdc.europa.eu/en/eaad/antibiotics/

Pages/factsExperts.aspx. Published 2014. Accessed July 11, 2019.

10. Falagas ME, Bliziotis IA. Fundamentals of antibiotics. In: McKean SC, Ross JJ, Dressler DD, Scheurer DB, eds. *Principles and Practice of Hospital Medicine.* 2nd ed. New York, NY: McGraw-Hill Education; 2016:1489-1497.
11. Barbut F, Maynard JL. Managing antibiotic associated diarrhoea: probiotics may help in prevention. *BMJ.* 2002;324(7350):1345.
12. Kapoor G, Saigal S, Elongavan A. Action and resistance mechanisms of antibiotics: A guide for clinicians. *J Anaesthesiol Clin Pharmacol.* 2017;33(3):300-305.
13. Hansen MP, Scott AM, McCullough A, et al. Adverse events in people taking macrolide antibiotics versus placebo for any indication. *Cochrane Database Syst Rev.* 2019;1(1):CD011825.
14. Antibiotic-associated diarrhea. Harvard Health Publishing website. www.health.harvard.edu/a_to_z/antibiotic-associated-diarrhea-a-to-z. Published February 2019. Accessed July 19, 2019.
15. Hooper DC, Shenoy ES, Varughese CA. Treatment and prophylaxis of bacterial infections. In: Jameson JL, Fauci AS, Kasper DL, Hauser SL, Longo DL, Loscalzo J, eds. *Harrison's Principles of Internal Medicine.* 20th ed. New York, NY: McGraw-Hill Education; 2018.
16. Kardas P. Comparison of patient compliance with once-daily and twice-daily antibiotic regimens in respiratory tract infections: results of a randomized trial. *J Antimicrob Chemother.* 2007;59(3):531-536.
17. Katzung BG. Chemotherapeutic drugs: Introduction. In: Katzung BG, ed. *Basic & Clinical Pharmacology.* 14th ed. New York, NY: McGraw-Hill Education; 2017:793-794.
18. Leekha S, Terrell CL, Edson RS. General principles of antimicrobial therapy. *Mayo Clin Proc.* 2011;86(2):156-167.
19. Letourneau AR. Beta-lactam antibiotics: Mechanisms of action and resistance and adverse effects. Up-to-Date website. www-uptodate-com.libproxy.chapman.edu/contents/beta-lactam-antibiotics-mechanisms-of-action-and-resistance-and-adverse-effects?search=antibiotics&source=search_result&selectedTitle=2~150&usage_type=default&display_rank=2. Published 2019. Accessed July 11, 2019.
20. Lewis T, Cook J. Fluoroquinolones and tendinopathy: a guide for athletes and sports clinicians and a systematic review of the literature. *J Athl Train.* 2014;49(3):422-427.
21. Morales DR, Slattery J, Pacurariu A, Pinheiro L, McGettigan P, Kurz X. Relative and absolute risk of tendon rupture with fluoroquinolone and concomitant fluoroquinolone/corticosteroid therapy: population-based nested case-control study. *Clin Drug Investig.* 2019;39(2):205-213.
22. Uses: Antibiotics. National Health Service website. www.nhs.uk/conditions/antibiotics/uses. Published 2019. Accessed July 11, 2019.
23. Pichichero ME. A review of evidence supporting the American Academy of Pediatrics recommendation for prescribing cephalosporin antibiotics for penicillin-allergic patients. *Pediatrics.* 2005;115(4):1048-1057.
24. Ross J. Is the "full course of antibiotics" full of baloney? Harvard Health Publishing website. www.health.harvard.edu/blog/is-the-full-course-of-antibiotics-full-of-baloney-2017081712253. Published August 17, 2017. Accessed July 18, 2019.
25. Sanchez GV, Fleming-Dutra KE, Roberts RM, Hicks LA. Core elements of outpatient antibiotic stewardship. *MMWR Recomm Rep.* 2016;65(No. RR-6):1-12.
26. Shybut T, Puckett E. Triceps ruptures after fluoroquinolone antibiotics: a report of 2 cases. *Sports Health.* 2017;9(5):474-476.
27. Shybut TB, Puckett ER. Triceps ruptures after fluoroquinolone antibiotics: a report of 2 cases. *Sports Health.* 2017;9(5):474-476.
28. Sutton SS, Bland CM. Antimicrobial principles. In: Sutton SS, ed. *McGraw-Hill's NAPLEX Review Guide.* 3rd ed. New York, NY: McGraw-Hill Education; 2018:184-196.
29. Tanne JH. FDA adds "black box" warning label to fluoroquinolone antibiotics. *BMJ.* 2008;337:a816.
30. Werth BJ. Overview of antibacterial drugs. Merck Manual Professional Version website. www.merckmanuals.com/professional/infectious-diseases/bacteria-and-antibacterial-drugs/overview-of-antibacterial-drugs?query=antibiotics. Published 2018. Accessed July 10, 2019.
31. Woodford N, Livermore DM. Infections caused by Gram-positive bacteria: a review of the global challenge. *J Infect.* 2009;59(Suppl 1):S4-16.
32. WHO model list of essential medicines, 2017. World Health Organization website. www.who.int/medicines/publications/essentialmedicines/en. Published 2017. Accessed November 26, 2018.

Chapter 11

1. COVID-19 and vascular disease. *EBioMedicine.* 2020;58:102966-102966.
2. Beasley MB, Travis WD. The respiratory system. In: Strayer DS, Rubin E, Saffitz JE, Schiller AL, eds. *Rubin's Pathology: Clinicopathologic Foundations of Medicine.* 7th ed. Philadelphia, PA: Wolters Kluwer Health; 2014: 679-750.
3. Bousquet J. Global initiative for asthma (GINA) and its objectives. *Clin Exp Allergy.* 2000;30 Suppl 1:2-5.
4. Bush LM. Streptococcal infections. Merck Manual Professional Version website. www.merckmanuals.com/professional/infectious-diseases/gram-positive-cocci/streptococcal-infections. Updated June 2019. Accessed September 1, 2019.
5. Camargo JCA, Rachelefsky G, Schatz M. Managing asthma exacerbations in the emergency department: summary of the National Asthma Education and Prevention Program expert panel. Report 3 guidelines for the management of asthma Exacerbations. *J Emerg Med.* 2009;37(2):S6-S17.

6. CDC on asthma control. Center for Disease Control and Prevention website. www.cdc.gov/asthma/default.htm. Published 2018. Accessed September 1, 2019.
7. CDC on flu treatment. Centers for Disease Control and Prevention website. www.cdc.gov/flu/index.htm. Published 2019. Accessed September 1, 2019.
8. Common cold and runny nose. Centers for Disease Control and Prevention website. www.cdc.gov/antibiotic-use/community/for-patients/common-illnesses/colds.html. Published 2019. Accessed September 1, 2019.
9. Symptoms of coronavirus. Centers for Disease Control and Prevention website. www.cdc.gov/coronavirus/2019-ncov/symptoms-testing/symptoms.html. Published 2020. Accessed November 5, 2020.
10. Cleary MA, Flanagan KW. *Acute and Emergency Care in Athletic Training*. Champaign, IL: Human Kinetics; 2020.
11. Cloutier MM, Baptist AP, Blake KV, et al. *2020 Focused Updates to the Asthma Management Guidelines: Clinician's Guide*. www.nhlbi.nih.gov/health-topics/all-publications-and-resources/clinician-guide-2020-focused-updates-asthma-management-guidelines. Published December 2020. Accessed March 5, 2021.
12. Delves PJ. Overview of allergic and atopic disorders. Merck Manual Professional Version website. www.merckmanuals.com/en-pr/professional/immunology-allergic-disorders/allergic,-autoimmune,-and-other-hypersensitivity-disorders/overview-of-allergic-and-atopic-disorders?query=Overview%20of%20Allergic%20and%20Atopic%20Disorders. Published 2018. Updated October 2020.
13. Diamond MS, Pierson TC. The challenges of vaccine development against a new virus during a pandemic. *Cell Host Microbe*. 2020;27(5):699-703.
14. Ebell MH, Call M, Shinholser J. Effectiveness of oseltamivir in adults: a meta-analysis of published and unpublished clinical trials. *Fam Pract*. 2013;30(2):125-133.
15. Fried MP. Sore throat. Merck Manual Professional Version website. www.merckmanuals.com/professional/ear,-nose,-and-throat-disorders/approach-to-the-patient-with-nasal-and-pharyngeal-symptoms/sore-throat?query=Strep%20Throat. Published 2018. Accessed September 1, 2019.
16. Fried MP. Sinusitis. Merck Manual Professional Version website. www.merckmanuals.com/professional/ear,-nose,-and-throat-disorders/nose-and-paranasal-sinus-disorders/sinusitis?query=sinusitis. Published 2019. Accessed September 1, 2019.
17. 2020 GINA Report, Global Strategy for Asthma Management and Prevention. Global Institute for Asthma website. https://ginasthma.org/gina-reports. Published 2020. Accessed March 5, 2021.
18. Hodder R, Lougheed MD, Rowe BH, FitzGerald JM, Kaplan AG, McIvor RA. Management of acute asthma in adults in the emergency department: nonventilatory management. *CMAJ*. 2010;182(2):E55-E67.
19. Katzung BG. Histamine, serotonin, & the ergot alkaloids. In: Katzung BG, ed. *Basic & Clinical Pharmacology*. 14th ed. New York, NY: McGraw-Hill Education; 2017.
20. Lougheed MD, Garvey N, Chapman KR, et al. Variations and gaps in management of acute asthma in Ontario emergency departments. *Chest*. 2009;135(3):724-736.
21. Miller MG, Weiler JM, Baker R, Collins J, D'Alonzo G. National Athletic Trainers' Association position statement: management of asthma in athletes. *J Athl Train*. 2005;40(3):224-245.
22. National Heart Lung and Blood Institute. *Expert Panel Report 3: Guidelines for the Diagnosis and Management of Asthma*. www.nhlbi.nih.gov/sites/default/files/media/docs/asthgdln_1.pdf. Published August 28, 2007. Accessed September 1, 2019.
23. National Heart Lung and Blood Institute. *Monitoring Your Asthma*. www.nhlbi.nih.gov/health-topics/all-publications-and-resources/lmbb-monitoring-your-asthma. Published March 2020. Accessed March 5, 2021.
24. Ortega VE. Asthma. Merck Manual Professional Version website. www.merckmanuals.com/professional/pulmonary-disorders/asthma-and-related-disorders/asthma?query=asthma. Updated July 2019. Accessed September 2, 2019.
25. Ortega VE, Genese F. Treatment of acute asthma exacerbations. Merck Manual Professional Version website. www.merckmanuals.com/professional/pulmonary-disorders/asthma-and-related-disorders/treatment-of-acute-asthma-exacerbations. Updated July 2019. Accessed September 2, 2019.
26. Sethi S. Community-acquired pneumonia. Merck Manual Professional Version website. www.merckmanuals.com/professional/pulmonary-disorders/pneumonia/community-acquired-pneumonia. Published 2019. Accessed August 31, 2010.
27. Sharkey KA, MacNaughton WK. Gastrointestinal motility and water flux, emesis, and biliary and pancreatic disease. In: Brunton LL, Hilal-Dandan R, Knollmann BC, eds. *Goodman & Gilman's: The Pharmacological Basis of Therapeutics*. 13th ed. New York, NY: McGraw-Hill Education; 2017:921-944.
28. Tesini BL. Common cold. Merck Manual Professional Version website. www.merckmanuals.com/professional/infectious-diseases/respiratory-viruses/common-cold. Published 2018. Accessed September 1, 2019.
29. Tesini BL. Influenza. Merck Manual Professional Version website. www.merckmanuals.com/professional/infectious-diseases/respiratory-viruses/influenza. Published 2018. Accessed August 31, 2019.
30. Tesini BL. Overview of viral respiratory infections. Merck Manual Professional Version website. www.merckmanuals.com/professional/infectious-diseases/respiratory-viruses/overview-of-viral-respiratory-infections?query=upper%20respiratory%20infection. Published 2018. Accessed August 31, 2019.
31. Tesini BL. Coronaviruses and acute respiratory syndromes (COVID-19, MERS, and SARS). Merck Manual

Professional Version website. www.merckmanuals.com/professional/infectious-diseases/respiratory-viruses/coronaviruses-and-acute-respiratory-syndromes-covid-19-mers-and-sars#v47572290. Published 2020. Accessed November 5, 2020.

32. Tamiflu (oseltamivir phosphate) information. US Food and Drug Administration website. www.fda.gov/drugs/postmarket-drug-safety-information-patients-and-providers/tamiflu-oseltamivir-phosphate-information. Published 2018. Accessed October 3, 2019.

33. FDA requires Boxed Warning about serious mental health side effects for asthma and allergy drug montelukast (Singulair); advises restricting use for allergic rhinitis. US Food and Drug Administration website. www.fda.gov/drugs/drug-safety-and-availability/fda-requires-boxed-warning-about-serious-mental-health-side-effects-asthma-and-allergy-drug#:~:text=FDA%20is%20requiring%20a%20Boxed%20Warning%20stating%20that%20serious%20neuropsychiatric,patients%20taking%20montelukast%20(Singulair). Updated March 13, 2020. Accessed March 5, 2021.

34. Asthma treatment. webMD website. www.webmd.com/asthma/asthma-treatments#1. Published 2019. Accessed October 3, 2019.

35. Coronavirus disease (COVID-19). World Health Organization website. www.who.int/emergencies/diseases/novel-coronavirus-2019/question-and-answers-hub/q-a-detail/q-a-coronaviruses. Published October 12, 2020. Accessed November 5, 2020.

Chapter 12

1. Altman L. No trace of heart medications in Gathers, autopsy indicates. *NY Times*. March 16, 1990:B9. www.nytimes.com/1990/03/16/sports/no-trace-of-heart-medication-in-gathers-autopsy-indicates.html.

2. Antithrombotic therapy. American Society of Hematology website. www.hematology.org/about/history/50-years/antithrombotic-therapy#:~:text=There%20are%20two%20classes%20of,clots%20from%20forming%20and%20growing. Published December 2008. Accessed November 30, 2020.

3. Bakris GL. Hypertensive emergencies. Merck Manual Professional Version website. www.merckmanuals.com/professional/cardiovascular-disorders/hypertension/hypertensive-emergencies?query=hypertensive%20disorders. Published 2018. Accessed September 4, 2019.

4. Benham MD, Fannell MW. Cardiac emergencies. In: Stone CK, Humphries RL, eds. *Current Diagnosis & Treatment: Emergency Medicine*. 8th ed. New York, NY: McGraw-Hill Education; 2017.

5. Bittl JA, Baber U, Bradley SM, Wijeysundera DN. Duration of dual antiplatelet therapy: a systematic review for the 2016 ACC/AHA guideline focused update on duration of dual antiplatelet therapy in patients with coronary artery disease: a report of the American College of Cardiology/American Heart Association task force on clinical practice guidelines. *Circulation*. 2016;134(10):e156-178.

6. Do your statins and grapefruit juice safely mix? Cleveland Clinic website. https://health.clevelandclinic.org/statins-grapefruit-safely-mix. Published 2016. Accessed September 10, 2019.

7. Amiodarone. Drugs.com. www.drugs.com/amiodarone.html. Published 2019. Accessed September 9, 2019.

8. Eschenhagen T. Treatment of ischemic heart disease. In: Brunton LL, Hilal-Dandan R, Knollmann BC, eds. *Goodman & Gilman's: The Pharmacological Basis of Therapeutics*. 13th ed. New York, NY: McGraw-Hill Education; 2017:489-506.

9. Eschenhagen T. Treatment of hypertension. In: Brunton LL, Hilal-Dandan R, Knollmann BC, eds. *Goodman & Gilman's: The Pharmacological Basis of Therapeutics*. 13th ed. New York, NY: McGraw-Hill Education; 2017:507-526.

10. Florek J, Girzadas D. Amiodarone. *StatPearls*. www.ncbi.nlm.nih.gov/books/NBK482154/. Published 2018. Accessed September 10, 2019.

11. Grapefruit juice and some drugs don't mix. U.S. Food and Drug Administration website. www.fda.gov/consumers/consumer-updates/grapefruit-juice-and-some-drugs-dont-mix. Updated July 18, 2017. Accessed September 10, 2019.

12. Gurgle HE, Blumenthal DK. Drug therapy for dyslipidemias. In: Brunton LL, Hilal-Dandan R, Knollmann BC, eds. *Goodman & Gilman's: The Pharmacological Basis of Therapeutics*. 13th ed. New York, NY: McGraw-Hill Education; 2017:605-618.

13. Harter K, Levine M, Henderson SO. Anticoagulation drug therapy: a review. *West J Emerg Med*. 2015;16(1):11-17.

14. Grapefruit juice and statins. Harvard Health Publishing website. www.health.harvard.edu/heart-health/grapefruit-juice-and-statins. Published April 2015. Accessed September 10, 2019.

15. Hilal-Dandan R. Renin and angiotensin. In: Brunton LL, Hilal-Dandan R, Knollmann BC, eds. *Goodman & Gilman's: The Pharmacological Basis of Therapeutics*. 13th ed. New York, NY: McGraw-Hill Education; 2017:471-488.

16. Hogg K, Weitz JI. Blood coagulation and anticoagulant, fibrinolytic, and antiplatelet drugs. In: Brunton LL, Hilal-Dandan R, Knollmann BC, eds. *Goodman & Gilman's: The Pharmacological Basis of Therapeutics*. 13th ed. New York, NY: McGraw-Hill Education; 2017:585-604.

17. Knollmann BC, Roden DM. Antiarrhythmic drugs. In: Brunton LL, Hilal-Dandan R, Knollmann BC, eds. *Goodman & Gilman's: The Pharmacological Basis of Therapeutics*. 13th ed. New York, NY: McGraw-Hill Education; 2017:547-572.

18. Levine GN, Bates ER, Bittl JA, et al. 2016 ACC/AHA guideline focused update on duration of dual antiplatelet therapy in patients with coronary artery disease: a report of the American College of Cardiology/American Heart Association task force on clinical practice guidelines. *Circulation*. 2016;134(10):e123-155.

19. Amiodarone (oral route). Mayo Clinic website. www.mayoclinic.org/drugs-supplements/amiodarone-oral-route/proper-use/drg-20061854. Published 2019. Accessed September 9, 2019.

20. Mitchell LB. Overview of arrhythmias. Merck Manual Professional Version website. www.merckmanuals.com/professional/cardiovascular-disorders/arrhythmias-and-conduction-disorders/overview-of-arrhythmias?query=Arrhythmias#v936653. Updated July 2019. Accessed September 4, 2019.

21. Arrhythmia. National Heart Lung and Blood Institute website. www.nhlbi.nih.gov/health-topics/arrhythmia. Published 2019. Accessed September 4, 2019.

22. Simon AM. Chest pain. In: Tintinalli JE, Stapczynski JS, Ma OJ, Yealy DM, Meckler GD, Cline DM, eds. *Tintinalli's Emergency Medicine: A Comprehensive Study Guide*. 8th ed. New York, NY: McGraw-Hill Education; 2016.

23. Simons J. The $10 Billion Pill. Hold the fries, please. Lipitor, the cholesterol-lowering drug, has become the bestselling pharmaceutical in history. Here's how Pfizer did it. *Fortune Magazine*. January 20, 2003. https://archive.fortune.com/magazines/fortune/fortune_archive/2003/01/20/335643/index.htm. Accessed September 4, 2019.

24. Sweis RN, Jivan A. Overview of acute coronary syndromes (ACS). Merck Manual Professional Version website. www.merckmanuals.com/professional/cardiovascular-disorders/coronary-artery-disease/overview-of-acute-coronary-syndromes-acs. Published 2018. Accessed September 4, 2019.

25. Sweis RN, Jivan A. Drugs for acute coronary syndromes. Merck Manual Professional Version website. www.merckmanuals.com/professional/cardiovascular-disorders/coronary-artery-disease/drugs-for-acute-coronary-syndromes. Published 2018. Accessed September 4, 2019.

26. Thanassoulis G, Afshar M. Atherosclerosis. Merck Manual Professional Version website. www.merckmanuals.com/professional/cardiovascular-disorders/arteriosclerosis/atherosclerosis?query=Atherosclerosis#v933891. Updated July 2019. Accessed September 5, 2019.

27. Thompson AD. Chest pain. Merck Manual Professional Version website. www.merckmanuals.com/professional/cardiovascular-disorders/symptoms-of-cardiovascular-disorders/chest-pain?query=chest%20pain. Published 2018. Accessed September 4, 2019.

28. Gathers died of diseased, scarred heart, autopsy shows. *United Press International*. March 15, 1990. www.upi.com/Archives/1990/03/15/Gathers-died-of-diseased-scarred-heart-autopsy-shows/6570637477200. Accessed August 30, 2019.

Chapter 13

1. American Diabetes Association. ADA position statement: Classification and diagnosis of diabetes, sec 2. In standards of medical care in diabetes. *Diabetes Care*. 2018;41(Supplement 1):S13-S27.

2. American Diabetes Association. ADA position statement: pharmacologic approaches to glycemic treatment. sec. 8. In standards of medical care in diabetes-2018. *Diabetes Care*. 2018;41(Supplement 1):S73-S85.

3. American Diabetes Association. *Low blood glucose (hypoglycemia)*. https://professional.diabetes.org/sites/professional.diabetes.org/files/pel/source/sci-advisor_2018_low_blood_glucose_hypoglycemia-newb-final.pdf. Published 2018. Accessed September 12, 2019.

4. Blood sugar and exercise. American Diabetes Association website. www.diabetes.org/fitness/get-and-stay-fit/getting-started-safely/blood-glucose-and-exercise. Published 2019. Accessed October 7, 2019.

5. Brutsaert EF. Diabetes mellitus (DM). Merck Manual Professional Version website. www.merckmanuals.com/home/hormonal-and-metabolic-disorders/diabetes-mellitus-dm-and-disorders-of-blood-sugar-metabolism/diabetes-mellitus-dm. Published 2019. Accessed September 11, 2019.

6. Brutsaert EF. Drug treatment of diabetes mellitus. Merck Manual Professional Version website. www.merckmanuals.com/professional/endocrine-and-metabolic-disorders/diabetes-mellitus-and-disorders-of-carbohydrate-metabolism/drug-treatment-of-diabetes-mellitus#v29299467. Published 2019. Accessed September 11, 2019.

7. Cleary MA, Flanagan KW. *Acute and Emergency Care in Athletic Training*. Champaign, IL: Human Kinetics; 2020.

8. Colberg SR, Sigal RJ, Fernhall B, et al. Exercise and type 2 diabetes. The American College of Sports Medicine and the American Diabetes Association: joint position statement. *Diabetes Care*. 2010;33(12):e147-e167.

9. Colberg SR, Albright AL, Blissmer BJ, et al. Exercise and type 2 diabetes: American College of Sports Medicine and the American Diabetes Association: joint position statement. Exercise and type 2 diabetes. *Med Sci Sports Exerc*. 2010;42(12):2282-2303.

10. Colberg SR, Sigal RJ, Fernhall B, et al. Exercise and type 2 diabetes: the American College of Sports Medicine and the American Diabetes Association: joint position statement executive summary. *Diabetes Care*. 2010;33(12):2692-2696.

11. Drug interactions between ciprofloxacin and Lantus. Drugs.com website. www.drugs.com/drug-interactions/ciprofloxacin-with-lantus-672-0-1344-803.html. Published 2019. Accessed May 25, 2021.

12. Jardiance. Drugs.com website. www.drugs.com/pro/jardiance.html. Published 2019. Accessed October 4, 2019.

13. Trulicity. Drugs.com website. www.drugs.com/pro/trulicity.html#s-34090-1. Published 2019. Accessed October 7, 2019.

14. Dungan K, DeSantis A. Glucagon-like peptide-1 receptor agonists for the treatment of type 2 diabetes mellitus. Up to Date website. www.uptodate.com/contents/glucagon-like-peptide-1-receptor-agonists-for-the-treatment-of-type-2-diabetes-mellitus. Published 2019. Accessed October 7, 2019.

15. Farrell PA. Diabetes, exercise and competitive sports. *Sports Science Exchange 90*. 2003;16(3). www.gssiweb.org/sports-science-exchange/article/sse-90-diabetes-exercise-and-competitive-sports#articleTopic_7. Accessed September 12, 2019.

16. Gabbay R, Wagner N, Kahn P. Expanding glucagon access and use in the prehospital setting. Journal of Emergency Medical Services website. www.jems.com/2018/08/17/expanding-glucagon-access-and-use-in-the-prehospital-setting. 2018. Accessed September 12, 2019.

17. Ghosh S, Collier A. Management of diabetes. In: Ghosh S, Collier A, eds. *Churchill's Pocketbook of Diabetes*. 2nd ed. Oxford: Churchill Livingstone; 2012:83-125.

18. Jimenez CC, Corcoran MH, Crawley JT, et al. National Athletic Trainers' Association position statement: management of the athlete with type 1 diabetes mellitus. *J Athl Train*. 2007;42(4):536-545.

19. Kennedy MSN, Masharani U. Pancreatic hormones and antidiabetic drugs. In: Katzung BG, ed. *Basic & Clinical Pharmacology*. 14th ed. New York, NY: McGraw-Hill Education; 2017;747-771.

20. Lisle DK, Trojian TH. Managing the athlete with type 1 diabetes. *Curr Sports Med Rep*. 2006;5(2):93-98.

21. 15/15 rule. MedlinePlus website. https://medlineplus.gov/ency/imagepages/19815.htm. Published 2018. Accessed December 30, 2019.

22. How to give an emergency glucagon injection to treat low blood sugar. Memorial Sloan Kettering Cancer Center website. www.mskcc.org/cancer-care/patient-education/glucagon-emergency-kit-low-blood-sugar-glucagon-injection#. Updated December 15, 2016. Accessed September 12, 2019.

23. Nathan DM. The diabetes control and complications trial/epidemiology of diabetes interventions and complications study at 30 years: overview. *Diabetes Care*. 2014;37(1):9-16.

24. Nathan DM. Diabetes: advances in diagnosis and treatment. *JAMA*. 2015;314(10):1052-1062.

25. Orchard TJ, Nathan DM, Zinman B, et al. Association between 7 years of intensive treatment of type 1 diabetes and long-term mortality. *JAMA*. 2015;313(1):45-53.

26. Perkins BA, Riddell MC. Type 1 diabetes and exercise: using the insulin pump to maximum advantage. *Can J Diabetes*. 2006;30(1):72-79.

27. Peters AL, Ahmann AJ, Battelino T, et al. Clinical practice guideline. Diabetes technology—continuous subcutaneous insulin infusion therapy and continuous glucose monitoring in adults: an endocrine society clinical practice guideline. *J Clin Endocrinol Metab*. 2016(11):3922.

28. Porth CM, Gaspard KJ. Diabetes mellitus and the metabolic syndrome. In: Porth CM, Gaspard KJ, eds. *Essentials of Pathophysiology: Concepts of Altered Health States*. 4th ed. Philadelphia, PA: Wolters Kluwer; 2015.

29. Powers AC, D'Alessio D. Endocrine pancreas and pharmacotherapy of diabetes mellitus and hypoglycemia. In: Brunton LL, Hilal-Dandan R, Knollmann BC, eds. *Goodman & Gilman's: The Pharmacological Basis of Therapeutics*. 13th ed. New York, NY: McGraw-Hill Education; 2017;863-886.

30. Selected antidiabetic agents/selected quinolones interactions. WebMD website. www.webmd.com/drugs/2/drug-13818/humalog-u-100-insulin-subcutaneous/details/list-interaction-details/dmid-1442/dmtitle-selected-antidiabetic-agents-selected-quinolones/intrtype-drug. Published 2018. Accessed October 3, 2019.

31. Diabetes. World Health Organization website. www.who.int/health-topics/diabetes. Published 2019. Accessed September 11, 2019.

Chapter 14

1. Pedialyte website. https://pedialyte.com. Published 2019. Accessed August 31, 2019.

2. Ansari P. Acute abdominal pain. Merck Manual Professional Version website. www.merckmanuals.com/professional/gastrointestinal-disorders/acute-abdomen-and-surgical-gastroenterology/acute-abdominal-pain. Published 2018. Accessed August 29, 2019.

3. Bartlett JG. Clinical practice. Antibiotic-associated diarrhea. *N Engl J Med*. 2002;346(5):334-339.

4. Boyce TG. Gastroenteritis. Merck Manual Professional Version website. www.merckmanuals.com/professional/gastrointestinal-disorders/gastroenteritis/gastroenteritis. Updated June 2019. Accessed August 29, 2019.

5. Burns C. Surgery for appendicitis? Antibiotics alone may be enough. Harvard Health website. www.health.harvard.edu/blog/surgery-for-appendicitis-antibiotics-alone-may-be-enough-2019010915692. Published January 9, 2019. Accessed September 1, 2019.

6. Centers for Disease Control and Prevention. Food poisoning symptoms. www.cdc.gov/foodsafety/symptoms.html. Published 2019. Accessed September 3, 2019.

7. Chey WD, Wong BC. American College of Gastroenterology guideline on the management of *Helicobacter pylori* infection. *Am J Gastrointerol*. 2007;102(8):1808-1825.

8. Cleary MA, Flanagan KW. *Acute and Emergency Care in Athletic Training*. Champaign, IL: Human Kinetics; 2020.

9. Corbett SW, Stack LB, Knoop KJ. Chest and abdomen. In: Knoop KJ, Stack LB, Storrow AB, Thurman RJ, eds. *The Atlas of Emergency Medicine*. 4th ed. New York, NY: McGraw-Hill Education; 2016;165-179.

10. Fiorini G, Zullo A, Vakil N, et al. Rifabutin triple therapy is effective in patients with multidrug-resistant strains of *Helicobacter pylori*. *J Clin Gastroenterol*. 2018;52(2):137.

11. Ford AC, Gurusamy KS, Delaney B, Forman D, Moayyedi P. Eradication therapy for peptic ulcer disease in *Helicobacter pylori*-positive people. *Cochrane Database Syst Rev*. 2016;4(4):CD003840.

12. Barbut F, Meynard JL. Managing antibiotic associated diarrhoea: probiotics may help in prevention. *BMJ*. 2002;324(7350):1345-1346.

13. Furyk JS, Meek RA, Egerton-Warburton D. Drugs for the treatment of nausea and vomiting in adults in the emergency department setting. *Cochrane Database Syst Rev.* 2015(9):CD010106.
14. Gisbert JP, Khorrami S, Carballo F, Calvet X, Gené E, Dominguez-Muñoz E. *H. pylori* eradication therapy vs. antisecretory non-eradication therapy (with or without long-term maintenance antisecretory therapy) for the prevention of recurrent bleeding from peptic ulcer. *Cochrane Database Syst Rev.* 2004;(2):CD004062.
15. Gordon DC. Acute abdominal pain. In: Sherman SC, Weber JM, Schindlbeck MA, Patwari RG, eds. *Clinical Emergency Medicine.* New York, NY: McGraw-Hill Education; 2014;112-117.
16. Greenberger NJ. Constipation. Merck Manual Professional Version website. www.merckmanuals.com/professional/gastrointestinal-disorders/symptoms-of-gi-disorders/constipation?query=constipation. Published 2018. Accessed August 29, 2019.
17. Greenberger NJ. Diarrhea. Merck Manual Professional Version website. www.merckmanuals.com/professional/gastrointestinal-disorders/symptoms-of-gi-disorders/diarrhea?query=diarrhea. Published 2018. Accessed August 29, 2019.
18. Greenberger NJ. Nausea and vomiting. Merck Manual Professional Version website. www.merckmanuals.com/professional/gastrointestinal-disorders/symptoms-of-gi-disorders/nausea-and-vomiting. Published 2018. Accessed August 29, 2019.
19. Hang BS, Bork S, Ditkoff J, Long B, Koyfman A. Nausea and vomiting. In: Tintinalli JE, Stapczynski JS, Ma OJ, Yealy DM, Meckler GD, Cline DM, eds. *Tintinalli's Emergency Medicine: A Comprehensive Study Guide.* 8th ed. New York, NY: McGraw-Hill Education; 2016.
20. Lacy BE, Hussain ZH, Mearin F. Treatment for constipation: New and old pharmacological strategies. *Neurogastroenterol Motil.* 2014;26(6):749-763.
21. Lacy BE, Mearin F, Chang L, et al. Bowel disorders. *Gastroenterology.* 2016;150(6):1393-1407.
22. The CODA Collaborative. A randomized trial comparing antibiotics with appendectomy for appendicitis. *N Engl J Med.* 2020;383:1907-1919.
23. Lynch K. Gastroesophageal reflux disease (GERD). Merck Manual Professional Version website. www.merckmanuals.com/professional/gastrointestinal-disorders/esophageal-and-swallowing-disorders/gastroesophageal-reflux-disease-gerd. Published 2019. Accessed August 29, 2019.
24. Moleski SM. Evaluation of the GI patient. Merck Manual Professional Version website. www.merckmanuals.com/professional/gastrointestinal-disorders/approach-to-the-gi-patient/evaluation-of-the-gi-patient. Published 2017. Accessed August 29, 2019.
25. Acid reflux (GER & GERD) in adults. National Institute of Diabetes and Digestive and Kidney Diseases website. www.niddk.nih.gov/health-information/digestive-diseases/acid-reflux-ger-gerd-adults. Published 2019. Accessed August 31, 2019.
26. Ogawa R, Echizen H. Clinically significant drug interactions with antacids: an update. *Drugs.* 2011;71(14):1839-1864.
27. Olsen KM, McCaleb RV. Evaluation of the gastrointestinal tract. In: DiPiro JT, Yee GC, Posey LM, Haines ST, Nolin TD, Ellingrod V, eds. *Pharmacotherapy: A Pathophysiologic Approach.* 11th ed. New York, NY: McGraw-Hill Education; 2020;461-462.
28. Poon SHT, Lee JWY, Man KNG, et al. The current management of acute uncomplicated appendicitis: should there be a change in paradigm? A systematic review of the literatures and analysis of treatment performance. *World J Emerg Surg.* 2017;12:46.
29. Sharkey KA, MacNaughton WK. Pharmacotherapy for gastric acidity, peptic ulcers, and gastroesophageal reflux disease. In: Brunton LL, Hilal-Dandan R, Knollmann BC, eds. *Goodman & Gilman's: The Pharmacological Basis of Therapeutics.* 13th ed. New York, NY: McGraw-Hill Education; 2017;909-920.
30. Sharkey KA, MacNaughton WK. Gastrointestinal motility and water flux, emesis, and biliary and pancreatic disease. In: Brunton LL, Hilal-Dandan R, Knollmann BC, eds. *Goodman & Gilman's: The Pharmacological Basis of Therapeutics.* 13th ed. New York, NY: McGraw-Hill Education; 2017;921-944.
31. Shelton KN, Clements JN. Naloxegol for managing opioid-induced constipation. *JAAPA.* 2017;30(9):51-53.
32. Uritsky TJ. Methylnaltrexone: peripherally acting micro-opioid receptor antagonist. *J Adv Pract Oncol.* 2019;10(1):62-67.
33. Vakil N. Drug treatment of gastric acidity. Merck Manual Professional Version website. www.merckmanuals.com/professional/gastrointestinal-disorders/gastritis-and-peptic-ulcer-disease/drug-treatment-of-gastric-acidity. Published 2018. Accessed August 29, 2019.
34. Vakil N. Overview of gastritis. Merck Manual Professional Version website. www.merckmanuals.com/professional/gastrointestinal-disorders/gastritis-and-peptic-ulcer-disease/overview-of-gastritis. Published 2018. Accessed August 29, 2019.
35. Vakil N. Peptic ulcer disease. Merck Manual Professional Version website. www.merckmanuals.com/professional/gastrointestinal-disorders/gastritis-and-peptic-ulcer-disease/peptic-ulcer-disease. Published 2018. Accessed August 29, 2019.
36. Vakil N. *Helicobacter pylori* infection. Merck Manual Professional Version website. www.merckmanuals.com/professional/gastrointestinal-disorders/gastritis-and-peptic-ulcer-disease/helicobacter-pylori-infection#v892052. Published 2018. Accessed August 29, 2019.
37. Vakil N. Overview of acid secretion. Merck Manual Professional Version website. www.merckmanuals.com/professional/gastrointestinal-disorders/gastritis-and-peptic-ulcer-disease/overview-of-acid-secretion. Published 2018. Accessed August 29, 2019.
38. Walfish AE, Ching Companioni RA. Ulcerative colitis. Merck Manual Professional Version website. www.mer-

ckmanuals.com/professional/gastrointestinal-disorders/inflammatory-bowel-disease-ibd/ulcerative-colitis. Published 2019. Accessed August 29, 2019.

39. Walfish AE, Ching Companioni RA. Overview of inflammatory bowel disease. Merck Manual Professional Version website. www.merckmanuals.com/professional/gastrointestinal-disorders/inflammatory-bowel-disease-ibd/overview-of-inflammatory-bowel-disease. Published 2019. Accessed August 29, 2019.
40. Walfish AE, Ching Companioni RA. Drugs for inflammatory bowel disease. Merck Manual Professional Version website. www.merckmanuals.com/professional/gastrointestinal-disorders/inflammatory-bowel-disease-ibd/drugs-for-inflammatory-bowel-disease. Published 2019. Accessed August 29, 2019.
41. Wiley JW, Chang L. Functional bowel disorders. *Gastroenterology.* 2018;155(1):1-4.

Chapter 15

1. Berbari EF, Kanj SS, Kowalski TJ, et al. 2015 Infectious Diseases Society of America (IDSA) clinical practice guidelines for the diagnosis and treatment of native vertebral osteomyelitis in adults. *Clin Infect Dis.* 2015;61(6):e26-46.
2. Bernhardt DT. Concussion medication. MedScape website. https://emedicine.medscape.com/article/92095-medication. Updated September 24, 2018. Accessed October 15, 2019.
3. Biundo JJ. Bursitis. Merck Manual Professional Version website. www.merckmanuals.com/professional/musculoskeletal-and-connective-tissue-disorders/bursa,-muscle,-and-tendon-disorders/bursitis. Published 2018. Accessed October 5, 2019.
4. Biundo JJ. Fibromyalgia. Merck Manual Professional Version website. www.merckmanuals.com/professional/musculoskeletal-and-connective-tissue-disorders/bursa,-muscle,-and-tendon-disorders/fibromyalgia. Published 2018. Accessed October 4, 2019.
5. Biundo JJ. Tendinitis and tenosynovitis. Merck Manual Professional Version website. www.merckmanuals.com/professional/musculoskeletal-and-connective-tissue-disorders/bursa,-muscle,-and-tendon-disorders/tendinitis-and-tenosynovitis. Published 2018. Accessed October 5, 2019.
6. Bobacz K. Pharmacologic treatment of hand-, knee- and hip-osteoarthritis. *Wien Med Wochenschr.* 2013;163(9-10):236-242.
7. Chaparro LE, Furlan AD, Deshpande A, Mailis-Gagnon A, Atlas S, Turk DC. Opioids compared to placebo or other treatments for chronic low-back pain. *Cochrane Database Syst Rev.* 2013(8):CD004959.
8. Cohen H. Controversies and challenges in fibromyalgia: a review and a proposal. *Ther Adv Musculoskel Dis.* 2017;9:115-127.
9. Febuxostat. Drugs.com website. www.drugs.com/ppa/febuxostat.html. Published 2019. Accessed October 31, 2019.
10. Toradol. Drugs.com website. www.drugs.com/toradol.html. Published 2019. Accessed October 31, 2019.
11. Colchicine. Drugs.com website. www.drugs.com/ppa/colchicine.html. Updated July 8, 2020. Accessed March 5, 2021.
12. Edwards NL. Gout. Merck Manual Professional Version website. www.merckmanuals.com/professional/musculoskeletal-and-connective-tissue-disorders/crystal-induced-arthritides/gout. Published 2018. Accessed October 4, 2019.
13. Gaskell H, Moore RA, Derry S, Stannard C. Oxycodone for pain in fibromyalgia in adults. *Cochrane Database Syst Rev.* 2016;9(9):CD012329.
14. Gusho CA, Jenson M. Patient-reported outcomes of short-term intra-articular hyaluronic acid for osteoarthritis of the knee: a consecutive case series. *Cureus.* 2019;11(6):e4972.
15. Harvard Health Publications. Osteoarthritis. Drugs.com website. www.drugs.com/health-guide/osteoarthritis.html. Published 2019. Accessed October 31, 2019.
16. Hochberg MC, Altman RD, April KT, et al. American College of Rheumatology 2012 recommendations for the use of nonpharmacologic and pharmacologic therapies in osteoarthritis of the hand, hip, and knee. *Arthritis Care Res (Hoboken).* 2012;64(4):465-474.
17. Kirthi V, Derry S, Moore RA. Aspirin with or without an antiemetic for acute migraine headaches in adults. *Cochrane Database Syst Rev.* 2013;4:CD008041.
18. Koes BW, van Tulder M, Lin CW, Macedo LG, McAuley J, Maher C. An updated overview of clinical guidelines for the management of non-specific low back pain in primary care. *Eur Spine J.* 2010;19(12):2075-2094.
19. Kontzias A. Osteoarthritis (OA). Merck Manual Professional Version website. www.merckmanuals.com/professional/musculoskeletal-and-connective-tissue-disorders/joint-disorders/osteoarthritis-oa. Published 2018. Accessed October 4, 2019.
20. Kontzias A. Rheumatoid arthritis (RA). Merck Manual Professional Version website. www.merckmanuals.com/professional/musculoskeletal-and-connective-tissue-disorders/joint-disorders/rheumatoid-arthritis-ra. Published 2018. Accessed October 4, 2019.
21. Marmura MJ, Silberstein SD, Schwedt TJ. The acute treatment of migraine in adults: The American Headache Society evidence assessment of migraine pharmacotherapies. *Headache.* 2015;55(1):3-20.
22. Complex regional pain syndrome. Mayo Clinic website. www.mayoclinic.org/diseases-conditions/complex-regional-pain-syndrome/diagnosis-treatment/drc-20371156. Published 2018. Accessed October 5, 2019.
23. Concussion. Mayo Clinic website. www.mayoclinic.org/diseases-conditions/concussion/diagnosis-treatment/drc-20355600. Published 2019. Accessed October 15, 2019.
24. Migraine. Mayo Clinic website. www.mayoclinic.org/diseases-conditions/migraine-headache/symptoms-

causes/syc-20360201. Published 2019. Accessed October 6, 2019.

25. McAlindon TE, Bannuru RR, Sullivan MC, et al. OARSI guidelines for the non-surgical management of knee osteoarthritis. *Osteoarthritis Cartilage.* 2014;22(3):363-388.

26. Moley PJ. Evaluation of neck and back pain. Merck Manual Professional Version website. www.merckmanuals.com/professional/musculoskeletal-and-connective-tissue-disorders/neck-and-back-pain/evaluation-of-neck-and-back-pain#v908411. Published 2019. Accessed October 5, 2019.

27. Moore RA, Derry S, Aldington D, Cole P, Wiffen PJ. Amitriptyline for fibromyalgia in adults. *Cochrane Database Syst Rev.* 2015;7:CD011824.

28. National Collaborating Centre for Chronic Conditions. *Osteoarthritis: National Clinical Guideline for Care and Management in Adults.* London, England: Royal College of Physicians; 2008. www.ncbi.nlm.nih.gov/pubmed/21290638. Accessed October 5, 2019.

29. Low back pain fact sheet. National Institute of Neurological Disorders and Stroke website. www.ninds.nih.gov/Disorders/Patient-Caregiver-Education/Fact-Sheets/Low-Back-Pain-Fact-Sheet#3102_7. Published 2014. Accessed October 5, 2019.

30. Complex regional pain syndrome fact sheet. National Institute of Neurological Disorders and Stroke website. www.ninds.nih.gov/Disorders/Patient-Caregiver-Education/Fact-Sheets/Complex-Regional-Pain-Syndrome-Fact-Sheet. Published 2017. Accessed October 5, 2019.

31. Orr SL, Friedman BW, Christie S, et al. Management of adults with acute migraine in the emergency department: The American Headache Society evidence assessment of parenteral pharmacotherapies. *Headache.* 2016;56(6):911-940.

32. Qaseem A, Wilt TJ, McLean RM, Forciea MA, Clinical Guidelines Committee of the American College of Physicians. Noninvasive treatments for acute, subacute, and chronic low back pain: a clinical practice guideline from the American College of Physicians. *Ann Intern Med.* 2017;166(7):514-530.

33. Ross JJ. Septic arthritis of native joints. *Infect Dis Clin North Am.* 2017;31(2):203-218.

34. Schmitt S. Acute infectious arthritis. Merck Manual Professional Version website. www.merckmanuals.com/professional/musculoskeletal-and-connective-tissue-disorders/infections-of-joints-and-bones/acute-infectious-arthritis. Published 2019. Accessed October 5, 2019.

35. Schmitt S. Osteomyelitis. Merck Manual Professional Version website. www.merckmanuals.com/professional/musculoskeletal-and-connective-tissue-disorders/infections-of-joints-and-bones/osteomyelitis. Published 2019. Accessed April 12, 2021.

36. Schmitt S. Prosthetic joint infectious arthritis. Merck Manual Professional Version website. www.merckmanuals.com/professional/musculoskeletal-and-connective-tissue-disorders/infections-of-joints-and-bones/prosthetic-joint-infectious-arthritis. Published 2019. Accessed October 5, 2019.

37. Silberstein S. Approach to the patient with headache. Merck Manual Professional Version website. www.merckmanuals.com/professional/neurologic-disorders/headache/approach-to-the-patient-with-headache#v1040037. Published 2018. Accessed October 4, 2019.

38. Silberstein SD. Migraine. Merck Manual Professional Version website. www.merckmanuals.com/professional/neurologic-disorders/headache/migraine#v27292163. Published 2018. Accessed October 4, 2019.

39. Silberstein SD. Tension-Type Headache. Merck Manual Professional Version website. www.merckmanuals.com/professional/neurologic-disorders/headache/tension-type-headache. Published 2018. Accessed October 4, 2019.

40. Singh JA, Saag KG, Bridges SL, Jr., et al. 2015 American College of Rheumatology guideline for the treatment of rheumatoid arthritis. *Arthritis Rheumatol.* 2016;68(1):1-26.

41. Smith MA. New guidelines for management of low back pain. In: DiPiro JT, ed. *Pharmacotherapy Updates.* New York, NY: McGraw-Hill; 2016.

42. Stephens G, Derry S, Moore RA. Paracetamol (acetaminophen) for acute treatment of episodic tension-type headache in adults. *Cochrane Database Syst Rev.* 2016;6:CD011889.

43. Urquhart DM, Hoving JL, Assendelft WJJ, Roland M, van Tulder MW. Antidepressants for non-specific low back pain. *Cochrane Database Syst Rev.* 2008;1:CD001703.

44. van Tulder MW, Touray T, Furlan AD, Solway S, Bouter LM. Muscle relaxants for non-specific low-back pain. *Cochrane Database Syst Rev.* 2003;2:CD004252.

45. Veys L, Derry S, Moore RA. Ketoprofen for episodic tension-type headache in adults. *Cochrane Database Syst Rev.* 2016;9:CD012190.

46. Villa-Forte A. Pain in and around a single joint. Merck Manual Professional Version website. www.merckmanuals.com/professional/musculoskeletal-and-connective-tissue-disorders/pain-in-and-around-joints/pain-in-and-around-a-single-joint. Published 2019. Accessed October 4, 2019.

47. Walitt B, Urrútia G, Nishishinya MB, Cantrell SE, Häuser W. Selective serotonin reuptake inhibitors for fibromyalgia syndrome. *Cochrane Database Syst Rev.* 2015;6:CD011735.

48. Watson J. Complex regional pain syndrome (CRPS). Merck Manual Professional Version website. www.merckmanuals.com/professional/neurologic-disorders/pain/complex-regional-pain-syndrome-crps?query=Complex%20regional%20pain%20syndrome. Published 2018. Accessed October 4, 2019.

49. Wolfe F, Clauw DJ, Fitzcharles MA, et al. 2016 revisions to the 2010/2011 fibromyalgia diagnostic criteria. *Sem in Arthritis Rheum.* 2016(3):319.

50. Headache disorders. World Health Organization website. www.who.int/en/news-room/fact-sheets/detail/headache-disorders. Published April 8, 2016. Accessed October 6, 2019.
51. Musculoskeletal conditions. World Health Organization website. www.who.int/news-room/fact-sheets/detail/musculoskeletal-conditions. Published 2019. Accessed October 4, 2019.

Chapter 16

1. Aaron DM. Candidiasis (mucocutaneous, moniliasis). Merck Manual Professional Version website. www.merckmanuals.com/professional/dermatologic-disorders/fungal-skin-infections/candidiasis-mucocutaneous#v964306. Published 2018. Accessed October 8, 2019.
2. Aaron DM. Overview of dermatophytoses. Merck Manual Professional Version website. www.merckmanuals.com/professional/dermatologic-disorders/fungal-skin-infections/overview-of-dermatophytoses?query=Tinea%20 corporis. Published 2018. Accessed October 8, 2019.
3. American Academy of Dermatology recommendation. Choosing Wisely website. www.choosingwisely.org/clinician-lists/american-academy-dermatology-oral-antibiotics-atopic-dermatitis. Published October 29, 2013. Accessed October 9, 2019.
4. Amerson EH, Burgin S, Shinkai K. Fundamentals of clinical dermatology: morphology and special clinical considerations. In: Kang S, Amagai M, Bruckner AL, et al., eds. *Fitzpatrick's Dermatology.* 9th ed. New York, NY: McGraw-Hill Education; 2019:1-17.
5. Beam JW, Buckley B, Holcomb WR, Ciocca M. National Athletic Trainers' Association position statement: management of acute skin trauma. *J Athl Train.* 2016;51(12):1053-1070.
6. Benedetti J. Urticaria (hives; wheals). Merck Manual Professional Version website. www.merckmanuals.com/professional/dermatologic-disorders/approach-to-the-dermatologic-patient/urticaria#v959353. Updated February 2019. Accessed October 8, 2019.
7. Benedetti J. Itching (pruritus). Merck Manual Professional Version website. www.merckmanuals.com/professional/dermatologic-disorders/approach-to-the-dermatologic-patient/itching#v958662. Updated February 2019. Accessed October 8, 2019.
8. Bush LM. Bacteremia. Merck Manual Professional Version website. www.merckmanuals.com/professional/infectious-diseases/biology-of-infectious-disease/bacteremia?query=bacteremia. Published 2018. Accessed October 9, 2019.
9. Molluscum contagiosum. Centers for Disease Control and Prevention website. www.cdc.gov/poxvirus/molluscum-contagiosum/index.html. Updated May 11, 2015. Accessed October 8, 2019.
10. Ringworm information for healthcare professionals. Centers for Disease Control and Prevention website. www.cdc.gov/fungal/diseases/ringworm/health-professionals.html. Published 2018. Accessed October 8, 2019.
11. Psoriasis. Centers for Disease Control and Prevention website. www.cdc.gov/psoriasis. Published 2018. Accessed October 8, 2019.
12. Candidiasis. Centers for Disease Control and Prevention website. www.cdc.gov/fungal/diseases/candidiasis. Published 2019. Accessed October 8, 2019.
13. Daum RS. Clinical practice. Skin and soft-tissue infections caused by methicillin-resistant Staphylococcus aureus. *N Engl J Med.* 2007;357(4):380-390.
14. Dhar AD. Overview of bacterial skin infections. Merck Manual Professional Version website. www.merckmanuals.com/professional/dermatologic-disorders/bacterial-skin-infections/overview-of-bacterial-skin-infections?query=Skin%20and%20soft-tissue%20 infections. Published 2019. Accessed October 9, 2019.
15. Dhar AD. Impetigo and ecthyma. Merck Manual Professional Version website. www.merckmanuals.com/professional/dermatologic-disorders/bacterial-skin-infections/impetigo-and-ecthyma. Published 2019. Accessed October 9, 2019.
16. Dinulos JGH. Molluscum contagiosum. Merck Manual Professional Version website. www.merckmanuals.com/professional/dermatologic-disorders/viral-skin-diseases/molluscum-contagiosum?query=molluscum%20 contagiosum. Published 2018. Accessed October 9, 2019.
17. Multum, C. Calamine (topical). Drugs.com website. www.drugs.com/mtm/calamine-topical.html. Published 2019. Accessed October 9, 2019.
18. Hydrocortisone (topical). Drugs.com website. www.drugs.com/ppa/hydrocortisone-topical.html. Published 2019. Accessed October 10, 2019.
19. Eichenfield LF, Tom WL, Berger TG, et al. Guidelines of care for the management of atopic dermatitis: section 2. Management and treatment of atopic dermatitis with topical therapies. *J Am Acad Dermatol.* 2014;71(1):116-132.
20. Feldman SR. Treatment of psoriasis in adults. UpToDate website. www-uptodate-com.libproxy.chapman.edu/contents/treatment-of-psoriasis-in-adults?search=psoriasis&source=search_result&selectedTitle=1~150&usage_type=default&display_rank=1#H902797172. Published 2019. Accessed October 8, 2019.
21. Fookes C. Topical steroids. Drugs.com website. www.drugs.com/drug-class/topical-steroids.html. Published June 20, 2018. Acccessed June 10, 2021.
22. Gonzalez ME. Contact dermatitis. Merck Manual Professional Version website. www.merckmanuals.com/professional/dermatologic-disorders/dermatitis/contact-dermatitis?query=Dermatitis. Published 2019. Accessed October 10, 2019.
23. Gonzalez ME. Atopic dermatitis (eczema). Merck Manual Professional Version website. www.merckmanuals.com/professional/dermatologic-disorders/dermatitis/atopic-dermatitis-eczema#v44326938. Published 2019. Accessed October 12, 2019.

24. Keloids. Harvard Health Publishing website. www.health.harvard.edu/a_to_z/keloids-a-to-z. Published June 17, 2020. Accessed November 13, 2020.

25. Kaye KM. Herpes simplex virus (HSV) infections (herpes labialis; herpetic gingivostomatitis). Merck Manual Professional Version website. www.merckmanuals.com/professional/infectious-diseases/herpesviruses/herpes-simplex-virus-hsv-infections?query=herpes. Published 2018. Accessed October 8, 2019.

26. Keri JE. Principles of topical dermatologic therapy. Merck Manual Professional Version website. www.merckmanuals.com/professional/dermatologic-disorders/principles-of-topical-dermatologic-therapy/principles-of-topical-dermatologic-therapy. Published 2019. Accessed October 8, 2019.

27. Kubo A, Amagai M. Skin barrier. In: Kang S, Amagai M, Bruckner AL, et al., eds. *Fitzpatrick's Dermatology.* 9th ed. New York, NY: McGraw-Hill Education; 2019:206-231.

28. Law RM, Law DTS. Dermatologic drug reactions and common skin conditions. In: DiPiro JT, Talbert RL, Yee GC, Matzke GR, Wells BG, Posey LM, eds. *Pharmacotherapy: A Pathophysiologic Approach.* 10th ed. New York, NY: McGraw-Hill Education; 2016:1591-1592.

29. Lawley LP, McCall CO, Lawley TJ. Eczema, psoriasis, cutaneous infections, acne, and other common skin disorders. In: Jameson JL, Fauci AS, Kasper DL, Hauser SL, Longo DL, Loscalzo J, eds. *Harrison's Principles of Internal Medicine.* 20th ed. New York, NY: McGraw-Hill Education; 2018.

30. Liu C, Bayer A, Cosgrove SE, et al. Clinical practice guidelines by the Infectious Diseases Society of America for the treatment of methicillin-resistant Staphylococcus aureus infections in adults and children. *Clin Infect Dis.* 2011;52(3):e18-55.

31. Lowy FD. Methicillin-resistant Staphylococcus aureus (MRSA) in adults: treatment of bacteremia. UpToDate website. www-uptodate-com.libproxy.chapman.edu/contents/methicillin-resistant-staphylococcus-aureus-mrsa-in-adults-treatment-of-bacteremia?topicRef=3176&source=see_link. Published 2019. Accessed October 9, 2019.

32. National Athletic Trainers' Association. Skin diseases in athletics: fact sheet. www.nata.org/sites/default/files/fact-sheet-skin-disease.pdf. Published 2010. Accessed October 8, 2019.

33. National Collegiate Athletic Association. *2017-2018 NCAA Sports Medicine Handbook.* 26th ed. 2017. www.ncaapublications.com. Accessed February 10, 2019.

34. Puri N, Talwar A. The efficacy of silicone gel for the treatment of hypertrophic scars and keloids. *J Cutan Aesthet Surg.* 2009;2(2):104-106.

35. Stevens DL, Bisno AL, Chambers HF, et al. Practice guidelines for the diagnosis and management of skin and soft tissue infections: 2014 update by the Infectious Diseases Society of America. *Clin Infect Dis.* 2014;59(2):147-159.

36. Waterbrook AL, Hiller K, Hays DP, Berkman M. Do topical antibiotics help prevent infection in minor traumatic uncomplicated soft tissue wounds? *Ann Emerg Med.* 2013;61(1):86-88.

37. Weidinger S, Novak N. Atopic dermatitis. *Lancet.* 2016;387(10023):1109-1122.

38. Weston WL, Howe W. Treatment of atopic dermatitis (eczema). UpToDate website. www-uptodate-com.libproxy.chapman.edu/contents/treatment-of-atopic-dermatitis-eczema?search=atopic%20dermatitis&source=search_result&selectedTitle=1~150&usage_type=default&display_rank=1. Published 2019. Accessed October 8, 2019.

39. Wilson EK, Deweber K, Berry JW, Wilckens JH. Cutaneous infections in wrestlers. *Sports Health.* 2013;5(5):423-437.

40. Zinder SM, Basler RS, Foley J, Scarlata C, Vasily DB. National Athletic Trainers' Association position statement: skin diseases. *J Athl Train.* 2010;45(4):411-428.

Chapter 17

1. American College of Obstetricians and Gynecologists. ACOG Committee opinion: physical activity and exercise during pregnancy and the postpartum period. *Obstet Gynecol.* 2015;126:e135-e142.

2. Anderson L. Types of birth control pills (oral contraceptives). Drugs.com website. www.drugs.com/article/birth-control-pill.html. Published 2018. Accessed November 19, 2019.

3. Anderson L. Permanent birth control methods. Drugs.com website. www.drugs.com/article/permanent-birth-control.html. Published 2018. Accessed November 19, 2019.

4. Anderson L. Hormonal birth control methods (non-pill options). Drugs.com website. www.drugs.com/article/hormonal-birth-control.html. Published 2018. Accessed November 19, 2019.

5. Andrews EB, Gilsenan AW, Midkiff K, et al. The US postmarketing surveillance study of adult osteosarcoma and teriparatide: study design and findings from the first 7 years. *J Bone Miner Res.* 2012;27(12):2429-2437.

6. Bush LM, Perez MT. Toxic shock syndrome (TSS). Merck Manual Professional Version website. www.merckmanuals.com/professional/infectious-diseases/gram-positive-cocci/toxic-shock-syndrome-tss?query=Toxic%20shock%20syndrome. Published 2019. Accessed November 19, 2019.

7. Cachay ER. Human immunodeficiency virus (HIV) infection. Merck Manual Professional Version website. www.merckmanuals.com/professional/infectious-diseases/human-immunodeficiency-virus-hiv/human-immunodeficiency-virus-hiv-infection?query=Acute%20HIV%20Infection. Published 2019. Accessed November 19, 2019.

8. Casey FE. Sterilization. Merck Manual Professional Version website. www.merckmanuals.com/professional/gynecology-and-obstetrics/family-planning/sterilization?query=permanent%20contraception. Published 2018. Accessed November 19, 2019.

9. Casey FE. Oral contraceptives. Merck Manual Professional Version website. www.merckmanuals.com/professional/gynecology-and-obstetrics/family-planning/oral-contraceptives?query=progestin%20oral. Published 2018. Accessed November 15, 2019.
10. Casey FE. Transdermal and vaginal ring hormonal contraceptives. Merck Manual Professional Version website. www.merckmanuals.com/professional/gynecology-and-obstetrics/family-planning/transdermal-and-vaginal-ring-hormonal-contraceptives. Published 2018. Accessed November 15, 2019.
11. Casey FE. Intrauterine device (IUDs; IUD). Merck Manual Professional Version website. www.merckmanuals.com/professional/gynecology-and-obstetrics/family-planning/intrauterine-device-iuds-iud. Published 2018. Accessed November 15, 2019.
12. US Medical Eligibility Criteria (US MEC) for Contraceptive Use, 2016. Centers for Disease Control and Prevention website. www.cdc.gov/reproductivehealth/contraception/mmwr/mec/summary.html. Published 2016. Accessed November 12, 2019.
13. CDC Contraceptive Guidance for Health Care Providers. Centers for Disease Control and Prevention website. www.cdc.gov/reproductivehealth/contraception/contraception_guidance.htm. Published 2017. Accessed November, 12, 2019.
14. Sexually Transmitted Disease Surveillance 2018. Centers for Disease Control and Prevention website. www.cdc.gov/std/stats18/natoverview.htm. Published 2018. Accessed November 12, 2019.
15. Di Luigi L, Sansone M, Sansone A, et al. Phosphodiesterase Type 5 Inhibitors, Sport and Doping. *Curr Sports Med Rep.* 2017;16(6):443-447.
16. Nexplanon. Drugs.com website. www.drugs.com/pro/nexplanon.html. Published 2018. Accessed November 19, 2019.
17. Vasectomy. Drugs.com website. www.drugs.com/health-guide/vasectomy.html. Published 2019. Accessed November 19, 2019.
18. Medications for birth control (contraception). Drugs.com website. www.drugs.com/condition/contraception.html. Published 2019. Accessed November 12, 2019.
19. Medications for endometriosis. Drugs.com website. www.drugs.com/condition/endometriosis.html. Published 2019. Accessed November 20, 2019.
20. Sinha S. Boniva. Drugs.com website. www.drugs.com/boniva.html. Published 2019. Accessed January 1, 2020.
21. Hormonal contraceptives. Drugs.com website. www.drugs.com/cg/hormonal-contraceptives.html. Published 2019. Accessed November 15, 2019.
22. Essure. Drugs.com website. www.drugs.com/mcp/essure. Published 2019. Accessed November 19, 2019.
23. Thornton P. NuvaRing. Drugs.com website. www.drugs.com/cdi/nuvaring.html. Published 2020. Accessed November 11, 2020.
24. Ethinyl estradiol/norelgestromin dosage. Drugs.com website. www.drugs.com/dosage/ethinyl-estradiol-norelgestromin.html. Published 2020. Accessed November 9, 2020.
25. Durbin K. Skyla. Drugs.com website. www.drugs.com/skyla.html. Published 2019. Accessed November 16, 2019.
26. Ekenros L, Hirschberg AL, Heijne A, Friden C. Oral contraceptives do not affect muscle strength and hop performance in active women. *Clin J Sport Med.* 2013(3):202.
27. Entringer S. Mirena. Drugs.com website. www.drugs.com/mirena.html. Published 2019. Accessed November 16, 2019.
28. Essure permanent birth control: information for health care providers. Food and Drug Administration website. www.fda.gov/medical-devices/essure-permanent-birth-control/essure-permanent-birth-control-information-health-care-providers. Published 2019. Accessed November 19, 2019.
29. Gavin L, MacKay AP, Brown K, et al. Sexual and reproductive health of persons aged 10-24 years—United States, 2002-2007. *MMWR Surveill Summ.* 2009;58(6):1-58.
30. Glass J. Viagra before a workout? Yup, it's a thing. *Men's Health.* October 1, 2018. www.menshealth.com/health/a23550766/viagra-before-workout. Accessed January 1, 2020.
31. Goje O. Pelvic inflammatory disease (PID). Merck Manual Professional Version website. www.merckmanuals.com/professional/gynecology-and-obstetrics/vaginitis,-cervicitis,-and-pelvic-inflammatory-disease-pid/pelvic-inflammatory-disease-pid?query=Pelvic%20Inflammatory%20Disease. Published 2019. Accessed November 19, 2019.
32. Harvard Health Publishing. Impotence (erectile dysfunction). Drugs.com website. www.drugs.com/health-guide/impotence-erectile-dysfunction.html. Published 2019. Accessed November 21, 2019.
33. Hirsch IH. Erectile dysfunction (impotence; ED). Merck Manual Professional Version website. www.merckmanuals.com/professional/genitourinary-disorders/male-sexual-dysfunction/erectile-dysfunction?query=erectile%20dysfunction. Published 2019. Accessed November 21, 2019.
34. IARC Working Group on the Evaluation of Carcinogenic Risks to Humans. Combined estrogen-progestogen contraceptives and combined estrogen-progestogen menopausal therapy. *IARC Monogr Eval Carcinog Risks Hum.* 2007;91:1-528.
35. Imam TH. Bacterial urinary tract infections (UTIs). Merck Manual Professional Version website. www.merckmanuals.com/professional/genitourinary-disorders/urinary-tract-infections-utis/bacterial-urinary-tract-infections-utis?query=Urinary%20Tract%20Infections. Published 2019. Accessed November 21, 2019.
36. Karaguzel G, Holick MF. Diagnosis and treatment of osteopenia. *Rev Endocr Metab Disord.* 2010;11(4):237-251.

37. Lindsay R, Cosman F. Osteoporosis. In: Jameson JL, Fauci AS, Kasper DL, Hauser SL, Longo DL, Loscalzo J, eds. *Harrison's Principles of Internal Medicine*. 20th ed. New York, NY: McGraw-Hill Education; 2018.

38. Liu JH. Endometriosis. Merck Manual Professional Version website. www.merckmanuals.com/professional/gynecology-and-obstetrics/endometriosis/endometriosis?query=endometriosis. Published 2019. Accessed November 20, 2019.

39. Toxic shock syndrome. Mayo Clinic website. www.mayoclinic.org/diseases-conditions/toxic-shock-syndrome/symptoms-causes/syc-20355384. Published 2017. Accessed November 19, 2019.

40. Urinary tract infection (UTI). Mayo Clinic website. www.mayoclinic.org/diseases-conditions/urinary-tract-infection/symptoms-causes/syc-20353447. Published 2019. Accessed November 21, 2019.

41. Osteoporosis. Mayo Clinic website. www.mayoclinic.org/diseases-conditions/osteoporosis/symptoms-causes/syc-20351968. Published 2019. Accessed December 4, 2019.

42. Mayo Clinic. Contraceptive sponge. Drugs.com website. www.drugs.com/mcp/contraceptive-sponge. Published 2019. Accessed November 19, 2019.

43. Endometriosis. Mayo Clinic website. www.mayoclinic.org/diseases-conditions/endometriosis/symptoms-causes/syc-20354656. Published 2019. Accessed November 20, 2019.

44. Mayo Clinic. Kidney stones. Drugs.com website. www.drugs.com/mcd/kidney-stones. Published 2019. Accessed November 21, 2019.

45. Estrogen and progestin oral contraceptives (oral route). Mayo Clinic website. www.mayoclinic.org/drugs-supplements/estrogen-and-progestin-oral-contraceptives-oral-route/description/drg-20069422. Published 2019. Accessed November 19, 2019.

46. Minisola S, Cipriani C, Grotta GD, et al. Update on the safety and efficacy of teriparatide in the treatment of osteoporosis. *Ther Adv Musculoskelet Dis.* 2019;11:1759720X19877994.

47. Moreira CA, Bilezikian JP. Stress fractures: concepts and therapeutics. *J Clin Endocrinol Metab.* 2017;102(2):525-534.

48. Morris SR. Human papillomavirus (HPV) infection. Merck Manual Professional Version website. www.merckmanuals.com/professional/infectious-diseases/sexually-transmitted-diseases-stds/human-papillomavirus-hpv-infection?query=human%20papillomavirus. Published 2019. Accessed November 19, 2019.

49. Multum C. Xulane (transdermal). Drugs.com website. www.drugs.com/mtm/xulane-transdermal.html. Published 2018. Accessed November 19, 2019.

50. Natalie EC, Aline GC, Barbara CS, John PB. Therapy of osteoporosis in men with teriparatide. *J Osteoporos.* 2011;2011(2):463675.

51. Guidelines for certified athletic trainers confronted with pregnancy in female student-athletes. National Collegiate Athletic Association website. www.ncaa.org/sites/default/files/MPP%2BTrainers.pdf. Published 2015. Accessed December 4, 2019.

52. Reproductive health. National Institute of Environmental Health Sciences website. www.niehs.nih.gov/health/topics/conditions/repro-health/index.cfm. Published 2019. Accessed November 13, 2019.

53. Osteoporosis. National Institute on Aging website. www.nia.nih.gov/health/osteoporosis. Published 2019. Accessed December 4, 2019.

54. Petroczi A, Naughton DP. Potentially fatal new trend in performance enhancement: a cautionary note on nitrite. *J Int Soc Sports Nutr.* 2010;7:25.

55. Preminger GM. Urinary calculi (nephrolithiasis; stones; urolithiasis). Merck Manual Professional Version website. www.merckmanuals.com/professional/genitourinary-disorders/urinary-calculi/urinary-calculi. Published 2018. Accessed November 21, 2019.

56. Rechichi C, Dawson B, Goodman C. Athletic performance and the oral contraceptive. *Int J Sport Physiol Performance.* 2009;4(2):151.

57. Nur U, El Reda D, Hashim D, Weiderpass E. A prospective investigation of oral contraceptive use and breast cancer mortality: findings from the Swedish women's lifestyle and health cohort. *BMC Cancer.* 2019;19(1):807.

58. Birth control. US Food and Drug Administration website. www.fda.gov/consumers/free-publications-women/birth-control. Published 2018. Accessed November 12, 2019.

59. Birth control and sterilization. WebMD website. www.webmd.com/sex/birth-control/birth-control-sterilization#1. Published 2019. Accessed November 19, 2019.

60. Workowski KA, Bolan GA. Sexually transmitted diseases treatment guidelines, 2015. *MMWR Recomm Rep.* 2015;64(Rr-03):1-137.

61. World Health Organization. *Selected Practice Recommendations for Contraceptive Use*. 3rd ed. Geneva, Switzerland: Author; 2016.https://apps.who.int/iris/bitstream/handle/10665/252267/9789241565400-eng.pdf;jsessionid=1BF744B8DAFA4F3CE427719B7870CD9F?sequence=1. Accessed November 12, 2019.

62. WHO model list of essential medicines. World Health Organization website. www.who.int/medicines/publications/essentialmedicines/en. Published 2017. Accessed November 26, 2018.

63. Emergency contraception. World Health Organization website. www.who.int/en/news-room/fact-sheets/detail/emergency-contraception. Published February 2, 2018. Accessed November 12, 2019.

64. Drugs.com website. Depo-Provera. 2021. https://www.drugs.com/depo-provera.html. Accessed June 10, 2021.

Chapter 18

1. American Psychiatric Association. *DSM-5 Attention Deficit/Hyperactivity Disorder Fact Sheet*. 2013. www.psychiatry.org/psychiatrists/practice/dsm/educational-resources/dsm-5-fact-sheets.

2. American Psychiatric Association Work Group on Eating Disorders. Practice guideline for the treatment of patients with eating disorders (revision). *Am J Psychiatry.* 2000;157(1 Suppl):1-39.
3. Attia E, Walsh BT. Introduction to eating disorders. Merck Manual Professional Version website.. www.merckmanuals.com/professional/psychiatric-disorders/eating-disorders/introduction-to-eating-disorders. Published 2018. Accessed October 16, 2019.
4. Barnhill JW. Overview of anxiety disorders. Merck Manual Professional Version website. www.merckmanuals.com/professional/psychiatric-disorders/anxiety-and-stressor-related-disorders/overview-of-anxiety-disorders. Published 2018. Accessed October 16, 2019.
5. Barnhill JW. Acute stress disorder (ASD). Merck Manual Professional Version website. www.merckmanuals.com/professional/psychiatric-disorders/anxiety-and-stressor-related-disorders/acute-stress-disorder-asd. Published 2018. Accessed October 16, 2019.
6. Bonci CM, Bonci LJ, Granger LR, et al. National Athletic Trainers' Association position statement: preventing, detecting, and managing disordered eating in athletes. *J Athl Train.* 2008;43(1):80-108.
7. Carr C, Davidson J. Mind, body and sport: The psychologist perspective. National Collegiate Athletic Association website. www.ncaa.org/sport-science-institute/mind-body-and-sport-psychologist-perspective. Published 2019. Accessed October 23, 2019.
8. Clayton PJ. Suicidal behavior. Merck Manual Professional Version website. www.merckmanuals.com/professional/psychiatric-disorders/suicidal-behavior-and-self-injury/suicidal-behavior. Published 2018. Accessed October 16, 2019.
9. Coryell W. Overview of mood Disorders. Merck Manual Professional Version website. www.merckmanuals.com/professional/psychiatric-disorders/mood-disorders/overview-of-mood-disorders. Published 2018. Accessed October 16, 2019.
10. Ekhart C, van Hunsel F, Scholl J, de Vries S, van Puijenbroek E. Sex differences in reported adverse drug reactions of selective serotonin reuptake inhibitors. *Drug Saf.* 2018;41(7):677.
11. First MB. Medical assessment of the patient with mental symptoms. Merck Manual Professional Version website. www.merckmanuals.com/professional/psychiatric-disorders/approach-to-the-patient-with-mental-symptoms/medical-assessment-of-the-patient-with-mental-symptoms. Published 2017. Accessed October 16, 2019.
12. First MB. Behavioral emergencies. Merck Manual Professional Version website. www.merckmanuals.com/professional/psychiatric-disorders/approach-to-the-patient-with-mental-symptoms/behavioral-emergencies. Published 2017. Accessed October 16, 2019.
13. Fookes C. Antidepressants. Drugs.com website. www.drugs.com/drug-class/antidepressants.html. Published 2018. Accessed October 16, 2019.
14. Fookes C. Anxiolytics, sedatives, and hypnotics. Drugs.com website. www.drugs.com/drug-class/anxiolytics-sedatives-and-hypnotics.html. Published 2019.
15. Gouttebarge V, Kerkhoffs G. Sports career-related concussion and mental health symptoms in former elite athletes. *Neurochirurgie.* 2020 Feb 1;S0028-3770(20)30008-4. Online ahead of print.
16. Hasin DS, O'Brien CP. DSM-5 criteria for substance use disorders: recommendations and rationale. *Am J Psychiatry.* 2013;170(8):834-851.
17. Kolar D, Keller A, Golfinopoulos M, Cumyn L, Syer C, Hechtman L. Treatment of adults with attention-deficit/hyperactivity disorder. *Neuropsychiatr Dis Treat.* 2008;4(2):389-403.
18. Kosten T. Overview of substance-related disorders. Merck Manual Professional Version website. www.merckmanuals.com/professional/psychiatric-disorders/substance-related-disorders/overview-of-substance-related-disorders. Published 2018. Accessed October 16, 2019.
19. Lester D. Mind, body and sport: Suicidal tendencies. NCAA Sport Science Institute website. www.ncaa.org/sport-science-institute/mind-body-and-sport-suicidal-tendencies. Published 2012. Accessed November 12, 2020.
20. St. John's wort. Mayo Clinic website. www.mayoclinic.org/drugs-supplements-st-johns-wort/art-20362212. Published 2017. Accessed November 12, 2020.
21. Mayo Clinic staff. Anxiety disorders. Drugs.com website. www.drugs.com/mcd/anxiety-disorders. Published 2019. Accessed October 16, 2019.
22. Adult attention-deficit/hyperactivity disorder (ADHD). Mayo Clinic website. www.mayoclinic.org/diseases-conditions/adult-adhd/symptoms-causes/syc-20350878. Published 2019. Accessed November 12, 2020.
23. Mental health conditions. National Alliance on Mental Illness website. www.nami.org/Learn-More/Mental-Health-Conditions. Published 2019. Accessed October 16, 2019.
24. National Center for Complementary and Integrative Health. *St. John's wort and depression.* https://files.nccih.nih.gov/s3fs-public/SJW_and_Depression_11-30-2015.pdf. Published September 2013.
25. Mental health medications. National Institute of Mental Health website. www.nimh.nih.gov/health/topics/mental-health-medications/index.shtml. Published 2016. Accessed October 18, 2019.
26. Mental illness. National Institute of Mental Health website. www.nimh.nih.gov/health/statistics/mental-illness.shtml. Published 2019. Accessed October 16, 2019.
27. Schuch LG, Yip A, Nouri KF, et al. Serotonin syndrome following an uncomplicated orthopedic surgery in a patient with post-traumatic stress disorder. *Mil Med.* 2016;181(9):e1185-1188.
28. Schwab RJ. Approach to the patient with a sleep or wakefulness disorder. Merck Manual Professional Version website. www.merckmanuals.com/professional/

neurologic-disorders/sleep-and-wakefulness-disorders/approach-to-the-patient-with-a-sleep-or-wakefulness-disorder. Published 2020. Accessed November 12, 2020.

29. Silverberg ND, Panenka WJ. Antidepressants for depression after concussion and traumatic brain injury are still best practice. *BMC Psychiatry.* 2019;19(1):100.
30. Stache S, Howell D, Meehan WP, III. Concussion management practice patterns among sports medicine physicians. *Clin J Sport Med.* 2016;26(5):381-385.
31. Sulkes SB. Attention-deficit/hyperactivity disorder (ADD, ADHD). Merck Manual Professional Version website. www.merckmanuals.com/professional/pediatrics/learning-and-developmental-disorders/attention-deficit-hyperactivity-disorder-add,-adhd?query=adhd. Published 2018. Accessed October 16, 2019.

Chapter 19

1. Bents RT, Marsh E. Patterns of Ephedra and other stimulant use in collegiate hockey athletes. *Int J Sport Nutr Exerc Metab.* 2006;13:251-265.
2. Bourne J. Backstrom, the Olympics, & the use of pseudoephedrine in hockey. www.thescore.com/wolymhm/news/439444. Published 2014. Accessed August 20, 2019.
3. Chesanow N. Faster, higher, stronger: a history of doping in sports. www.medscape.com/features/slideshow/history-of-doping-in-sports. Published July 28, 2016. Accessed March 20, 2019.
4. Connor JM, Mazanov J. Would you dope? A general population test of the Goldman dilemma. *Br J Sports Med.* 2009;43(11):871-872.
5. Delanghe JR, Bollen M, Beullens M. Testing for recombinant erythropoietin. *Am J Hematol.* 2008;83(3):237-241.
6. Implementation of the Anabolic Steroid Control Act of 2004. Drug Enforcement Administration website. www.deadiversion.usdoj.gov/fed_regs/rules/2005/fr1216.htm#:~:text=Congress%20enacted%20the%20Anabolic%20Steroid,signed%20on%20October%2022%2C%202004.&text=Elimination%20of%20the%20need%20to,Schedule%20III%20of%20the%20CSA. Published November 23, 2005. Accessed March 5, 2021.
7. Drugs banned in sport. Drugs.com website. www.drugs.com/wada. Published 2017. Accessed July 11, 2019.
8. Epogen. Drugs.com website. www.drugs.com/epogen.html. Published 2018. Accessed August 22, 2019.
9. Schedule 3 (III) drugs. Drugs.com website. www.drugs.com/schedule-3-drugs.html. Published 2019. Accessed July 13, 2019.
10. Farzam K, Arif J. Beta blockers. *StatPearls.* www.ncbi.nlm.nih.gov/books/NBK532906. Published 2019. Accessed August 3, 2019.
11. Fishman MP, Lombardo SJ, Kharrazi FD. Vitamin D deficiency among professional basketball players. *Orthop J Sports Med.* 2016;4(7):1-5.
12. Gheorghiev MD, Hosseini F, Moran J, Cooper CE. Effects of pseudoephedrine on parameters affecting exercise performance: a meta-analysis. *Sports Med Open.* 2018;4(1):44.
13. Graham MR, Baker JS, Evans P, Hullin D, Thomas NE, Davies B. Potential benefits of recombinant human growth hormone (rhGH) to athletes. *Growth Horm IGF Res.* 2009;19(4):300-307.
14. Gronbladh A, Nylander E, Hallberg M. The neurobiology and addiction potential of anabolic androgenic steroids and the effects of growth hormone. *Brain Res Bull.* 2016;126(Pt 1):127-137.
15. Gugliotta T. Close call. *ESPN the Magazine.* April 3, 2000. www.espn.com/magazine/vol3no7gugliotta.html.
16. Harris W. 10 performance-enhancing drugs that aren't steroids. Beta blockers. How Stuff Works website. https://science.howstuffworks.com/10-performance-enhancing-drugs8.htm. Published 2012. Accessed August 4, 2019.
17. Why the FDA banned ephedra. Harvard Health Publishing website. www.health.harvard.edu/staying-healthy/ephedra-ban. Published 2004. Accessed August 20, 2019.
18. Hass CJ, Collins MA, Juncos JL. Resistance training with creatine monohydrate improves upper-body strength in patients with Parkinson disease: a randomized trial. *Neurorehabil Neural Repair.* 2007;21(2):107-115.
19. Henrotin Y, Marty M, Mobasheri A. What is the current status of chondroitin sulfate and glucosamine for the treatment of knee osteoarthritis? *Maturitas.* 2014;78(3):184-187.
20. Hoffman J, Ratamess N. Medical issues associated with anabolic steroid use: are they exaggerated? *J Sports Sci Med.* 2006(2):182.
21. Jacobs PL, Mahoney ET, Cohn KA, Sheradsky LF, Green BA. Oral creatine supplementation enhances upper extremity work capacity in persons with cervical-level spinal cord injury. *Arch Phys Med Rehabil.* 2002;83(1):19-23.
22. Jerosch J. Effects of glucosamine and chondroitin sulfate on cartilage metabolism in OA: outlook on other nutrient partners especially omega-3 fatty acids. *Int J Rheumatol.* 2011;2011:969012.
23. Kersey RD, Elliot DL, Goldberg L, et al. National Athletic Trainers' Association position statement: anabolic-androgenic steroids. *J Athl Train.* 2012;47(5):567-588.
24. Kicman A. Pharmacology of anabolic steroids. *Br J Pharmacol.* 2008;154(3):502-521.
25. Montero D, Breenfeldt-Andersen A, Oberholzer L, et al. Erythropoiesis with endurance training: dynamics and mechanisms. *Am J Physiol Regul Integr Comp Physiol.* 2017;312(6):R894-R902.
26. O'Brien M, McDougall JJ. Cannabis and joints: scientific evidence for the alleviation of osteoarthritis pain by cannabinoids. *Curr Opin Pharmacol.* 2018;40:104-109.
27. Ogan D, Pritchett K. Vitamin D and the athlete: risks, recommendations, and benefits. *Nutrients.* 2013;5:1856-1868.

28. Oliver JM, Anzalone AJ, Turner SM. Protection before impact: the potential neuroprotective role of nutritional supplementation in sports-related head trauma. *Sports Med.* 2018;48(Suppl 1):39-52.
29. Oransky I. Why would an Olympian shooter take propranolol? *Scientific American.* August 15, 2008. www.scientificamerican.com/article/olympics-shooter-doping-propranolol. Accessed August 5, 2019.
30. Pavlovic R, Nenna G, Calvi L, et al. Quality traits of "cannabidiol oils": cannabinoids content, terpene fingerprint and oxidation stability of European commercially available preparations. *Molecules.* 2018;20(23):5.
31. Petersen SG, Saxne T, Heinegard D, et al. Glucosamine but not ibuprofen alters cartilage turnover in osteoarthritis patients in response to physical training. *Osteoarthritis Cartilage.* 2010;18(1):34-40.
32. Powers ME. Ephedra and its application to sport performance: another concern for the athletic trainer? *J Athl Train.* 2001;36(4):420-424.
33. Pugmire L. Sports deaths put national spotlight on ephedra controversy. *LA Times.* March 1, 2003. www.latimes.com/archives/la-xpm-2003-mar-01-na-ephsport1-story.html. Accessed August 20, 2019.
34. Rawson ES, Miles MP, Larson-Meyer DE. Dietary supplements for health, adaptation, and recovery in athletes. *Int J Sport Nutr Exerc Metab.* 2018;28(2):188-199.
35. Saugy M, Robinson N, Saudan C, Baume N, Avois L, Mangin P. Human growth hormone doping in sport. *Br J Sports Med.* 2006;40(Suppl 1):i135-139.
36. Siebert DM, Rao AL. The use and abuse of human growth hormone in sports. *Sports Health.* 2018;10(5):419-426.
37. Sleivert G, Burke V, Palmer C, et al. The effects of deer antler velvet extract or powder supplementation on aerobic power, erythropoiesis, and muscular strength and endurance characteristics. *Int J Sport Nutr Exerc Metab.* 2003;13:251-265.
38. Effects of performance-enhancing drugs. US Anti-Doping Agency website. www.usada.org/substances/effects-of-performance-enhancing-drugs. Published 2019. Accessed August 22, 2019.
39. Willis KS, Smith DT, Broughton KS, Larson-Meyer DE. Vitamin D status and biomarkers of inflammation in runners. *Open Access J Sports Med.* 2012;3:35-42.
40. Blood doping. World Anti-Doping Agency website. www.wada-ama.org/en/questions-answers/blood-doping. Published 2019. Accessed August 22, 2019.
41. EPO detection. World Anti-Doping Agency website. www.wada-ama.org/en/questions-answers/epo-detection. Published 2019. Accessed August 3, 2019.
42. Who we are. World Anti-Doping Agency website. www.wada-ama.org/en/who-we-are. Published 2019. Accessed June 9, 2019.

Chapter 20

1. Abuhasira R, Shbiro L, Landschaft Y. Medical use of cannabis and cannabinoids containing products—Regulations in Europe and North America. *Eur J Intern Med.* 2018;49:2-6.
2. Anderson L. Synthetic cannabinoids (synthetic marijuana, spice, K2). Drugs.com website. www.drugs.com/illicit/synthetic-marijuana.html. Published 2018. Accessed November 1, 2019.
3. Aviram J, Samuelly-Leichtag G. Efficacy of cannabis-based medicines for pain management: a systematic review and meta-analysis of randomized controlled trials. *Pain Physician.* 2017;20(6):E755-E796.
4. Badowski ME. A review of oral cannabinoids and medical marijuana for the treatment of chemotherapy-induced nausea and vomiting: a focus on pharmacokinetic variability and pharmacodynamics. *Cancer Chemother Pharmacol.* 2017;80(3):441-449.
5. Bell J. Opinion: Don't hold your breath for quick NFL action to allow medical marijuana. *USA Today Sports.* May 22, 2019. www.usatoday.com/story/sports/nfl/columnist/bell/2019/05/22/nfl-medical-marijuana-not-immediate-horizon-players/1197332001. Accessed August 1, 2019.
6. Brents LK. Marijuana, the endocannabinoid system and the female reproductive system. *Yale J Biol Med.* 2016;89(2):175-191.
7. Brown P. Quality focus: certificates of analysis. Nutraceuticals World website. www.nutraceuticalsworld.com/issues/2008-11/view_columns/quality-focus-certificates-of-analysis. Published November 1, 2008. Accessed June 24, 2019.
8. Outbreak of lung injury associated with e-cigarette use, or vaping. Centers for Disease Control and Prevention website. www.cdc.gov/tobacco/basic_information/e-cigarettes/severe-lung-disease/healthcare-providers/index.html. Published 2019. Accessed November 1, 2019.
9. Cone EJ, Bigelow GE, Herrmann ES, et al. Non-smoker exposure to secondhand cannabis smoke. I. Urine screening and confirmation results. *J Anal Toxicol.* 2015;39(1):1-12.
10. Corroon J, Phillips JA. A cross-sectional study of cannabidiol users. *Cannabis Cannabinoid Res.* 2018;3(1):152-161.
11. Devinsky O, Cross JH, Laux L, et al. Trial of cannabidiol for drug-resistant seizures in the Dravet syndrome. *N Engl J Med.* 2017;376(21):2011-2020.
12. Multum C. Cannabidiol. Drugs.com website. www.drugs.com/mtm/cannabidiol.html. Published 2018. Accessed October 28, 2019.
13. Cannabis. Drugs.com website. www.drugs.com/npp/marijuana.html. Published 2018. Accessed October 24, 2019.
14. Marijuana. Drugs.com website. www.drugs.com/mca/marijuana. Published 2019. Accessed October 28, 2019.
15. Fischer B, Jeffries V, Hall W, Room R, Goldner E, Rehm J. Lower Risk Cannabis Use Guidelines for Canada (LRCUG): a narrative review of evidence and recommendations. *Can J Public Health.* 2011;102(5):324-327.
16. Fischer B, Russell C, Sabioni P, et al. Lower-Risk Cannabis Use Guidelines: A comprehensive update of evidence and recommendations. *Am J Public Health.* 2017;107(8):e1-e12.

17. Fisher E, Eccleston C, Degenhardt L, et al. Cannabinoids, cannabis, and cannabis-based medicine for pain management: a protocol for an overview of systematic reviews and a systematic review of randomised controlled trials. *Pain Rep.* 2019;4(3):e741.
18. FDA approves first drug comprised of an active ingredient derived from marijuana to treat rare, severe forms of epilepsy. U.S. Food and Drug Administration website. www.fda.gov/news-events/press-announcements/fda-approves-first-drug-comprised-active-ingredient-derived-marijuana-treat-rare-severe-forms. Published 2018. Accessed October 24, 2019.
19. FDA warns company marketing unapproved cannabidiol products with unsubstantiated claims to treat cancer, Alzheimer's disease, opioid withdrawal, pain and pet anxiety. U.S. Food and Drug Administration website. www.fda.gov/news-events/press-announcements/fda-warns-company-marketing-unapproved-cannabidiol-products-unsubstantiated-claims-treat-cancer. Published July 23, 2019. Accessed July 31, 2019.
20. Fookes C. Antidepressants. Drugs.com website. www.drugs.com/drug-class/antidepressants.html. Published 2018. Accessed October 16, 2019.
21. Gilron I, Blyth FM, Degenhardt L, et al. Risks of harm with cannabinoids, cannabis, and cannabis-based medicine for pain management relevant to patients receiving pain treatment: protocol for an overview of systematic reviews. *Pain Rep.* 2019;4(3):e742.
22. Gloss D, Vickrey B. Cannabinoids for epilepsy. *Cochrane Database Syst Rev.* 2014;2014(3):CD009270.
23. Häuser W, Finn DP, Kalso E, et al. European Pain Federation (EFIC) position paper on appropriate use of cannabis-based medicines and medical cannabis for chronic pain management. *Eur J Pain.* 2018;22(9):1547-1564.
24. Hazekamp A, Ware MA, Muller-Vahl KR, Abrams D, Grotenhermen F. The medicinal use of cannabis and cannabinoids—an international cross-sectional survey on administration forms. *J Psychoactive Drugs.* 2013;45(3):199-210.
25. Herrmann ES, Cone EJ, Mitchell JM, et al. Non-smoker exposure to secondhand cannabis smoke II: Effect of room ventilation on the physiological, subjective, and behavioral/cognitive effects. *Drug Alcohol Depend.* 2015;151:194-202.
26. Huestis MA, Mazzoni I, Rabin O. Cannabis in sport: anti-doping perspective. *Sports Med.* 2011;41(11):949-966.
27. Isabel Fraguas-Sanchez A, Isabel Torres-Suarez A. Medical use of cannabinoids. *Drugs.* 2018;78:1665-1703.
28. Perrine CG, Pickens CM, Boehmer TK, et al. Characteristics of a multistate outbreak of lung injury associated with e-cigarette use, or vaping—United States, 2019. *MMWR.* 2019;68(39):860-864. www.cdc.gov/mmwr/volumes/68/wr/pdfs/mm6839e1-H.pdf. Accessed October 29, 2019.
29. Mackie K. Cannabinoid receptors: where they are and what they do. *J Neuroendocrinol.* 2008;20(s1):10-14.
30. Melville NA. Seizure disorders enter medical marijuana debate. *Medscape Medical News.* August 14, 2013. www.medscape.com/viewarticle/809434. Accessed October 28, 2019.
31. Memedovich KA, Dowsett LE, Spackman E, Noseworthy T, Clement F. The adverse health effects and harms related to marijuana use: an overview review. *CMAJ Open.* 2018;6(3):E339-E346.
32. Synthetic cannabinoids (K2/Spice). National Institute on Drug Abuse website. www.drugabuse.gov/publications/drugfacts/synthetic-cannabinoids-k2spice. Published 2018. Accessed November 1, 2019.
33. NIH research on marijuana and cannabinoids. National Institute on Drug Abuse website. www.drugabuse.gov/drugs-abuse/marijuana/nih-research-marijuana-cannabinoids. Published 2018. Accessed October 24, 2019.
34. Marijuana research report. National Institute on Drug Abuse website. www.drugabuse.gov/publications/research-reports/marijuana/letter-director. Published 2019. Accessed October 24, 2019.
35. O'Brien M, McDougall JJ. Cannabis and joints: scientific evidence for the alleviation of osteoarthritis pain by cannabinoids. *Curr Opin Pharmacol.* 2018;40:104-109.
36. O'Malley GF, O'Malley R. Marijuana (cannabis). Merck Manual Professional Version website. www.merckmanuals.com/professional/special-subjects/recreational-drugs-and-intoxicants/marijuana-cannabis?query=cannabis. Published 2018. Accessed October 24, 2019.
37. Osborne H. Charlotte Figi: the girl who is changing medical marijuana laws across America. *International Business Times.* June 20, 2014. www.ibtimes.co.uk/charlotte-figi-girl-who-changing-medical-marijuana-laws-across-america-1453547. Accessed October 28, 2019.
38. Owens B. The professionalization of cannabis growing. *Nature.* 2019;572(7771):S10-S11.
39. Pavlovic R, Nenna G, Calvi L, et al. Quality traits of "cannabidiol oils": cannabinoids content, terpene fingerprint and oxidation stability of European commercially available preparations. *Molecules.* 2018;20(23):5.
40. Pellechia T. Legal cannabis industry poised for big growth, in North America and around the world. *Forbes.* March 1, 2018. www.forbes.com/sites/thomaspellechia/2018/03/01/double-digit-billions-puts-north-america-in-the-worldwide-cannabis-market-lead/#5146ee866510. Accessed August 1, 2019.
41. Centers for Disease Control and Prevention. *2018 Annual Surveillance Report of Drug-Related Risks and Outcomes: United States.* www.cdc.gov/drugoverdose/pdf/pubs/2018-cdc-drug-surveillance-report.pdf. Published 2018. Accessed May 5, 2019.
42. Rey JM, Martin A, Krabman P. Is the party over? Cannabis and juvenile psychiatric disorder: the past 10 years. *J Am Acad Child Adolesc Psychiatry.* 2004;43(10):1194-1205.
43. United Nations Office on Drugs and Crime. *Market Analysis of Plant-Based Drugs: Opiates, Cocaine, Can-*

nabis. World Drug Report 2017. Vienna, Austria: Author; 2017. www.unodc.org/wdr2017/field/Booklet_3_Plant-based_drugs.pdf. Accessed October 28, 2019.

44. What you need to know (and what we're working to find out) about products containing cannabis or cannabis-derived compounds, including CBD. U.S. Food and Drug Administration website. www.fda.gov/consumers/consumer-updates/what-you-need-know-and-what-were-working-find-out-about-products-containing-cannabis-or-cannabis. Published 2019. Accessed October 24, 2019.
45. Ware MA, Jensen D, Barrette A, Vernec A, Derman W. Cannabis and the health and performance of the elite athlete. *Clin J Sport Med*. 2018;28(5):480-484.
46. Whiting PF, Wolff RF, Deshpande S, et al. Cannabinoids for medical use: a systematic review and meta-analysis. *JAMA*. 2015;313(24):2456-2473.
47. Wilsey B, Atkinson JH, Marcotte TD, Grant I. The medicinal cannabis treatment agreement: providing information to chronic pain patients through a written document. *Clin J Pain*. 2015;31(12):1087-1096.
48. World Anti-Doping Agency. *World Anti-Doping Code International Standard Prohibited List*. www.wada-ama.org/sites/default/files/resources/files/2021list_en.pdf. Montreal, Canada: Author; 2021. Accessed May 10, 2021.
49. Zeiger JS, Silvers WS, Fleegler EM, Zeiger RS. Cannabis use in active athletes: behaviors related to subjective effects. *Plos One*. 2019;14(6):e0218998.

Chapter 21

1. Alquraini H, Auchus RJ. Strategies that athletes use to avoid detection of androgenic-anabolic steroid doping and sanctions. *Mol Cell Endocrinol*. 2018;464:28-33.
2. American College Health Association. ACHA Guidelines. Drug education and testing of student athletes. www.acha.org/documents/resources/guidelines/ACHA_Drug_Education_and_Testing_of_Student_Athletes_Feb2009.pdf. Published February 2009. Accessed August 17, 2019.
3. American Society for Addiction Medicine. Drug Testing: A White Paper of the American Society of Addiction Medicine (ASAM). Chevy Chase, MD: Author; 2013.
4. Badoud F, Guillarme D, Boccard J, et al. Analytical aspects in doping control: challenges and perspectives. *Forensic Sci Int*. 2011;213(1-3):49-61.
5. Brown P. Quality focus: certificates of analysis. Nutraceuticals World website. www.nutraceuticalsworld.com/issues/2008-11/view_columns/quality-focus-certificates-of-analysis. Published November 1, 2008. Accessed June 24, 2019.
6. Burnsed B. NCAA increases THC testing threshold. NCAA website. www.ncaa.org/about/resources/media-center/news/ncaa-increases-thc-testing-threshold. Published June 20, 2019. Accessed January 25, 2021.
7. Butch A. Sports drug testing laboratories. AACC website. www.aacc.org/publications/cln/articles/2014/january/sports-drug. Published January 1, 2014. Accessed April 4, 2019.
8. Centers for Substance Abuse Treatment. *Substance Abuse: Clinical Issues in Intensive Outpatient Treatment*. Treatment Improvement Protocol (TIP) Series, No. 47. Rockville MD: Substance Abuse and Mental Health Services Administration; 2006. www.ncbi.nlm.nih.gov/books/NBK64093.
9. Chesanow N. Faster, higher, stronger: a history of doping in sports. www.medscape.com/features/slideshow/history-of-doping-in-sports. Published 2016. Accessed March 20, 2019.
10. Drug test detection time. Confirm BioSciences website. www.confirmbiosciences.com/knowledge/terminology/drug-test-detection-time. Published 2019. Accessed May 21, 2019.
11. Drug Free Sport website. www.drugfreesport.com. Published 2018. Accessed March 25, 2019.
12. Ehrlich NEP. The athletic trainer's role in drug testing. *J Athl Train*. 1986;21(3):225-226.
13. Associated Press. MLB, union agree to opioid testing; marijuana removed as 'drug of abuse.' *ESPN*. December 12, 2019. www.espn.com/mlb/story/_/id/28283499/mlb-union-agree-opioid-testing-marijuana-removed-drug-abuse. Accessed January 4, 2020.
14. Information for consumers on using dietary supplements. U.S. Food and Drug Administration website. www.fda.gov/food/dietary-supplements/information-consumers-using-dietary-supplements. Published 2018. Accessed June 9, 2019.
15. Drug testing student athletes: Is it legal? Find Law website. https://education.findlaw.com/higher-education/drug-testing-student-athletes-is-it-legal.html. Updated June 20, 2016. Accessed April 5, 2019.
16. Geyer H, Schanzer W, Thevis M. Anabolic agents: recent strategies for their detection and protection from inadvertent doping. *Br J Sports Med*. 2014;48(10):820-826.
17. Heck J. Drug testing. *J Athl Train*. 1993;28(3):197-198.
18. Hendrickson B. NCAA Committee adjusts marijuana testing threshold. www.ncaa.org/about/resources/media-center/news/ncaa-committee-adjusts-marijuana-testing-threshold. Published January 25, 2013. Accessed April 9, 2019.
19. Drug testing reform. International Paruresis Association website. https://paruresis.org/drug-testing-reform. Published 2019. Accessed August 19, 2019.
20. Kuoch KLJ, Meyer D, Austin DW, Knowles SR. A systematic review of paruresis: Clinical implications and future directions. *J Psychosom Res*. 2017;98:122-129.
21. Labbate LA. Paruresis and urine drug testing. *Depress Anxiety*. 1996;4(5):249-252.
22. The real Whizzinator. Massive Dynamics website. https://realwhizzinatorxxx.com. Published 2019. Accessed August 19, 2019.
23. NATA Board of Directors. Summary of actions: Proceedings of the Board of Directors National Athletic Trainers' Association. *JNATA*. 1985;20(3):260-280.

24. National Collegiate Athletic Association. *NCAA Division I Manual: 2018-2019*. https://web3.ncaa.org/lsdbi/reports/getReport/90012. Published 2018. Accessed May 26, 2019.
25. NCAA drug testing program. National Collegiate Athletic Association website. www.ncaa.org/sport-science-institute/ncaa-drug-testing-program. Published 2018. Accessed May 8, 2019.
26. National Collegiate Athletics Association. *2018-19 NCAA Banned Drugs*. www.ncaa.org/sites/default/files/2018-19NCAA_Banned_Drugs_20180608.pdf. Published 2018. Accessed June 9, 2019.
27. NCAA Sport Sciences Institute. *NCAA Drug-Testing Program 2019-2020*. https://ncaaorg.s3.amazonaws.com/ssi/substance/2019-20SSI_DrugTestingProgramBooklet.pdf. Published 2019. Accessed July 23, 2019.
28. NCAA doping, drug education, and drug testing task force. NCAA website. www.ncaa.org/sport-science-institute/ncaa-doping-drug-education-and-drug-testing-task-force. Published 2013. Accessed March 24, 2019.
29. NSF International Certified for Sport website. www.nsfsport.com. Published 2019. Accessed June 12, 2019.
30. Patrick D. DeMont redeemed after 29 years. ESPN.com. www.espn.com/talent/danpatrick/s/2001/0202/1057642.html. Published December 6, 2001. Accessed March 27, 2019.
31. Schaffner K. Drug testing. *J Athl Train*. 1993;28(2):102.
32. Sears E. Behind the 'masking' drug that got Robinson Cano banned. *New York Post*. May 15, 2018. https://nypost.com/2018/05/15/behind-the-masking-drug-that-got-robinson-cano-banned. Accessed April 13, 2019.
33. Shirazi A, Tricker R. Current drug education policies in NCAA institutions: perceptions of head athletic trainers. *J Drug Education*. 2005;35:29-46.
34. Professional sports leagues steroid policies. Sports Reference website. In. Vol 2019. https://www.sports-reference.com/blog/professional-sports-leagues-steroid-policies/. Accessed March 18, 2021.
35. Starkey C, Abdenour TE, Finnane D. Athletic trainers' attitudes toward drug screening of intercollegiate athletes. *J Athl Train*. 1994;29(2):120-125.
36. Stern D. Testimony delivered to United States House Commerce, Trade and Consumer Protection Subcommittee hearings on steroids. NBA website. www.nba.com/news/stern_050518.htm. Published 2015. Accessed May 8, 2019.
37. Substance Abuse and Mental Health Services Administration. *Clinical Drug Testing in Primary Care Technical Assistance*. Publication series TAP 32. https://store.samhsa.gov/system/files/sma12-4668.pdf. Published 2012. Accessed June 9, 2019, 2019.
38. Thevis M, Opfermann G, Schanzer W. Urinary concentrations of morphine and codeine after consumption of poppy seeds. *J Anal Toxicol*. 2003(27):53-56.
39. Thompson C. How to pass a drug test using these detox drinks. *Vice*. February 16, 2018. www.vice.com/en_us/article/59kymq/we-tested-drinks-that-say-theyll-help-you-pass-a-drug-test. Accessed August 19, 2019.
40. Tsitsimpikou C, Tsarouhas K, Spandidos DA, Tsatsakis AM. Detection of stanozolol in the urine of athletes at a pg level: The possibility of passive exposure. *Biomed Rep*. 2016;5(6):665-666.
41. Ubha R. Maria Sharapova banned for two years over meldonium drug use. *CNN*. June 8, 2016. www.cnn.com/2016/06/08/tennis/maria-sharapova-two-year-ban-tennis-meldonium/index.html. Updated July 1, 2016. Accessed April 13, 2019.
42. Vernec AR. The Athlete Biological Passport: an integral element of innovative strategies in antidoping. *Br J Sports Med*. 2014;48(10):817-819.
43. Wood RI, Stanton SJ. Testosterone and sport: current perspectives. *Horm Behav*. 2012;61(1):147-155.
44. TUE physician guidelines. Medical information to support the decisions of TUE. World Anti-Doping Agency website. www.wada-ama.org/sites/default/files/resources/files/wada-tpg-medical-info-female-to-male-transsexual-athletes_1.3_en.pdf. Published 2016. Accessed June 22, 2019.
45. Who we are. World Anti-Doping Agency website. www.wada-ama.org/en/who-we-are. Published 2019. Accessed June 9, 2019.

Chapter 22

1. Continuum of depth of sedation: definition of general anesthesia and levels of sedation/analgesia. American Society of Anesthesiologists website. www.asahq.org/standards-and-guidelines/continuum-of-depth-of-sedation-definition-of-general-anesthesia-and-levels-of-sedationanalgesia. Published 1999. Accessed January 4, 2019.
2. American Society of Anesthesiologists Committee. Practice guidelines for preoperative fasting and the use of pharmacologic agents to reduce the risk of pulmonary aspiration: application to healthy patients undergoing elective procedures: an updated report by the American Society of Anesthesiologists Task Force on Preoperative Fasting and the Use of Pharmacologic Agents to Reduce the Risk of Pulmonary Aspiration. *Anesthesiology*. 2017;126(3):376-393.
3. Arnaldo JH, Marques de Almeida A, Fávaro E, Sguizzato GT. The influence of tourniquet use and operative time on the incidence of deep vein thrombosis in total knee arthroplasty. *Clinics (Sao Paolo)*. 2012;67(9):1053-1057.
4. Astur DC, Aleluia V, Veronese C, et al. A prospective double blinded randomized study of anterior cruciate ligament reconstruction with hamstrings tendon and spinal anesthesia with or without femoral nerve block. *Knee*. 2014;21(5):911-915.
5. Baca QJ, Schulman JM, Strichartz GR. Local anesthetic pharmacology. In: Golan DE, Armstrong E, Armstrong A, eds. *Principles of Pharmacology: The Pathophysiologic Basis of Drug Therapy*. 4th ed. Philadelphia, PA: Wolters Kluwer; 2016;167-182.

6. Butterworth JF, Mackey DC, Wasnick JD. The practice of anesthesiology. In: *Morgan & Mikhail's Clinical Anesthesiology.* 6th ed. New York, NY: McGraw-Hill Education; 2018.
7. Dingus S. Former Vikings Sharrif Floyd's $180M lawsuit reveals nightmare of "never event" surgery. Advocacy for Fairness in Sports website. http://advocacyforfairnessinsports.org/current-litigation/sharrif-floyd-v-dr-andrews-medical-malpractice/former-vikings-sharrif-floyds-180m-lawsuit-reveals-nightmare-of-never-event-surgery. Published November 7, 2018. Accessed February 13, 2019.
8. Dolk A, Cannerfelt R, Anderson RE, Jakobsson J. Inhalation anaesthesia is cost-effective for ambulatory surgery: a clinical comparison with propofol during elective knee arthroscopy. *Eur J Anaesthesiol.* 2002;19(2):88-92.
9. Eikaas H, Raeder J. Total intravenous anaesthesia techniques for ambulatory surgery. *Curr Opin Anaesthesiol.* 2009;22(6):725-729.
10. Eilers H, Yost S. General anesthetics. In: Katzung BG, ed. *Basic & Clinical Pharmacology.* 14th ed. New York, NY: McGraw-Hill Education; 2017;440-458.
11. Folsom AR, Tang W, Roetker NS, et al. Prospective study of sickle cell trait and venous thromboembolism incidence. *J Thromb Haemost.* 2015;13(1):2-9.
12. Gadsen J. Indications for peripheral nerve blocks. *New York School of Regional Anesthesia.* 2018;2018(November 26). www.nysora.com/indications-for-peripheral-nerve-blocks.
13. Graham WC, Flanigan DC. Venous thromboembolism following arthroscopic knee surgery: a current concepts review of incidence, prophylaxis, and preoperative risk assessment. *Sports Med.* 2014;44(3):331-343.
14. Joshi G, Gandhi K, Shah N, Gadsden J, Corman SL. Peripheral nerve blocks in the management of postoperative pain: challenges and opportunities. *J Clin Anesth.* 2016;35:524-529.
15. Katzung BG. *Basic & Clinical Pharmacology.* 14th ed. New York, NY: McGraw-Hill Education; 2018.
16. Trevor AJ, Katzung BG, Kruidering-Hall M. *Katzung & Trevor's Pharmacology: Examination & Board Review.* 12th ed. New York, NY: McGraw-Hill Education; 2018.
17. Latifzai K, Sites BD, Koval KJ. Orthopaedic anesthesia—part 2. Common techniques of regional anesthesia in orthopaedics. *Bull NYU Hosp Jt Dis.* 2008;66(4):306-316.
18. Lau BC, Jagodzinski J, Pandya NK. Incidence of symptomatic pulmonary embolus and deep vein thrombosis after knee arthroscopy in the pediatric and adolescent population. *Clin J Sport Med.* 2019;29(4):276-280.
19. Le-Wendling L, Bihorac A, Baslanti TO, et al. Regional anesthesia as compared with general anesthesia for surgery in geriatric patients with hip fracture: does it decrease morbidity, mortality, and health care costs? Results of a single-centered study. *Pain Med.* 2012;13(7):948-956.
20. Lopez B, Giordano C. Anesthetics. In: Whalen K, Feild C, Radhakrishnan R, eds. *Lippincott Illustrated Reviews: Pharmacology.* 7th ed. Philadelphia, PA: Wolters Kluwer; 2018;161-179.
21. Mariano E. Chapter 1 The Practice of Anesthesiology. In: Butterworth IV JF, Mackey DC, Wasnick JD. eds. Morgan & Mikhail's Clinical Anesthesiology, 6e. McGraw-Hill; Accessed May 25, 2021. https://accessmedicine-mhmedical-com.libproxy.chapman.edu/content.aspx?bookid=2444&sectionid=189634971
22. Mulroy MF, Larkin KL, Hodgson PS, Helman JD, Pollock JE, Liu SS. A comparison of spinal, epidural, and general anesthesia for outpatient knee arthroscopy. *Anesth Analg.* 2000;91(4):860-864.
23. O'Holleran JD, Altchek DW. The thrower's elbow: arthroscopic treatment of valgus extension overload syndrome. *HSS J.* 2006;2(1):83-93.
24. Patel HH, Pearn ML, Patel PM, Roth DM. General anesthetics and therapeutic gases. In: Brunton LL, Hilal-Dandan R, Knollmann BC, eds. *Goodman & Gilman's: The Pharmacological Basis of Therapeutics.* 13th ed. New York, NY: McGraw-Hill Education; 2017;387-404.
25. Pignatti M, Zanella S, Borgna-Pignatti C. Can the surgical tourniquet be used in patients with sickle cell disease or trait? A review of the literature. *Expert Rev Hematol.* 2017;10(2):175-182.
26. Runner RP, Boden SA, Godfrey WS, et al. Quadriceps strength deficits after a femoral nerve block versus adductor canal block for anterior cruciate ligament reconstruction: a prospective, single-blinded, randomized trial. *Orthop J Sports Med.* 2018;6(9):2325967118797990.
27. Shaikh SI, Nagarekha D, Hegade G, Marutheesh M. Postoperative nausea and vomiting: A simple yet complex problem. *Anesth Essays Res.* 2016;10(3):388-396.
28. Tubben RE, Murphy PB. *Epidural Blood Patch.* Treasure Island, FL; StatPearls: 2019.
29. Turnbull DK, Shepherd DB. Post-dural puncture headache: pathogenesis, prevention and treatment. *Br J Anaesth.* 2003;91(5):718-729.
30. Uribe AA, Arbona FL, Flanigan DC, Kaeding CC, Palettas M, Bergese SD. Comparing the efficacy of IV ibuprofen and ketorolac in the management of postoperative pain following arthroscopic knee surgery. a randomized double-blind active comparator pilot study. *Front Surg.* 2018;5:59.
31. Weibel S, Rucker G, Eberhart LH, et al. Drugs for preventing postoperative nausea and vomiting in adults after general anaesthesia: a network meta-analysis. *Cochrane Database Syst Rev.* 2020;10:CD012859.
32. Wouden J, Miller KW. General anesthetic pharmacology. In: Golan DE, Armstrong E, Armstrong A, eds. *Principles of Pharmacology: The Pathophysiologic Basis of Drug Therapy.* 4th ed. Philadelphia, PA: Wolters Kluwer; 2016;265-288.

Index

Note: The italicized *f* and *t* following page numbers refer to figures and tables, respectively.

D

E

T

U

V

W

Y

Z

About the Authors

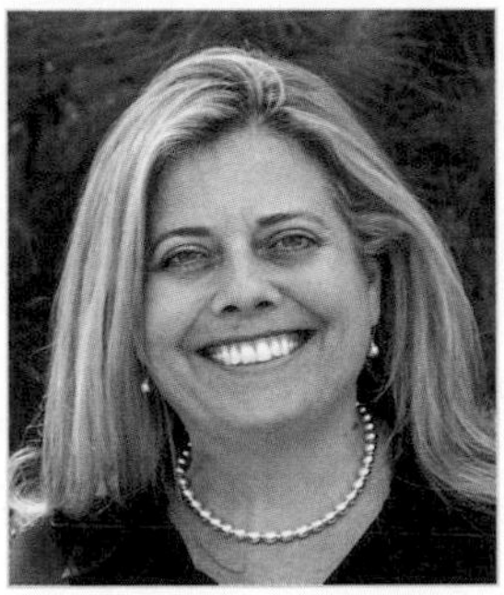

Michelle Cleary, PhD, ATC, is an associate professor in the physician assistant studies program in the Crean College of Health and Behavioral Science at Chapman University. Prior to joining Chapman in 2012, Cleary taught at Temple University, where she earned her doctorate, and at Florida International University and the University of Hawaii. She is certified as an athletic trainer by the Board of Certification (BOC). She has 20 years of experience teaching in accredited athletic training programs.

In addition to numerous journal articles and book chapters, Cleary has written two national position statements for the National Athletic Trainers' Association (NATA), has served on several NATA committees, and received the Most Distinguished Athletic Trainer award from NATA in 2019. Cleary wrote *Acute and Emergency Care in Athletic Training* with Katie Walsh Flanagan. She is the chair of the Research and Grants Committee of the Far West Athletic Trainers' Association and is also an active member of the California Athletic Trainers' Association, receiving the Outstanding Service Award in 2015. Her clinical experience includes time as an athletic trainer at the high school, NCAA Division I, and international/Olympic levels.

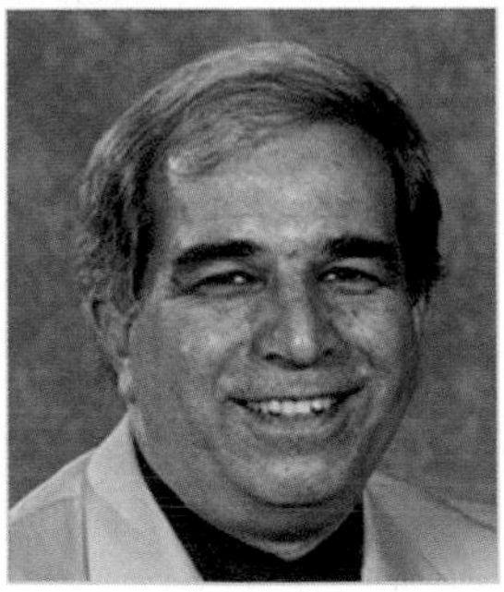

Thomas E Abdenour, DHSc, ATC, CES, received his doctorate degree in health science from A.T. Still University in 2011. He is a member of the National Athletic Trainers' Association (NATA) and is currently on the NATA's Foundation Board. Abdenour was inducted into the NATA Hall of Fame in 2007 and received the Most Distinguished Athletic Trainer award from NATA in 2014. He contributed to the 2009 NATA consensus statement *Managing Prescription and Non-Prescription Medication in the Athletic Training Facility.*

Abdenour is best known for his work in the National Basketball Association, where he spent 23 years as the head athletic trainer for the Golden State Warriors. In 1990, he was recognized as the Athletic Trainer of the Year by the National Basketball Athletic Trainers Association. Abdenour served as athletic trainer for the gold-medal-winning USA men's basketball team at the 2000 Summer Olympics in Sydney, Australia. He also founded the Champion Guidance Center for Men in Oakland, California, to support underprivileged men. Following his time with the Golden State Warriors, he served as the head athletic trainer at San Diego State University. While at San Diego State University, he was an approved clinical instructor and an adjunct faculty member in the department of exercise and nutrition science.

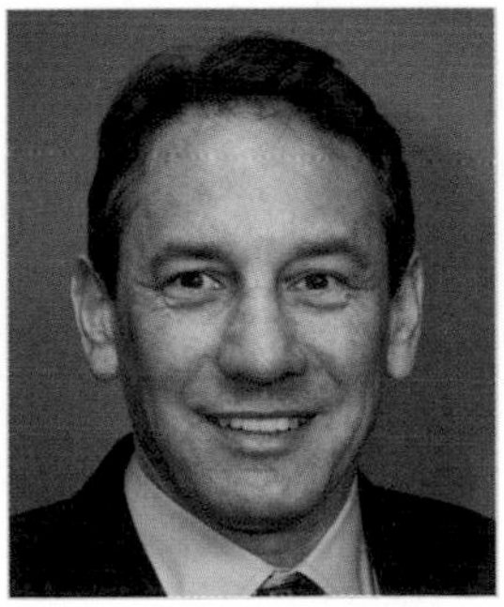

Michael Pavlovich, PharmD, earned his doctor of pharmacy degree in 1989 from the University of the Pacific. He is currently the president and owner of Westcliff Compounding Pharmacy. Pavlovich was an American Pharmacists Association (APhA) trustee from 2008 to 2014 and served in the APhA House of Delegates for more than 25 years. He received the Distinguished Achievement Award in Specialized Pharmacy Practice from APhA in 2012 and was recognized for his influence on the practice of pharmaceutical compounding and sports medicine. He is a past president of the California Pharmacists Association and a past board member of Pharmaceutical Care Network.

Prior to his employment at Westcliff Compounding Pharmacy, Pavlovich was the chief pharmacist for SportPharm, which revolutionized athletic trainers' capacity to manage prescription medications under the guidance of a team physician. He served as team pharmacist on the U.S. Olympic medical team at the 2008 Summer Olympics in Beijing, China. Pavlovich also contributed to the 2009 NATA consensus statement *Managing Prescription and Non-Prescription Medication in the Athletic Training Facility.* Many of his core recommendations for medication management in the athletic training clinic are still being followed today.